Mine Health and Safety Management

Edited by Michael Karmis

Published by the
Society for Mining, Metallurgy, and Exploration, Inc.

SME gratefully acknowledges the monetary contribution made by the Western Mining Resource Center, Mine Safety and Health Training Program at the Colorado School of Mines toward the production of this publication.

Society for Mining, Metallurgy, and Exploration, Inc. (SME)
8307 Shaffer Parkway
Littleton, Colorado, USA 80127
(303) 973-9550 / (800) 763-3132
www.smenet.org

SME advances the worldwide minerals community through information exchange and professional development. SME is the world's largest association of minerals professionals.

ISBN 0-87335-200-9

Library of Congress Cataloging-in-Publication Data

Mine health and safety management / edited by Michael Karmis.
  p. cm.
 Includes bibliographical references and index.
 ISBN 0-87335-200-9
 1. Miners--Health and hygiene. 2. Mine safety. 3. Mineral industries--Management. I. Karmis, Michael.

RC965.M48 M56 2001
618.9'803'088622--dc21

                  2001049135

Contents

Figures

Tables

Editorial Board

Preface

The twentieth century marked an era of great progress in mine health and safety. According to the National Safety Council's statistics of selected industries, mining now rates near the top of the safer industries. Engineering and technical developments have contributed a great deal to the improvements in mining health and safety. These same statistics also show an asymptotic trend, indicating that lower incident rates must come from operational systems that include both engineering and behavioral health and safety practices. Behavioral methods, aimed at human behavior in the workplace, may be the key to further improvements. Health and safety is everyone's responsibility, requiring the involvement of the employee and the commitment of management, leading to what H.L. Boling terms in his chapter a "behavior-based safety process."

Continual improvement in health and safety relies on understanding concepts and, as T.M. Smith pointed out, "the people within the process are the best qualified to improve the process."[1] Accepting the simple premise that "you can't improve what you don't understand," our comprehension must include communications and assessment leading to effective measurement and, therefore, to management. As a result, health and safety management is an integral component of a company's business plan. Furthermore, management actions must include infusing values and concepts, institutionalizing continuous improvement, communicating assessment, and managing improvement. Accountability, responsibility, empowerment, and assessment, then, are the keys. Health and safety management is a common framework that connects business planning, implementation, measurement, and performance improvement.[2]

In his *Safety in the Next Millennium* presentation, H.L. Boling states:

> The road map to success will include a process that ensures safe production is continuous, consistent and uncompromising. It will take integrating management's involvement into an unwavering commitment to people and the safe production process; then, consistently following it up with action and example.

According to Boling, the five principles of safety are:

1. All accidents are preventable.
2. All levels of management are responsible for safety.
3. All employees have the responsibility to themselves, their coworkers, and their family to work safely.
4. To eliminate accidents, management must ensure that all employees are properly trained on how to perform every task safely and efficiently.
5. Every employee must be involved in every area of the safety and production process.

---

1. Smith, T.M. 1992. Beyond your expectation: the next TQM step for the health and safety professional. *Proceedings 23rd Annual Institute on Mining Health, Safety and Research.* Edited by M. Karmis et al. Blacksburg, VA. August 24–26. 61–66.
2. Duke Energy, Environmental, Health and Safety, http://www.duke-energy.com/internet/stewardship/environment/ehsoperations.asp, April 13, 2000.

Jobs are only as safe or unsafe as we choose to make them. Therefore, accident prevention programs must identify reasons for unsafe conditions and/or behaviors and seek to redesign the work environment and/or unsafe behaviors. Upper management and employee commitment are vital in achieving good health and safety performance, let alone attaining what Scott Geller refers to in his chapter as "actively caring for a total safety culture."

A few years ago, in planning a health and safety meeting, Carl Metzgar—another great contributor to this book—articulated, in his usual eloquent manner, the need for education and training. He pointed out that the two are complementary but not the same, just as questions are as important as answers. He reminded us of this simple rhyme:

I keep six honest serving men
(They taught me all I knew):
Their names are What and Why and
When and How and Where and Who
                    –R. Kipling

It takes a lot of questions to develop and implement innovative health and safety programs. As George Germain notes in his chapter, "education" and "training" represent the difference between *knowledge* and *skills*. However, he stresses that more emphasis should be placed on similarities, since the main focus of both is *learning*. For practical purposes, learning involves the affective, cognitive, and behavioral domains—in other words, attitudes, knowledge, and skills.

This book is intended for use by undergraduate and graduate students in the minerals disciplines, practicing engineers and supervisors, health and safety professionals, and the research community. The book is divided into three parts. Part A deals with effective health and safety management systems. Part B focuses on building a health and safety culture. Finally, Part C concentrates on safety and health hazard anticipation, identification, evaluation, and control. The book's main purpose is to present aspects of management, leadership, regulation, and compliance that pertain to mining health and safety. Its main emphasis is on instilling concepts of a "safety culture" and fostering the ability to recognize and manage health and safety responsibilities and requirements.

As the editor of this book, I must acknowledge the contributing authors and editorial board members who truly represent leadership in the mining industry through health and safety programs, concepts, and management. They did an outstanding job in developing the book's layout, identifying the main themes and, of course, writing individual chapters. Thanks are also due to the many anonymous reviewers who verified the text's accuracy and quality. Margaret Radcliffe showed great leadership in acting as coordinator. She provided timely communications, and, most important, countless hours of work to ensure the compatibility of the final draft. The SME publishing staff, under the leadership of Jane Olivier, contributed the final link. They conducted a thorough editing of the text, assured quality and consistency, and led the publishing effort with great enthusiasm and professionalism.

Michael Karmis
Stonie Barker Professor, Department of Mining and Minerals Engineering
Director, Virginia Center for Coal and Energy Research
Virginia Tech, Blacksburg, Virginia

CHAPTER 1

History and Overview of Mine Health and Safety

R. Larry Grayson
Associate Director, Office for Mine Safety and Health Research
National Institute for Occupational Safety and Health, Washington, D.C.

Bruce Watzman
Vice President, Health and Safety
National Mining Association, Washington, D.C.

INTRODUCTION

Land ownership or control, agriculture, and mining have been the basis for wealth since time immemorial. Mining can be traced back to China circa 1100 B.C. (Cassidy 1981), as well as to most other ancient societies. Throughout history, the wealth generated by city–states or nations made them powerful and capable of consolidating their domestic power base and dominating rival states. Their wealth was coveted by stronger states, leading to incessant conflicts. Gold, silver, copper, precious stones, salt, granite, marble, and other minerals and rocks were not only sources of wealth, but they also sustained the will of the rulers and spurred the development of society.

The states, and the nobility, owned almost all land. They were responsible for the health and safety of their subjects, often slaves, who mined the materials. Until well after the Middle Ages, the welfare of people at work was generally ignored. People were tools used by nobility to generate wealth, maintain infrastructure, and fight wars. Generally speaking, the health and safety of miners, as for all workers, was not important.

In western cultures, the rights of citizens beyond nobility evolved after the Middle Ages and a greater distribution of wealth began as people gained the privilege, and eventually the right, to own land, establish businesses, and create their own wealth. Gradually, corporations were formed to control and perpetuate businesses. Among corporate responsibilities was the protection of workers' health and safety, a responsibility that would one day be embraced fully in modern society.

Commercial coal mining began in the United States in 1750 in Virginia (Cassidy 1981). With commercialization came the responsibility of a mining company for the health and safety of its employees. Unfortunately, at this time, the "rabble hypothesis" persisted across businesses; in other words, workers were considered unmotivated and unthinking tools. Owners and managers still did not place much emphasis on the welfare of workers. This was the picture in mining as well.

As mining was growing in the United States, a powerful nation was evolving. This nation had a conscience and was founded on the rights of its people to pursue life, liberty, and property. From a historical perspective, the U.S. government has defended the rights of people, at work as well as elsewhere. In many industries, an unacceptable toll on human life evolved as the industrial revolution progressed. As society advanced and the public became aware of the plight of workers, the government took action to protect them, often in response to outrage. In this chapter, we will review the evolution of efforts to protect miners' health and safety.

TABLE 1.1   Number of documented mine disasters[*] in the United States (Anon. 1997)

Period	Coal Mines	Noncoal Mines	Total
Through 1875	19	4	23
1876–1900	101	17	118
1901–1925	305	51	356
1926–1950	147	23	170
1951–1975	35	9	44
1976–present	13	1	14

*Disasters are defined by five or more deaths occurring from a single event

EARLY LEGISLATION

According to *Senate Report No. 95–181* (1977), "As early as 1865, a bill was introduced in the Congress to create a Federal Mining Bureau." It further states that "little was done until a series of serious mine disasters occurred after the turn of the century, causing public demand for Federal action to stop excessive loss of life."

In 1870, the first legislation on mine health and safety was passed in Pennsylvania (Pennsylvania Public Law 3) in response to outrage about the extent of death and injury. As shown in Table 1.1 (Anon. 1997), mine disasters were just beginning to become visible in the United States before 1875, and Pennsylvania took early action to "stem the tide." The Pennsylvania Act was "an act providing for the health and safety of persons employed in coal mines." It also formed the basis for eventual legislation in other states, as well as for federal legislative actions.

In 1891, Congress passed the first federal legislation to establish coal mine safety standards and inspections, but only in the territories (*House of Representatives Report No. 95–312* 1977). By this time, coal mine disasters were becoming much more frequent and nationally more visible (again refer to Table 1.1). In effect, early legislation was driven by tragedy in coal mines. By comparison, legislation to protect the health and safety of noncoal miners wasn't passed until 1966, at which time there were twice as many noncoal miners as coal miners.

By 1900, the U.S. industrial revolution was in high gear. Soon thereafter, national production was redoubled to support the World War I effort. As shown in Table 1.1, mine disasters were appallingly frequent between 1901 and 1925. During this period, the worst decade for mining fatalities occurred immediately before the Organic Act, which established the Bureau of Mines (Public Law 61–179 1910). The best available records indicate that 3,242 deaths occurred in coal mines in 1907, the worst single year in history, in which 18 coal mine disasters and two noncoal mine disasters were chronicled. The worst coal mine disaster in U.S. history occurred that year in Monongah, West Virginia, purportedly claiming the lives of 358 miners (Mine Safety and Health Administration [MSHA] 1999). Most historical accounts indicate that this number may have been even higher. The Organic Act was responsive to "Bloody December" in 1907 when four major coal mine disasters claimed 692 miners' lives, but even more, because of a privately funded study that "showed that a *single* Pennsylvania county logged 528 fatal mine-related accidents in a one-year period. Five thousand other mine workers in the county were maimed or totally disabled during the same year" (Traweek 1994). The government's role, however, was limited to research and investigation, not inspection and enforcement.

HISTORICAL FATALITY EXPERIENCE

Noncoal mining fatality records have been historically less certain than those for coal, especially prior to 1958 when the Department of the Interior first required all metal and nonmetal mine operators to report fatalities (*House of Representatives Report No. 95–312* 1977). After the establishment of the Bureau of Mines, fatality statistics certainly became more reliable in coal mining. Table 1.2 gives documented deaths for coal and noncoal mining in 5-year increments beginning with 1911.

The average number of miners employed is also given in Table 1.2, which allows the periodic fatality incident rate to be calculated. Until approximately 1971, the U.S. mining fatality experience was dominated by coal mining. Since then, the fatality experience of coal and noncoal mining is comparable in terms of the number of fatalities, but the fatality incident rate has generally been higher for underground coal mining until recently.

TABLE 1.2   U.S. 5-year mine fatality experience since 1911*

Time Period	Avg. Coal Fatals/Yr	Avg. Other Fatals/Yr	Avg. Total Fatals/Yr	Avg. Workers/Yr (000s)	Avg. Fatals/100 Miners
1911–1915	2,516	813	3,329	1,011.3	0.329
1916–1920	2,419	764	3,183	1,015.4	0.313
1921–1925	2,215	482	2,697	1,013.0	0.266
1926–1930	2,235	463	2,698	905.0	0.298
1931–1935	1,241	181	1,422	699.5	0.203
1936–1940	1,265	269	1,534	761.9	0.201
1941–1945	1,311	270	1,581	676.0	0.234
1946–1950	870	185	1,055	661.3	0.160
1951–1955	522	168	690	532.0	0.130
1956–1960	380	167	547	480.0	0.114
1961–1965	274	175	449	423.7	0.106
1966–1970	246	180	426	390.1	0.109
1971–1975	151	171	322	396.2	0.081
1976–1980	131	122	253	521.2	0.049
1981–1985	107	70	177	439.2	0.040
1986–1990	68	54	122	357.1	0.034
1991–1995	51	48	98	338.6	0.029

*Data before 1931 were obtained from Adams and Kohlos 1941; Adams and Wrenn 1941; and Reese, Wrenn, and Reid 1955. Data after 1930 were obtained from MSHA 1999

Generally, the fatality incident rate declined steadily over the years since 1911, but it dropped most rapidly after World War II (1946–1950) and following the passage of the Federal Coal Mine Health and Safety Act of 1969 (1971–1975) and the Federal Mine Safety and Health Amendments Act of 1977 (1976–1980). There were a few exceptions where progress stalled; however, as we will discuss in greater detail, a combination of factors has led to enormous strides in increased safety in the twentieth century.

FEDERAL LEGISLATIVE HISTORY—POSTORGANIC ACT

In response to continuing fatalities, as highlighted in *House of Representatives Report No. 91–563* (1969), the inadequacy of the Organic Act in curbing mine disasters (primarily in coal mines) became a growing concern through the 1920s and 1930s. It became apparent that coal mines required close scrutiny and that federal inspectors were needed. Congress addressed this "deliberate omission" by passing Public Law 49 (1941), in which "Federal inspectors were given authority to enter and inspect for health and safety hazards all anthracite, bituminous coal, and lignite mines in the United States." This law was referred to as the Federal Coal Mine Health and Safety Act. Inspection authority was housed in the Bureau of Mines, but the agency still "lacked authority to establish standards or to enforce compliance with standards."

In 1947, safety standards would first appear for bituminous coal and lignite mines with the enactment of Public Law 80–328 (MSHA 1999), but no enforcement provisions were granted. Although this act allowed federal inspectors to notify mine operators and state agencies of violations, it still contained no enforcement provisions. The law expired after 1 year because it was primarily directed toward information-gathering (*Senate Report No. 95–181* 1977).

Following another disaster in 1951 at a West Frankfort, Illinois, coal mine, in which 119 miners died in an explosion, public outrage was renewed. This led to enactment of Public Law 82–552 in 1952 (*House of Representatives Report No. 91–563* 1969). MSHA summarizes this act as follows (MSHA 1999):

- Emphasized prevention of major disasters
- Annual inspections required at underground coal mines
- Mandatory safety standards instituted for underground coal mines, with more stringent standards for "gassy" mines

- Federal inspectors given authority to issue orders of withdrawal in situations of imminent danger as well as notices of violation
- Mandated orders of withdrawal where less serious violations were not properly corrected. Enforcement of federal standards by state inspectors allowed under state plan system
- Anthracite mines covered, all surface coal mines exempted, along with all mines employing fewer than 15.

Ramani and Mutmansky (1999) also cite the following practices as having a significant long-term effect:

- The elimination of black powder
- The adoption of systematic roof-control plans
- The installation of main ventilation fans
- The elimination of underground smoking and open-flame lamps
- The required use of rock dusting
- The use of water sprays for dust reduction
- The mandatory use of pre-shift examinations for mine gases.

The 1952 law had serious deficiencies and unintentionally spurred a tremendous restructuring of the industry, a move geared toward small mines employing 14 or fewer miners. Again, the focus was primarily on underground coal mines. A task force was established to study the situation, and legislative action would continue as disasters persisted.

In 1961, emphasis shifted to noncoal mining. Public Law 87–300 sanctioned a Mine Safety Board to investigate mine safety in the noncoal sectors. This act resulted from growing evidence of deaths, serious injuries, and dangerous conditions in metal and nonmetal mines. The board submitted its report in 1963 after an 18-month study, which was primarily responsible for enactment of the Metal and Nonmetallic Mine Safety Act (Public Law 89–577) in 1966 (*House of Representatives Report No. 95–312* 1977). The study corroborated suspected conditions and serious outcomes and highlighted "the ineffectiveness of State and local efforts to reduce mine health and safety hazards."

MSHA summarizes the salient features of the Metal and Nonmetallic Mine Safety Act as follows (MSHA 1999):

- Procedures for developing safety and health standards for metal and nonmetal mines are instituted
- Standards could be advisory or mandatory
- One annual inspection is required for underground mines
- Federal inspectors are given the authority to issue notices of violation and orders of withdrawal
- Enforcement of federal standards by state inspectors is allowed under the state plan system
- Education and training programs are expanded.

Other mining-related legislation in 1966 (Public Law 89–376), responsive to recommendations of the coal mine task force report, extended the provisions of the 1952 act to coal mines that employed 14 or fewer miners. It also empowered bureau inspectors to issue withdrawal orders whenever repeated unwarrantable failures to comply with safety standards were discovered. However, federal emphasis was still on coal mine disasters, leaving as much as 90% of injury and fatality incidents to be addressed by state law and the federal safety code. This inadequacy was soon addressed because of public outrage generated by yet another coal mine disaster, along with an intolerable non-disaster death toll.

As MSHA states (MSHA 1999), "the death of 222 miners in 1967, 311 in 1968, the Farmington disaster, and the death of over 170 miners in non-disaster type accidents since Farmington now surrounds the consideration of" the Federal Coal Mine Health and Safety Act of 1969 (Public Law 91–173). Seventy-eight miners died in the Farmington, West Virginia, explosion, which galvanized Congress to take swift action. MSHA summarizes the major provisions of the 1969 act as follows:

- Enforcement powers in coal mines increased vastly
- Surface mines covered
- Four annual inspections required for each underground coal mine

- Stricter standards for gassy mines abolished, but additional inspections required in these mines
- Miners given right to request a federal inspection
- State enforcement plans discontinued
- Mandatory fines for all violations
- Criminal penalties for knowing and willful violations. Safety standards for all coal mines strengthened
- Health standards adopted
- Procedures incorporated for developing new health and safety standards
- Training grant program instituted
- Benefits provided to miners disabled by blacklung disease.

A nonlegislative administrative action from 1973 deserves mention at this point. In response to the Sunshine mine disaster in 1972, the Department of Interior created the Mining Enforcement and Safety Administration (MESA; *House of Representatives Report No. 95–312* 1977)—the precursor agency to MSHA—primarily because of "heavy criticism for not having promulgated and enforced sufficient lifesaving standards to protect metal and nonmetal miners from...disasters." This agency assumed the enforcement activities formerly performed by the Bureau of Mines and was physically located away from the bureau. This action emphasized another shift toward focusing more on non-coal mining.

Congress then scrutinized weaknesses of the 1966 Federal Metal and Nonmetallic Mine Safety Act. The conflicting role of the bureau had been addressed in the 1973 administrative decision to separate enforcement and inspection from research, which often focused on production and productivity. The criticism that led to establishing MESA was reinforced strongly by the visibility of the following two other noncoal disasters:

- The 1968 Cargill salt mine fire in Belle Isle, Louisiana, where 21 miners perished
- The 1971 Barnett fluorspar-lead-zinc complex in Rosiclare, Illinois, where seven miners died.

As mentioned earlier, the Sunshine silver mine fire in Kellogg, Idaho, occurred in 1972, claiming the lives of 91 miners. In addition to the impact of the disasters, Congress began scrutinizing safety statistics more closely and found the following, for different periods in the 1970s:

- The average fatality rate for all metal and nonmetal miners had jumped to more than 75% of that for all coal miners
- The rates for casualties among metal and nonmetal miners in three areas surpassed those for their coal mining counterparts
- The fatality rate for surface metal and nonmetal miners had exceeded that for surface coal miners
- Nonfatal disabling injury rates for underground metal and nonmetal miners had exceeded those for underground coal miners.

The combined effect of these statistics led to passage of the Federal Mine Safety and Health Amendments Act of 1977 (Public Law 95–164). MSHA summarizes the major provisions of the 1977 act as follows (MSHA 1999):

- Placed coal mines, metal, and nonmetal mines under a single law, with enforcement provisions similar to the 1969 act. Separate safety and health standards were retained
- Moved enforcement agency to Department of Labor, renamed it MSHA
- Required four annual inspections at all underground mines, two at all surface mines
- Eliminated advisory standards for metal and nonmetal mines
- Discontinued state enforcement plans in metal and nonmetal sectors
- Provided for mandatory miner training
- Required mine rescue teams for all underground mines
- Increased involvement of miners and their representatives in health and safety activities.

With the mining fatality experience and U.S. legislative history having set the stage, we will now assess the progress of mine health and safety over the past century. It will be presented from a broader historical sense, integrating key economic and political events to better frame the perspective on progress. Next, we will look at prospects for progress in the new century and the impediments that must be overcome.

A PERSPECTIVE ON PROGRESS

As we consider progress to date, a broad view of health and safety statistics is a good starting point for assessing overall progress in addressing workplace health and safety problems. There are a number of "yardsticks" by which such an assessment can be made, including calculating rates for:

- Fatalities
- Serious injuries and disabilities
- Lost-time injuries
- Disabling disease, which often causes or contributes to death.

Generally, fatality reduction is the most reliable statistic and measure of progress, especially since 1958 for the noncoal sectors, and we will use it here as the principal basis of comparison. Using injury or disease statistics makes sense only when reliable tracking systems are in place, along with standard definitions, which are stable over time. This didn't occur in the mining industry until after 1986, for injuries, when the MSHA definition of accident last changed.

Progress in Reducing Fatalities

Based on statistics gathered during a long period of time and presented in Table 1.2, we can see a tremendous reduction in fatalities in both the coal and noncoal sectors. These numbers refer to fatalities and incident rates based on total employees. Specifically, a comparison of the average number of fatal mining incidents per year is given near the beginning of the century, just after establishment of the U.S. Bureau of Mines in 1910, and near the end of this century. These comparative statistics follow:

- For 1911–1920
  - Total mining fatalities: 3,256 per year
  - Coal mining fatalities: 2,468 per year
- For 1991–1995
  - Total mining fatalities: 98 per year
  - Coal mining fatalities: 51 per year.

Ramani and Mutmansky (1999) highlight the tremendous success in preventing coal mining deaths by stating that "Coal mining fatalities have dropped to one-sixtieth of what they were at the beginning of the century even though coal production during the same period rose by a factor of five."

An examination of the fatal incident rate (IR) for the same time frames reveals the following average statistics:

- For 1911–1920:
  - 1.0 million miners employed in the industry
  - 32.1 fatals/10,000 workers; IR = 0.321
- For 1991–1995:
  - 338,000 miners employed in the industry
  - 2.9 fatals/10,000 workers; IR = 0.029.

These statistics show an order of magnitude improvement in the fatal IR over 8.5 decades. Here the fatal IR for a period gives the annual average number of fatalities per 100 workers. Prior to 1970, employee hours worked—the denominator used today for incident rates—cannot be reliably determined.

Detailed Assessment, 1911–1970   To present more detailed and concrete evidence of progress over time, one of the best indicators is a periodic improvement in the rate of change of the fatal IR with respect to time. On a plot of the fatal IR by 5-year periods, this gives the slope of the curve at any point in time. From one period to another, it gives the change rate for improvement or regression. Based on statistics given in Table 1.2, for specific periods of interest, the fatal IR change rate is shown in Table 1.3. The base period for calculations was 1911–1915, during which the fatal IR was 0.329. Each period's rate of change is based on the statistics from the previous 5-year period. Table 1.3 also gives the percentage change in the number of fatalities for both coal and noncoal sectors, which is another measure of progress. However, these latter measures do not reflect the mining activity or the numbers of miners employed, both of which have a significant impact on fatality statistics. The rate of change of the fatal IR accounts for the level of mining activity reflected through total employment and thus gives a better measure of progress. As we explore later, historical events can well be related to milestones in progress or reversals of progress.

As Table 1.3 shows, a modest reduction of 9.4% occurred in the total mining fatal IR during four 5-year periods following the establishment of the U.S. Bureau of Mines in 1910. After an initial reduction of 4.9% in the incident rate from the 1911–1915 period to the 1916–1920 period, and of 15.0% from 1916–1920 to 1921–1925, the tide turned and the incident rate increased by 12.0% in the 1926–1930 period. The proportion of fatalities for the coal sector increased from 75% to nearly 83% over the 20-year period. Reflective of these proportions, the number of fatalities in noncoal mining fell 43.1%, while they were reduced in coal by only 11.2%. As we saw in Table 1.2, mining employment dropped approximately 10% to about 900,000.

A drastic reduction of fatalities occurred during the next 5-year period, 1931–1935, which saw a 31.9% decrease in the fatal IR. This may be because of the economic depression, which brought layoffs, and the miners that were retained were undoubtedly the hardest and most conscientious workers (Grayson 1999; Ramani and Mutmansky 1999). Another probable cause of the improvement was the industry's implementation of technological change, which has generally been evolutionary rather than revolutionary. Based on this premise, the early technological developments of the Bureau of Mines, such as permissible explosives, safety electrical systems, better understanding of the explosibility of methane and coal, and rock dusting (Ramani and Mutmansky 1999), were not well implemented for a decade or two. In the 1930s, technology improvements included loaders, introduced in 1914, and chain conveyors, used as early as 1902, which became more broadly adopted and possibly began to reduce some hazards to miners. By 1935, for example, 13.5% of underground coal was loaded mechanically (Peele 1941).

Whatever the causes, tremendous reductions were achieved for both sectors, although coal continued to account for 87% of the fatalities. Coal fatalities dropped 44.5% from 2,235 to 1,241 per year in the previous 5-year period (as shown in Table 1.2). Noncoal fatalities dropped 60.9% from 463 to 181. Although total mining employment dropped 22.7% to 700,000, this was definitely a breakthrough period for mine health and safety as the major improvement in the fatal IR shows.

This success was followed by a stagnant period of no change in 1936–1940, and a consequent refocusing by Congress as disasters continued. When war broke out and an influx of new miners replaced those fighting for our nation's principles, mining suffered a 16% increase in the fatal incident

TABLE 1.3 Coal and noncoal fatality change, total mining fatal IR rate of change, and average change in employment, 1911–1970

Period	Coal Mining Fatality Change %	Noncoal Mining Fatality Change %	Total Mining IR Rate of Change %	Avg. Change in Employment %
1911–1930	−11.2	−43.1	−9.4	−10.5
1931–1935	−44.5	−60.9	−31.9	−22.7
1936–1940	+1.9	+48.6	No Change	+8.9
1941–1945	+3.6	+0.4	+16.0	−11.3
1946–1950	−33.6	−31.5	−31.6	−2.2
1951–1955	−40.0	−9.2	−18.8	−19.6
1956–1960	−27.2	−0.6	−12.3	−9.8
1961–1965	−27.9	+4.8	−7.0	−11.7
1966–1970	−10.2	+2.9	+2.8	−7.9

rate. Total employment also dropped 11.3%, an event that resulted in a higher proportion of inexperienced miners. At this time, coal accounted for nearly 83% of the fatalities.

Following World War II, the third greatest reduction (31.6%) in the mining fatal IR occurred during the next 5-year period of 1946–1950. This was clearly a breakthrough period, as experienced miner war heroes returned to their jobs. Technology progressed as well, as rubber-tired face haulage was introduced in coal mines, roof bolting was emerging, tungsten-carbide cutting elements were placed in fortified holders, and AC power began supplanting DC power (Anon. 1990; Crickmer and Zegeer 1981; Gregory 1980; and Green 1986). Ramani and Mutmanksy (1999) note the impact of the budding social revolution of the late 1930s and the catalytic role of the United Mine Workers of America led by John L. Lewis. Coal fatalities fell from 1,311 per year to 870 (a 33.6% reduction) while noncoal fell from 270 to 185 (a 31.5% reduction). Despite tremendous improvements, many miners were still dying on the job. Employment held fairly constant, dropping only 2.2% to 661,000.

From this point, the fatal IR dropped in successive periods but at a decreasing rate, from a reduction of 31.6%, as just mentioned, to 18.8% to 12.3% to 7% during the period between 1961 and 1965. Employment dropped as well by 19.6%, 9.8%, and 11.7%, respectively. Technological developments stagnated during the recession of the 1950s and 1960s. For example, although the Lee Norse prototype "continuous miner" was developed in 1941 and the "Joy ripper miner" in 1948, a continuous miner section wasn't established until 1964 (Anon. 1990; Crickmer and Zegeer 1981; and Green 1986). Joy introduced the first rubber-tired, all-wheel-drive shuttle car in 1966. Notably, widespread use of continuous miners didn't occur until 1970.

Coal accounted for a continually decreasing proportion of fatalities, dropping from 83% to 76% to 70% to 61%. The number of coal fatalities likewise dropped from 870 per year to 522 to 380 to 274, while noncoal held steady over the three periods at 168, 167, and 175, respectively. Continuous improvement was occurring during each 5-year period, but again, at a decreasing rate. This was a portentous sign of loss of intensity and Congress called for closer scrutiny of the noncoal sector.

Things changed drastically between 1966 and 1970. The visibility of and public outrage over the Farmington disaster fueled the fire for significant change. During that 5-year period, the statistics reveal that the fatal IR increased by 2.8%, even as coal's proportion of fatalities continued to decrease, down to 57% of total fatalities. But because of Farmington, the 1969 Federal Coal Mine Health and Safety Act became law.

Have the Acts Been Effective?   The 1969 act was intended to reduce the incidence of coal mine deaths and injuries, especially fatalities from explosions and fires as well as deaths and disabilities from blacklung disease. To spur improvements, significant regulations were introduced, as described earlier.

As shown in Table 1.4, in the first 5-year period following the 1969 act, the fatal IR dropped 25.7% and coal fatalities dropped from 246 per year to 151, a 38.6% reduction while employment held steady. Also for the first time, coal accounted for less than half of the nation's mining fatalities, at 46.9%. Unfortunately, another highly visible mining disaster occurred during this period, this time in the noncoal sector, as the Sunshine silver mine fire grabbed national headlines. As mentioned earlier, this, coupled with closer congressional scrutiny of noncoal safety statistics, was the primary impetus for enactment of the 1977 Federal Mine Health and Safety Amendments Act.

A logical question arises. Have the acts been effective? We all know the answer, but many of us have challenged each other's role in achieving improvements, such as government, operators, labor, and research institutions. Nonetheless, the answer is an unequivocal, "Yes." However, a proper perspective on attribution of their effectiveness requires an evaluation of the quite complex interrelationships

TABLE 1.4   Fatal IR rate of change, 1971–1995

Period	Coal Mining Fatality Change %	Noncoal Mining Fatality Change %	Total Mining IR Rate of Change %	Avg. Change in Employment %
1971–1975	−38.6	−5.0	−25.7	+1.6
1976–1980	−13.2	−28.7	−39.5	+31.5
1981–1985	−18.3	−42.6	−18.4	−15.7
1986–1990	−36.4	−22.9	−15.0	−18.7
1991–1995	−25.0	−11.1	−14.7	−5.2

they evoked. No doubt, the improvements achieved resulted from strong and sustained efforts by mine operators, organized labor, academic institutions, and research and enforcement agencies of the government.

Studying the magnitude of fatalities doesn't give the right answer to this question either. The more accurate answer is that the single greatest change in the fatal IR in this century occurred during the next 5-year period, 1976–1980, with a 39.5% reduction (see Table 1.4). Fatalities in coal decreased from 151 per year to 131 (13.2%), while for noncoal they decreased from 171 to 122 (28.7%). These achievements occurred, by the way, when the employment in mining increased by 31.5%, nearly a third, primarily in the coal sector in response to the oil embargo. Coal's proportion of the fatalities also increased, rising above 50% again to 51.8%. At the same time, innovations in continuous mining included:

- Use of cabs and canopies on face equipment
- Incorporation of automated temporary roof support systems on roof bolting machines
- Adoption of remote control for continuous miners
- Development of integrated continuous miners roof bolters.

As another example, longwall mining boomed in the mid-1970s after introduction of shields, which were developed by the Russians. In 1973, there were 40 longwall faces, none with shields, and by 1985, there were 118 longwall faces, 110 of which were equipped with shields.

The success of reducing the fatal IR continues from this point on, with no more reversals in improvements. Of course, continuous improvement in every facet of business is the hard rule now rather than the exception. The final three full 5-year periods show reductions in the fatal incident rate of 18.4%, 15.0%, and 14.7%, respectively. The coal proportion of fatalities was reduced concurrently from 61% to 56% to 52%—to less than half again today.

Two more noteworthy successes deserve attention. During the period from 1986 to 1990, each sector averaged fewer than 100 fatalities per year for the first time this century. Remarkably, for the first time, total fatalities in mining averaged fewer than 100 per year during the period from 1991 to 1995. These are excellent achievements considering the continued success in reducing the fatal IR.

Progress in Reducing Injuries and Diseases of the Lung

Progress has been achieved on other fronts as well, although accurate historical accounts are relatively recent (beginning in 1958 for noncoal). Some statistics were accumulated nonetheless, and these are summarized in Table 1.5 (MSHA 1999). These figures can be kept in good perspective, especially for the large increases in the 1971–1975 and 1976–1980 periods, by recalling that more stringently monitored accident reporting accompanied passage of the 1969 and 1977 acts.

Once again, remember that the MSHA definition of "accident" changed with the 1977 act, and, given a year for the changes to be fully implemented, Table 1.6 provides a new definition-related perspective on improvement in the nonfatal injury rate. Note that rates increased for a year or two for the different sectors, until equilibrium on reporting was reached and new regulations were relatively consistently enforced. After the break-in period, the rates began dropping each year until 1986, when the definition of "accident" was changed. The increases beginning in 1986 also resulted from a General Accounting Office (GAO) study (1987), which detected underreporting of accidents (primarily in small mines). After 3 more years of adjustment, improvement of the nonfatal injury rate began again. For the period from 1989 to 1995, the nonfatal injury rate dropped from 12.39 per 100 miners to 9.90 for underground coal mining, from 6.75 to 4.64 for underground metal/nonmetal mining, from 3.54 to 2.52 for surface coal mining, and from 4.65 to 3.12 for surface metal/nonmetal mining.

Table 1.7 provides summary statistics for all major safety measures—the number of fatalities, the fatal IR, the number of nonfatal days lost (NFDL) accidents, the NFDL IR, the total accident IR (MSHA reportable by definition), and the overall severity measure (SM). It also shows these measures for all mining sectors separately, broken down by underground and surface mining. This table gives good safety performance comparisons among sectors and among mine types. Table 1.8 gives the number of mines and miners for each sector and mine type for comparison purposes.

The discussion to this point has addressed the safety experience in the industry. Equally important is the health-related experience. One measure for the coal sector is the incidence of cases of coal workers' pneumoconiosis (CWP) and progressive massive fibrosis (PMF). From 1970 to 1995, the prevalence of CWP and PMF among miners, based on the statutory operator-sponsored x-ray program, dropped from 11% to 3% (U.S. Department of Labor 1996). Further, as noted by Ramani and Mutmansky (1999), "The total prevalence of PMF has decreased even more dramatically, from about 1% to less than 0.1%." However, it should be noted that participation of miners in the x-ray program was optional, and it is not known how representative the prevalence rates are of the entire industry. Nevertheless, it is clear that significant progress has been made in miners' health as well. It is also clear that more needs to be done to eliminate CWP and PMF.

TABLE 1.5   Injuries for coal and noncoal mining by 5-year period, 1936–1998 (MSHA 1999)

Year	NFDL IR U/G Coal	NFDL IR U/G/NM	NFDL IR Surface Coal	NFDL IR Surface M/NM
1978	10.41	9.74	3.52	4.12
1979	11.88	10.67	3.52	4.26
1980	12.13	9.39	3.48	3.62
1981	10.88	8.58	3.43	3.17
1982	9.94	5.80	3.27	2.51
1983	8.25	5.96	2.71	2.80
1984	8.28	5.26	2.66	2.80
1985	7.40	4.86	2.72	2.74
1986	8.05	5.35	3.21	3.19
1987	12.19	5.70	3.39	3.88
1988	12.93	6.73	3.51	4.33
1989	12.39	6.75	3.54	4.65
1990	12.15	6.31	3.57	4.60
1991	12.28	5.87	3.34	4.32
1992	11.61	4.80	3.17	4.28
1993	10.18	5.37	2.61	3.71
1994	11.08	5.69	3.12	3.72
1995	9.90	4.64	2.52	3.12

TABLE 1.6   Comparison of nonfatal days lost (NFDL) incident rates for U.S. underground and surface mines by coal and metal/nonmetal sectors (Reich and McAteer 1997a, b, c, d, e)

Year	NFDL IR U/G Coal	NFDL IR U/G/NM	NFDL IR Surface Coal	NFDL IR Surface M/NM
1978	10.41	9.74	3.52	4.12
1979	11.88	10.67	3.52	4.26
1980	12.13	9.39	3.48	3.62
1981	10.88	8.58	3.43	3.17
1982	9.94	5.80	3.27	2.51
1983	8.25	5.96	2.71	2.80
1984	8.28	5.26	2.66	2.80
1985	7.40	4.86	2.72	2.74
1986	8.05	5.35	3.21	3.19
1987	12.19	5.70	3.39	3.88
1988	12.93	6.73	3.51	4.33
1989	12.39	6.75	3.54	4.65
1990	12.15	6.31	3.57	4.60
1991	12.28	5.87	3.34	4.32
1992	11.61	4.80	3.17	4.28
1993	10.18	5.37	2.61	3.71
1994	11.08	5.69	3.12	3.72
1995	9.90	4.64	2.52	3.12

TABLE 1.7   U.S. fatalities, nonfatal days lost (NFDL) injuries, total accident incident rates (IRs), and severity measures for underground and surface mines by sector, 1995 (Reich and McAteer 1997a, b, c, d, e)

Sector	No. Fatals	Fatal IR	No. NFDL	NFDL IR	Total IR	Overall SM
Coal Underground	25	.05	5,426	10.57	13.50	772
Coal Surface	10	.03	942	2.75	4.06	288
Metal Underground	3	.04	422	5.79	9.75	498
Metal Surface	5	.03	469	2.52	4.23	290
Nonmetal U/G	3	.08	146	3.83	6.34	712
Nonmetal Surface	3	.05	137	2.41	4.19	433
Stone Underground	0	0	75	3.71	5.53	122
Stone Surface	11	.04	1,201	4.15	6.86	345
Sand/Gravel Surface	4	.02	881	3.56	5.62	269
Sand/Gravel Dredge	2	.04	182	3.77	6.10	335

TABLE 1.8   Number of mines and employees at U.S. mines in 1995 (Reich and McAteer 1997a, b, c, d, e)

Mining Sector	U/G Mines	Surface Mines	U/G Miners	Surface Miners
Coal	1,081	1,275	51,777	33,875
Metal	118	176	7,560	17,509
Nonmetal	57	570	3,904	5,832
Stone	102	3,296	1,940	29,028
Sand and Gravel*	—	6,021	—	32,970

*Includes 824 dredge operations employing 4,669 miners

INDUSTRY'S MARCH TOWARD CONTINUOUS IMPROVEMENT

This century has realized a tremendous continuation of improvements in mine health and safety. There have also been phenomenal productivity improvements, cost reductions, and successes in reducing both disease and injury. Undoubtedly operators, labor, manufacturers, and service companies have all worked hard to help achieve these successes; they have even, in many cases, assimilated into their culture the approaches used to attain them. At critical historical junctures, government certainly has played a major role, through inspection, enforcement, health and safety knowledge, and technology development as the result of research. Academia, too, has had an important role, especially through research and education of generations of mining engineers and mine managers.

The road to achieving these successes has not been easy, or straightforward over time. In a democracy, many political convolutions are involved in reaching a negotiated consensus in legislation and rulemaking at any point in historical time. As a nation, the U.S. citizenry has furnished the impetus for major change in mine health and safety performances, in essence, providing a national conscience to ensure safe and healthful workplaces for miners. Leaders of Congress, government agencies, labor organizations, and mining companies have taken turns in driving the success. The successive initiatives have created the industry's current march toward continuous improvement. This movement embraces mine health and safety as a cornerstone for successful mine operations. Improvements in all areas reduce costs and control losses of life, property, time, and information.

OVERVIEW OF CHALLENGES TO FURTHER PROGRESS

As mentioned earlier, the industry today focuses on continuous improvement in all areas of business, including:

- Fatalities
- Disabilities
- Injuries
- First aid cases

- Disease
- Regulatory compliance
- Productivity
- Costs.

The safety and health statistics presented previously do show that significant progress has been made, but mining continues to be one of the highest risk occupations in our nation. Our goal must be to make mining a model of excellence in all respects—a shining image of accomplishment.

Impediments to Continuous Improvement and Prospects for the Future

Next we will take a look at the current impediments to further progress in reducing the risks of miners in this industry. Fatality problem areas include powered haulage, ground control, and working around equipment/machinery. Injury-rate problem areas include handling materials, maintenance and repair, construction work, roof bolting, and other targeted tasks such as working on or around conveyor belts. General areas of concern with respect to fatalities and serious injuries, which demand special focus, are small mines and contractors employed at mine sites.

The list of lingering health-related impediments includes CWP, silicosis, hearing loss, and musculoskeletal disorders, which are just now being recognized and defined as a distinct problem.

We also need to recognize some emerging realities as we work toward continuous improvement in mining in the next century. These include:

- Conditions will degrade rather than improve
- We will mine deeper, thinner seams and orebodies
- We will encounter more discontinuous reserves
- New miners will join the workforce
- The industry will face even tougher competition
- Fewer companies will exist, but they will be multinationals.

Hence, to continue improvements, the industry must:

- Seek new mining methods and new technologies
- Organize and manage work more effectively
- Demand more health and safety features on mining equipment
- Ensure that best work practices are integral in accomplishing work
- Seek breakthroughs in handling some of the most persistent problems
- Incorporate health, safety, and environmental aspects in every facet of planning
- Set goals and objectives systematically to drive continuous improvements across the board.

Reduction in the cost of production, through, for example, increased productivity, will drive these imperatives. Change clearly stepped up to an unprecedented level in the last decade before the twenty-first century, and it will likely continue to accelerate. As an industry, we must act proactively and change commensurately.

SUMMARY

Our industry can be proud of the progress that we made in this century. Our milestones include continuous improvement in health and safety statistics virtually since World War II, a significant movement toward integrating health and safety into our business culture, and meeting significant challenges successfully. In this sense, this industry is both robust and mature. However, mining remains dangerous in relative terms, a fact that will never vanish.

The prospects for progress are bright. We believe that the industry shall again succeed in overcoming the impediments to further advancement in the next century. In our opinion, the best path for success in the next round of challenges is extensive partnerships in research and development—linking operators, labor, academia, and government. This approach will allow us to share limited resources to overcome common challenges.

REFERENCES

Adams, W.W., and M.E. Kohlos. 1941. *Metal- and Nonmetal-Mine Accidents in the United States During the Calendar Year 1939 (Excluding Coal Mines)*. Bureau of Mines Bulletin 440. Washington, DC: U.S. Government Printing Office. Table 34.

Adams, W.W., and V.E. Wrenn. 1941. *Quarry Accidents in the United States During the Calendar Year 1939*. Bureau of Mines Bulletin 438. Washington, DC: U.S. Government Printing Office. Table 40.

Anon. 1990. *Encyclopedia Britannica*. 15th ed. Chicago: Encyclopedia Britannica. (various articles on mining).

———. 1996. *Work-Related Lung Disease Surveillance Report.* Department of Health and Human Services (NIOSH) Publication No. 96-134. Washington, DC: U.S. Government Printing Office. 447 pp.

———. 1997. Historical data on mine disasters in the United States. *The Guardian.* 28(2): 5. London, U.K.: National Mine Rescue Association.

Cassidy, S.M. 1981. History of coal mining. *Elements of Practical Coal Mining*. 2nd ed. Edited by D.F. Crickmer and D.A. Zegeer. New York: Society of Mining Engineers–American Institute of Mining Engineers (SME-AIME).

Crickmer, D.F., and D.A. Zegeer. 1981. *Elements of Practical Coal Mining*. New York: AIME.

Federal Coal Mine Health and Safety Act. Public Law 91–173. 1969.

Federal Mine Safety and Health Amendments Act. Public Law 95–164. 1977.

GAO. 1987. *Mine Safety: Inspector Hiring, Penalty Assessments, and Injury Reporting.* Briefing Report to the Honorable Howard M. Metzenbaum, U.S. Senate. Washington, DC: GAO. 9 pp.

Grayson, R.L. 1999. Mine health and safety: progress and prospects for the future. *Mining Engineering.* 51(6): 63–65.

Green, P. 1986. Modern deep mining: revolutionary, evolutionary. *Coal Age.* 91(6): 59–65.

Gregory, C.E. 1980. *A Concise History of Mining*. New York: Pergamon Press.

House of Representatives Report No. 91–563. 1969. Ninety-first Congress, First Session. October 13.

House of Representatives Report No. 95–312. 1977. Ninety-fifth Congress, First Session. May 13.

MSHA. 1999. Web site: www.msha.gov.

Organic Act. Public Law 61–179. 1910.

Peele, R. 1941. *Mining Engineers' Handbook*. 3rd ed. New York: John Wiley and Sons.

Ramani, R.V., and J.M. Mutmansky. 1999. Mine health and safety at the turn of the millennium. *Mining Engineering.* 51(9): 25–30.

Reese, S.T., V.E. Wrenn, and E.J. Reid. 1955. *Injury Experience in Coal Mining, 1952: Analysis of Mine Safety Factors, Related Employment, and Production Data*. Bureau of Mines Bulletin 559. Washington, DC: U.S. Government Printing Office. Tables 51 and 52.

Reich, R.B., and J.D. McAteer. 1997a. *Injury Experience in Coal Mining, 1995*. Mine Safety and Health Administration IR 1242. Washington, DC: U.S. Government Printing Office. 16, 285.

———. 1997b. *Injury Experience in Metallic Mineral Mining, 1995*. Mine Safety and Health Administration IR 1243. Washington, DC: U.S. Government Printing Office. 14, 192.

———. 1997c. *Injury Experience in Nonmetallic Mineral Mining (Except Stone and Coal), 1995*. Mine Safety and Health Administration IR 1244. Washington, DC: U.S. Government Printing Office. 14, 241.

———. 1997d. *Injury Experience in Stone Mining, 1995*. Mine Safety and Health Administration IR 1245. Washington, DC: U.S. Government Printing Office. 14, 413.

———. 1997e. *Injury Experience in Sand and Gravel Mining, 1995*. Mine Safety and Health Administration IR 1246. Washington, DC: U.S. Government Printing Office. 14, 82.

Senate Report No. 95–181. 1977. Ninety-fifth Congress, First Session, May 16.

Traweek, W. 1994. Presentation at the National Safety Council Annual Conference and Exhibition, Mining Section Session. Orlando, FL.

U.S. Department of Labor. 1996. *Report of the Advisory Committee on the Elimination of Pneumoconiosis among Coal Mine Workers.* Washington, DC: MSHA.

CHAPTER 2

Health and Safety Management

Tom A. Hethmon
Director, Occupational Health and Safety
Phelps Dodge Corporation, Phoenix, Arizona

Charles W. Doane
Manager, Safety Systems
Phelps Dodge Corporation, Phoenix, Arizona

THE IMPORTANCE OF HEALTH AND SAFETY MANAGEMENT IN MINING

From the earliest written records on human occupation, mining has been characterized as a dangerous trade with a high probability of injury, illness, or worse (Agricola 1556). This characterization developed over thousands of years during which life was fragile for those who removed and processed ore. Regrettably, mining accidents were often viewed as one of the tragic costs of extracting the materials necessary for the development of modern life.

Today, mining is among the safest industries in the United States as reflected by comparable industry fatality and injury rates (National Safety Council [NSC] 1998). These improvements are the result of a number of factors, including:

- Improved mining methods, such as increased automation and other procedures, which have limited the interaction between man, machine, and mined material (see Figure 2.1)
- Routine general education and specialized hazard training for workers
- Broader understanding and application of health and safety management systems and techniques
- Greater recognition of the moral imperative to protect the industry's greatest asset—its people.

Although these improvements are laudable, miners in the United States and abroad continue to be injured, develop occupational disease, and, in 60 instances in 1998, die on the job (Mine Health and Safety Administration [MSHA] 1999).

For students or practitioners of mining health and safety, there is no more important knowledge than a clear understanding of the value of human life and health and the irreversible consequences that result from a loss of either. This fundamental awareness drives mine owners, managers, and workers to establish priorities that facilitate a safe, healthy, and profitable workplace. But it is not enough to work hard in the present to preserve the future. We must also learn from the past to secure future outcomes. The twenty-first century mine operator must fight the stigma of the inherent hazard and inevitable link to occupational illness and injury. However, this is simpler said than done and represents a significant challenge.

For example, in 1998 an employee with more than 20 years of experience with a large mining company known for its strong health and safety culture suffered a bilateral amputation of the hands. This incident involved work deemed to be safe, and the job had been done without incident for many years. The pain and suffering of the worker, his team members and family, and the community in which he lives continues to be felt. The man and his family must manage the lifelong consequences, including quality-of-life issues and the ability to provide financially for his family.

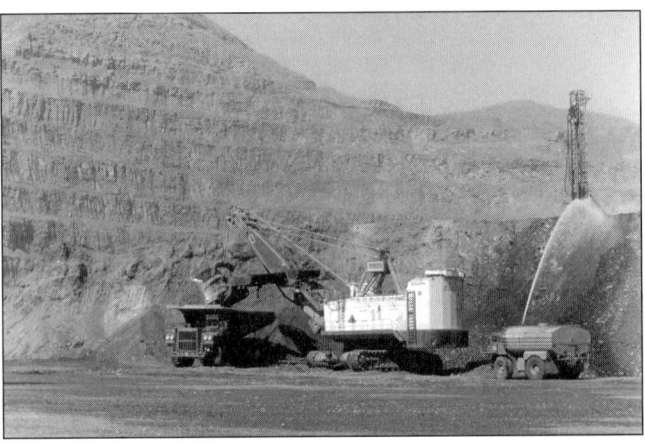

FIGURE 2.1   Open pit mine operations

Unfortunately, similar scenarios have occurred in many industries, affecting the lives of thousands of people and costing companies billions of dollars in lost revenue and other costs. In the United States in 1997 alone, more than 5,000 people lost their lives in work-related incidents and more than 3.8 million suffered disabling injuries. In that same year, workplace injuries and illnesses resulted in a direct cost to U.S. industry of nearly $128 billion, with estimated total costs—direct and indirect—of a staggering $600 billion (NSC 1999).

With such profound statistics, there can be little doubt that health and safety is a critical function for any mining organization. Beyond its moral imperative, successful health and safety programs make good business sense. In recognition of this perspective, mining managers and health and safety practitioners must have a clear understanding of what is required to manage these programs effectively. The goal of this text is to provide students and professionals alike with insights into health and safety management practices.

A mining health and safety agenda is not substantially different from those practiced in other industries. Certainly the engineering aspects of mining are somewhat different and some administrative practices relating to health and safety are unique, but the principles presented in this text and many developments in mining health and safety are not mutually exclusive of approaches in other industries. Therefore, we must not ignore best practices from other industries just because they function differently from mining.

A broad spectrum of approaches to health and safety management may be found in the mining industry. At one end of the continuum are companies that believe that there is a high probability of injury and illness associated with mining and that formal intervention can limit but not prevent such events. This approach generally views health and safety as an ancillary function within the organization and as a cost of doing business. With this type of thinking, the purpose of health and safety is to minimize loss and address regulatory compliance.

On the other end of the spectrum are organizations that have adopted a proactive and comprehensive view of health and safety based on the belief that all injuries and illnesses are preventable. They intend to achieve a high degree of integration of the health and safety function into the organization's business plan. They view health and safety as a critical obligation as well as a primary indicator of operational excellence.

Fortunately, the proactive philosophy has become more prevalent in the mining industry and those companies that disregard the welfare of their employees are increasingly rare. In the last decade, the focus on workplace health and safety has risen significantly through media exposure, and a growing number of companies recognized the benefits of effective health and safety management. They acknowledge that when managed at a high level, health and safety optimizes workforce effectiveness and productivity and represents an opportunity to have a positive impact on stockholder value. In addition, prospective employees prefer to work for organizations that value and protect their workers.

As a result, companies that make health and safety a priority are more likely to recruit quality employees.

Often overlooked as a human right, the ability to work in a safe environment should be central to the development of effective health and safety measures. This kind of employee protection is not a benefit, but a fundamental right. No person or organization is justified in placing an individual in a situation of potential injury, or in failing to develop controls for effectively managing risk and hazards. This moral obligation is a driving force in progressive companies that promote health and safety. Not only does it make good business sense, but first and foremost it shows genuine concern for the well-being of employees. Within such organizations, health and safety is viewed not only as a priority, but a core value that guides other business priorities—priorities can change; values don't.

THE EVOLUTION OF HEALTH AND SAFETY MANAGEMENT

The modern safety movement reflects the lessons learned during the last 150 years of industrial development. Researcher Carl Mussacchio wrote, "the late 19th century hatched new industries like a brooding hen, and because industry was new, safety techniques were primitive" (Mussacchio 1975). During this period, concern for working conditions and employee safety was vocalized only in a few basic industries such as steel, coal, textiles, and railway. A scattering of small labor organizations demanded action to curbing employee injuries. In 1867, Massachusetts instituted the first state factory inspection requirements in the United States. In 1882, the Joliet Works of Illinois Steel Company first introduced plant-safety functions—many historians agree that this was the birthplace of the American industrial-safety movement (Pope 1990).

During the 1800s and early 1900s, Americans were generally unaware of how many workers were being killed and disabled annually in industrial accidents. The Russell Sage Foundation, founded in 1905, sought to determine the extent of workplace injuries by means of its "Pittsburgh Survey," a survey instrument used initially in the greater Pittsburgh area. The results were shocking as the Sage investigators identified 526 on-the-job fatalities and 500 disabling injuries within a 1-year period in a single county.

The Pittsburgh Survey is credited with instigating the formation of a safety establishment and the advent of organized safety programs within U.S. industry. Published in 1907, the survey findings set off a chain reaction of legislation and industry development:

1908	Congress enacted the first Workers Compensation law for federal employees.
1910	The U.S. Bureau of Mines was established.
1910–1915	State safety and industrial hygiene departments were established in many jurisdictions.
1911	The American Society of Safety Engineers was established.
1911–1915	New York was the first state to pass Workers Compensation laws.
1912	The National Council for Industrial Safety (the forerunner of NSC) was organized.

"In a sense, those pioneers who enacted national safety movements were fanatics and extremists. They were a handful of professional safetymen, a few management leaders, some public officials and some insurance men. These were the few to whom so many owe so much today" (Meyer 1987).

In 1911, the United States held its first national conference on industrial diseases. In 1912, the U.S. Public Health Service, established in 1902, was expanded to include an occupational health division. In 1916, the American Occupational Medical Association was chartered. For the first time in our history, occupational health was being systematically addressed. It was during this period that the occupational medicine pioneer, Alice Hamilton, began her work characterizing the potential health hazards of the trades in the United States, including mining (Hamilton 1943).

Organized industrial safety programs became more prevalent in the 1920s (see Figure 2.2). Companies began competing for safety awards for working without a lost-time accident. In 1926, Carnegie Steel Company boasted 2.6 million man-hours without a lost-time injury. Illinois Steel recorded 3 million man-hours and Clark Thread Company more than 10 million. In 1926, the NSC reported 24,000 industrial fatalities and more than 3 million nonfatal injuries, with an average national injury rate of 31.9 per 100 workers (Petersen 1989).

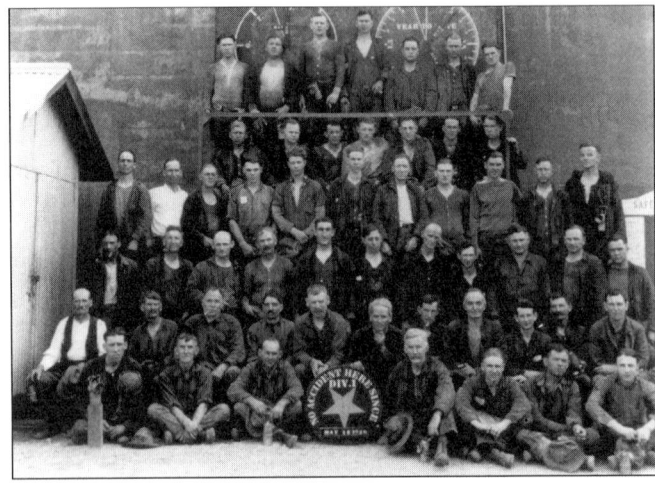

FIGURE 2.2   Miner's safety performance recognition, circa 1920s

In 1931, H.W. Heinrich published *Industrial Accident Prevention*. This work outlined his "domino theory of accident prevention." Heinrich identified five factors that result in injury, and likened them to dominoes:

1. Environment
2. Fault of the individual
3. Unsafe act or condition
4. Accident
5. Injury.

Knocking over the first causes a chain reaction that ends in an injury. Heinirch also proposed that 88% of all injuries were caused by unsafe acts, unsafe conditions accounted for only 10%, and accident reduction could best be accomplished by controlling unsafe acts with safety rule enforcement, discipline, and safety education.

Heinrich's work was the forerunner of the widely held philosophy that proactive safety was centered in the "three Es"–"engineering, education, and enforcement"–a viewpoint that has lasted nearly four decades. The idea that 85% of accidents were caused by unsafe acts and only 15% by hazardous conditions resulted in nearly universal adherence in safety management circles and the emphasis appeared appropriate (Petersen 1989). This observation was subsequently validated by other organizations, although with different numerical ratios (e.g., DuPont).

Enacted in 1941, Public Law 49 of the Seventy-Seventh Congress gave the U.S. Bureau of Mines authority to make "annual or necessary inspections and investigations." In 1952, Public Law 552 of the Eighty-Second Congress exempted mines employing less than 15 and gave the Bureau of Mines closure and withdrawal authority. In 1952, the Federal Coal Mine Safety Act authorized annual inspections in underground mines. The act sanctioned civil penalties for failure to cooperate with inspectors. During the 1950s, the national average injury rate for general industry dropped to below 7 injuries per 100 workers per year. However, prevailing wisdom concluded that virtually all safety engineering had progressed as far as could be expected. Greater emphasis was placed on engaging production supervision in day-to-day safety management activities and recognizing the importance of senior management support (Pope 1990). Educational courses for management, "tailgate" talks with employees, and in some companies joint management–union safety committees were all part of safety education and motivation.

During the 1960s accident frequency rates suddenly increased nearly 33%. In response, Congress became actively involved in enacting legislation to place controls on workplace safety. The first federal statute to include noncoal mines was the 1966 Federal Metal and Nonmetallic Mine Safety Act. The Federal Coal Mine Health and Safety Act of 1969 (Public Law 91–173) preceded the Occupational

Safety and Health Act (OSHA). Amended by Public Law 95–164 in 1977, it was called the Federal Mine Safety and Health Act of 1977. In the 1970s, OSHA was passed during the Nixon administration as a promulgation of safety and health standards. OSHA ensured workplace safety in general industry. But despite an increased role for government in workplace safety, incident rates continued their upward trend. By the end of the 1980s, the average national injury rate for general industry exceeded 13 per 100 workers (Pope 1990). As the number of injuries escalated, many companies began to look beyond traditional safety management techniques, such as Heinrich's model with its predominate focus on engineering, protective equipment, enforcement of rules, and safety committees. A focus on safety management systems became more prevalent, emphasizing increased involvement in safety at all levels of the organization.

The most significant trend in the last 20 years has been the development of mechanisms to address management and worker behavior relating to safety in addition to the physical environment. Any study of the development of health and safety methods in the last century must acknowledge that the concepts of safe and unsafe behavior are not new. The following text extracted from a safety and accident prevention course from a large metal mining company in 1920 proves this (Gidley):

> If a miner, by expenditure of a definite amount of energy in a certain way, can show a greater advantage than that obtained by expending the same energy in another way, then the first way must be considered the more efficient, if the conditions are unchanged in other aspects; but if, in saving the energy, he runs greater risk of injury, the gain in efficiency and safety is not sound and real, but only temporary and illusionary. Another characteristic among miners is the willingness to assume risks if time and energy may be saved. This trait is daily in evidence. Men are prone to take chances by assuming risks regardless of efforts advanced for their safety. Whether this is recklessness, ignorance, carelessness, lack of forethought or something else, the desire to perform a certain piece of work without using the necessary precautions for safety have a decided bearing on the cause of accidents.

However, an approach that could affect behavior modification was not well understood at the time. Today, the three Es of safety have been modified to include attention to social issues such as:

- Empowering workers
- Adopting progressive labor practices
- Instilling health and safety as a personal and organizational value
- Developing positive worker attitudes and a focus on behavior modification, most commonly in the form of behavior observation and feedback systems
- Conducting analyses of ergonomics and human factors.

THE IMPACT OF MINE HEALTH AND SAFETY REGULATIONS

Both society at large and the industry in general take a negative view of corporate executives who exclude occupational health and safety as an integral part of their business responsibilities. Many U.S. mining companies maintain substantial health and safety programs with senior management providing leadership and significant resources. Companies recognize the value of their employees and their obligation to maintain safe workplaces, as well as the potential costs associated with failure to control their facilities. But companies are also influenced by the need for regulatory compliance. Failure to adhere to applicable regulations can result in financial impacts such as citations, fines, and civil and, in extreme cases, criminal liability. Both MSHA and OSHA have played a significant role in influencing the industry to establish formal, minimum standards. Some countries with extensive mining industries, such as Brazil and Mexico, have mining-specific regulations. They also have health and safety mandates in their national constitutions to recognize the potential toll on national welfare as well as the importance of working men and women.

By its nature, government regulation is often reactive in its development, with many of the current mining health and safety regulations resulting from the industry's past performance. New regulations are developed based on identified patterns of hazards, death, injury, or illness. Regulations are developed to prevent recurrence. Although regulations help, the correlation between improved worker protection and regulatory enforcement is not clear. No research unequivocally establishes this relationship. The correlation between the introduction of new regulations and a decrease in incidence rates is difficult to separate from influences such as:

- Increased management and labor involvement
- Changing social mores
- Improved mining equipment and practices.

At a minimum, mining health and safety regulations play an important role. However, comprehensive compliance with all regulations is no assurance of an injury- and illness-free workplace. Therefore, regulations notwithstanding, it remains the responsibility of management and workers alike to strive for this goal.

SAFETY VERSUS OCCUPATIONAL HEALTH

In many mining companies, the term "safety" implies an organizational function that may include safety and occupational health and/or industrial hygiene. The primary focus of management today is safety, or preventing negative, generally irreversible, events of acute duration. The outcomes of safety-related events are usually visible and can evoke strong emotions if the results are severe.

Occupational illnesses and diseases tend to be chronic and are generally characterized by temporary or permanent physical dysfunction. With the exception of some symptoms, they are not generally visible. Therefore, safety overrides health in mining because occupational ailments take years to develop and management observes less physical trauma, if they witness anything at all. Despite this long-held bias, recognition is now emerging. Experts now see that occupational illness and disease do result in significant emotional and financial toll to workers, their families and communities, and their employers. Effective health and safety management must include acknowledging the importance of occupational health hazards and the proportionate application of resources to address those issues (Cralley 1988).

ELEMENTS OF HEALTH AND SAFETY MANAGEMENT

Ask 100 mining health and safety professionals what they believe are the core elements of effective mine health and safety management and you're likely to get 100 different answers. The question of what represents the most effective method is a subject of ongoing debate because the fundamental nature of injuries and illness in the mining industry involves the convergence of many factors including:

- Geology
- Extractive and processing technologies
- Individual and organizational characteristics and behavior
- Micro- and macroeconomics.

The fact that human loss continues in the industry also indicates that no single correct health and safety method has been defined and no absolute consensus has been established. However, there are obvious predominate patterns in the types of activities conducted in almost all mines to safeguard miners and those who support them, such as contractors and vendors. These include, but are not limited to, mechanisms that:

Identify, Correct, and Prevent Hazards

This may include:

- Auditing procedures for physical hazards and work practice deviations and behaviors
- Engineering for safe design
- Review of hazardous material storage, handling, and use
- Process safety management
- Incident reporting and analysis.

Educate and Train Personnel in Hazard Recognition, Control, and Work Practices

The education (general knowledge and information) and training (specific instruction) of new miners, process workers, and managers include:

- Site-specific hazards
- Regulatory requirements
- Health and safety responsibilities
- Standard work practices (codes of safe practice plus job safety analysis)
- Rules and procedures
- Specialized training and periodic refresher training to renew skills and knowledge. This ensures that workers recognize the hazards to which they may be exposed and understand the processes and systems that are in place to prevent injury.

Facilitate Commitment and Involvement

The sharing of values, empowerment, responsibility, accountability, attitude, cooperation, and reinforcement among all levels of an organization from the CEO to the most junior position democratizes health and safety. This implies that the necessary culture is established and that the expectations and actions necessary for effective health and safety management are understood.

However, it would be grossly simplistic to suggest that these three elements in and of themselves offer sufficient guidance for health and safety management. Research and anecdotal experience both suggest that effective health and safety management involves all personnel regardless of position or experience. It must be recognized that some activities have more impact than others.

Research conducted by the National Institute for Occupational Safety and Health (NIOSH) in the 1970s suggests that companies with low accident trends show certain attributes more predominately that those with high accident rates. Determined through a questionnaire study of 192 companies (Cohen et al. 1975), these characteristics include a more stable workforce with:

- Demographics such as mature, married employees with extensive work experience
- An emphasis on balancing engineering and nonengineering approaches to accident prevention
- More frequent but less formal audits of the physical conditions of the workplace
- A more humanistic approach to discipline for rules violations
- Greater emphasis on job health and safety training and supplemental modes of training for production personnel
- More use of health and safety incentive programs
- Greater utilization of outside influences in heightening health and safety awareness
- Greater management emphasis on and commitment to health and safety.

In 1987, the U.S. Bureau of Mines conducted a 3-year analysis of 10 mining companies and 62 underground coal mines to evaluate the effect of management practices on coal mine health and safety. The bureau concluded that senior management's commitment is critical to establishing strong health and safety performance. This resolve was expressed in ways that were unique to specific companies as well as common to the industry. The three primary indicators of commitment are:

- A complete sequence of activities and processes for managing health and safety that could be tracked and reinforced in a participative environment
- A strong element of advocacy by one or more key management officials
- The employees' view that the company's approach to safety and worker protection is unique.

Other attributes of companies with good health and safety performance include:

- Health and safety/productivity incentives
- Discipline policies
- Incident investigation processes
- Effective broad-based communication systems
- Positive labor-management relations.

The research also notes a positive correlation between health and safety performance and productivity. In other words, safe and healthy mines are productive mines (Gaertner et al. 1987).

Still other research suggests a relationship between health and safety management and organizational characteristics and practices. Sanders, Paterson, and Peay, working with the National Academy of Science (NAS), identified specific management practices that contributed to decreased injury rates, including:

- High employee morale
- Decentralized decision making
- Innovative and flexible management relative to the introduction of new procedures and initiatives (Sanders et al. 1976; NAS 1976). This research may be more than 20 years old, but the conclusions still have merit for the future development of good health and safety management systems.

THE SYSTEMS MODEL OF HEALTH AND SAFETY MANAGEMENT

When viewed as a total system, health and safety management involves three broad and interrelated domains as depicted in the fundamental model shown in Figure 2.3.

This model is based on two underlying premises:

1. Health and safety is affected by all aspects of the design and workings of an organization.
2. The design and management of health and safety systems must integrate all three domains in proportions that reflect an organization's unique characteristics. In other words, no one system is universally effective.

Ultimately, the system should be measurable, modifiable, perceived to be positive by those it affects, and as simple as possible. And though no one system will work effectively in all organizations, some basic tenets are universal (Peterson 1996):

- Health and safety is a management function and should be led and managed accordingly. This necessitates a high degree of management commitment and involvement.
- Unifying elements produce a set of defined responsibilities and accountability for those activities at all levels of the organization.
- Incidents, injuries, and illnesses are an indication of a problem in the system, not simply human error.
- Performance goals must reflect management objectives.

People

People are at the core of health and safety. As research and experience indicates, most safety incidents are behavior related. It has been said that safety is a continuous battle with human nature but a fight that can be won with an appropriate investment in understanding people with all their capabilities, limitations, and behaviors. As such, successful health and safety management must be centered on people (Geller 1996)—both labor and management. However, the human element is very complicated and dynamic, requiring constant attention and feedback.

Every individual is unique. Designing systems that motivate not only individuals but an entire workforce, then, is one of the most significant challenges facing companies today. The complexities of such a task become apparent given an understanding of the variances between individual personalities and their likes and dislikes. What might inspire one person may have no value to another. One

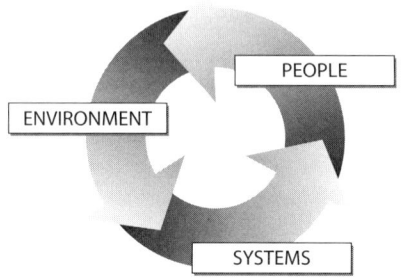

FIGURE 2.3   The systems model of health and safety management

size does not fit all. Hence, the keys to enrolling workers and management into a vision of an organization that does not accept injury as part of the job are creativity, imagination, and the development of diverse systems, creating a net wide enough to capture an entire workforce. Many factors must be considered in designing systems that will optimize results by focusing on the human domain. The most important elements are listed below.

- Age
- Attitude
- Behavior
- Communication
- Complacency
- Empowerment
- Expectations
- Experience

- Health
- Knowledge
- Language
- Leadership
- Motives
- Needs
- Perception
- Personality

- Physical capability
- Responsibility
- Risk perception
- Skills
- Stress
- Values.

Environment

This domain relates to the physical work space including the materials and mechanisms found therein. These are the elements of mining that can be seen and must be controlled, or at least understood, to the point of predicting how they will affect work and workers (American Institute of Mine Engineering 1992; NSC 1992; Hethmon and Dotson 1997). It must be realized that studies indicate that behavior contributes to the vast majority of accidents, but almost without exception, environmental conditions also play a contributory role.

As such, identifying and abating physical hazards is a fundamental safety principle. The mining environment can be vast, whether it is an underground or open pit mine. Unless the mechanism employed to review hazards is comprehensive, critical portions may be overlooked. Many physical hazard audit programs fall short in placing boundaries around the perceived workplace and failing to recognize the full scope of work conducted at any one time. This is particularly true for employees working alone, for nonstandard work, and for infrastructure support activities, such as geology, engineering, electrical, and road maintenance. To effectively control environmental factors and minimize potential for injury and illness, a broad and comprehensive view must be applied. The contribution of all possible influences must be considered and assessed, including the following list of items.

- Ergonomics
- Exposure controls
- Facility design
- Geology
- Guarding
- Housekeeping
- Human factors
- Materials

- Mine design and layout
- Processes and process design
- Time of day/night
- Tools and equipment
- Transportation
- Utilities
- Weather.

Systems

These are the processes by which things get done. They include health and safety regulatory compliance activities, production and maintenance methods, interaction between entities within the organization, proactive and reactive health and safety practices, social processes and programs, human resource activities, communication mechanisms, intrinsic and extrinsic rewards, and measurement systems. The list goes on (see pg. 26) (NSC 1992; McSween 1995).

Organizations are designed for the results they obtain, whether it's production, safety, or quality. Results are determined in large part by the systems that have been implemented based on the organization's design and how those systems are managed.

In addition to design, a major failing of many otherwise effective systems is the lack of a renewal phase or process. To be successful, systems must periodically be reevaluated to determine if they are adding value, addressing problems, and contributing to continuous improvement. Proper feedback provides a mechanism to enhance systems, correct those yielding poor results, and eliminate those that are ineffective. Although many mechanisms to assess system effectiveness exist, some of the most practical and telling are perception surveys, dialogues with critical individuals, cost-benefit analyses, and careful visual evaluations of the system in operation.

- Accountability
- Behavior modification
- Change management
- Communication
- Consistency
- Contractors
- Contracts administration
- Counseling and discipline
- Culture[1]
- Emergency response
- Enrollment
- Goals, vision, and mission
- Hazard abatement and control
- Hazard identification
- Health and safety staffing
- Hiring practices
- Incident investigation
- Industrial hygiene

- Information management
- Leadership
- Motivation and reward
- Occupational medicine
- Performance appraisal
- Performance measurement
- Policies, procedures, and rules
- Process safety
- Procurement
- Programs[2]
- Recognition
- Resources
- Safety engineering
- Strategic planning
- Supervision
- Teams
- Training and education
- Wellness.

SYSTEM FAILURES AND INJURY DYNAMICS IN MINING

Although many theories attempt to explain accident and injury causation, every accident falls into one of the following categories:

1. An object strikes a person.
2. A person contacts an object.

An object may be mobile, immobile, large as a multimillion pound shovel, solid, liquid, or even electromagnetic in nature, including any combination thereof. Sometimes autonomous physiological and biomechanical processes result in injury and illness (e.g., repetitive motion disorders). However, the vast majority of injuries in the mining industry can be categorized by one of these two causes. Looking beyond the proximal cause, we can find a universe of root causation associated with both injuries and illnesses. Adding to root causation are operational and organizational variables specifically associated with mining. Some characteristics that contribute to the potential for injury and illness are unique to the mining industry, such as extracting, transporting, and processing large volumes of ore–geological properties and geophysical forces. Mined material prices are not easily influenced by the producer who often must employ increasing numbers and sizes of extractive and process equipment to optimize economies of scale. The operation and interaction of workers with such large pieces of equipment increases the hazard potential (see Figure 2.4).

It is a common misconception that injuries, particularly fatalities and life-threatening incidents, result from a single major breakdown in the safety process. In reality, most incidents (including those with major ramifications) result from simple safety system failures. One has only to study the root causes of such incidents as the Scofield Mine disaster of 1900 (Scofield, Utah), the July 1942 explosion at the

---

1. Organizational culture is the accumulation of what is discussed, written, assumed, valued, and acted on.
2. Programs generally refer to the standard health and safety processes used to address specific hazards or operating activities (e.g., energy control, electrical systems, confined space entry, conveyance, cranes, forklifts, hearing conservation, material handling, explosives, machine guarding, respiratory protection, welding, haulage, fire control, hazardous materials, and job safety analysis).

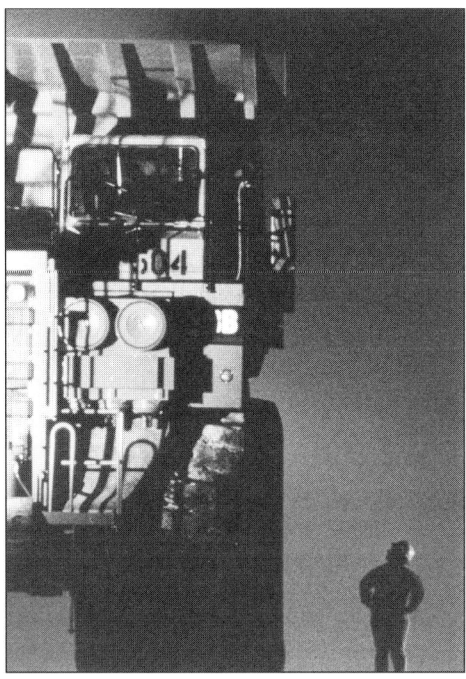

FIGURE 2.4   The size of mobile mine equipment continues to increase

Scotts Run mines (West Virginia), the Braden (El Tiente, Chile) mine fire and explosion in 1945, the 1968 Belle Isle salt mine (Louisiana) fire, the Sunshine mine (Coeur d'Alene, Idaho) fire in May 1972, and the Dongcun coal mine disaster in Datong, China, in July 1996, to understand this point. Although the emphasis on safety at each of these mines varied widely, none was believed to lack the basic elements of a safety program. Yet an analysis of these events highlights the variety of small miscalculations, oversights, and errors, including lack of clarity about job responsibilities, organizational restructuring that failed to identify needed safety resources, management assumptions that were never validated, failure of management communication, inadequate training, violation of established safety systems and procedures, failure to conduct required safety audits, and failure to learn lessons from prior safety events. Like dominoes, the small failures affect other variables that ultimately contribute to the negative event and outcome.

In his study of major incidents resulting from minor failures, Pybus (1996) offers the following advice:

1. Ignore small accidents at your peril—they signal worse things to come.
2. Know the worst that can happen and the risk of it happening.
3. Have formal controls over those factors you can't afford to have go wrong.
4. Don't expect people to do the right things unless they know they are.
5. Don't expect people to do the right things unless they have the right resources.
6. Don't expect people to do the right things if there are conflicts of interest.
7. You will never know how well or how poorly things are working unless you check carefully. Make clear that you want to hear the bad news as well as the good news.
8. Without clear lines of responsibility and accountability, you will lose control.

Another important misunderstanding that leads to the failure of health and safety systems is that major elements of traditional safety programs often do not work as assumed. Hansen concluded that research conducted by NIOSH indicated that many traditional safety program elements did not correlate with safety effectiveness and results in terms of safety incidents. These traditional safety elements include:

- Committees
- Staff

- Meetings
- Training
- Inspections
- Rules
- Records.

In some cases, the companies with the worst safety records had the best safety committees and staff. Factors found to correlate with better incident statistics included management and cultural factors such as management involvement, financial support, management/labor relations, attitudes toward employees, supervisor interactions, planning, and job quality (Hansen 1993).

The prevention of injury and illness and the development of a business culture centered on health and safety must come from a paradigm of authentic caring, which includes listening actively, encouraging self-efficacy, removing barriers, and coaching performance (Blair 1996). The traditional safety paradigm of top-down control where management makes all the decisions, establishes the rules, and is responsible for making changes when necessary has proven to be less successful in developing such cultures. In these environments, employee knowledge about work conditions and safety problems is not integrated into decision making and problem solving and effective change is not obtained (Blair 1996).

Yet another potential management system error is the assumption that places blame for health and safety problems on people. For example, incidents are the result of unsafe acts and behaviors, which should be expanded to include the uncommon understanding that incidents are also the result of flawed organizational values, decisions, and practices. Progressive safety cultures tend to supplement or replace traditional safety management philosophy with systems thinking. For example, organizational problems related to poor performance (management involvement, lack of resources, lack of worker empowerment, poor communication, lack of clear goals, and lack of accountability) should be identified and addressed, rather than focusing solely on (Hansen 1995):

- Worker attitudes
- Rote obedience to health and safety rules
- Reactive fixes and accident analyses focused on root causes of accidents (which are often deeply imbedded in the organization) rather than proactive planning and consequence analysis.

ESTABLISHING HEALTH AND SAFETY PERFORMANCE GOALS

A critical function in health and safety management is the process of defining acceptable performance standards. Goal setting involves the goal itself, and the rate of progress toward the goal. Given the moral imperative of protecting human lives, most organizations maintain a goal of zero injuries and illness, although some believe it is not possible to completely eliminate mining injuries and illnesses. Some companies elect to have zero as an ultimate goal, but may not recognize it formally in their annual goal-setting agenda. Other companies recognize zero as their goal both internally and publicly. Less variation occurs in the identification of optimal goals, but much greater differences arise in organizations about the rate of progress. Two general perspectives relate to the rate of progress in health and safety performance goals: continuous incremental improvement and immediate attainment (zero incidents).

The continuous improvement approach defines some degree of incremental improvement on an annual basis; zero implies the immediate elimination of injuries or illnesses. Continuous improvement, regardless of its rate, indirectly acknowledges that a certain percentage of the workforce will be hurt each year. Choosing between these options is often unsatisfactory because continuous improvement in essence budgets for injuries and illness while zero often invites failure if but a single injury occurs.

As companies struggle with these issues, the obvious question must be asked: "Although zero is always the most desirable outcome, is it possible?" Achieving zero incidents can be an intimidating and difficult goal, but it is neither impossible nor unrealistic. Zero has been accomplished by organizations on a small scale (Nelson 1996). In fact, many companies at any given time are already at zero;

that is, the periods without injury or illness are far longer than those periods that include an incident. The more realistic challenge, then, is sustaining zero rather than obtaining zero.

The key to eliminating injury and illness is more of a mental challenge than a physical one. Nelson reports several construction companies that have gone well over a year without a recordable injury and some mining companies that have completed an entire year without an injury. Many corporations report individual plants around the globe going 1, 2, 3, or even 4 years without a single injury. So what is the key to zero, and how can it be sustained?

Developing a road map or strategic plan to zero begins with the fundamentals. An organization must manage its basic health and safety systems efficiently and continuously. Companies that have reached zero indicate that they constantly look for opportunities to improve basic programs (Nelson 1996). Many of the essential components of a health and safety program are presented in the following chapters of this book, including:

- Cause and effect of loss
- Behavior modification
- Engineering
- Regulations
- Education and training
- Inspections
- Auditing and hazard identification
- Incident reporting and analysis
- Communications
- Task analysis and observation
- Dealing with emergencies
- Working with contractors
- Risk analysis
- Hazard control
- Industrial hygiene
- Specific hazard issues such as:
    - Ground control
    - Fires
    - Explosives
    - Haulage
    - Electrical safety.

Beyond these basics, other elements must also be put in place. As we discussed earlier, successful health and safety cultures must be rooted in:

- Management involvement
- Caring, open communication
- Mutual respect and trust
- Health and safety as an individual and organizational value
- Worker empowerment.

These elements are difficult to develop in any organization, which may suggest why large mining companies have found zero difficult to obtain. Conversely, no research or laws prohibit success. Norman George, director of manufacturing for Hoechst Roussel Pharmaceuticals, Inc., says, "People's attitudes toward safety clearly influence their behaviors. To achieve zero injuries in the workplace, no matter the size, people must believe that they are responsible for their safety and the safety of their co-workers." Therein lies the challenge. Accepting personal responsibility for safety means not transferring responsibility to a coworker, a supervisor, a specific professional, or the corporation. It is an empowering approach that says: "If I take responsibility for my safety, I can reduce workplace hazards. This will benefit me, my coworkers, my family, and my life" (Topf 1995).

ROLES, RESPONSIBILITIES, AND ACCOUNTABILITY

Every individual plays a role in health and safety, but the ultimate responsibility lies with both senior and line management. Management at these levels must recognize and actively support the system by providing the necessary resources and leadership. Too often, safety is isolated from the mainstream of an organization and left to staff members (most often the health and safety professionals) who may lack the authority and the organizational influence to effect change. As a staff function, health and safety may be limited in its ability to identify and resolve management oversights that contribute to accident causation. To succeed, safety must be viewed as a line management function with the line managers held responsible and accountable for performance (Hansen 1995).

When health and safety is addressed like other line functions, such as production, maintenance, and quality, it stops being viewed as ancillary to the organization's core work. When health and safety management is identified as a line function, it is planned, organized, staffed, directed, and controlled accordingly. As a result, accountability, performance, and rewards are more clearly understood.

The importance of accountability and responsibility, along with the expectation of roles, cannot be overstated. Senior management's role is to ensure that health and safety is integrated into the business from the top down and to provide visible leadership for the function. Middle management's role is to ensure the effective administration of the health and safety system by making sure that subordinates perform effectively as well as modeling the behaviors and actions consistent with defined goals. Line management—including supervisors and team coordinators or coaches in high-performance or self-directed teams—should perform the activities that drive performance and optimize interaction with workers. Finally, the health and safety professional should be a technical resource responsible for providing strategic and tactical support to management and workers. Above all else, every employee is responsible for working safely, actively participating in the health and safety process, and providing feedback to management.

THE HEALTH AND SAFETY PROFESSIONAL

In the last decade or two there have been two general paths for the development of U.S. mining health and safety professionals:

1. Those who acquire formal, academic education
2. Those who develop on-the-job expertise.

Only a few U.S. academic programs specialize in educating students in mine health and safety methods. More commonly, a wide selection of community colleges and 4-year institutions offer undergraduate and graduate degrees in safety engineering, health and safety management, and industrial hygiene, among other disciplines.

Each path has advantages and disadvantages. The academically trained professional normally lacks experience upon leaving school and therefore is armed with knowledge and untested theories. These individuals face challenges in the mine environment that would otherwise be known only through experience. They are often characterized as lacking real world knowledge compared with health and safety professionals who are selected from the working ranks. These seasoned mine workers learn health and safety management "in the trenches." However, they may be viewed as lacking an adequate understanding of the technical aspects of the profession. These candidates typically have a limited understanding of health and safety in a broader context. In general, both of these broad stereotypes are inaccurate to one degree or another. The quality and effectiveness of health and safety professionals depends more on their personal motivation and their desire to actively advocate for the protection of their coworkers than any other criteria. Regardless of their background, mining health and safety professionals must develop an understanding of organizational and individual behavior and how those issues relate to health and safety. The ability to communicate effectively is also important.

The number of mining health and safety professionals in the mining industry who acquire professional credentials is growing. Organizations that offer professional certifications require candidates to meet specific education and experience requirements and successfully complete one or more examinations. Some certifications call for a college degree as a minimum educational requirement. Maintenance of certification usually requires adherence to a code of ethics and the accumulation of professional development credits. Both safety specialists and industrial hygienists now have a variety of certification plans available to them, including:

- The Board of Certified Safety Professionals (BCSP)
- Associate Safety Professional (ASP)
- Certified Safety Professional (CSP)
- American Board of Industrial Hygiene (ABIH)
- Industrial Hygienist In Training (IHIT)
- Certified Industrial Hygienist (CIH).

In addition, these certifications are offered under the Joint Occupational Health and Safety Technologist Committee (a joint ABIH-BCSP organization).

- Certified Occupational Health and Safety Technologist (COHST)
- International Society of Mine Safety Professionals (ISMSP)
- Associate Mine Safety Professional (AMSP)
- Certified Mine Safety Professional (CMSP).

Other certification plans are available in Canada, Great Britain, South Africa, and elsewhere. Professional certification in health and safety should not be viewed as a measure of professional effectiveness but as a base measure of technical competence.

MANAGING CHANGE

The ability to recognize change, and its inevitability, as well as having a mechanism in place to address change in health and safety, is a key hallmark of successful management systems. Change is constant in the mining industry beginning with the mining process itself and moving through variations in personnel, mine ownership, operating philosophies, resources, weather, and the economies that drive the demand for mined products. Although these changes are not unique to mining, the industry is more prone to change at all levels compared with general and service industries in the United States. These change stimuli can originate internally or externally, but all have the same effect on complicated management systems such as health and safety: They disrupt the status quo and make it more difficult to establish and maintain equilibrium and predictability.

Take the example of a company with a health and safety management system that emphasizes a high degree of accountability for supervisors who must continuously communicate with workers about safety-related issues. The company historically adheres to the traditional philosophy of management by objectives, also known as command and control. If the company adopts a new management approach by introducing self-directed teams, the traditional supervisor's role would be altered to ensure that the same communications continue. Unless these issues are recognized in advance, the impact on safety management can be significant and negative.

Change of this nature can have a significant impact on performance as workers are distracted by new patterns of work, new environments or people, and altered resources. Several important factors arise for the mining health and safety professional to consider in managing change.

People naturally resist change, but often they are less resistant if they have a hand in designing or facilitating it. Change can provoke apprehension and fear that leads to coping strategies such as denial and resistance, both passive and active. If not addressed, these reactions may undermine the effort at hand. Concern and distraction is most often fueled by a lack of information. As we stated previously, effective communication in health and safety management is essential.

Change-management strategies that support health and safety are not always formal programs. They frequently scan the organization and environment for planned or pending change. Then they ensure that the plan is either consistent with existing health and safety systems or that methods are appropriately amended appropriately to be compatible. Some changes are clearly improvements; others must be implemented without adversely affecting performance. Health and safety programs that reflect an organization's culture and demonstrate the flexibility to change along with the organization will have a greater chance for consistent long-term success.

MEASURING HEALTH AND SAFETY PERFORMANCE

In a recent marketing ploy, a delivery company boasted that on-time deliveries improved by a remarkable 85%. In the wake of such bravado, the company failed to inform potential customers that the meaning of on time had expanded from 2 to 4 hours as the maximum allowable time lapse between when delivery was promised and the actual delivery time. No actual change occurred, but the external perception of performance was significantly enhanced.

The development and tracking of metrics is the only objective measure of health and safety performance and progress. The two types of performance metrics are:

- Outcome or results-based measures
- Process or activity-related measures.

"What gets measured gets done" is an adage that is as applicable to health and safety performance as it is to any other business function.

Ironically, the most frequently tracked metric in the mining industry is incidence rates, such as reportable and lost-time injuries—a measure that generally provides little perspective on systematic problems in health and safety. In fact, the vast majority of U.S. mining companies in the United States measure performance using incidence rates. Such data indicate the number of injuries on the job during a specified period. This information provides a basis for comparison with other companies. Unfortunately, injury rates are weak predictors that provide only a general indication of future performance. They do not furnish any warning of the probability of a major incident because the underlying causes of such events—inadequate leadership, deficient procedures, and lack of employee involvement—are not effectively addressed within injury rate measures.

There clearly is a need to use outcome measures ("downstream" or "trailing" metrics) as a tool to compare results with other organizations. Using injury rates as an exclusive measurement tool is inadequate for three reasons (Pybus 1996):

1. Outputs result from a combination of many cultural and system inputs.
2. Output is subject to natural variation. In other words, do nothing different and it may still vary over time.
3. Exclusive focus on output measures can facilitate complacency and impulse reaction.

As illustrated in the following simplistic model (Figure 2.5), outputs depend on both the existing culture of an organization and the systems established within that culture.

To utilize outputs as a measure of performance that will indicate how the system can be improved, it is important to understand the influence that the culture and systems have on the result. The most effective and consistent means to improve output performance is focusing on upstream factors that directly influence outcomes. Once understood, organizations can implement change to upstream processes that have a higher probability of affecting output performance.

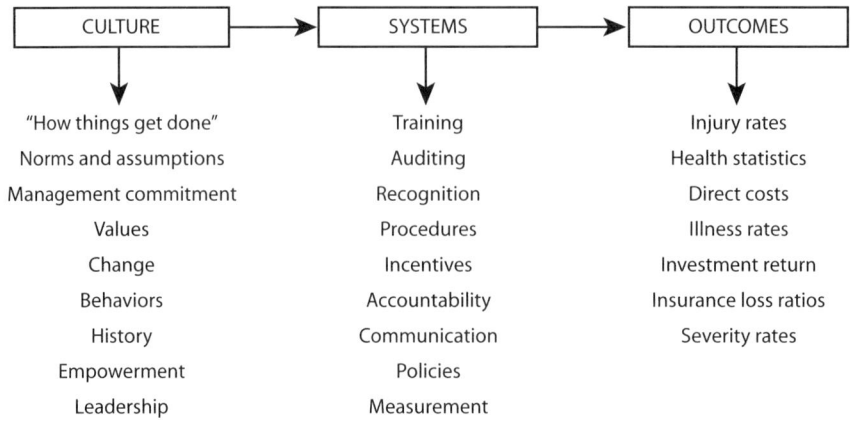

FIGURE 2.5 Simple model of outcomes dependent on culture and systems

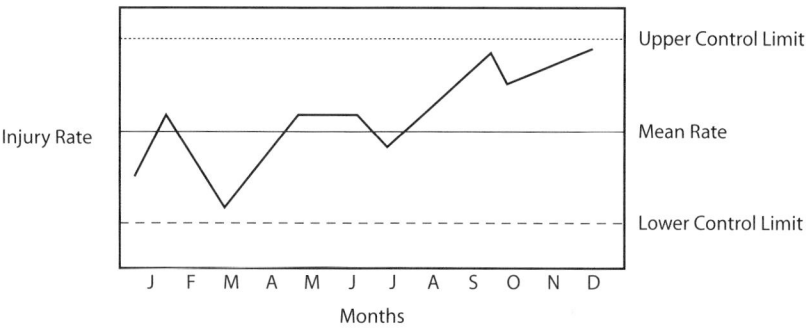

FIGURE 2.6   Statistical control chart with incident rate variation

Historical injury rates do not indicate if improved performance resulted from proactive strategies or chance. Consider the scenario of an employee walking beneath loose rock in an underground drift. When the ceiling collapses, the employee's position determines whether the incident results in property damage, minor injury, a lost-time injury, or a fatality. In other words, chance is a predominant factor in determining outcome, but injury rates do not reflect this. Because safety incidents are complex, with varying causal factors, they make weak statistical tools for determining overall program performance. By relying on such measures, it is very difficult to ascertain if a safety objective has been achieved (Espisito 1993).

Health and safety performance, as measured by injury rates, is naturally variable. There can be minimal change in management activities, yet performance can and often does vary naturally between limits that are statistically defined by past performance. Figure 2.6 represents monthly fluctuations of the mean incident rate, which is the average of all monthly rates.

To clearly understand safety performance, injury rates must be viewed in relation to the control limits of health and safety systems. Upper and lower control limits are calculated using standard statistical methods based on historical monthly incident rates. For this reason, it is not statistically meaningful to take action for a higher than average rate—one that was measured, for example, during the month of September—even though it may vary considerably from the previous month's rate. Attempting to determine when safety performance is outside the control of implemented systems is impossible without using control limits as external parameters (Pybus 1996).

Failure to recognize this natural variation can lead to organizational complacency when incident rates are below normal, and impulse reactions when the rates rise above average. Indeed, random process variation accounts for these extremes. Management representatives can become frustrated in their apparent inability to control output results. Perceived problems based on short-term trends lead to energy and resources being expended by hopping from one issue to another (Pybus 1996).

To effectively measure safety performance that yields a balanced view of progress and simultaneously provides real control over that progress, it is critical to recognize that outputs are the result of a combination of many cultural and systemic factors. A balanced measurement portfolio with clear and useful information about the culture, systems, and outputs catalyzes subsequent improvements in all three measures.

Developing appropriate criteria for health and safety performance is not an easy task. Theorists and scholars have grappled with this issue for decades (Petersen 1989). However, general guidelines that can effectively measure upstream systems have been proposed and implemented in progressive mining companies. Such procedures provide meaningful predictions of output safety performance. The scope of measurements should include employee involvement in safety, supervisor and management performance, and system effectiveness.

Employee participation is key to eliminating the potential for injury and illness. Measurement tools may include:

- Percentage of safe on-the-job behaviors, measured against a prescribed list of behaviors
- Number of hours spent in health and safety training on a regular basis
- Participation in health and safety audits and incident investigation

- Number of times employee leads health and safety meetings
- Completion of corrective actions from audits/investigations within specified time limits
- Reporting and investigating near-miss incidents
- Completion of job safety analyses specific to job tasks
- Amount of time spent observing fellow employee behavior
- Maintaining work area in a clean and organized manner
- Number of safety suggestions implemented within the workplace
- Reporting/correcting unsafe conditions.

Measurement is more crucial at the supervisor/management level as these individuals have a broad span of control and influence over the entire workforce and, hence, a direct impact on overall safety. Such measurements might include:

- Number of health and safety audits conducted in a prescribed time period
- Number of health and safety meetings held
- Quality of health and safety meetings held, determined by employee perception
- Percentage of incident investigations completed within a prescribed period of time
- Percentage of action items from audits or investigations corrected within an allotted time
- Number of one-on-one safety contacts between employees
- Percentage of safe behaviors within a group of miners or workers
- Number of MSHA/OSHA citations per inspector day
- Percentage of employees with complete and current health and safety training
- Number of deficiencies within department/division as determined by external auditors
- Number of near miss (a.k.a. "near hit") incidents reported and investigated
- Number of hours spent in health and safety management training
- Frequency of health and safety communications within the department/division
- Percentage of department/division health and safety goals obtained
- Number of hours employees within the department/division participated in safety training
- Percentage of time spent in health and safety related activities.

Companies sometimes implement a health and safety system and expect the process to flourish without instituting measures to determine if any actual impact is being made. System measurement can include:

- A trend analysis of repeated incidents
- Reduction in the number of corrective actions identified in health and safety audits
- Improvement in percentage of safe behaviors within the organization
- Number of health and safety suggestions received
- Average time to correct health and safety work orders
- Quality of health and safety training as identified by post-training exams
- Number of near misses reported and investigated
- Level of involvement of contractors in the health and safety system
- Workers Compensation costs.

THE FUTURE

The future of health and safety management in mining is directly related to economic and technological shifts in the industry. These changes could take many different forms but are likely to be driven by several common factors:

- Economic globalization
- Automation of the mining process
- Increasing knowledge in the general population and among mine workers resulting in part from access to the Internet

- Increasing use of international health and safety management systems
- Increasing integration of health and safety into mine business planning
- Most significant, increasing social pressure to reduce disability and the loss of human life.

As quality orebodies become more scarce and difficult to mine in the United States, the industry is focusing attention on new mines abroad. This economic pattern is already apparent. In the last 10 years, a significant decrease in new domestic mines has been matched by a corresponding increase in the number of foreign mines opened by American mining companies (E & MJ International Directory of Mining 1997). The potential impact of increasing globalization on mining health and safety management includes the need to adapt processes and systems to the culture in question, yet remain consistent with the company's domestic policies. Therefore, mining companies must implement their health and safety policies abroad. However, language, cultural differences, hierarchical relationships, regulatory policies, and perspectives on acceptable levels of risk may vary from U.S. standards.

Sustainable development is a relatively new idea that implies that companies must attempt to "meet the needs of the present without compromising the ability of future generations to meet their own needs" (World Commission on Environment and Development 1997). The aim of sustainable development is to minimize the impact of industrial activity on the world's resources, but it is also viewed as a tool to more effectively integrate the environmental, health, and safety processes into corporate strategies by ensuring that business decisions have a minimal impact on the resources of the organization and its surrounding community.

As mining equipment becomes larger in order to optimize mine plans and leverage economies of a scale, there is a proportionate decrease in the degree of direct control a miner can have on the operation of shovels, haulage trucks, and the like. This can lead to an increased risk of injury and/or property loss if even larger pieces of equipment cannot be adequately managed. Other trends include a movement toward more autonomous mining equipment. Sometime in the near future, longwall mining machines and haulage trucks in open pit mines will operate nearly autonomously, without a direct operator. This autonomy would be expected to result in a decrease in human loss if the separation between man and equipment were sufficient; however, this protection is gained at the potential price of diminished need for mine equipment operators. Other developments in autonomous mining that may impact the health and safety of miners have to do with in situ mining technology.

The advent of the Internet has led to a revolution in information and information technology. Ten years ago, information about health and safety in the mining industry was accessible almost exclusively through written documents and some limited databases. In contrast, an ever-growing volume of electronic information about all aspects of mine health and safety is available today. For instance, the regulatory compliance record and incident and severity rates of companies under MSHA jurisdiction are readily available through MSHA's Web page. Various online discussions provide a public forum for addressing all aspects of health and safety management. Policies and procedures from public and private organizations are shared on the Internet, as well as information from advocacy groups and trade associations. Research no longer exclusively requires a trip to a library, but a visit to a virtual library that results in a more informed public, including mine workers.

The popularity of international environmental, health, and safety management systems has risen in recent years and is a trend that should be expected to continue for a long time. The foremost example of this trend is the International Standards Organization (ISO) Standard 14001 for environmental management (American Industrial Hygiene Association 1996). The goal of ISO is to reduce the number of standards necessary to compete in the world marketplace. By developing consensus standards, manufacturers no longer must comply with 100 or more individual country standards. In addition to ISO, there is

- The American National Standards Institute (ANSI)
- South Africa's National Occupational Safety Association (NOSA) Mining 5-Star System
- The OSHA Voluntary Protection Program (VPP) in the United States
- The joint British Standards Institute and Health and Safety Executive HS (G) 65 (BS 8800)
- The American Industrial Hygiene Association (AIHA) occupational health and safety management system.

As performance improves in the mining industry, companies are increasingly integrating health and safety into their business plans. Mining companies now connect the dots between policy enforcement, organization and operations, and health and safety outcomes. Specialized strategic planning processes that emphasize social and technical aspects of an organization facilitate this alignment and are likely to be ever more prominent (Pasmore 1978).

Perhaps the most significant factor affecting future health and safety management paradigms in the United States and abroad is the increasing societal pressure to reduce disability and loss of human life. This is often combined with a greater effectiveness of management systems in the United States. As third-world countries gain economic parity with second-world countries and eventually with current world economic powers, there will be a greater recognition that disability and death are not an acceptable trade-off for growth. A direct relationship exists between economic empowerment and social advocacy. With an abundance of low-cost labor, some countries lack sufficient health and safety policies and enough capital for equipment. Yet safe production and the preservation of life are just as important there as in the United States.

INFORMATION AND RESOURCES

There is an abundance of information and other resources available to the student or practitioner of health and safety management in the mining industry:

- U.S. Department of Labor, Mine Safety and Health Administration (MSHA)
  4015 Wilson Blvd.
  Arlington, VA 22203
  703/235-1452
  URL: www.msha.gov

- U.S. Department of Labor, Occupational Health and Safety Administration (OSHA)
  200 Constitution Avenue
  Washington D.C. 20210
  202/693-1999
  URL: www.osha.gov

- National Mining Association (NMA)
  1130 17th Street NW
  Washington, D.C. 20036
  202/463-2625
  URL: www.nma.org

- National Safety Council (NSC)
  1121 Spring Lake Drive
  Itasca, IL 60143
  800/621-7619
  URL: www.nsc.org

- American Board of Industrial Hygiene (ABIH)
  6015 W. St Joseph, Suite 102
  Lansing, MI 48917
  517/321-2638
  URL: www.abih.org

- American Society of Safety Engineers (ASSE)
  1800 E. Oakton Street
  Des Plains, IL 60018
  847/699-2929
  URL: www.asse.org

- American Industrial Hygiene Association (AIHA)
  2700 Prosperity Avenue, Suite 250
  Fairfax, VA 22031
  703/849-8888
  URL: www.aiha.org

- Board of Certified Safety Professionals (BCSP)
  208 Burwash Avenue
  Savoy, IL 61874
  217/359-9263
  URL: www.bcsp.com
- Montana Tech University
  1300 West Park Street
  Butte, MT 59701
  800/455-8324
  URL: www.mtech.edu
- Virginia Polytechnic Institute and State University (Virginia Tech)
  Blacksburg, VA 24061
  540/231-6671
  URL: www.vt.edu
- Office of Special Programs and Continuing Education (SPACE)
  Mine Safety and Health Training Program
  Colorado School of Mines
  Golden, CO 80401-1887
  Phone: 303/279-0773 or 303/273-3982
  Fax: 303/279-0866 or 303/273-3314
  URL: www.mines.edu/Outreach/Cont_Ed/msht.htm
- University of Arizona
  Tucson, AZ 85721
  520/621-2211
  URL: www.uoa.edu
- National Occupational Safety Association (NOSA)
  508 Proes Street
  Arcadia, Pretoria
  P.O. Box 26434, Arcadia, 0007
  +27 12 303-9700 or 083 917 NOSA
  URL: www.nosa.co.za
- National Institute of Occupational Safety and Health (NIOSH)
  Office of Mining Health & Safety Research
  URL: www.cdc.gov/niosh

  Pittsburgh Research Laboratory
  P.O. Box 18070
  Pittsburgh, PA 15236
  412/386-6556

  Spokane Research Laboratory
  315 E. Montgomery Avenue
  Spokane, WA 99207
  509/354-8000
- International Labour Organization (ILO)
  Geneva, Switzerland
  4122-799-6111
  URL: www.ilo.org
- International Society of Mine Safety Professionals (ISMSP)
  P.O. Box 70
  Pima, AZ 85543
  520/485-0711

REFERENCES

Agricola, G. 1950. *De Re Metallica*. [Circa 1556]. 1912 translation of the original text. New York: Dover Publications.

American Industrial Hygiene Association. 1996. *New Frontiers in Occupational Health and Safety: A Management Systems Approach and the ISO Model*. Edited by C.F. Redinger and S.P. Levine. Fairfax, VA: AIHA Publications.

American Institute of Mine Engineering. 1992. *SME Mining Engineering Handbook*. 2nd ed. Volumes 1 and 2. Littleton, CO: Society for Mining, Metallurgy, and Exploration.

Blair, E.H. 1996. Achieving a total safety paradigm through authentic caring and quality. *Professional Safety* (41)5: 24–27.

Cohen A., M. Smith, and H.H. Cohen. 1975. *Safety Program Practices in High Versus Low Accident Rate Companies–An Interim Report (Questionnaire Phase)*. Cincinnati: U.S. Department of Health, Education and Welfare, NIOSH.

Esposito, P. 1993. Applying statistical process control to safety. *Professional Safety* 38(2): 18–23.

——. 1997. *E & MJ International Directory of Mining*. Chicago: Intertec Publishing.

Gaertner, G.H. et al. 1987. *Determining the Effects of Management Practices on Coal Miners' Safety*. Prepared under Westat Incorporated contract no. J0145029. Rockville, MD: U.S. Bureau of Mines.

Geller, S. 1996. *The Psychology of Safety*. Radnor, PA: Chilton Book Company.

Gidley, W.W. 1920. *Practical Mining Course, Safety and Accident Prevention*. Bisbee, AZ: Phelps Dodge Corporation.

——. 1998. *Industrial Hygiene Management*. Edited by J.T. Garrett, L.J. Cralley, and L.V. Cralley. New York: John Wiley & Sons.

Hamilton, A. 1943. *Exploring the Dangerous Trades*. Boston: Little, Brown & Company.

Hansen, L. 1993. Safety management: a call for revolution. *Professional Safety* 38(3): 16–21.

——. 1995. Re-braining corporate safety and health. *Professional Safety* 40(10): 24–29.

Heinrich, H.W. 1931. *Industrial Accident Prevention*. New York: McGraw-Hill.

Hethmon, T., and K. Dotson. 1997. Chapter 15: surface mining. In *Encyclopedia of Occupational Health and Safety*. 4th ed. Geneva: International Labour Office.

McSween, T.E. 1995. *The Values-Based Safety Process: Improving Your Safety Culture with a Behavioral Approach*. New York: Van Nostrand Reinhold.

Meyer, R.L. 1987. A look at the First Congress. *Safety and Health* 135(2): 22–23.

MSHA. 1999. *The Number of Operator Injuries, Injury-Incident Rates: Average Numbers of Employees and Employee Hours by Work Location and Mineral Industry*. Arlington, VA: MSHA.

Mussacchio, C. 1975. The industrial revolution: what price for progress? *Occupational Hazards* 45.

NAS. 1982. Committee on underground coal mine safety. In *Toward Safer Underground Coal Mines*. New York: NAS.

Nelson, A.J. 1996. Remarkable zero injury performance. *Professional Safety* 41(1): 22–25.

NSC. 1992. *Accident Prevention Manual for Business & Industry: Engineering and Technology*. 10th ed. Edited by P.M. Laing. Des Plaines, IL: NSC.

——. 1995. *Accident Facts*. Des Plaines, IL: NSC.

Pasmore, W.A., and J.J. Sherwood. 1978. *Socio-Technical Systems: A Source Book*. San Diego: University Associates.

Petersen, D. 1989. *Techniques of Safety Management*. 3rd ed. Goshen, NY: Aloray.

——. 1996. *Safety by Objectives–What Gets Measured and Rewarded Gets Done*, 2nd ed. New York: Van Nostrand Reinhold.

Pope, W.C. 1990. *Managing for Performance Perfection*. Weaverville, NC: Bonnie Brae Publications.

Pybus, R. 1996. *Safety Management: Strategy and Practice*. Oxford: Linacre House.

Sanders, M.S., T.V. Patterson, and J.M. Peay. 1976. *The Effect of Organizational Climate and Policy on Coal Mine Safety*. Naval Weapons Support Center. Applied Science Department.

Topf, M.D. 1995. Change in attitude fosters responsibility for safety. *Professional Safety* 40(12): 24–27.

The World Commission on Environment and Development. 1992. *Sustainable Development*. Geneva: The World Commission on Environment and Development.

CHAPTER 3

Causes and Effects of Loss

Carl R. Metzgar
Chairman, Metzgar Consulting Group
Winston-Salem, North Carolina

> *Every human being is a more complex system than any other system to which he belongs.*
> *—Alfred North Whitehead*

INTRODUCTION

Loss control is an activity driven by people. It is just as subject to fashion, fad, and whim as any other people-driven activity. A downgrading incident can be isolated, described, and shown to degrade health, physical well-being, or condition of a person. Equipment is downgraded when it is damaged; processes are downgraded when they are interrupted. Downgrading incidents are inescapable when the unqualified are allowed to exercise judgment and make decisions. To rationally approach the challenge of loss control, managers need a sound theory from which to develop strategies. William Haddon Jr.'s "Energy Transfer Theory" and his accompanying "10 Strategies for Loss Reduction" combine to make a solid foundation for loss control policies. After defining loss and technology's contribution to severity, Haddon's 10 strategies will be introduced as a framework for thinking toward action. Loss-control theories help prevent injury and property damage.

DEFINITION OF LOSS

"Loss" is the word of choice because "safety" and "accident" are confusing words for communicating a precise or useful definition between people or levels, in the traditional hierarchical organization as well as in the new "team" organizations. Safety and accident are ordinary words used by people with diverse interests in a special way. Using these ordinary words in a special way without explaining the new or different way the words are being used may promote misunderstanding. For example, to a vice-president, the term "safety program" means a printed book with administration procedures. To a truck driver, "safety program" means having brakes that work. Therefore, "safety" and "accident" do not have the same meaning for the regulator and the regulated. The differences in understanding between management and labor are significant and sometimes troublesome as well. Forty years ago, Gibson suggested (1961, p. 301):

> The term 'accident,' it seems to me, refers to a makeshift concept with a hodgepodge of legal, medical, and statistical overtones. Two of its meanings are incompatible. Defined as a harmful encounter with the environment, a danger not averted, an accident is a psychological phenomenon, subject to prediction and control. But defined as an unpredictable event, it is by definition uncontrollable. The two meanings are hopelessly entangled in the common usage. There is no hope of defining it for research purposes. Hence I suggest that the word be discarded in scientific discussion.

Just as "accident" cannot be defined for research purposes, neither can it be defined for loss-control management purposes. Loss control in mining can be every bit as scientific a discipline as pure or applied research. A "loss" is more easily agreed upon. *The New Shorter Oxford English Dictionary* says a "loss is a diminution of one's possessions or advantages; detriment or disadvantage involved in being deprived of something, or resulting from a change of condition." Loss can also include the failure to take advantage of something or a failure to gain or obtain.

The diminution of a possession, detriment, or disadvantage represents something tangible. The loss can relate to health, well-being, particular injury, or property damage. Something is gone, diminished, or damaged in a loss. A loss results in harm.

For consideration here, then, a loss is the result of interrupted practices or procedures that can lead to personal injury or property damage. A disruption in a process is also a loss. A loss is harm to a person, to an organization, or both (Bird 1986).

EFFECTS OF LOSS

To be understood for critical evaluation, losses have to be identified, named, and described. Losses cost injury, pain, mental anguish, money, and effort. When losses are understood, the means to prevent them are more rationally generated. Without enlightened diagnosis of errors, disciplined treatment of causes is not likely to follow.

Losses fall into three categories: personal, economic, and speculative. Although personal and economic losses can be separated for the convenience of description and analysis, they are never isolated. Speculative losses are a separate category and extremely difficult to deal with. Because losses are always dynamic, they have effects on each other.

Personal Loss

Personal loss comprises injury or injuries, their physical manifestations, and the elusive but real pain and psychological involvement of the victim and associated people. Injuries vary—from unattended minor cuts, abrasions, and dust in the eyes—to fractures, avulsions, enucleations, and fatalities. Each injury represents a unique loss. Only the magnitude changes. Often an incident's magnitude depends on a fraction of an inch or second. Personal identity disappears in the abstraction of statistics. Manipulation of statistics and press releases has no effect on the miner whose back hurts.

Serious injuries involve much more than tissue damage. Serious injuries have an impact on the mental condition of the victim, family, coworkers, and friends. The Workers Compensation system takes care of the physical damage with medical payments for care and scheduled payments for disability with indemnity payments for loss of work time. But despite emerging research, no system currently quantifies or indemnifies pain in an acceptable way to all interested parties. So far, Workers Compensation does not pay for claims of pain. Injured workers and the people surrounding them experience other feelings that can also be counted as losses.

Economic Loss

Some losses generated by personal injury are quantifiable and count as insurable losses, such as medical expenses and lost wages. Permanent partial or total disabilities fall into this category as well. An amputated finger is an example of a permanent partial disability, or one that lasts a lifetime, but is limited in scope. Bilateral blindness is an example of a permanent total disability. Although differing among the states, these definitions are fairly well established. Ways to evaluate and compensate for disabilities that do not heal or recover completely have been agreed on. Each state has its own statutory limits.

Downgrading incident property damage losses are economic losses and are generally underreported. In the case of property damage, the labor and parts costs can usually be located fairly easily if management wants them accumulated. Rather than referring to them as property damage, the maintenance budget absorbs many downgrading incident charges as ordinary wear and tear. A downgrading incident represents management failure, whereas wear and tear are predictable, calculated, and prepared for. Not all managements are comfortable quantifying their failures. Ignoring property damage does not change the size of the loss, it only allows for the misdirection of time and other resources. The lack of an appropriate response to property damage is responsible for reductions in profitability.

In the case of charges resulting from a power interruption, for example, the difficulty in recovering the costs often keeps the costs from being gathered. When power is interrupted and the processing plant goes down with loaded belts, screens, and crushers, the true cost of lost production and restarting the plant is minimized or downplayed. There may not have been any injury or property damage from the power outage, but the productive process has been interrupted, which carries a cost. Other examples of interruption include regulatory inspections, plant visitations, delayed arrival of equipment, or traffic delays that keep delivery trucks from arriving to haul away product. Difficulty with railroads about the availability of cars on a timely basis is often a serious disruption in the peak season. These losses, which are demonstrable facts that can be supported, can be quantified if it is determined that they should be. However, speculative losses are much more difficult to deal with.

Speculative Losses

Speculative losses waste the most time, generate the most conversation, and are the most difficult to capture. They defy quantification. Speculative losses are "imaginary horribles" with questionable bases and they produce heat but no light. This is the fear of the unknown moved to the verbal level. Workers are more afraid of insignificant unquantified risk, like the radio frequency field around a handheld radio, than they are of the risks of not locking out equipment "just this one time" in situations known to be hazardous. Conversations are wasted but the concern is a speculative cost that can't be pinned down. There are unknown costs in trying to explain away unjustified fears. Idle speculations have blind people in a dark room searching for a black cat that isn't there. In response to the fact that not all costs are easily recovered, various ratios have been devised to inflate the verifiable incident charges to justify loss control budgets. One example is the 1:29:300 fatality-to-injury to no-injury episodes (Heinrich 1959). The value of the ratios is questionable and they can be distorted and misused (Metzgar 1999). If the real costs are accurately accumulated, there is no need to take an uninformed guess at speculative costs. The time spent by bystanders and others—the "standing around time" associated with a downgrading incident represents a loss. That time can't be quantified yet it remains a cost. Another critical but impossible to quantify loss is the damage to individual and group morale.

A supervisor's time is always listed as a cost of doing an investigation for minor or serious injuries. Every conversation has at least one other person who contributes to the cost as well. In the case of a fatality, more company and outside people are always involved than in less serious incidents.

For example, an actual 1996 Mine Safety Health Administration (MSHA) fatality report lists 22 people involved in the investigation: eight representatives from the company, one from the independent contractor, six from the county fire and police departments, and three from the fire and rescue group. MSHA had four people in attendance at one time or another. Granted that a fatality should get a lot of attention, but 22 people spending time on the investigation represents a lot of unmanaged cost. Include staging and travel time, and the cost becomes significant.

Emotional, rational, and irrational responses abound in downgrading incident situations. Conversations with emergency medical service (EMS) professionals reveal that there is no typical victim or typical response to injury no matter how serious or minor. Neither is there a typical witness, family member, coworker, supervisor, manager, or friend. When there is only property damage, behavior levels return to normal rather quickly, even when the loss is sizable. But injury complicates everyone's relationships and responses and the complications continue for a long time. These very human complications become a part of the cost picture, although they are difficult to measure.

In the cases that find their way to litigation, the additional monetary and other costs add up quickly. Legal proceedings, whether in the administrative or court systems, also take a long time and aggravate the relationships between all the parties.

Personal, economic, and speculative costs have to be dealt with when there is a downgrading incident. These costs are some of the effects of loss. The downgrading incident, something that has gone wrong, is the basis for these costs. The incidents are what are to be avoided. Loss-control activities and better management offer some devices to avoid the costs. There are many precursors to a loss and they start to fall into place long before a damaging energy transfer occurs. However the beginning moment of an energy transfer is only one point of concentration for loss prevention efforts. There are multiple moments for intervention to limit losses.

ENERGY TRANSFER AS THE CAUSE OF LOSS

Activity, whether natural or manmade, depends on energy flows. When there is activity, there is energy transferring from one place or condition to another. The energy can be controlled for productive use and generate a positive result, as in using a crusher to make little stones out of boulders or it can remain uncontrolled and be the cause of loss, as in a runaway truck. The first statement of the energy transfer insight as the cause of injury came in 1961 when Gibson said, "Injuries to a living organism can be produced only by some energy interchange" (Gibson 1961, p. 297).

In 1963, Haddon published his more detailed statement of the energy transfer theory (p. 636):

> Accidents, at least those of concern to the medical profession, are defined in effect by the unexpected occurrence of injury. The first [hereafter called Type I] of these comprises all injuries caused by interference with normal whole body or local energy exchange. At the whole body level, examples of injuries due to such interference with normal energy exchange include the results of suffocation by mechanical or chemical means for example, by drowning, strangulation, carbon monoxide inhalation and cyanide poisoning....
>
> The second [hereafter called Type II] and more important group of injuries compromises all those in which the damage is caused by the delivery to the body of amounts of energy in excess of corresponding local or whole body injury thresholds. The types of energy which can be delivered, however, are but few in number, and each produces highly specific lesions. Foremost are injuries due to the delivery of mechanical energy. The impacts of moving objects such as bullets, hypodermic needles, knives, and falling objects and those produced when a moving body collides with relatively stationary structures, as in falls, plane crashes, and auto crashes illustrate this group. The energy transferred injuriously may also be thermal, as in the case of first, second, and third degree burns; electrical, as in electrocution; or, it may be ionizing radiation.... Finally, chemical energy may also be transferred in excess of body thresholds, and this group of injuries includes all those due to plant and animal toxins, and to inorganic and organic compounds.... Viewed in this light, the fundamental problem in the prevention of injury is the prevention of such abnormal energy exchanges, and research in accident causation and prevention can and must be analyzed in similar terms.

Despite Haddon's use of the word accident, the search is not for accidents. We saw earlier in this chapter that there is no agreement about what accidents are. The search is for energy exchange from some source to a human body or physical structure. Gibson and Haddon were thinking in terms of injury, but the theory can and should be extended to property damage and loss to process as well. In the Type II cases, the energy transfer is large enough to do damage to the human body or physical structure. The Type I kind of injury to the body is able to interfere with the normal energy transfers within the body. In 1997, there were 489 times the number of Type I injuries as Type II injuries in mining in the United States.

This entry of energy into loss-control programming is most revealing. Although loss control is a human endeavor, there is a lot of room for a scientific method and its application. One of the more significant challenges of scientific loss control is that the researchers or loss-control professionals are inside the very process they are trying to observe and control. Loss control is an experiment in process, in a system that is in flux.

Energy is abstract in quantity and quality. In physics, energy is divided into nine forms. Energy is gravitational, kinetic, heat, elastic, electrical, chemical, radiant, nuclear, or mass. There are useful formulas for handling each one. Energy is productive when it is under control. Out of control energy is either wasted or loss producing. The well-known physicist Richard Feynman said, "It is important to realize that in physics today, we have no knowledge of what energy is" (Feynman 1963, p. 71). We can calculate it, we can measure its effects, and we can make it do work. Despite its abstract nature, however, the idea of energy transfer is a useful injury prevention construct.

Haddon (1963) reduces the abstract energy forms to five with common names relevant to loss control: mechanical, thermal, electrical, ionizing radiation, and chemical energy. Suzan Baker charts mechanical energy as responsible for 74% of accidental deaths in 1986 in the United States (Baker 1992, p. 5). The population of the United States makes a very large general sample. Forms of energy other than mechanical are responsible for the remaining 26% of fatalities.

Mining experience can fit into Haddon's categories of mechanical, thermal, electrical, chemical, and ionizing radiation. The following data are from MSHA's *Informational Reports for 1998* for fatalities and lost workday injuries reported in 1997 (MSHA 1998). To arrive at a meaningful sample, it is necessary to combine fatalities and lost workday injuries because there are so few fatalities in modern mining in the United States. Fatality experience is only representative of fatalities and cannot be projected as typical of the total injury experience, which also includes non-fatal injuries. Without doubt, each fatality is a tragedy. However, the fatalities total is not large enough for balanced analysis of the injury experience in the U.S. mining industry. Here are the percentages for 1997:

Type	Percentage of Occurrence
Haddon Type I (interference with normal energy exchange)	0.2
Haddon Type II (energy transfer beyond the body threshold)	
Mechanical	95.76
Thermal	1.61
Electrical and radiation, including UV and ionizing	1.37
Chemical	1.04

It is interesting to note that the percentages of the "other" and "unclassified categories," which are left out of the MSHA list, are greater than Type I, thermal, electrical and radiation, and chemical cases combined. Type I shown, with the addition of "other" and "unclassified," make up a small percentage of injuries. Mechanical energy transfer should be the principal area for loss-control practice.

Another of Haddon's penetrating observations was that each kind of energy transfer produced its own particular and peculiar injuries (Haddon 1967). Mechanical injury produces tearing, breaking, crushing, and displacement injuries that are the result of impact from moving objects like falling rock, being caught in pinch points, or moving vehicles. Thermal injury produces inflammation, charring, and coagulation from first-, second-, and third-degree burns. Electrical energy injuries can interfere with nerve and muscle function and cause charring and coagulation. Ionizing radiation can disrupt cellular and subcellular components of the body. Chemical energy injuries can destroy or damage the body in particular response to the attacking chemical.

Baker's data are for fatalities in the general population. The MSHA data are for fatalities and lost workday injuries in the mining industry. This could be seen as a comparison of wheelbarrows and dump trucks, but the point is to demonstrate that the experience in the mining industry, in particular, is radically different from the experience of the U.S. population in general. With 95% of mining injuries caused by mechanical energy, the area for concentrating of effort has been isolated. If prevention work is to be pertinent, the area of focus will have to be subdivided for analysis, but the mechanisms for correction can be narrowed down. The abstract, statistically generated fact has to be translated into particular countermeasures where workers work.

Later Haddon published another very significant observation (1968, p. 1435–1436):

> The most common and universal fallacy in the field, whether viewed within a descriptive or etiologic framework, is one which is so ingrained that it is seldom explicitly recognized. It involves the assumption that the priority rank of countermeasures, in terms of their ability to influence the end results of concern, must parallel the ranking, in order of their relative contributions, of causes influencing those end results. In its most common form, it states that because drivers cause most accidents, programs correspondingly must be concerned with drivers. In the real world, there is no basis for making this assumption, especially since in numerous areas of the field it leads to demonstrably false conclusions.

Two major thinking tools are now in place for progress in injury prevention. First is the theory that injury results only when there is an energy transfer beyond the ability of the body or structure to resist it. The second tool is the idea that the priority rank of countermeasures does not have to match the relative contributions of causes. Useful and effective countermeasures can be implemented before all the particulars of the causes are known. It is also important to remember that single countermeasures are not usually 100% effective. Therefore it is wise to use multiple countermeasures. The loss-control manager has to use a wardrobe approach to correction programming. Countermeasures, like clothes, have to be mixed, matched, and adjusted to the geography and the season.

Haddon worked primarily in pedestrian, automobile, and highway loss control. Because of his training, education, and position, Haddon was able to throw off the dead end of blaming the driver for his injury. Yes, the driver was often responsible for the collision, but changing all the behaviors of all the drivers was not one of the options. With no change in human nature in 2000 years, the prospect for radical driver behavioral change on a large scale was dismal. The driver is often alone or unwilling to be influenced by a passenger. There are great areas for fresh thought and action in considering the jumps from the "particular" to the "general" and back again in driver behavior. The 10 Haddon strategies were not put forward to eliminate all crashes but rather to reduce the harmful effects of crashes that did occur. Haddon was searching for actions that would reduce the effects of collisions. In the mining environment, peers and supervisors are present to contribute support for behavioral and environmental change. It may not be possible to eliminate all losses. but countermeasures are available to keep injuries less serious and losses smaller.

Gibson, the first person to advance the energy transfer theory, went on to other things and did nothing with his idea (Guarnieri 1992, p. 152). Haddon was appointed the first director of the National Highway Safety Bureau, Federal Highway Administration, U.S. Department of Transportation in 1966 and served until 1969. In this position he was able to promote his ideas. His implemented ideas were effective in reducing the severity of traffic injuries. These same ideas for damage control are transferable to the technology in the mining industries.

TECHNOLOGY-DRIVEN INJURY SEVERITY

Any workplace is designed for production. In mining, large amounts of energy are used. For example, fuel, electricity, and explosives are major budget items and management expends a lot of mental energy to ensure that these resources are used effectively. Any failure to achieve the efficient use of energy is a downgrading incident.

The fuel and electricity are used to power large pieces of equipment with the capacity to transform and transfer a lot of energy to do a great deal of work. When this energy is misdirected, it can harm people and equipment. As any emergency room physician can attest, the human body has marvelous recovery capacity. The troublesome tradeoff is that it is easy to injure the human body. For example, it only takes 5 seconds of exposure for water at 140°F to cause a full thickness burn to adult skin (Withers 1984). If the burn area is relatively small, full recovery is a reasonable expectation.

The actual number of fatalities in mining has been declining for years. Reliable detailed data for accurately evaluating the severity of injuries in the face of declining frequency do not exist. However, a very useful hypothesis has been proposed to explain the severity of injuries. Based on the acceptance of Haddon's energy transfer theory of injury causation Kriebel suggested, "that injury severity is a function of the maximum amount of harm the technology can produce" (1982, p. 212). For example, the crushing power of a belt going over a head pulley will determine the severity of the injury to a hand that gets caught.

Physical guards placed between workers and pinch points have been a most effective method for reducing the frequency of injuries. Guarding has been so successful that other countermeasure strategies have been neglected. "Frequency of injuries is determined largely by the nature of interactions between workers and production processes" (Kriebel 1982, p. 209). For example, if workers contact the pinch point where a conveyor belt goes over an idler or head or tail pulley, the resulting injury is usually serious. Each year this type of incident causes one or more fatalities in mining and processing industries.

No one denies the effectiveness of guards. When guards are in place, they prevent contact and the resulting injury. Guarding, then, reduces injury frequency. The energy in a head pulley and a belt going over it is more than enough to tear skin and break bones. The mechanical energy present is not changed by the presence of a guard. When the guard is in place the worker is separated from the harm, but the energy is still a real and present danger. The energy is separated from the worker, but the same amount of energy is available to do harm if the pinch point is contacted. A guarded head pulley represents an energy hazard impeded by a barrier. If the guard is missing or the worker achieves access to the pinch point, the injury or damage to the worker is as serious as ever. We can see then, that guarding reduces frequency, not severity—the guard has had no effect on the technology or the quantity of energy available.

HADDON'S 10 STRATEGIES FOR PREVENTING LOSS

The Haddon countermeasure strategies follow in order, along with Metzgar mining industry examples of how to apply the concept in each case (Haddon 1980; Metzgar 1996, 1997.)

1. To prevent the creation of the hazard in the first place. *Example*: Do not build a stockpile beyond the height at which it becomes a hazard to people and equipment.

2. To reduce the amount of hazard brought into being. *Example*: Limit the amount of explosives stored in magazines and limit quantities of caps and primers.

3. To prevent the release of the hazard that already exists. *Example:* Attach safety cables to conveyer belt counter weights so if the belt breaks the weight will only fall a short distance, be contained, and do no damage.

4. To modify the rate or spatial distribution of release of the hazard from its source. *Example:* Install controls on the discharge gates of a storage bin or pressure relief valves that bleed off pressure before it accumulates and bursts a tank.

5. To separate, in time or space, the hazard and that which is to be protected. *Example:* Reposition a muffler or exhaust pipe on a loader so the noise source is removed from the operator.

6. To separate the hazard and that which is to be protected by interposition of a material barrier. *Example:* Siting guards on head and tail pulleys.

7. To modify relevant basic qualities of the hazard. *Example:* Use different voltages for electrical control and power circuits.

8. To make what is to be protected more resistant to damage from the hazard. *Example:* Use hard surface welding of loader bucket lips.

9. To begin to counter the damage already done by the environmental hazard. *Example:* Relocate a road so operations can continue, offer first aid training, plan for an emergency response.

10. To stabilize, repair, and rehabilitate the objects of the damage. *Example:* Retrain a worker in a new job if his injury prevents him from doing his old job.

These ten strategies fall into three categories: "precontact" (1–3), "contact" (4–8), and "postcontact" (9 and 10). The highest level of senior management has the most effect on large amounts of energy at the precontact stage. Supervisors farther down the chain of command have their influence closer to the moment and place of contact. Senior management has to provide the resources and decision-making framework if the strategies in the 4–8 contact zone are to work well. Senior management has to provide the resources to be effective in the postcontact stage. Preplanning is most effective in taking advantage of the countermeasures in the postcontact or recovery phase of the incident sequence. Senior management has to be so clear and unequivocal in its policies and follow-up that middle managers are not tempted to project expectations that frustrate the stated goals of the president down the chain of command.

PREDICTION—THE FLAWED KEY TO PREVENTION

Effective application of countermeasure strategies depends on accurate observation and acute analysis, the same qualities necessary for doing good science. The expectation of science is that it be able to predict. Management has the same expectation of the loss-control function. W.I.B. Beverridge, in his book *The Art of Scientific Investigation*, which outlines suggestions for how to do research in the broad field of biology, has a specific comment for the loss-control worker (1957):

> *A difficulty we are always up against is that we have to argue from past and present to the future. Science, to be of value, must predict. We have to reason from data obtained in the past by experiment and observation, and plan accordingly for the future.*

This presents special difficulties in loss control. Simply observing a process or situation can change the circumstances and influence the results. The very fact that a process or situation is being observed to prepare for modification often changes the process. Prediction in detail is most difficult, yet that is what is expected of the loss-control practitioner and supervisor. The arrival of the next downgrading incident in particular is unknown. That causes apprehension and a challenge to confidence in the loss-control practitioner or production supervisor. Mineral reserves can be core sampled and the prospective yield known within predictable limits, but even exhaustive pre-evaluation of a workforce cannot predict any individual's action.

The desire for prediction is widespread. After all, science is expected to be able to predict. Management expects loss-control specialists to be capable of predictions, forgetting the difference between the general and the particular. General industry experience is not transferable to a particular company or plant. A well-known economist wrote the following about economic prediction (Heilbroner 1991).

> It is not that people necessarily place much confidence in what economists have to say; it is that they have a profound human need to hear utterances about the future, plausible or not. Seen from this point of view, economic predictions, like those of the ancient seers and sibyls, serve two functions. To the naïve they hold out hope that foreknowledge will help the hearer to escape a dire fate or make a fortune. To the knowing they provide reassurance that the future is not just chance and contingency. The human psyche can tolerate a great deal of prospective misery, but it cannot bear the thought that the future is beyond all power of anticipation.

Managers want to know what's going to happen. What applies in economics applies in loss control—probabilities become certainties when the samples get large enough. The samples simply do not get large enough for accurate prediction of injuries for a company, let alone in a single plant. Thus, predicting from the generalities of industry exposure to the particular is not possible. General population certainties are not transferable to a particular plant. The loss-control manager can't predict, for example, which worker on which day at which plant will have the downgrading incident.

Countermeasures are like a three-deck screen. The first deck takes out the big easy problems. The second countermeasure takes out the midsize problems and the third deck screen gets the last good product. That leaves all the material that passed through every screen and remains to be sorted out. Some workers and some situations pass through all the countermeasure screens.

ACTIVE VERSUS PASSIVE COUNTERMEASURES

A further distinction and explanation of countermeasures is included in two kinds of corrective actions. Haddon distinguishes between active and passive countermeasures (1980). It is important in loss-control management to respect the significant difference between active and passive countermeasures if maximum effects of the selected countermeasures are to be achieved. In the automobile collision field, for example, features such as seat belts, soft rounded interior surfaces, and air bags are designed to prevent large amounts of energy from being transferred to small areas of the body, successfully reducing the severity of injuries. In the mining environment, it is often necessary to deal with large amounts of energy being delivered to relatively small areas of the body. Although there are challenges in applying the energy transfer theory, the effort will be rewarded with fewer and less serious injuries.

The physical plant is the environment in which the worker has to function. Countermeasure strategies have to compensate for errors in design, in judgment, and in action. The strategies must also adapt to errors in procedures. A misguided policy or procedure can be as devastating to a smooth manufacturing process as a short circuit is to the smooth flow of electricity. The need to deal with this complex task is the argument for using a variety of the countermeasures in combination and at the right time. One of the curious anomalies of loss control is that, more often than not, we do not know which countermeasure was the effective one in a given situation.

Haddon never claimed that his strategies represented an effective "cookbook." He claimed only that they were an aid to cognition, judgment, consideration of actual and possible control programs, and teaching (1980). He also did not suggest that the strategies could determine policy—but if the policy were to result in improvements, then using the strategies as a starting point would help in the

injury reduction process. Haddon also made the point that the analysis of countermeasure application could start before all the causes are known. When it comes to countermeasures, the primary
question is "What works?" We have not been so effective in reducing losses that we must exhaust all
the subtleties of causation before we can start to make corrections.

The air bag is a passive countermeasure in the automobile world. This factory-installed safety
feature is expected to deploy when needed with no action required on the part of the driver or passenger. The device is expected to function even when the driver does nothing.

In a plant, a circuit breaker is a passive safety device. The electric current, the motor, the load,
and the circuit breaker determine when the current is to be interrupted. There is no worker standing
by to evaluate the motor and then break the circuit. Effectiveness depends on correct installation and
maintenance, not personal intervention.

Seat belts in private vehicles or company-owned loaders and haul trucks are active countermeasures. Even though the belts are installed at the factory, the driver or passenger has to actively buckle
the belt for it to be effective. In this case, effectiveness depends on an individual's activity.

Similarly, when a welder steps to the side of the oxygen bottle (out of the line of fire of the pressure reducer's adjusting stem) to open the valve, he or she is using an active countermeasure.

INJURY OR DISEASE?

Injury or disease results when one or more parts of the body are damaged by an outside force. Haddon
suggested that injury occurs where the damage is manifested in the period from an instant to 48 hours,
whereas disease is damage that manifests itself in an interval greater than 48 hours (Haddon 1980).
Some energies can cause either or both injury and disease. A worker can shock the spine in a fall or a
jump, a single experience that causes an instant *injury*. On the other hand, the vibrations experienced
while driving a truck over a long period of time transmit small shocks (therefore energy) to the spine,
which can accumulate and result in the same back condition. But in this example, the time elapsed
causes a *disease*.

The loss in these two examples is back pain or damage. Only the amount of time it takes to see
the result is different. Thus the result is the same but the cause is either a disease process or an injury
process.

APPEARANCE AND REALITY

It would be refreshing if loss control were as rational as this background and layout of strategies
would suggest, but it doesn't work that way. In the natural flow of life the important often gets over-
run, buried, and ignored by the misevaluation of the immediate. Potential problems have to be
emphasized time after time. No matter how physically close, loss potential is always intellectually
remote. As Zweig wrote (1927, 1955):

> Most people have very little imagination. They are hardly moved by anything which does not directly
> touch them, which does not positively hammer its message upon their senses; but even a trifle, should
> it happen under their very eyes, and within the immediate range of their feelings, will instantly kin-
> dle in them a disproportionate amount of passion. We may say that the rarity of their interest is
> compensated by an inappropriate and exaggerated vehemence when their interest is at last aroused.

Many people follow the responses of others rather than determining what their own response
should be. For example, people who are ordinarily reasonable may reflect the response of the media
rather than think or act for themselves. The statement "We hope to learn something from this incident
so that it never happens again" has been repeated countless times. Once this mantra has been stated,
when the actual investigation is done, it may be so short, biased, and controlled that nothing is ever
learned. The public pontificators may be the same decision makers who make certain that the investigation stops before the cause is discovered.

SEPARATION IN TIME AND PLACE OF CAUSE AND EFFECT

The important feature of the following example is that countermeasure actions have to be taken at appropriate times at appropriate levels in the hierarchy to be effective and to anticipate what can happen as a plan evolves. Anticipation is a very important countermeasure. Countermeasures are most effective in the precontact phase of an incident or potential incident.

Imagine, if you will, an 85-ton haul truck that crashed into a highwall. The driver had a broken leg and developed back problems. The truck was nearly totaled. At the top of the ramp the slope was 19% for about 60 yards. The ramp slope changed to 10% for 200 yards. At the bottom of this ramp there was a nearly 90° turn at the base of the highwall. It is very likely that the driver did not use the engine, transmission, and retarder correctly, although that fact was never clearly and firmly established. A series of "why" questions is in order.

Why was the truck on a 19% grade? Because the operation was running out of material that could be mined. Although the mining plan was well developed, the operation was rapidly exhausting the available reserves. The mine's management thought that to keep operating, "We have to get that material!"

If the mining plan was well developed, why were adequate reserves not available? Because stripping of new reserves was way behind schedule.

Why was the stripping behind schedule? Because the area to be stripped was under an old plant and a stockpile area that had been replaced, and the old plant had to be disassembled.

Why was the disassembly behind schedule? Because the new plant had not been completed on time.

Why was the new plant behind schedule? Because the board of directors failed to approve the capital project in time for all the subsequent actions to be completed on schedule. The capital request had been submitted on time and in good order by the local and division management.

Now, fit this sequence on the grid of the 10 Haddon strategies.

This downgrading incident could have been prevented in the precontact stage, by not allowing the situation to develop in the first place, by never putting a loaded truck on a 19% grade. This countermeasure was available only to the most senior members of management. The front line supervisor had no influence on the most significant cause of this injury. The root cause of this injury, property damage, and loss to process incident, then, was years and miles from the time and place of the energy transfer incident.

This is a large and dramatic example. Many smaller examples have the same sort of factual trail but cause smaller losses. It takes a lot of small losses to add up to a big loss. However, the small losses are taking place every day and involve much more than the worker and his supervisor. The greater the amount of energy involved, the more important it is for the intervention to take place at a very high level in the organization and very early in the work or planning phase for the effective use of the 10 strategies.

SUMMARY

In mining, there are technical failures and people failures. People are responsible for both the technical and human failures and can be far removed in time and place, and people are ultimately responsible for the technology in mining and mineral processing. Neutralizing downgrading incidents takes the practicality of a good theory. Observation and management of energy transfers are a sound beginning for loss reduction. The energy transfer theory is practical for guiding these observations. Downgrading incidents are inescapable when the unqualified are allowed to exercise judgments and make decisions. To minimize the number and size of failures it takes policy and procedures of the most enlightened kind. Prior Planning Prevents Predictable Poor Performance. There is no substitute for effective follow-up for locating and effectively controlling energy transfers.

REFERENCES

Baker, S.P., et al. 1992. *The Injury Fact Book*. New York: Oxford University Press.

Beverridge, W.I.B. 1957. *The Art of Scientific Investigation*. New York: W.W. Norton & Company.

Bird, F.E., Jr., and G.L. Germain. 1986. *Practical Loss Control Leadership*. Loganville, GA: Institute Publishing.

Brown, L., editor. 1993. *The New Shorter Oxford English Dictionary on Historical Principles*. Oxford: Clarendon Press.

Feynman, R.P. 1963. *Six Easy Pieces*. Reading, MA: Addison-Wesley.

Gibson, J.A. 1961. The contribution of experimental psychology to the formulation of the problem of safety—a brief for basic research. *Behavioral Approaches to Accident Research*. New York: Association for the Aid of Crippled Children. 77–89. Reprinted in *Accident Research: Methods and Approaches*. 1964. Edited by W. Haddon, Jr., et al. New York: Harper & Row. 296–304.

Guarnieri, M. 1992. Landmarks in the history of safety. *Journal of Safety Research* 23: 151–158.

Haddon, W. 1963. A note concerning accident theory and research with special reference to motor vehicle accidents. *Annals of The New York Academy of Sciences* 107: 635–646.

——. 1967. The prevention of accidents. In *Textbook of Preventative Medicine*. Edited by Clark & MacMahon. Boston: Little Brown. 591–621.

——. 1980. Advances in the epidemiology of injuries as a basis for public policy. *Public Health Reports* 95: 411–421.

Heilbruner, R. 1991. Economic predictions. *The New Yorker* 67(20): 70–77.

Heinrich, H.W. 1959. *Industrial Accident Prevention: A Scientific Approach*. New York: McGraw-Hill.

Kriebel, D. 1982. Occupational injuries: factors associated with frequency and severity. *International Archives of Occupational and Environmental Health* 50: 209–218.

Metzgar, C. 1996. A roadblock and a practical bypass. *Mine Safety and Health News* 3(21): 599–603.

——. 1997. Different look, new view. *Pit and Quarry* 90(1): QS6–QS9.

——. 1999. Always read the references. *Journal of Safety Management* (in press).

MSHA. 1998. *Injury Experience in Stone Mining, 1997; Injury Experience in Sand and Gravel Mining, 1997; Injury Experience in Nonmetallic Mining (Except Stone and Coal), 1997; Injury Experience in Metallic Mineral Mining, 1997; Injury Experience in Coal Mining, 1997*. MSHA. U.S. Department of Labor.

Withers, B.F., and S.P. Baker. 1984. Epidemiology and prevention of injuries. *Emergency Medical Clinics of North America* 2(4): 701–715.

Zweig, S. 1927, 1955. Twenty-four hours in a woman's life. In *Stories and Legends*. Translated by E. Paul and C. FitzGibbon. London: Cassell and Company Limited.

CHAPTER 4

Measurement Techniques in Safety Management

Robert M. Arnold
Newmont Gold, Indonesia

INTRODUCTION

One of the most rewarding experiences in safety management is watching what happens when management is given valid, relevant, and practical data on their efforts to prevent accidents. Traditionally a lot of attention is paid to accident frequency and severity rates. The importance of these measurements in a safety management program is a given. It is exciting, however, to see the improvements that take place when management is simply made aware of how it's doing in its efforts to prevent accidents. Having the right measurements does indeed bring about improvement. In other words, the measurement itself motivates action. When properly done, safety measurements guide the implementation of solid programs for preventing accidents. And safety measurements do lead to improved performance. Peter Drucker, a leading expert on management systems, said, "The measurement used determines what one pays attention to." With this in mind, we can see that when we measure the right things, we identify where we are and what we need to do to get us where we want to be.

Louis A. Allen, a leading management expert and consultant, said that "Everything that exists, exists in a certain amount and can be measured." This includes the efforts that an operation makes to prevent accidents. Measuring safety performance is not complicated. In this chapter we present ways to measure **effort,** or work being done to prevent accidents, as well as the **results** of those efforts. The chapter also presents ways to measure and summarize accident **causes**. In summary, we will look at three types of safety measurements:

1. Measurements of results (injuries/illnesses/and other types of accidents frequency rates)
2. Measurements of causes (the immediate and underlying causes of accidents)
3. Measurements of effort (the work being done to prevent accidents and reduce harm).

When we measure something accurately, we learn more about its true nature. The tools and techniques found in this chapter will help you to accurately measure that something called Safety and Health. Measuring your safety and health programs effectively will move you a step closer to knowing their true nature and how to manage them. Any successful accident prevention program uses all three types of safety measurements—**results, causes**, and **effort**.

MEASUREMENTS OF RESULTS

There are various ways to measure the results of work being done to prevent accidents. The effects of having an accident include, for example, injuries, illnesses, anguish suffering, financial losses, increased insurance costs, poor productivity, absenteeism, production delays, high labor costs, machinery downtime, and poor community image. Two types of measurements of results are commonly used. The first, and by far the most common, tracks **accident frequency and severity rates**. The second type measures **attitudes** such as employee perceptions of the company's commitment to accident prevention. Many factors affect perceptions, but one of the most important factors is what the company is doing to prevent accidents

MEASUREMENTS OF RESULTS—ACCIDENTS

Accidents are most often measured as frequency and severity rates. Frequency rates are used rather than the actual number of accidents because they show how many accidents occurred per a fixed number of employees or hours. This allows a site to compare its performance to past performance with a certain degree of confidence. To illustrate, let's assume that last year your site had 80 injuries that were serious enough to require reporting them to government authorities. At the end of the current year, you're summarizing your data, and discover that your site had 100 reportable accidents and dangerous occurrences. If you're looking at the numbers alone, it appears that your programs performed more poorly this year than last. But this perception would change if you knew that this year your site had 75% more employees this year than last. Knowing this would allow you to conclude that instead of getting worse, your programs were actually getting better. In reality your number of accidents increased by only 20% while employee exposure hours increased by 75%. Based on accident rates, not actual numbers, your program improved. It is important to use rates rather than actual numbers for this reason.

To calculate accident frequency rates for injuries, near-miss accidents, and property damage accidents, you need to know

- The number of accidents that have occurred
- The number of employee hours worked.

The calculations follow:

Frequency rate = number of accidents × 200,000 divided by the total employee hours worked. North Americans use 200,000 hours as a base, the Europeans tend to use 100,000 hours, and still others use 1,000,000 hours in their rate calculations. The reason 200,000 hours is used in North America is because it roughly equals the number of hours worked by 100 employees during a normal work year. Using 200,000 as a base makes it easy to estimate the site's frequency rate by simply knowing the number of employees at work. For example, if your site has 200 employees and you had six recordable injuries, you have a frequency rate of about 3; if you had 400 employees with six recordable injuries, you have an accident rate of about 1.5. Commonly used frequency and severity rates are:

- Lost-time injury/illness frequency rate
- Recordable injury/illness frequency rate
- Disabling injury/illness frequency rate
- Medical aid frequency rate
- First aid or minor injury/illness frequency rate
- Disabling injury/illness severity rate
- Property damage frequency rate
- Property damage severity rate (monetary)
- All accident frequency rate
- Near-miss frequency rate.

The following formulas are used to calculate the various frequency rates:

$$\text{Lost-time injury/illness frequency rate} = \frac{(\text{lost-time accidents}) \times 200,000}{\text{employee hours worked}}$$

$$\text{Recordable injury/illness frequency rate} = \frac{(\text{number of recordable injuries}) \times 200,000}{\text{employee hours worked}}$$

$$\text{Disabling injury/illness frequency rate} = \frac{(\text{number of disabling injuries}) \times 200{,}000}{\text{employee hours worked}}$$

$$\text{Medical aid frequency rate} = \frac{(\text{number of medical injuries}) \times 200{,}000}{\text{employee hours worked}}$$

$$\text{First aid/minor injury frequency rate} = \frac{(\text{number of first aid/minor injuries}) \times 200{,}000}{\text{employee hours worked}}$$

$$\text{Property damage frequency rate} = \frac{(\text{number of property damage accidents}) \times 200{,}000}{\text{employee hours worked}}$$

$$\text{All accident frequency rate} = \frac{(\text{number of accidents}) \times 200{,}000}{\text{employee hours worked}}$$

$$\text{Near-miss frequency rate} = \frac{(\text{number of near misses}) \times 200{,}000}{\text{employee hours worked}}$$

Frequency rates tell how many accidents took place per 200,000 hours worked. They do not tell how serious the accidents were. For example, one lost-time accident may involve a day off and another may require 10 days away from work. For this reason, another accident rate was created, called an accident severity rate. To calculate an accident severity rate you need to know the number of work days lost and the number of employee hours worked. The formula for calculating a severity rate is:

$$\text{Accident severity rate} = \frac{(\text{total days lost}) \times 200{,}000}{\text{employee hours worked}}$$

Property damage severity rates can also be calculated by determining the total cost of property damage accidents × 200,000, divided by the total employee hours worked.

Not only do base rate numbers change from country to country, but definitions of the types of accidents may also vary from country to country. It is important to know what definitions are being used for such things as lost time, recordables, first aid cases, and others if you are planning to compare accident frequency rates. For example, the definition of a recordable injury and illness in the United States may be different from the definition used in Canada, Latin America, Asia, or the United Kingdom. In areas where no clearly defined definitions exist, the site must develop its own. This is usually what has to take place in cases of property damage and process interruptions.

REASONS FOR USING ACCIDENT FREQUENCY AND SEVERITY RATES

There are many good reasons for using accident frequency and severity rates. As mentioned earlier, these measurements of results are part of any effective safety management program. When accident frequency and severity rates are properly used, they can lead to an increased commitment to preventing accidents. Several of the most obvious benefits of frequency and severity rates are:

- They indicate the results of the site's efforts to prevent accidents and when correctly used can lead to accident prevention.
- They motivate management.
- They are well accepted.
- They are easy to calculate.
- They are easy to understand.
- They have been used for a long time and have established credibility.
- They are good for self-comparison and trend analysis.
- They form a practical basis for employee recognition programs.
- They can be used to gain a positive image for the organization or units within the organization.

DISADVANTAGES OF ACCIDENT FREQUENCY AND SEVERITY RATES

Frequency and severity rates have limitations and they can lead to a cover-up mentality or even to underreporting of what is taking place in the workplace. In the long run, such covering up actually harms a site's accident prevention efforts. If not properly understood, accident frequency rates can lead to a very reactionary approach that is based on a statistically insignificant number. Only through understanding the problems associated with accident frequency and severity rates can you be able to overcome their limitations and take full advantage of their benefits. Several problems associated with using frequency rates include:

- Accidents are relatively rare events and so frequency rates based on them may not be statistically valid (an in-depth discussion on accident statistics is covered later in this chapter).

- Frequency rates are reactive, not predictive; in other words, they do not measure the level of safety protection at the site, they measure the level of "un-safety" protection at the site. This is very significant.

- Frequency rates are easily manipulated by how one chooses to define such things as a lost workday, a recordable accident, and so forth.

- They are easily biased by such things as using onsite versus external medical personnel, labor agreements, local Workers Compensation payments and laws, and the use of light work duty programs.

- When too much focus is placed on them, they encourage a false sense of security or the other extreme, an overreaction.

There are several ways to overcome these limitations and put accident frequency and severity rates to good use in your organization.

- First and foremost, management must clearly understand and appreciate what accident frequency rates are and how they should be used. This is done only by educating members of management on safety measurement techniques so they can understand the strengths and weaknesses of results, measurements, causes, and effects. Once they understand the potential and how to interpret and use all three types of measurements, they will be more likely to employ a balanced and professional approach to using accident statistics.

- Make sure you use as many rates as practical when drawing conclusions and interpreting your site's performance. Do not depend on a single rate to indicate how well or how poorly safety programs are working.

- Use rates primarily for self-comparison, not for comparisons to other organizations. It is not known what biases exist in these other organizations about how rates are generated.

- Finally, use statistical control techniques. Too often small changes in accident rates evoke an overreaction by site personnel. Valuable time and effort go into correcting a problem that does not exist or that does not deserve the attention it is given. Accidents are fairly rare events and small changes in accident rates may have little to do with changes in the overall level of control or effectiveness of the site's safety program. Indeed, these changes may not even be statistically significant.

Statistical control charts help the site to identify what is meaningful versus what is not statistically valid or random. These charts enable the user to focus attention on real, significant variations as opposed to imagined problems or special cases.

Control charts plot what are called upper and lower control limits and the organization's average accident rate. These control limits indicate a level within which variations of accident rates are not considered significant (when following certain rules of interpretation). Accident rates higher than the upper control limit and lower than the lower control limit are generally considered statistically valid. Accident rates within the control limits often indicate that there is no statistically significant change in the organization's accident prevention programs based on the accident rates analyzed. Figure 4.1 illustrates a statistical control chart. One way to develop a statistical chart with upper and lower control limits is as follows:

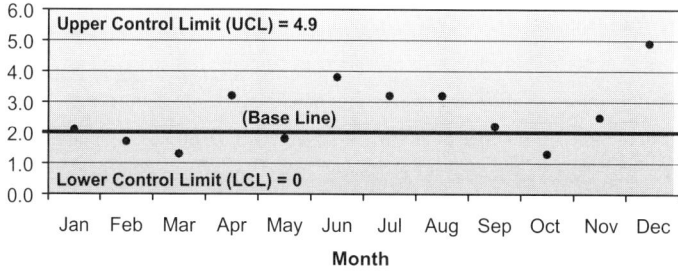

FIGURE 4.1   Universal Copper and Metals Mine accident frequency rate control chart

- Establish a base rate by taking the average of the previous 5 years' (60 months') accident rate being analyzed.
- Take the square root of this average and multiply this by two. Add this number to the average rate and this number becomes the upper control limit. Subtract it from the average and you have the lower control limit. Statistical control charts have three lines on them, an average or base rate, an upper control limit, and a lower control limit.

The following illustrates how this calculation works:

1. Establish a base rate by averaging the frequency rates from the preceding 60-month period. *Example:*

   - Last year's rate—2.0
   - Two years previous—3.0
   - Three years previous—1.0
   - Four years previous—3.0
   - Five years previous—1.0
   - Total—10.0.

   The average is 10.4 divided by 5, or 2.1.

2. Establish upper and lower limits by determining the positive and negative value of 2 times the square root of the base rate. *Example:*

   The square root of 2.0 is 1.40. Two times this is 2.8. Therefore 2.8 plus 2.1 (the base rate) is 4.9 and 2.0 minus 2.8 is a negative 0.8. The upper control limit is 4.9 and the lower control limit is 0, since it is impossible to have a negative accident rate. Figure 4.1 illustrates what this control chart would look like. The points have been added to illustrate the current year's monthly frequency rates.

This is a very basic method for calculating upper and lower control limits. Other methods can also be used to calculate these limits. To ensure that the statistical control charts are as reliable as practical, keep several guidelines in mind. First, use accident rates that have as many sets of data as possible. For example, an all injury/illness frequency rate works better than a lost time frequency rate. Second, try to use at least twenty sets of data in calculating the base rate or average. In our example we only used five data points for practical purposes. However, they represented 60 individual monthly frequency rates.

Interpreting statistical control charts properly helps to reduce the over-reaction to accident rates that are not statistically valid. Figure 4.2 lists several guidelines to help you interpret the data provided by statistical control charts.

MEASUREMENTS OF RESULTS—ATTITUDE

Another measurement of results takes a look at attitudes. Attitudes about safety, to a certain extent, result from the efforts the site puts into preventing accidents. They reflect pride, disappointment, or confidence, among others, in the site's program. For this reason, measuring people's attitudes regarding

---

A process is out of control … when one of the following happens:

1. One or more points fall outside the control limit. (December's rate in Figure 4.1).

2. When dividing the chart into three equal zones on either side of the base line:

   - Two out of three consecutive points in the closest zone (same side). January through March of Figure 4.1.

   - Four out of five consecutive points in the middle zone (same side). April through July of Figure 4.1.

3. Nine consecutive points on the same side of the base rate are significant.

4. Six consecutive points are increasing or decreasing.

FIGURE 4.2   Rules for interpreting statistical control charts

the site's safety programs are measurements of results. Some believe that attitudes cannot be measured; only behaviors can be measured. Others believe behaviors reflect attitudes and that by measuring behaviors we are indirectly measuring attitudes. Regardless of your perceptions as to which leads to which, it is important to give people opportunities to express their feelings about the effectiveness of the safety program.

Perception surveys are commonly used to measure attitudes. They tell us what people's impressions are, and provide information needed to address fundamental program problems. They are a true indicator of how well the site's programs are reaching employees.

To conduct effective perception surveys, keep several guidelines in mind:

- When asking questions, make sure they relate to the people being asked. For example don't ask an employee if he feels that the mine manager supports safety effectively in his normal work activities such as staff meetings, and so forth. The average worker wouldn't have any idea how to answer this with any degree of reliability. However, they can provide meaningful perceptions about whether they feel that the senior manager supports the safety program on the shop floor by giving talks, making inspections, and so forth. Even though management and nonmanagement may have common perceptions about many issues, other issues should be targeted to one group or the other. For example, you might want to know how management feels about the level of employee commitment to the site's safety programs and vice versa.

- When conducting surveys, make sure to ask several questions that assess the same issue in different ways so that comparisons can be made. This technique assists in determining whether the information obtained is valid or invalid.

- When recording perceptions use a five- to seven-point scale ranging from strong disagreement with the statement (lowest number) to strong agreement with the statement (highest number). This type of scale is called a Likert scale.

- Use appropriate random sampling techniques when assessing employee perceptions. This means that you need to sample appropriate numbers of employees; for example, with small numbers of employees this might mean all employees, whereas with large numbers of employees, such as several hundred, this might mean taking only a small proportion (e.g., 15%–25% of employees). This also means that all shifts and all occupations should be represented.

- Write a statement and ask employees how well they agree with it. For example, "Management shows a high degree of commitment to the site's safety program by participating regularly in safety inspections in my work area." Ask employees if they strongly agree, somewhat agree, don't know, disagree, or strongly disagree. Each response can have a number assigned to it like five for strongly agree and one for strongly disagree. This allows the survey results to be quantified.

- Use techniques to ensure anonymity of the survey participants.

- Request information on the survey that permits you to analyze data by employee groups if needed such as production, maintenance, nonmanagement, management/supervision, work shift, and so forth.

Figure 4.3 is a sample employee perception survey that illustrates many of the characteristics mentioned.

MEASUREMENTS OF CAUSES

Measurements of causes relate to the factors that lead to accidents. They include both immediate causes, such as substandard acts and substandard conditions, and their underlying causes, such as individual and work factors. Individual factor causes include inadequate knowledge, skill, motivation, and capability. Work factors include such things as inadequate training, supervision, design, purchasing, inspections, and so forth. If not controlled, the two types of causes—immediate and underlying—can lead to accidents.

Measurements of causes usually refer to measuring substandard acts and site conditions. These types of causes immediately precede an accident. These substandard acts and site conditions are usually identified in large numbers and therefore need to be measured appropriately to enable good use of the data. There are two common ways of doing this. The first, and by far the most common, is to identify the immediate causes from investigation reports; the second is to determine the substandard acts (behaviors) and conditions that could result in an accident.

Acts and conditions such as these can be detected either before or after accidents occur. Job observations and behavior sampling are the two most common techniques used to identify substandard acts. Planned general inspections, like those regular inspections of working areas with hazards being documented, are very common ways to identify substandard conditions before accidents take place. All three techniques—inspections, observations, and behavior sampling—yield information before accidents occur. These measurements are before the loss, and preventive in nature.

It is especially important to identify and evaluate the *underlying* causes to prevent substandard acts and conditions from occurring. Some ways to identify evident causes before they result in accidents are relatively simple. However, short of doing systems audits, it is more difficult to identify underlying causes before accidents. The most practical way to do this is to properly train those who investigate accidents in investigation techniques and accident causation. In addition, it helps to have a quality control process in place to measure whether or not these causes are identified appropriately.

As with frequency and severity rates, statistics can be helpful in analyzing and interpreting which of the accident causes are the most significant. The statistical technique suggested for use with accident frequency and severity rates was control charts. For analyzing accident causes, we suggest a "Pareto" chart. Pareto charts illustrate which problems are occurring at what frequency in a single glance. They allow you to identify, at a glance, the most common problems, helping you to focus efforts on problems leading to greatest results. Pareto charts are easy to make. They are bar charts, or histograms, that illustrate acts and conditions occurring at the site. To construct a Pareto chart you simply list the type of act or condition on the horizontal axis of the chart and the frequency in terms of percentages of occurrences on the vertical axis. The acts or conditions are then graphed in descending order from the most frequent to the least frequent starting from the left. Figure 4.4 is a sample chart.

Measurements of causes are part of any successful safety and health program and are very common, especially measurements of immediate causes of accidents such as acts and conditions. Although these types of measurements of causes are useful, they are reactive and after the fact. Measurements of causes focusing on underlying causes of accidents, while still post-event and reactive, do focus attention on the work needed to prevent substandard acts and conditions from occurring and are therefore more valuable. Measurements of causes fall just short of directly measuring effort being placed into preventing accidents. Measurements of effort are described in the section that follows.

UNIVERSAL COPPER AND METALS
SAFETY PROGRAM ATTITUDE SURVEY

Date _____

❏ Management   ❏ Staff

❏ Production   ❏ Shift

❏ Maintenance   ❏ Other

Safety is a key element of the way we do business here at Universal Metals. To help us understand how we are doing, what improvements we need to make and how far we have to go, we would like to have you circle or mark the answer which best reflects what you think about our Safety programs. When you are done, please place the survey in the envelope provided and return it to Human Resources. Do not put your name on the survey. When we get the form back, we will provide you with a summary of the results and ask you to help us make the improvements necessary to our Safety programs.

Handling Safety issues is primarily the line manager's responsibility.

Disagree Strongly	Disagree	Neutral	Agree	Agree Strongly
❏	❏	❏	❏	❏

If all Safety rules and procedures are complied with, it is inevitable that productivity will suffer.

Disagree Strongly	Disagree	Neutral	Agree	Agree Strongly
❏	❏	❏	❏	❏

Most accidents which happen at the site are simple in nature and impractical to prevent.

Disagree Strongly	Disagree	Neutral	Agree	Agree Strongly
❏	❏	❏	❏	❏

Proper safety management is important to the site's senior management.

Disagree Strongly	Disagree	Neutral	Agree	Agree Strongly
❏	❏	❏	❏	❏

Safety is given equal consideration with production at this site.

Disagree Strongly	Disagree	Neutral	Agree	Agree Strongly
❏	❏	❏	❏	❏

There are situations in which a supervisor should have the authority to suspend Safety rules and procedures in favor of completing the task.

Disagree Strongly	Disagree	Neutral	Agree	Agree Strongly
❏	❏	❏	❏	❏

There are situations in which a supervisor should have the authority to suspend Safety rules and procedures in favor of completing the task.

Disagree Strongly	Disagree	Neutral	Agree	Agree Strongly
❏	❏	❏	❏	❏

The Safety responsibilities of my job are clearly spelled out for me.

Disagree Strongly	Disagree	Neutral	Agree	Agree Strongly
❏	❏	❏	❏	❏

The Safety training I have received is adequate for me to meet my responsibilities.

Disagree Strongly	Disagree	Neutral	Agree	Agree Strongly
❏	❏	❏	❏	❏

The Safety attitude of those who report to me is good.

Disagree Strongly	Disagree	Neutral	Agree	Agree Strongly
❏	❏	❏	❏	❏

FIGURE 4.3   Universal Copper and Metals Safety Program attitude survey

The overall quality of Safety is above average.

Disagree Strongly	Disagree	Neutral	Agree	Agree Strongly
❏	❏	❏	❏	❏

In my area of responsibility, minor injuries, property damage accidents, environmental spills and near misses are reported properly and promptly.

Disagree Strongly	Disagree	Neutral	Agree	Agree Strongly
❏	❏	❏	❏	❏

Knowledge of the site's Safety program and expectations is essential to any manager at any level.

Disagree Strongly	Disagree	Neutral	Agree	Agree Strongly
❏	❏	❏	❏	❏

The Safety department gives proper and timely response to my injuries.

Disagree Strongly	Disagree	Neutral	Agree	Agree Strongly
❏	❏	❏	❏	❏

Positive reinforcement (commendation) for a job well done is just as important as punishment when a worker violates rules and procedures.

Disagree Strongly	Disagree	Neutral	Agree	Agree Strongly
❏	❏	❏	❏	❏

Management puts so much pressure on production performance that Safety suffers.

Disagree Strongly	Disagree	Neutral	Agree	Agree Strongly
❏	❏	❏	❏	❏

Management practices what it preaches regarding Safety.

Disagree Strongly	Disagree	Neutral	Agree	Agree Strongly
❏	❏	❏	❏	❏

The Safety meetings are beneficial.

Disagree Strongly	Disagree	Neutral	Agree	Agree Strongly
❏	❏	❏	❏	❏

An overload of paperwork is a major problem with the implementation of our Safety programs.

Disagree Strongly	Disagree	Neutral	Agree	Agree Strongly
❏	❏	❏	❏	❏

What are the three best aspects of the site's Safety program?

1.

2.

3.

What are the three biggest problems with the site's Safety program?

1.

2.

3.

FIGURE 4.3   Universal Copper and Metals Safety Program attitude survey (continued)

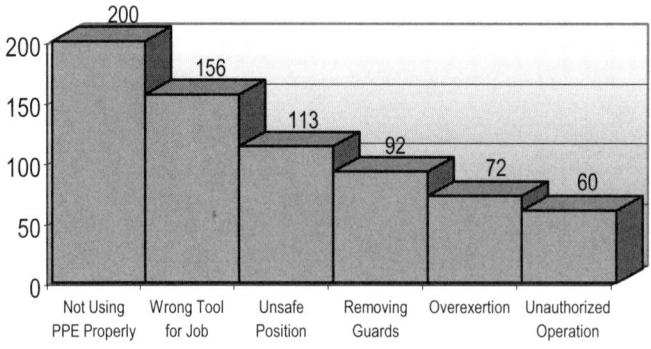

FIGURE 4.4   Universal Copper and Metals substandard acts

MEASUREMENTS OF EFFORT

While measurements of results are common and an important part of any successful safety and health program, to be proactive and preventive you must consider different measurements such as effort being put forth to prevent accidents. These types of measurements are called measurements of effort and assess the amount of control that exists within the system. Measurements of effort evaluate:

- Whether your safety system has the proper elements to ensure accidents are prevented
- Whether it defines appropriate roles and responsibilities for doing work required to make the elements effective
- Whether the roles and responsibilities are in place and working.

One of our challenges as safety and health professionals is to ensure that safety programs have the right elements or activities to prevent accidents. An indication of the features common to successful safety programs is found by looking at the elements emerging in international standards documents such as the International Standards Organization's (ISO) 14001, Environmental Management Systems. In addition, government programs are focusing on self-regulation and world-class management practices such as the U.S. Occupational Safety and Health Administration's (OSHA) Voluntary Protection Program (VPP). The elements of ISO14001 and OSHA's VPP programs are illustrated in Figure 4.5.

With information gained by research conducted in the 1980s, practical experience in safety management systems auditing, and trends in codes, regulations, and industry standards, elements common to successful safety programs can be identified as follows:

- Planning and leadership
- Training and communications
- Job and operation analysis and control
- Change management
- Purchasing systems
- Work rules and operating permits
- Inspections
- Occupational health and hygiene systems
- Personal protective equipment (PPE)
- Accident investigation and analysis
- Emergency preparedness
- Audits and reviews.

Two types of measurements of effort, routine checks and management systems audits, are described in the following section.

ISO 14001	OSHA VPP
1. **Environmental Policy**	1. **Management Leadership & Employee Involvement** Commitment Organization Responsibility Accountability Resources Planning Contract Workers Employee Involvement Annual Evaluation of Your Safety and Health Program Employee Notification
2. **Planning** Environmental Aspects Objectives and Targets Management Program	2. **Worksite Analysis** Pre-use Analysis Comprehensive Surveys Self Inspections Routine Hazard Analysis Employee Reports of Hazards Accident Investigations Pattern Analysis
3. **Implementation and Operation** Structure and Responsibilities Training, Awareness, and Competence Communication Documentation Document Control Operational Control Emergency Preparedness	3. **Hazard Prevention and Control** Professional Expertise Safety and Health Rules PPE Emergency Preparedness Preventive Maintenance Medical Program
4. **Checking and Corrective Action** Monitoring and Measurement Nonconformance and Corrective Action Records Management Systems Audit	4. **Safety and Health Training**
5. **Management Review**	5. **Safety and Health Training**

FIGURE 4.5 Management system elements of ISO's 14001 and OSHA's VPP

MEASUREMENTS OF EFFORT—ROUTINE CHECKS

Routine measurements of work to prevent accidents should be done fairly frequently and kept simple. They measure indicators of how well the site's safety program is working. Here is how they are done.

1. Select practical activities for the work site to be effective, like:
   - Conducting supervisor inspections
   - Holding safety meetings
   - Complying with PPE requirements
   - Reporting and promptly investigating accidents

   - Completing job observations
   - Ensuring that requirements for carrying out this work are established at clearly defined frequencies.

2. Define a practical frequency of carrying out routine measurements. They are usually done at 1-, 2-, or 3-month intervals.

3. Determine the percentage compliance to the site's requirements for each activity.

4. Summarize the measurements by areas of accountability, such as departments, so that managers are aware of their performance and can take appropriate actions to reinforce good performance or to correct deficiencies.

5. Communicate the findings to appropriate personnel, such as the accountable managers and *their* managers.

Figure 4.6 is a form used to summarize routine measurements. You will note that Universal Copper and Metals Mine chooses to measure such things as inspections, safety talks, and spot job observations. Each issue is very operationally focused and has significant impact at the working level.

If done in the manner described, these measurements are simple to carry out, require very little effort to complete, and are an excellent way to determine if safety programs are in place and working throughout the site. Management does indeed attach increased importance to anything that is quantified, and the quantification process alone motivates improvement.

MEASUREMENTS OF EFFORT—MANAGEMENT SYSTEMS AUDITS

Although routine measurements of effort are important, they do not provide an in-depth evaluation of work being done to prevent accidents. Management systems audits provide this in-depth analysis. They take more time to complete but they measure the site's complete safety management system, rather than just indicators. They complement routine measurements.

Too often, safety audits are based on subjective criteria and opinions. These subjective results lead to inconsistencies and wasted effort. Decision makers need more professional and objective

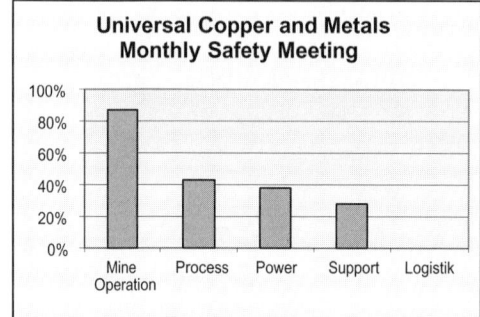
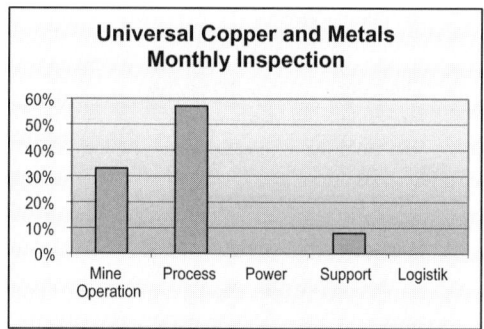
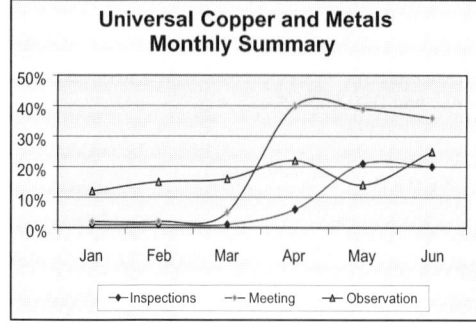
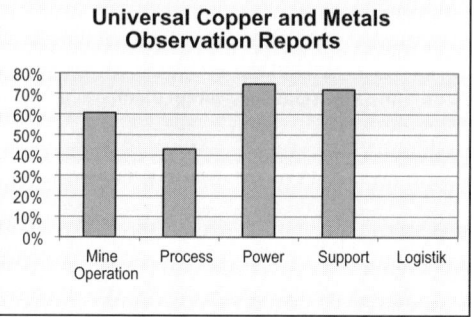

FIGURE 4.6   **Universal Copper and Metals Mine monthly reports**

information from their safety staff. Several practical ways to overcome this subjectivity and inconsistency and bring more reliability to the audit process are

- Develop an objective management systems audit
- Use a reliable audit process
- Ensure that competent people conduct the audits.

DEVELOPING AN OBJECTIVE AUDIT

Here is how to ensure your audit process is objective:

- Divide the safety system into its component parts or elements. The elements common to successful safety systems have been listed earlier.
- Using knowledgeable and experienced people, assign weightings or value factors for each element such that when added together they total 100. The weightings should reflect the importance of each element in comparison to other elements for preventing accidents.
- Ask enough questions to ensure that the work in the element is properly assessed.
- Ensure that each question is quantified or weighted properly by using the advice of knowledgeable and experienced people.
- Devise a system for objectively issuing points for the questions asked.
- Quantify results and record findings.

Keys to keeping the audit practical and effective are to control the number of questions being asked and to avoid being overly prescriptive. Being too prescriptive simply means asking too many detailed questions rather than allowing flexibility to meet the intent of the audit's requirement in a manner that best suits their needs. Keep your audit document simple and straightforward.

Use a Reliable Audit Process

Putting a reliable audit process into place is the second way to keep the audit objective. A good audit process has two parts. The first assesses and defines the site's formal programs, such as those with documented procedures, work methods, and processes. The second involves verifying that those procedures, methods, and processes are in place at the working level.

Defining what the safety program requirements are involves interviewing the most knowledgeable people at the site as well as reviewing appropriate policies, procedures, roles, and responsibilities. As noted, this part of the audit also includes checking records that document and define program requirements such as procedures, rule booklets, policies, surveys, and so forth.

Emphasize Verification

The second part of the audit requires you to verify that what is alleged is actually in place. This type of verification involves reviewing records, interviewing employees, and checking worksite conditions. The emphasis of the audit should be on the verification phase.

Use a Qualified Auditor

The third technique to guarantee audit reliability is to ensure that the audit is conducted by competent people. Although competency is a difficult characteristic to define, auditors must have several characteristics before they qualify:

- They must be properly trained and experienced in conducting management systems audits.
- They should have some technical knowledge and skill in the areas they are evaluating.
- They must know the intent of the audit instrument being used.
- They must have the proper demeanor to conduct audits of this type. The audit process is evaluating systems and working processes, as carried out by people. Management systems auditors need excellent people, listening, and time management skills.
- Finally, they must be unbiased. This means they should have at least a minimum amount of vested interest in the results.

Team audits are popular because it is rare to find all of these attributes in a single person. Team audits generally include staff safety professionals, operating managers, topic experts, employees, third party professionals, and others.

USING MEASUREMENTS OF EFFORT

Management systems audits and routine measurements provide information necessary to develop short- and long-range plans for improvement. They form an important part of an overall improvement process. Because many do not understand an improvement process, the most typical aspects of such a process are listed below.

- Orienting and training key site personnel on their roles and responsibilities in the safety program
- Developing and committing to a 3- to 5-year plan for long-term improvement
- Training and developing safety personnel in a management systems approach
- Conducting management systems audits as well as routine evaluations of the safety program
- Developing action plans to address audit findings
- Conducting introductory training for line managers
- Developing safety management roles and responsibilities and program requirements
- Providing in-depth training for on-site experts
- Developing reference material to aid personnel in implementing and managing the program.

In summary, "If you can't measure it, you can't manage it." Safety professionals and managers must measure safety performance in a balanced way, rather than simply measuring results. The latter measures how unsafe a site may be, but reveals very little about what needs to be done to prevent accidents from occurring. A balanced safety measurement program must be used to prevent accidents, not to react to them.

CHAPTER 5

Applications of Behavioral Science to Improve Mine Safety

E. Scott Geller, Ned Carter,[1] Jason DePasquale, Charles Pettinger, and Joshua Williams
Virginia Polytechnic Institute and State University, Blacksburg, Virginia

As discussed in other chapters of this text, engineering intervention—ranging from improved lighting to vehicle and machinery design—has improved mine safety dramatically. However, because the environmental context of both surface and underground mining is often hazardous, continuously changing, and sometimes unpredictable, it's impossible to protect the miner completely with environmental manipulations. Therefore, mining experts have pointed out the need to complement technological advancements with a focus on the human dimensions of safety, including the application of employee surveys, training series, incentive programs, and feedback presentations (Langton 1995; Peters 1995; Peters, Bockosh, and Fotta 1997). In fact, the U.S. Bureau of Mines referred to the need to apply fundamental psychological principles in the enhancement of miners' ability to recognize and react appropriately to threats in their risky work environment (Kowalski, Folta, and Barrett 1995). The question remains as to what these fundamental psychological principles are. This chapter answers this important question.

H.L. Boling (1995) establishes the psychological focus of this chapter by pointing out that, "Today the progressive, productive and safe companies around the world have one common denominator, an innovative safety program that is behavior-based" (p. 2). The term "behavior-based safety" has become quite popular among safety professionals, consultants, and members of safety steering committees. It is commonly used to reflect a proactive upstream approach to safety by focusing attention on at-risk behaviors that can lead to an injury and on safe behaviors that can contribute to injury prevention. Beyond this general definition, however, there seems to be substantial misperception, misunderstanding, and misapplication.

A number of recent books detail the principles and procedures of behavior-based safety, and they provide solid evidence for the success of this approach to injury prevention (e.g., Geller 1996a, 1998a, 1998d; Krause 1995; Krause, Hidley, and Hodson 1996; McSween 1995; Sulzer-Azaroff 1998). Each of these books is consistent with regard to certain basic principles and methods, as well as the beneficial outcomes of behavior-based safety. We offer a brief review of these principles, procedures, and benefits here, and recommend these texts for follow up and continued learning. We start with a definition and rationale for three basic principles of the behavior-based approach.

---

1. Contributed while on leave from The Department of Occupational and Environmental Medicine, University Hospital, Uppsala, Sweden.

PRINCIPLE 1: FOCUS INTERVENTION ON OBSERVABLE BEHAVIOR

The behavior-based approach is founded on behavioral science as conceptualized and researched by B.F. Skinner (1938, 1953, and 1974). Experimental behavior analysis, and later applied behavior analysis, emerged from Skinner's research and teaching. He laid the groundwork for numerous therapies and interventions to improve the quality of life of individuals, groups, and entire communities (Geller, Winett, and Everett 1982; Goldstein and Krasner 1987; Greene et al. 1987). Whether working one-on-one in a clinical setting or with work teams throughout an organization, the intervention procedures always target specific behaviors in order to produce constructive change. In other words, the behavior-based approach focuses on observing what people do, analyzes why they do it, and then applies a research-supported intervention strategy to improve their actions.

Whatever intervention strategy is used to improve a human aspect of safety, the process should target behavior. Whether using training, feedback, injury investigation, coaching, or incentives to benefit safety, focus on behavior. Why? First, because you can be objective and impersonal about behavior. You can talk about behavior independently from people's opinions, attitudes, and feelings. Behavior varies according to factors in the external world, including equipment design, management systems, behaviors shown by others, and various social dynamics. Open discussions about the environmental and interpersonal determinants of safe versus at-risk behavior can lead to practical modifications of the work culture to encourage safe behavior and discourage at-risk behavior.

Behavior-based intervention *acts people into thinking differently,* whereas person-based intervention *thinks people into acting differently.* The person-based approach is used successfully by many psychiatrists and clinical psychologists in professional therapy sessions, but it is not cost-effective in a group or organizational setting. To be effective, person-focused intervention requires extensive one-on-one interaction between a client and a specially trained intervention specialist. Even if time and facilities were available for an intervention to focus on internal and nonobservable attitudes and person states, few safety professionals or consultants have the education, training, and experience to implement such an approach. Internal person factors can be improved indirectly, however, by directly focusing on behaviors in certain ways.

The key is to focus on behavior and you'll be on the right track, whatever the intervention approach. It's **behavior-based** commitment, **behavior-based** goal-setting, **behavior-based** feedback, **behavior-based** training, **behavior-based** recognition (Geller 1997a), **behavior-based** incentives and rewards (Geller 1996b), and so on.

PRINCIPLE 2: LOOK FOR EXTERNAL FACTORS TO IMPROVE PERFORMANCE

Internal person dimensions like attitudes, perceptions, and cognitions are difficult to define objectively and change directly. So stop trying! Most of us don't have the education, training, experience, nor time to deal with people's attitudes or person states directly. Instead, you should look for external factors influencing behavior independent of individual feelings, preferences, and perceptions. When you empower people to analyze behavior from a systems perspective and implement interventions to improve behavior, you will indirectly improve their attitude, commitment, and internal motivation.

In the first widely used American textbook in psychology, *Principles of Psychology*, William James (1890) explained the reciprocity between behavior and attitude as follows:

> Sit all day in a moping posture, sigh, and reply to everything with a dismal voice, and your melancholy lingers ... If we wish to conquer undesirable emotional tendencies in ourselves, we must ... go through the outward movements of those contrary dispositions which we prefer to cultivate.

Careful observation and analysis of ongoing work practices can pinpoint many potential causes of safe and at-risk behaviors. Those causes external to people–including reward and punishment contingencies, policies, or supervisory behaviors–can often be altered to improve both behavior and attitude. In contrast, internal person factors are difficult to identify, and if defined, they are even more difficult to change directly. So with behavior-based safety the focus is placed on external factors–environmental conditions and behaviors–that can be changed upstream from a potential injury.

PRINCIPLE 3: FOCUS ON POSITIVE CONSEQUENCES TO MOTIVATE SAFETY IMPROVEMENT

The ABC contingency is a basic tenet of behavior-based safety:

- A stands for activator, or the antecedent events that direct behavior.
- B stands for the desired behavior.
- C refers to consequence, or to the environmental stimuli that motivate behavior.

We do what we do to gain a positive consequence or to escape or avoid a negative consequence. And, we stop doing what we're doing when our behavior results in immediate negative consequences.

The most powerful motivating consequences are soon and certain. That's why most at-risk behavior occurs. Compared to safe behavior, at-risk behavior provides the worker with such soon and certain consequences as comfort, convenience, perceived efficiency, and faster job completion.

As this third principle indicates, using positive over negative consequences is critically important. It's relevant to attitude, and to many other internal dimensions of people. Think about it. How does a reward, personal recognition, or a group celebration make you feel, compared to reprimand or criticism? Both consequences can have a significant impact on behavior. The difference lies in the accompanying attitude or feeling state.

As detailed elsewhere (Geller 1996a, 1997a, and 1998d), when positive recognition is delivered correctly, it does more than increase the frequency of the behavior it follows. It also increases the likelihood that other safe behaviors will occur, and that positive recognition will be used more often to benefit both behavior and attitude. The popular common sense belief that we learn more from our mistakes than our achievements is wrong. We learn more from our successes. So recognizing safe behavior facilitates more learning and positive motivation than criticizing at-risk behavior. Remember that only with positive consequences can you improve both behavior and attitude at the same time.

DON'T RELY ON COMMON SENSE

More explanations for these and additional principles of behavior-based safety are presented elsewhere (Geller 1997b, 1998c). These three principles are most critical with regard to the development of interventions to improve the human dynamics of mine safety. Do they sound like plain old common sense to you? If so, we're glad. But we must warn you that others will not necessarily feel the same without appropriate education, training, or experience. Common sense or intuition is often incorrect. What sounds good to one person will not necessarily sound right to another. Consider, for example, the following common-sense strategies people have implemented in an attempt to deal with the human dynamics of safety.

- Punish a person who returns to work after a lost-time injury.
- Implement a safety incentive program whereby everyone in an organization gets a prize if no one reports an injury.
- Set up a Safe Employee of the Month Program in which one individual in a large facility is publicly recognized for having the best safety attitude.
- Establish an observation system whereby employees must observe one unsafe condition or behavior each day and stop it.
- Invite a motivational speaker to address all employees with themes like:
  - Try Harder.
  - Change Your Attitude About Safety.
  - Self-Affirmation Is the Key to Motivation.
  - Safety Awareness and a Positive Attitude Are Keys to Behavior Change.
- Post signs with slogans like:
  - Think Safety.
  - Safety Is a Condition of Employment.
  - Zero Accidents Is Our Goal.

 – Safety Is a Priority.

 – All Injuries Are Preventable.

Do any of these psychological tactics sound familiar? All these strategies are ineffective and run counter to the three behavior-based principles described above. Some of these techniques can actually do more harm than good to the human dynamics of industrial safety and health. Yet I'm sure you've seen, perhaps even experienced, some of these intervention approaches. Why? Because they seemed like good common sense to someone.

It takes empirical investigation, not common sense, to guide the development and implementation of an improvement intervention, whether repairing a bridge, constructing a building, or administrating an incentive/reward process. "Contrary to popular belief, there is not too little common sense in business, there is too much" (Daniels 1994, p. 10).

Behavior-based safety, as reflected in the three principles described here, is based on more than 40 years of rigorous research. And with additional research, the methods and tools of behavior-based safety will continue to improve. Let's consider a general behavioral safety method that has been used by several researchers to evaluate the effectiveness of specific intervention techniques to prevent injury (e.g., Fellner and Sulzer-Azaroff 1984; Geller 1988; Komaki, Heinzmann, and Lawson 1980; Ludwig and Geller 1997; Sulzer-Azaroff and DeSantamaria, 1980). It has also been used by numerous organizations to improve safety performance (cf. Geller 1996a, 1998d).

THE "DO IT" PROCESS

The "DO IT" process puts people in control of improving behaviors, thereby preventing injuries. It is a general method for solving the behavioral dimensions of safety problems. It provides objective data for exploring why certain safety-related behaviors occur or don't occur and for evaluating the impact of interventions designed to increase safe behavior or decrease at-risk behavior. If an intervention does not produce a desired effect, it is either refined or replaced with a completely different approach to behavior change.

"D" for Define

The process begins by defining certain behaviors with which to work. These are the targets of the behavior improvement process. They are safe behaviors that need to increase or at-risk behaviors that need to decrease. Because avoiding at-risk behaviors often requires certain safe behaviors, safe targets might be behaviors that substitute for particular at-risk behaviors. On the other hand, a safe target behavior can be defined independently of an associated at-risk behavior. The definition of a safe target might be as basic as using certain personal protective equipment (PPE) or walking within designated pedestrian walkways. Or the safe target could be a process requiring a particular sequence of safe behaviors, as when lifting, parking a truck for unloading, or locking out energy sources.

Deriving a precise definition of a DO IT target is facilitated by developing a checklist that can be used to evaluate whether a certain target behavior or process is being performed safely. Just developing such behavioral definitions can lead to valuable learning. When people get involved in developing a behavioral checklist, they own a training process that can improve human dynamics on both the outside (behaviors) and the inside (feelings and attitudes) of people.

"O" for Observe

When people observe each other for certain safe or at-risk behaviors, they realize that everyone engages in at-risk behavior, sometimes without even knowing it. The purpose of the observation stage is not fault-finding, but it is a fact-finding process to discover behaviors and conditions that need to be changed or continued in order to prevent injuries.

Behavioral observations are done only with the awareness and permission of the person under observation. Unannounced observations might give a more realistic picture of at-risk behaviors, but such audits reduce interpersonal trust and give the impression that behavior-based safety is a negative or "gotcha" program. And from a behavior-change perspective, observations without permission cannot raise safety "mindfulness" (Geller 1999a; Langer 1989). It's likely that the mindfulness developed and increased from up-front and voluntary behavioral observation process is critical for behavior change and injury prevention.

It's easy to fall into a mindless job routine, becoming incapable of handling unexpected events in a safe and timely manner. And some mindless behavior can put a person in immediate risk for personal injury. We need to understand that this can happen to anyone and that a concerted effort to increase mindfulness on the job is warranted. Behavior-based observation and feedback provides the mechanism for making this happen.

To develop an observation process, teams of workers need to decide:

- What kind of checklist will be used during observations?
- Who will conduct the behavioral observations?
- How often will the observations be conducted?
- How will data from the checklist be summarized and interpreted?
- How will people be informed of the results from an observation process?

There is not one generic observation procedure for all situations, and customization and refinement should never stop. It's often advantageous to begin with a limited number of behaviors and a relatively simple checklist. This reduces the possibility that some people will feel overwhelmed at the start. Starting small also enables the broadest range of voluntary participation and offers numerous opportunities to successively improve the process by expanding its coverage of both behaviors and work areas.

"I" for Intervene

During this stage, interventions are designed and implemented in an attempt to increase safe behavior and/or decrease at-risk behavior. As reflected in Principle 2 above, intervention means changing external conditions of the system to make safe behavior more likely than at-risk behavior. When designing interventions, Principle 3 is your guide. Specifically, the most motivating consequences are soon, certain, and sizable. And, of course, positive consequences are preferable to negative consequences.

The process of observing and recording the frequency of safe and at-risk behavior on a checklist provides an opportunity to give individuals and groups valuable behavior-based feedback. When the results of a behavioral observation are shown to individuals or groups, they receive the kind of information that enables practice to improve performance. Considerable research has shown that providing workers with feedback about their safe and at-risk behaviors is a very cost-effective intervention approach for improving safety performance (e.g., Geller 1996a; Krause et al. 1996; Reber, Wallin, and Chhokar 1990; Sulzer-Azaroff and DeSantamaria 1980; McAfee and Winn 1989; Petersen 1989).

In addition to behavioral feedback, researchers have found a number of other intervention strategies to be effective at increasing safe work practices. These include worker-designed safety slogans, "near hit" and corrective action reporting, safe behavior promise cards, individual and group goal-setting, actively caring thank-you cards, and safety coaching, as well as incentive/reward programs for individuals or groups. These are described elsewhere (Geller 1996a and 1998d), and some have been applied in mining settings (Fox, Hopkins, and Anger 1987; Rhoton 1980). Later in this chapter we offer guidelines for matching the intervention strategy with the behavioral target and situation.

"T" for Test

The test phase of DO IT provides work teams with the information they need to refine or replace a behavior-change intervention, thereby improving the process. If observations show a lack of significant improvement in the target behavior, the work team analyzes and discusses the situation, and either refines the intervention or chooses another approach. On the other hand, if the target reaches the desired frequency level, the participants can turn their attention to another set of behaviors. They might add new critical behaviors to their checklist, expanding their domain of behavioral observations. They might design a new intervention procedure to focus only on new behaviors.

Every time the participants evaluate an intervention approach, they learn more about how to improve safety performance. They have essentially become behavioral scientists, using the DO IT process to:

- Diagnose a human dynamics problem.
- Monitor the impact of a behavior-change intervention.
- Refine interventions for continuous improvement.

Such testing results in motivating consequences that support this learning process and keep the participants involved.

Let's consider some basic principles about behavior-change techniques that can facilitate the development of the most effective intervention for a particular situation. First, it's important to understand the difference between other-directed, self-directed, and automatic behavior (Watson and Tharp 1993).

THREE TYPES OF BEHAVIOR

On-the-job behavior starts out as other-directed, in the sense that we follow someone else's instructions. Such direction can come from a training program, an operation manual, or a policy statement. After learning what to do, essentially by memorizing or internalizing the appropriate instructions, our behavior enters the self-directed stage. In other words, we talk to ourselves or formulate an image before performing a behavior to activate the right response. Sometimes we talk to ourselves after performing a behavior to reassure ourselves that we performed correctly or to figure out ways to do better next time. At this point we're usually open to corrective feedback if it's delivered well by a person we trust.

Some behaviors, performed frequently and consistently over a period of time, become automatic. A habit is formed. Some habits are good and some are not, depending on their short- and long-term consequences. If implemented correctly, rewards, recognition, and other positive consequences can facilitate the transfer of behavior from the self-directed phase to the habit phase.

Of course self-directed behavior is not always desirable. When we take a short cut, for example, we intentionally choose to ignore a safety precaution to perform more efficiently or with more comfort or convenience. In this state, people are consciously incompetent. Attempts to change self-directed behavior from incompetent to competent is often difficult, because it usually requires a relevant change in personal motivation.

Before a bad habit can be changed to a good one, the target behavior must become self-directed. In other words, people need to become aware of their undesirable habit (as in at-risk behavior) before adjustment is possible. Then, if the person is motivated to improve, their new self-directed behavior can become automatic.

Let's see what kinds of behavior-based interventions are appropriate for the three transitions alluded to above.

- Turning a risky habit (when the person is unconsciously incompetent) into safe self-directed behavior.
- Changing risky self-directed behavior (when the person is consciously incompetent) to safe self-directed behavior.
- Turning safe self-directed behavior (when the person is consciously competent) into a safe habit (unconscious competence).

THREE KINDS OF INTERVENTION STRATEGIES

Behavior-based safety trainers and consultants teach the ABC model (or three-term contingency) as a framework to understand and analyze behavior or to develop interventions for improving behavior. As given in Principle 3, the A stands for activators or antecedent events that precede behavior B, and C refers to the consequences following behavior and produced by it. Activators direct behavior; consequences motivate behavior.

Activators and consequences are external to the performer (as in the environment), or internal (as in self-instructions or self-recognition). They can be intrinsic or extrinsic to a behavior, meaning that they provide direction or motivation naturally as a task is performed (as in a computer game), or they are added to the situation extrinsically to improve performance. An incentive/reward program is external and extrinsic. It adds an activator (an incentive) and a consequence (a reward) to the situation to direct and motivate desirable behavior (Geller 1996b).

Instructional Intervention

An instructional intervention is typically an activator or antecedent event used to get new behavior started or to move behavior from the automatic (habit) stage to the self-directed stage. Or it is used to improve behavior already in the self-directed stage. The aim is to get the performer's attention and instruct him or her to transition from unconscious incompetence to conscious competence. You assume that the person wants to improve, so external motivation is not needed—only external and extrinsic direction.

This type of intervention consists primarily of activators, as exemplified by education sessions, training exercises, and directive feedback. Because your purpose is to instruct, the intervention comes before the target behavior and focuses on helping the performer internalize your instructions. As we've all experienced, this type of intervention is more effective when the instructions are specific and given one-on-one. Role-playing exercises give instructors opportunities to customize directions specific to individual attempts to improve. Plus, they allow participants the chance to receive rewarding feedback for improvement.

Supportive Intervention

Once a person learns the right way to do something, practice is important so the behavior becomes part of a natural routine. Continued practice leads to fluency and in many cases to automatic or habitual behavior. This is an especially desirable state for safety-related behavior. But perfect practice does not come easily, and benefits greatly from supportive intervention. We need support to reassure us that we are doing the right thing and to encourage us to keep going.

While instructional intervention consists primarily of activators, supportive intervention focuses on the application of positive consequences. Thus, when we give people rewarding feedback or recognition for particular safe behavior, we are showing our appreciation for their efforts and increasing the likelihood they will perform the behavior again. Each occurrence of the desired behavior facilitates fluency and helps to build a good habit.

After people know what to do, then they need to perform the behavior correctly many times before it can become a productive habit. Therefore, the positive reinforcement we give people for their safety-related behavior can go a long way toward facilitating fluency and a transition to the automatic or habit stage. Such supportive intervention is often most powerful when it comes from one's peers.

Note that supportive intervention is typically not preceded by a specific activator. In other words, when you support self-directed behavior you don't need to provide an instructional antecedent. The person knows what to do. You don't need to activate desired behavior with a promise (an incentive) or a threat (a disincentive). The person is already motivated to do the right thing.

Motivational Intervention

When people know what to do and don't do it, a motivational intervention is needed. In other words, when people are consciously incompetent about safety-related behavior, they require some external encouragement or pressure to change. Instruction alone is obviously insufficient because they knowingly do the wrong thing. In safety we refer to this as taking a calculated risk.

We usually take calculated risks or shortcuts because we perceive the positive consequences of the at-risk behavior to be more powerful than the negative consequences. This is because the positive consequences of comfort, convenience, and efficiency are immediate and certain, while the negative consequences of at-risk behavior (such as an injury) are improbable and seem remote. Furthermore, the safe alternative is relatively inconvenient, uncomfortable, or inefficient—negative consequences that are both immediate and certain. As a result, we often need to add both activators and consequences to the situation to move people from conscious incompetence to conscious competence.

An incentive/reward program is useful here. Such a program attempts to motivate a certain target behavior by promising people a positive consequence if they perform it. The promise is the incentive and the consequence is the reward. In safety, this kind of motivational intervention is much less common than disincentives and penalties. This is when a rule, policy, or law threatens to give people a negative consequence (a penalty) if they fail to comply or take a calculated risk.

Often a disincentive/penalty intervention is ineffective, because like an injury, the negative consequence or penalty seems remote and improbable. The behavioral impact of these enforcement programs is enhanced by increasing the severity of the penalty and "catching" more people taking calculated risks. But the large-scale implementation of this kind of intervention can seem inconsistent and unfair. And because threats of punishment appear to challenge individual freedom and choice (Skinner 1971), this approach to behavior change can backfire and activate more calculated risk taking, even sabotage, theft, or interpersonal aggression.

Motivational intervention is clearly the most challenging, requiring enough external influence to get the target behavior started without triggering a desire to assert personal freedom. Remember the objective is to motivate a transition from conscious incompetence to a *self-directed* state of conscious competence. Powerful external consequences might improve behavior only temporarily, as long as the behavioral intervention is in place. Hence the individual is consciously competent, but the excessive outside control makes the behavior entirely other-directed. Excessive control on the outside of people can limit the amount of control or self-direction they develop on the inside.

Long-term implementation of a motivational intervention, coupled with consistent supportive intervention, can lead to good habits. In other words, with substantial motivation and support, other-directed safe behavior can transition to unconscious competence without first becoming self-directed.

In Summary

Figure 5.1 reviews this intervention information by depicting relationships between four competency states (unconscious incompetence, conscious incompetence, conscious competence, and unconscious competence) and four intervention approaches (instructional intervention, motivational intervention, supportive intervention, and self-management). When people are unaware of the safe work practice (i.e., they are unconsciously incompetent), they need repeated instructional intervention until they understand what to do. Then, as depicted at the far left of Figure 5.1, the critical question is whether they perform the desired behavior. If they do, the question of behavioral fluency is relevant. A fluent response becomes a habit or part of a regular routine, and thus the individual is unconsciously competent.

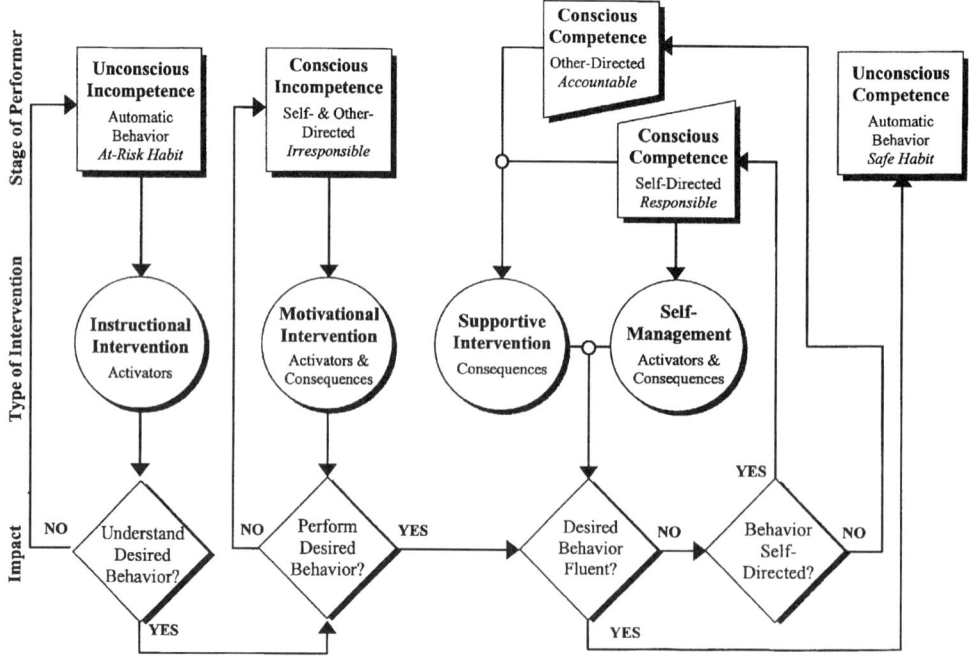

FIGURE 5.1   The flow of behavior change

When workers know how to perform a task safely but don't, they are considered consciously incompetent or irresponsible. This is when an external motivational intervention can be useful, as discussed earlier. Then when the desired behavior occurs at least once, supportive intervention is needed to get the behavior to a fluent state.

Most employees need supportive intervention for their safe behavior. In other words, most experienced workers know what to do in order to prevent injury on their jobs, and they have performed their jobs safely one or more times. But the safe way might not be habitual. The individual is consciously competent but needs supportive recognition or feedback for response maintenance and increased fluency.

Figure 5.1 illustrates a distinction between conscious competence/other-directed and conscious competence/self-directed. If a safe work practice is self-directed, the employee is considered responsible and self-management intervention is relevant. As detailed elsewhere (Watson and Tharp 1997), the methods and tools of effective self-management are derived from behavioral science research and are perfectly consistent with the principles of behavior-based safety.

In essence, self-management involves the application of the DO IT process (described previously) to one's own behavior. An individual defines one or more target behaviors to improve, monitors these behaviors, manipulates relevant activators and consequences to increase desired behavior and decrease undesired behavior, and tracks continual change in the target behaviors to determine the impact of the self-management process. See Geller (1998a) and Geller and Clarke (1999) for details regarding the application of self-management techniques for injury prevention.

ACCOUNTABILITY VERSUS RESPONSIBILITY

From the perspective of large-scale safety and health promotion, the differentiation in Figure 5.1 between accountability and responsibility is critical. People often use the words accountability and responsibility interchangeably. Whether you hold someone accountable or responsible for getting something done, you mean the same thing. You want that person to accomplish a certain task, and you intend to make sure that it happens. However, let's consider the receiving end of this situation. How does a person feel about an assignment—does he or she feel accountable or responsible? A distinction is evident.

When held accountable, you are asked to reach a certain objective or goal, often within a designated time period. But you might not feel responsible for meeting the deadline. Or, you might feel responsible enough to complete the assignment, but that's all. You do only what is required and no more. In this case, accountability is the same as responsibility.

There are times, however, when you extend your responsibility beyond accountability. You do more than what is required. You go beyond the call of duty as defined by a particular accountability system. This is often essential when it comes to industrial safety and health. To improve safety beyond the current performance plateau experienced by many companies, workers need to extend their responsibility for safety beyond that for which they are held accountable. They need to transition from an other-directed state to a self-directed state.

Many mining tasks are accomplished by a lone worker. There's no supervisor or coworker around to hold the employee accountable for performing the job safely. So the challenge for safety professionals and corporate leaders is to build the kind of work culture that enables or facilitates responsibility or *personal* accountability for safety. An accountability system is needed that encourages personal involvement and commitment for safety. Then you'll start a spiral of accountability feeding responsibility, feeding more involvement and more responsibility, ultimately resulting in people becoming totally committed to achieving an injury-free workplace. Psychological research on relationships between environmental conditions or contingencies (as in an accountability system) and people's feeling states (like personal accountability or responsibility) suggests five general ways to make this happen. (More details are given in Geller 1998a.)

Decrease Top-Down Controls for Safety

Mine safety often becomes a confrontation between a rule enforcer and a rule breaker. As such, safety is viewed as compliance with certain safety policies and mandates. One person holds another accountable for at-risk behavior, as in: "I saw what you did." Safety becomes a gotcha game, one dictated by Mine

Safety and Health Administration (MSHA) standards and unwittingly supported by corporate rules and regulations. Then the primary job of safety personnel is to check for worker compliance with safety procedures and to correct incidences of noncompliance. Making safety a priority means increasing enforcement of safety policies. This climate leads to fault finding and punishment contingencies that prevent the development of personal accountability.

Promote Fact Finding   If you want to increase people's responsibility for safety, you need to focus on fact finding, not fault finding. An injury or a near hit results from several causes, some of which have nothing to do with the person directly involved. Improving safety depends on discovering all the factors that contribute to injury potential. We can't do this if the work context makes people unwilling or frightened to discuss an incident openly because they're afraid of being blamed or punished. Removing fear of failure is critical to developing internal feelings of personal accountability (cf. Geller 1999c).

Decrease Punishment   In many work cultures, holding people accountable means punishing them for their mistakes. This can impede responsibility for reporting errors, calculated risks and near hits, and for looking for ways to reduce them. Geller (1996a, 1998a, and 1998d) has outlined various situations in which punishment is not desirable and discussed why mistakes and human errors never warrant punishment. Here we want to make the point that punishment procedures typically stifle the openness and interpersonal trust needed to conduct a responsible incident analysis and derive an effective corrective action plan.

Increase Feelings of Empowerment

From a psychological perspective, empowerment is not *holding* people accountable to do more. It is *feeling* empowered or responsible to do more. Employees need to be asked, "What will it take to make you feel more empowered or personally responsible for safety around here?" Seeking frank answers to this question and then actively working toward the changes requested will probably do more to increase employee involvement, commitment, and responsibility for safety than anything else.

The type of accountability system in place to evaluate the safety performance of individuals, work teams, and the entire work force influences whether people feel empowered and responsible to improve safety. Research indicates that for an accountability system to promote personal responsibility it needs to:

- Be proactive.
- Promote the reporting of all injuries, near hits, and property damage incidents.
- Distinguish between the journey (process goals) and the destination (outcome goals or vision).
- Hold people accountable for results they can control.
- Use recognition, rewards, and celebrations to shape process behaviors.
- Consider environment, behavior, and person factors in all incident investigations.
- Include daily audits of work practices and environmental conditions, as well as periodic assessments of perceptions and person states, through interviews, focus group meetings, and plant-wide surveys.

Help People Feel Important

When people's feelings of importance related to safety increase, their personal responsibility for safety also increases. So a rationale for decreasing top-down control over safety is that enforcement or punishment procedures decrease the recipient's sense of importance. And the strategies reviewed above for increasing feelings of empowerment also enhance personal perceptions of importance.

When people have choices in a situation they feel more important. And when their sense of importance is increased, they want to get more involved and make more choices. That's why it's important to first teach everyone the theory and principles behind a new process, and then help teams to customize specific procedures for their work areas. Choice is motivating in itself and promotes a sense of ownership of methods and tools. This leads naturally to both personal and interpersonal accountability for making the process work.

Cultivate Belonging and Interpersonal Trust

According to a recent study of 20 companies in the midst of implementing some form of behavior-based safety program, trust in management's ability to support the process was a critical determinant of employee involvement (DePasquale and Geller in press; Geller et al. 1998). Furthermore, building a spirit of community or belonging among coworkers will increase their sense of personal responsibility for industrial safety and health. The improvement of work practices requires interpersonal observation and feedback. But for this to happen, people need to adopt a collective win/win perspective instead of the individualistic win/lose orientation common in many work settings. People who feel a sense of belonging, trust, and win/win interdependency with their coworkers will also feel responsible for their coworkers' safety.

Ways to measure and increase interpersonal trust in a work setting are detailed elsewhere (Geller 1998b and 1999b). Here we review key points from these sources. Remember that a "we–they" mentality inhibits trust building. People need to appreciate and respect each other's differences and work interdependently. Their participation is critical for the organization's synergistic success. But building the kind of belonging and trust needed to break down independent perspectives and we–they barriers is ongoing and never-ending. You can help make this happen by promoting the following "C-words" in yourself and in others.

Communication   How we interact with others is obviously a key determinant of interpersonal trust. What people say and how they say it influences our trust in both their capabilities and their intentions. An individual's expertise is displayed by the person's spoken or written words and by the confidence and credibility linked to the words. You've probably noticed many times that the way something is said, including intonation, pace, facial expressions, hand gestures, and overall posture, has a greater impact than what was actually said. And, you've certainly experienced personal feelings of trust toward another person change as the result of how that individual communicated information.

We can get others to trust our knowledge, skill, or ability by our actions. Presenting our case with clarity, confidence, and charisma certainly helps. But what about trust in intentions? Do you know people who have impressive credentials and communicate elegantly, but something makes you suspicious about their intentions? You believe they know what to do, but you're not convinced they will do what they say. They have the right talk but give the impression they don't walk it.

One of the most powerful communication strategies for increasing trust in intention is active listening. When you listen to others first before communicating your own perspective, you not only increase the chance they will reciprocate and listen to you, you also learn how to present your message for optimal understanding, appreciation, and buy-in.

Caring   When you take the time to listen to other people's perspectives, you send a most important message that you care about them. And when people believe you care about them, they will care about what you tell them. They trust you will look out for them when applying your knowledge, skills, or abilities. They trust your intentions because they believe you care.

You also communicate caring and build interpersonal trust when you ask questions. We're not talking about the typical general questions we often ask people we haven't seen for awhile. We ask, "How are you doing?" and we get the standard reply "I'm doing fine, how about you?" No, we're referring to informed inquiry about a particular task or set of circumstances. Questions targeting a specific aspect of a person's job send the signal you care about him or her. This communication is more than a general greeting. It's a statement of genuine interest in a person's behavior and feelings. It's especially powerful when it reflects active caring about health and safety.

To show caring with specific behavior-based questions, you need to take the time to learn what others are doing. This comes from active listening and behavior-based observation. You've heard the phrase "walk the talk." Well, here we're talking about "hearing the talk, and watching the walk." This shows you care and gives you an opportunity to "talk the walk" so people will trust your intentions.

Candor   We trust people who are frank and open with us. They don't beat around the bush. They get right to the point, whether asking for a favor or giving us behavioral feedback. And when these individuals don't know an answer to a question, they don't ignore us or hem and haw about possibilities. They tell us outright when they don't know, and they tell us that they'll get back to us later. And when they get back to us soon with an answer, our trust in both their intention and ability increases.

The second definition of "candor" in the *American Heritage Dictionary* (1991) reflects another important aspect of trust building—"freedom from prejudice" (p. 233). When people's interactions with you reflect prejudice or the tendency to evaluate or judge another person on the basis of a stereotype or a preconceived notion about group characteristics, you have reason to mistrust these individuals, both in their ability to evaluate others and in their intentions to treat people fairly. And your trust in these persons decreases even when the prejudice is not directed toward you.

When a person gives an opinion about another because of race, religion, gender, age, sexual orientation, or birthplace, you should doubt this individual's ability to make people-related decisions. You should wonder whether their intentions to perform on behalf of another individual will be biased or tainted by a tendency to prejudge people on the basis of overly simple and usually inaccurate stereotypes.

Consistency   Perhaps the quickest way to destroy interpersonal trust is to not follow through on an agreement. How often do we make a promise we don't keep? Most promises are behavior-consequence contingencies. We specify that a certain consequence will follow a certain behavior. Whether the consequence is positive or negative, trust decreases when the behavior is not rewarded or punished as promised.

One problem with punishment contingencies is that they are difficult to implement fairly and consistently. It's easy to state a policy that anyone not using appropriate PPE will be written up, but it's quite difficult or impossible to carry out this contingency consistently for a large workforce. What about safety incentive programs that offer everyone rewards when no injuries occur over a designated period and participants observe coworkers getting hurt but not turning in an injury report? And, how about a safe employee of the month program that selects winners according to nonobjective criteria or that doesn't consider everyone consistently as a potential award recipient? You risk the possibility of reducing trust every time you implement a contingency (such as a punishment policy or incentive program) that is not administered fairly and consistently.

Commitment   People who are dependable and reliable are not only show consistency, they demonstrate commitment. When you follow through on a promise or pledge to do something, you send others the message that they can count on you. You can be trusted to do what you say you will do. Making a commitment and honoring it builds trust in both intention and ability.

Telling a personal anecdote to illustrate a point is often a good way to demonstrate commitment for something. And when this commitment is consistent with the theme of your speech or written presentation, your credibility increases. The audience has reason to trust your intentions to give accurate and useful information.

Consensus   Demonstrating personal commitment to a mission, purpose, or goal helps to build group consensus. And when a group reaches consensus, all group members agree on a decision or course of action and are willing to support it. Leaders or group facilitators who develop consensus among people are trusted. This is the opposite of top-down decision making, and it is not the same as negotiating, calling for a vote and letting the majority win, or working out a compromise between two differing sets of opinions.

Whenever the results of a group decision come across as win–lose, some mistrust is going to develop. A majority might be pleased, but others will be discontent and might actively or passively resist involvement. And even the winners could feel lowered interpersonal trust. "We won this decision, but what about next time?" And without solid backup support of the decision, the outcome will be less than desired. "Without everyone's buy-in, commitment, and involvement, we can't trust the process to come off as expected."

So how can group consensus be developed? How can the outcome of a heated debate on ways to solve a problem be perceived as a win–win solution everyone supports? How can a win–lose compromise or negotiation perceived to depreciate interpersonal trust be avoided? Solutions are more easily spoken than accomplished. Consensus building takes time and energy and requires candid, consistent, and caring communication among all members of a discussion or decision-making group (Geller 1998b; Rees 1997). In other words, when people demonstrate the C-words discussed here for building trust in interpersonal dialogue, they also develop consensus and more interpersonal trust regarding a particular decision or action plan.

Building consensus around a group process or action plan is not easy. There's no quick fix to doing this. It requires plenty of interpersonal communication, including straightforward opinion sharing, intense discussion, emotional debate, active listening, careful evaluation, methodical organization, and systematic prioritizing. But on important matters, the outcome is well worth the investment. When you develop a solution or process that every potential participant can get behind and champion, you have cultivated the degree of interpersonal trust needed for total involvement. Involvement in turn builds personal commitment, more interpersonal trust, and even more involvement.

Character   This final C-word for trust building means different things to many people. But generally, a person with character is considered honest, ethical, and principled. People with character are credible or worthy of another's trust because they display confidence and competence in following a consistent set of personal beliefs. They are believable and trusted because they know who they are, they know where they want to go, and they know how to get there.

A person with character practices all the strategies discussed here for cultivating a trusting culture. This C-word, then, epitomizes interpersonal trust from both an intention and capability perspective. We'd like to add a few additional trust-building methods, however, that especially fit this category, although they do overlap with other C-words discussed here.

First, individuals with character are willing to admit vulnerability. They realize that they aren't perfect and need behavioral feedback from others. They know their strengths and weaknesses and find exemplars to model. By actively listening to others and observing their behaviors, individuals with character learn how to improve their own performance. And if they're building a high performance team, they can readily find people with knowledge, skills, and abilities to complement their own competencies. They know how to make diversity work for them, their group, and the entire organization.

Having the courage to admit your weaknesses means that you're willing to recognize when you've made a mistake and to ask for forgiveness. There is probably no better way to build trust between individuals than to own up to an error that might have affected another person. Of course you should also indicate what you will do better next time or ask for specific advice on how to improve. This kind of vulnerability enables you to heed the powerful enrichment principle we learned from Frank Bird, "good better best, never let us rest, until our good is better and our better best" (Bird and Germain 1987, p. 111).

And what is your trust level for a group leader who not only admits failure but continually seeks ways to improve? This is the kind of person you want on your team. You can openly discuss your own incompetencies or insecurities with this person without fear of ridicule or reprisal. Indeed, you trust that this person will appreciate your desire to improve and will offer the guidance you need to do better. You also trust this individual to maintain the confidentiality of any disclosure of personal failure or vulnerability.

Building interdependent trust and belonging should be part of the mission statement for every corporate endeavor that involves people. It should influence almost every conversation we have with coworkers. It is a continuous journey, essential to cultivating an organization of individuals and teams whose personal and shared accountabilities for safety and health are sufficient to achieve a "Total Safety Culture." The seven C-words reviewed here are easy to remember, and although their meanings overlap to some extent, each offers distinct directives for trust-building behavior.

SUMMARY AND CONCLUSIONS

This chapter began with a review of three basic principles that define a behavioral science approach to improving the human element of mining safety, including a rationale for using a behavior-based approach. Then a basic framework for implementing a behavior management system was introduced. It was called DO IT for the four basic processes of behavior-based safety:

1. Define target behaviors to support or improve.
2. Observe critical behaviors to help people become more mindful of safe versus at-risk work practices and to provide constructive behavioral feedback.
3. Intervene for instruction, support, motivation, or safety self-management.

4. Test the impact of the intervention process to verify the beneficial influence of the behavior-based procedures and learn how to continuously improve the behavior management system.

Our subsequent discussion of a distinction between accountability and ways to develop personal responsibility went beyond the test phase of a DO IT process. For example, issues of empowerment, belonging, and interpersonal trust implicate subjective feeling states that are difficult or impossible to measure. This might seem problematic for managers inspired by the popular management principle, "You can only manage what you can measure."

There are some things we should do, however, because they are right. Many of the recommendations given here for developing an accountability system that promotes personal responsibility cannot be readily monitored nor measured, but you need to have faith in the research-supported theory that promoting feelings of empowerment, trust, and belonging are important for safety improvement (cf. Geller 1996a, 1998a, and 1999b). This is like taking vitamin pills regularly without noticing any measurable consequences.

We are motivated by consequences, however, so let's consider certain benefits you can expect to gain from a successful behavior-based safety management process as reviewed in this chapter. Since most injuries are caused in part by at-risk behavior, a reduction in at-risk behavior and an increase in safe behavior will lead to injury prevention. However, we'd like you to consider five other benefits that result from people contributing interdependently to an effective behavior-based safety process. These outcomes are critically important and relate to much more than safety. In fact, they can benefit every important function of your organization. In explaining these we'll review most of the key psychological principles covered in this chapter.

Benefit 1: It Focuses Evaluation on the Right Numbers

How is safety performance measured at most mining facilities? It's measured by final outcomes—injuries that occur during the year. Companies keep score by trying to improve their incident rate. Do workers walk around the job thinking about lowering the company's incident rate? Can they relate to that? Of course not. It's too abstract and remote. And it's not really under the workers' immediate control.

Top management needs to keep worrying about the outcome numbers, but not the people doing the jobs on the floor. They need to focus on the process—the day-to-day operations. That's what they can control, and that's the focus of behavior-based safety. When workers concentrate on what they can actually **do** for safety, they'll reach the outcome everyone wants—fewer injuries.

Benefit 2: It Builds Positive Attitudes

Have you ever noticed how safety-related conversations often resemble an adult-child confrontation? One person holds another accountable for at-risk behavior, as in "I saw what you did." Then safety becomes a "gotcha game," reinforced by MSHA regulations and corporate rules. This heavy-handed approach only diminishes a person's feelings of empowerment, importance, belonging, and interpersonal trust.

Behavior-based safety focuses on the use of rewards, positive feedback, and interpersonal recognition to motivate and support safe behavior. This encourages people to get involved in a safety improvement process because they want to, not because they feel threatened and think they have to. Thus, through behavior-based safety people act themselves into a positive attitude.

Benefit 3: It Increases Personal Responsibility for Safety

When people have tools they can use on a daily basis to prevent injuries, and they have support to use these tools, they have real control over safety. If they're held accountable for process numbers they can control, and they believe their efforts will prevent workplace injuries, they'll feel responsible and do more than required. They'll feel empowered and want to get involved in an improvement process.

Benefit 4: It Facilitates Interpersonal Coaching and Teamwork

Imagine a workplace where everyone coaches each other about the safest way to perform a job. When workers depend on others in this way to improve safety, they understand teamwork. They appreciate how everyone's safe and at-risk behavior influences the safety of everyone else. With this interdependent attitude, they're willing to use behavior-based coaching to actively care for their coworkers.

The five letters of COACH reflect the main ingredients of behavior-based coaching: **C** is for **care**. Know I care and you'll care what I know. **O** is for **observe**. I care so much I'm willing to watch you work, so I can give you behavior-based feedback. **A** is for **analyze**. I'll think about my observations to understand barriers to safe behavior. **C** is for **communicate**. I'll recognize and support the safe behavior I see, and I'll give corrective feedback for at-risk behaviors in a way that is accepted by the person I observe. **H** is for **help**. Behavior-based coaching helps increase safe behavior and decrease at-risk behavior, thus preventing injuries. It also helps to build interpersonal trust and an interdependent mindset.

Benefit 5: It Teaches and Promotes Systems Thinking

It's easy to get bogged down with handling immediate short-term demands—like production deadlines—and lose sight of the bigger picture. Systems thinkers take a broad and long-term perspective. They look beyond immediate payoffs, like the ease, speed, or comfort they get by taking a risky shortcut. They consider the possibility of a bigger payoff in the distant future. They realize that safe behavior teaches others by example and protects them from injury.

Systems thinkers understand the link between behavior and attitude. A small change in behavior can result in a beneficial change in attitude, followed by more behavior change and then more attitude change—eventually resulting in total commitment. So behavior-based safety sets the stage for systems thinking and interdependent teamwork, and this can lead ultimately to a Total Safety Culture.

REFERENCES

American Heritage Dictionary. 1991. 2nd college ed. New York: Houghton Mifflin.

Bird, F.E., Jr., and G.L. Germain. 1987. *Commitment*. Loganville, GA: International Loss Control Institute.

Boling, H.L. 1995. Building a positive safety culture that is behavior based. In *Proceedings of the Twenty-Sixth Annual Institute of Mining Health, Safety, and Research*. Edited by G.R. Tinner, A. Bacho, and M. Karmis. Blacksburg, VA: Virginia Polytechnic Institute and State University.

Daniels, A.C. 1994. *Bringing Out the Best in People*. New York: McGraw-Hill.

DePasquale, J.D., and E.S. Geller. Critical success factors for behavior-based safety: A study of 20 industry-wide applications. *Journal of Safety Research*, in press.

Fellner, D.J., and B. Sulzer-Azaroff. 1984. Increasing industrial safety practices and conditions through posted feedback. *Journal of Safety Research* 15: 7–21.

Fox, D.K., B.L. Hopkins, and W.K. Anger. 1987. The long-term effects of a token economy on safety performance in open pit mining. *Journal of Applied Behavior Analysis* 20: 215–224.

Geller, E.S. 1988. A behavioral science approach to transportation safety. *Bulletin of the New York Academy of Medicine* 64: 632–661.

——. 1996a. *The Psychology of Safety: How to Improve Behaviors and Attitudes on the Job*. Boca Raton, FL: CRC Press.

——. 1996b. The truth about safety incentives. *Professional Safety* 41(10): 34–39.

——. 1997a. Key processes for continuous safety improvement: behavior-based recognition and celebration. *Professional Safety* 42(10): 40–44.

——. 1997b. What is behavior-based safety, anyway? *Occupational Health and Safety* 66(1): 25–35.

——. 1998a. *Beyond Safety Accountability: How to Increase Personal Responsibility*. Neenah, WI: J.J. Keller and Associates.

——. 1998b. *Building Successful Safety Teams: Together Everyone Achieves More*. Neenah, WI: J.J. Keller and Associates.

——. 1998c. Principles of behavior-based safety. *Proceedings of the ASSE Behavioral Safety Symposium, Light Up Safety in the New Millennium*. 3–24.

——. 1998d. *Understanding Behavior-Based Safety: Step-By-Step Methods To Improve Your Workplace.* 2nd ed. Neenah, WI: J.J. Keller and Associates.

——. 1999a. Are you mindful or mindless when working? *Industrial Safety and Hygiene News* 33(7): 16–17.

——. 1999b. Interpersonal trust: key to getting the best from behavior-based safety coaching. *Professional Safety* 44(4): 16–19.

——. 1999c. What's wrong with 'accident investigations'? *Industrial Safety and Hygiene News* 33(2): 12, 14.

Geller, E.S., T.E. Boyce, J.H. Williams, C.B. Pettinger, J.P. DePasquale, and S.W. Clarke. 1998. Researching behavior-based safety: a multi-method assessment and evaluation. In *Proceedings of the American Society of Safety Engineers*. 537–559.

Geller, E.S., and S.W. Clarke. 1999. Safety self-management: a key behavior-based process for injury prevention. *Professional Safety* 44(7): 29–33.

Geller, E.S., R.A. Winett, and P.B. Everett. 1982. *Environmental Preservation: New Strategies for Behavior Change*. New York: Pergamon Press.

Goldstein, A.P., and L. Krasner. 1987. *Modern Applied Psychology*. New York: Pergamon Press.

Greene, B.F., R.A. Winett, R. Van Houten, E.S. Geller, and B.A. Iwata, editors. 1987. *Behavior Analysis in the Community: Readings from the Journal of Applied Behavior Analysis*. Lawrence, KS: Society for the Experimental Analysis of Behavior.

James, W. 1890. *Principles of Psychology*. New York: Doves.

Komaki, J., A.T. Heinzmann, and L. Lawson. 1980. Effect of training and feedback: component analysis of a behavioral safety program. *Journal of Applied Psychology* 65(3): 261–270.

Kowalski, K.M., B. Fotta, and E.A. Barrett. 1995. Modifying behavior to improve miners' hazard recognition skills through training. In *Proceedings of the Twenty-Sixth Annual Institute of Mining Health, Safety, and Research*. Edited by G.R. Tinner, A. Bacho, and M. Karmis. Blacksburg, VA: Virginia Polytechnic Institute and State University.

Krause, T.T. 1995. *Employee-Driven Systems for Safe Behavior: Integrating Behavioral and Statistical Methodologies*. New York: Van Nostrand Reinhold.

Krause, T.R., J.H. Hidley, and S.J. Hodson. 1996. *The Behavior-Based Safety Process: Managing Involvement for an Injury-Free Culture*. 2nd ed. New York: Van Nostrand Reinhold.

Langer, E.J. 1989. *Mindfulness*. Reading, MA: Perseus Books.

Langton, J.F. 1995. Update on MSHA's health and safety initiatives. In *Proceedings of the Twenty-Sixth Annual Institute of Mining Health, Safety, and Research*. Edited by G.R. Tinner, A. Bacho, and M. Karmis. Blacksburg, VA: Virginia Polytechnic Institute and State University.

Ludwig, T.D., and E.S. Geller. 1997. Managing injury control among professional pizza deliverers: Effects of goal setting and response generalization. *Journal of Applied Psychology* 82: 243–261.

McAfee, R.B., and A.R. Winn. 1989. The use of incentives/feedback to enhance workplace safety: A critique of the literature. *Journal of Safety Research* 20: 7–19.

McSween, T.E. 1995. *The Values-Based Safety Process: Improving Your Safety Culture with a Behavioral Approach*. New York: Van Nostrand Reinhold.

Peters, R.H. 1995. Encouraging self-protective employee behavior: what do we know? In *Proceedings of the Twenty-Sixth Annual Institute of Mining Health, Safety, and Research*. Edited by G.R. Tinner, A. Bacho, and M. Karmis. Blacksburg, VA: Virginia Polytechnic Institute and State University.

Peters, R.H., G.R. Bockosh, and B. Fotta. 1997. "Overview of U.S. Research on Three Approaches to Ensuring That Coal Miners Work Safely: Management, Workplace Design, and Training." Paper presented at the Japan Technical Cooperation Center for Coal Resources Development.

Petersen, D. 1989. *Safe Behavior Reinforcement*. Goshen, NY: Aloray.

Reber, R.A., J.A. Wallin, and J.S. Chhokar. 1990. Improving safety performance with goal setting and feedback. *Human Performance* 3(1): 51–61.

Rees, F. 1997. *Teamwork from Start to Finish*. San Francisco: Jossey-Bass.

Rhoton, W.A. 1980. A procedure to improve compliance with coal mine safety regulations. *Journal of Organizational Behavior Management* 2(4): 243–249.

Skinner, B.F. 1938. *The Behavior of Organisms: An Experimental Analysis*. Acton, MA: Copley Publishing Group.

——. 1953. *Science and Human Behavior*. New York: Macmillan.

——. 1971. *Beyond Freedom and Dignity*. New York: Alfred A. Knopf.

——. 1974. *About Behaviorism*. New York: Alfred A. Knopf.

Sulzer-Azaroff, B. 1998. *Who Killed My Daddy? A Behavioral Safety Fable*. Cambridge, MA: Cambridge Center for Behavioral Studies.

Sulzer-Azaroff, B., and M.C. De Santamaria. 1980. Industrial safety hazard reduction through performance feedback. *Journal of Applied Behavior Analysis* 13: 287–295.

Watson, D.L., and R.G. Tharp. 1997. *Self-Directed Behavior: Self-Modification for Personal Adjustment*. 7th ed. Pacific Grove, CA: Brooks/Cole Publishing Company.

CHAPTER 6

Engineering for Health and Safety

Roger L. Brauer, Ph.D., C.S.P., P.E.
Executive Director, Board of Certified Safety Professionals, Tolono, Illinois

FUNDAMENTALS OF SAFETY AND HEALTH ENGINEERING

Safety engineering is the application of engineering principles and practices to the protection of people, property, and the environment. Safety engineering differs from many other engineering disciplines. At the applied level, there are minimal overlaps among civil, mechanical, electrical, industrial, chemical, and other engineering areas of practice. Safety engineering differs because it requires some knowledge of all of the other engineering specialties. One must know about structures, machines, energy systems, electronics and computers, processes of various kinds, transportation systems and equipment, mechanics of fluids and gases, and biological processes, for example.

Complete knowledge of all engineering disciplines is not possible for any safety engineer. A safety engineer will often depend on assistance from other engineering specialists. However, sufficient knowledge of each area is necessary to effectively communicate about safety and health matters. The role of communicator on the technical aspects of safety and health is crucial for safety engineers.

To be effective in safety and health, one must be able to recognize (and sometimes anticipate), evaluate, and control hazards and manage the surrounding processes. Safety engineering focuses on prevention and design. The engineering process must prevent injuries and illnesses and avoid loss of property or environmental damage by preventing accidents or incidents. This is accomplished by eliminating or minimizing hazards and contributing elements that can lead to accidents or cause injury.

Many divide the kinds of preventive actions necessary to achieve optimum safety and health in the workplace into two classes: engineering controls and administrative controls. Administrative controls involve policy, procedures, employment and job assignment practices, procurement and contracts, training, culture, and similar business and management practices. Engineering controls involve design of equipment, processes, vehicles, tools, buildings, and sites. Although engineers may be involved in both areas, safety engineering emphasizes engineering controls.

Basic Concepts

Figure 6.1 illustrates one safety engineering concept, which is actually a combination of two concepts that have existed in safety for many years. Some see limitations for each in dealing with safety and health, but they are useful to illustrate the important roles for safety engineering.

In the first concept, William Heinrich argues that accidents are caused by unsafe acts and conditions. He and others differ significantly with regard to the relative importance of unsafe acts and unsafe conditions or their combinations. The other concept covers the three Es of safety: Engineering, Education, and Enforcement.

Education is a primary approach to preventing unsafe acts. Education extends well beyond the classroom and into coaching and other means to affect changes in people's behavior. Details about these approaches appear in other chapters.

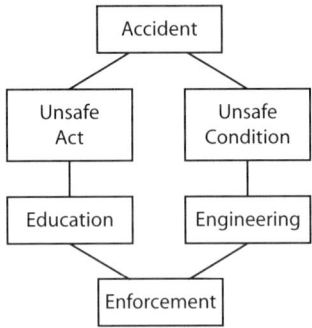

FIGURE 6.1   Although the primary role of safety engineering is to prevent unsafe conditions, it must reflect the hundreds of design standards for safety (enforcement) and reduce the opportunity for errors and unsafe acts by users through designs that reflect human limitations and capabilities

Most would agree that the primary focus of safety engineering is to prevent unsafe conditions. By eliminating hazards altogether, by reducing the severity of a hazard, or by reducing the likelihood that conditions will lead to an undesired event, accidents can be prevented.

Enforcement involves activities designed to ensure that a wide range of standards intended to achieve safety and health are actually applied. Standards include laws, regulations, and standards promulgated by governments at any level. Standards include voluntary and consensus standards. Standards also include standards of practice, procedures, and practices that comprise commonly used business practices or commonly used procedures in a particular craft or profession. Education and engineering are both vehicles for enforcing standards.

Looking once again at Figure 6.1, we can see that engineering cannot be limited to simply preventing unsafe conditions. Engineering also plays a vital role in preventing unsafe acts. Designing for people is a critical part of this. Safety engineering must recognize the capabilities and limitations of people. They come in different sizes; are different ages; have differing experiences, knowledge, and skills; and differ in capability. Many design decisions affect what people do and how well they perform. Designing for people must eliminate the likelihood of unsafe acts or reduce the danger if an unsafe act occurs.

Engineering Strategies

A general strategy for safety engineering appears in Figure 6.2. This strategy provides a sequence of choices in dealing with designs for safety and health.

In evaluating design options, the first priority is to eliminate a hazard or unsafe condition. If a hazard is eliminated, the potential for harm or loss is gone. Education and enforcement become irrelevant. For example, it is well known that manual materials handling is a major source of injury. If equipment or operations designs eliminate manual handling, the potential source of injury is gone, and there is no need to train the operator in proper lifting.

Unfortunately, eliminating hazards is not always possible. The next priority, then, seeks to reduce the hazard level. Changing a design to reduce the severity is one approach. Another is reducing the likelihood of occurrence. Redundancy is one way to help reduce this probability. It is important, particularly for hazards with high severity, to incorporate various forms of redundancy so that the failure of a single component or a human error alone cannot trigger a dangerous event. Analysis for single point failures, ending in serious consequences is critical.

The next priority in the sequence is to provide safety devices, or features that prevent people from being exposed to a hazard. Safety devices are automatic and require no action on the part of a person. Safety devices do not eliminate hazards. Examples of safety devices are interlocks, dead-man switches, guards, fences, automatic fire doors, some types of fire sprinklers, and automatic air brakes that activate when there is a break in an air line. A significant problem with many safety devices is that people intentionally disable them and fail to reinstall or activate them after service or maintenance.

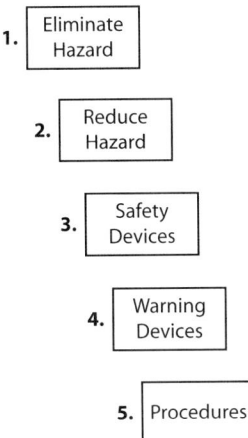

FIGURE 6.2   The Hazard Control Priority Tree provides an orderly strategy for selecting controls for hazards

The next level of priority is application of warning devices. These do not eliminate hazards. They do not provide protection. They require human perception (usually visual or auditory) and a proper response. The sequence between hazard and protection is very complex and offers many opportunities for failure. The following sequence is typically involved in making warning devices effective:

1. The hazard must be recognized in design or by some sensor.
2. The hazard must be differentiated from other hazards or conditions.
3. The warning must be given.
4. The warning device must operate.
5. The warning must be sensed by a person.
6. The warning must be perceived and understood relative to competing information or backgrounds.
7. The person receiving the information must know what action is required.
8. The person must take the protective action.
9. The correct action must be completed in a timely manner.

Failure in any of these steps makes warnings ineffective.

The final priority and last choice in reducing danger is use of procedures—actions that must be completed. They require learning, understanding, and often practice to achieve an acceptable performance level. Procedures do not eliminate hazards. They require human performance. Design of procedures is critical and must reflect human characteristics, capabilities, and limitations. Using personal protective equipment (PPE) is an example of a procedure.

Energy Management

Another useful concept in safety engineering involves energy management in design. From physics, we know that energy takes several forms in materials and objects, such as potential, kinetic, thermal, and internal (such as the fuel value of a material). Hazards are related to the amount of energy, the release of energy, and the rate at which energy is released. William Haddon offered a series of strategies having to do with energy, energy transfer, and potential or actual release of energy (1970). Although his ideas evolved from vehicle accidents and the design of vehicles, passenger protection, and highways, the strategies can apply in many different settings. The list below summarizes his strategies.

- Prevent the marshaling of energy.
- Reduce the amount of energy marshaled.
- Prevent the release of energy.
- Modify the rate at which energy is released from its source or modify the spatial distribution of the released energy.

- Separate in space or time the energy being released from the structure that can be damaged or the human who can be injured.
- Separate the energy being released from a structure or person that can suffer loss by interposing a barrier.
- Modify the surfaces of structures that come into contact with people or other structures.
- Strengthen the structure or person susceptible to damage.
- Detect damage quickly and counter it with continuation or extension.
- During the period following damage and the return to normal conditions, take measures to restore a stable condition.

Haddon argued that any measure that prevents injury or damage is satisfactory. However, it makes good sense to apply strategies that are at the top of the list, particularly when the amount of energy is large.

Continuous Improvement and Reengineering

American business has rediscovered the concepts of quality and continuous improvement as promoted by Deming (1986), Juran (1992), and others. The point to be made here is that errors (of which accidents and incidents are a part) are a component of the management process. Preventing them through engineering, administration, and other means is also a part of the management process.

Another popular business concept today is reengineering (see, for example, Hammer and Champy 1993). The business management process is a major element of this philosophy. A major difference between reengineering and the quality philosophies is scale. Continuous improvement achieves change incrementally; reengineering achieves change in large, comprehensive process modifications.

Safety engineering may be involved in either discipline and both philosophies are useful for achieving safety objectives. Very often, the way a company does business requires safety engineering. It is important to note that safety and safety engineering are not separate endeavors within an organization. They are part of responding to external and internal customers, reducing process times, reducing errors, and minimizing variability. Safety and safety engineering are part of the bottom line and profitability. They are not just humanitarian or public relations matters.

HAZARD RECOGNITION, EVALUATION, AND CONTROL

To be effective in preventing illness and injury or damage to property and the environment, one must have an understanding of the hazard restraint control options. One must be able to evaluate hazards and controls in various ways. Hazards need to be evaluated to determine what factors are related to an undesired event. There is a need to evaluate the risk associated with each hazard event (likelihood of the event occurring and the extent or severity of results). There is a need to identify and evaluate each control option. It is important to estimate the cost to implement control(s) and the cost and risk reduction that the controls can achieve. One must estimate the potential effectiveness of the control(s).

Other chapters address some aspects of hazard recognition, evaluation, and control. This chapter covers selected topics as examples.

Structures and Mechanics

Structural safety is critical in most mining operations, whether surface or underground. Because mining involves the removal and movement of soil, rocks, and minerals, a basic knowledge of soil mechanics is essential. Closely related are the mechanics of structures and structural components used to prevent collapse of mines and mine surfaces. These structures and components involve materials of various kinds and are subjected to many kinds of structural loads. Very often mining must also deal with surface and ground water, which require an understanding of fluid mechanics.

Fundamental to all these materials and structures is an understanding of their static and dynamic behaviors and properties. Understanding the failures in structures and materials relies on analysis of these properties and behaviors.

Stress   Stress is the load per unit area applied to some material. There are several forms of loading and stress: tension, compression, shear, bending, and torsion. Figure 6.3 illustrates these different kinds of stress.

Tension   Tension and tensile stress involve forces that tend to pull a material apart. Some materials have very little tensile strength. Concrete, glass, and other brittle materials usually have very limited tensile strength. They will crack and break easily under tensile load. Most soils are likely to fail under tensile loads compared to ductile materials, such as metals. Ductile materials will elongate under tensile load and tend to lose strength as the cross-sectional dimensions get smaller during elongation. A chain or rope has high tensile strength but has virtually no compression strength.

Compression   Compression and compression stress involve forces acting to compress or bear on a material. Rock and concrete are much stronger under compression loads than under tensile loads. Some soils have high compression load strength and others do not. Wood and some plastics have limited compression strength and tend to deform or crush under local loads. If restrained, fluids have high compression strength but have virtually no tension strength.

Shear   Shear and shear stress involve opposing forces acting in opposite directions but not in direct alignment with each other. Cutting and tearing actions involve shear. Fluids and materials that act much like fluids (sand and some other loose or wet soils) have very little shear capacity.

Bending   Bending can only occur if a structural element is restrained at one location or end and a load is placed lateral to the material at some point other than the restrained end. Bending involves a torsional load combined with a tensile or compression load. Bending infers some deflection in the material due to the loading. Bending produces compression on one side of the bend and tension on the other. Bending can occur with one end restrained (cantilever load) or with both ends restrained or supported (simple beam).

Torsion   Torsion and torsion stress involve rotational loads on a material. A section of the material must be retrained in order for a torsional load to be applied. A torsional failure on a shaft will create a somewhat spiraled break compared to a bending failure for the same material. Compare the difference in fractures between a piece of chalk when you simply bend it in your hands and when you hold one end tight and twist the other end.

Stresses are related to actual loads using formulas with the following form:

$$L = SA \qquad\qquad (EQ\ 6.1)$$

where L is the load or total force, S is the load per unit area, and A is the area over which the load is applied. The capacity of a material to carry or withstand any type of loading is determined from data tables. One must compare the actual stress to that identified in tables for a particular type of load to

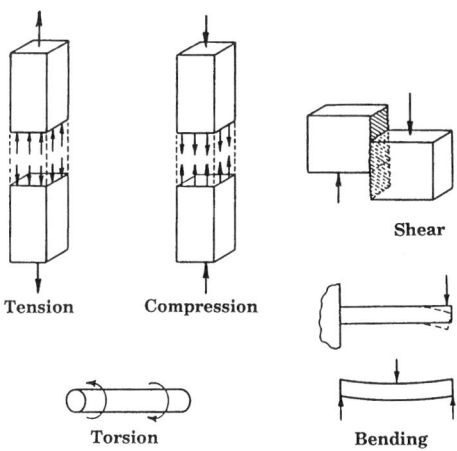

FIGURE 6.3   Design of structures affects how loads transfer from one element to another and have an impact on the likelihood of failure

determine if failure is likely for a material. Often a factor of safety is added to Equation 6.1. The factor of safety is an adjustment to help define what load a material can carry safely. The values vary by types of materials. The factor of safety recognizes that many materials are not homogeneous.

When looking up the load carrying properties of materials, it is important to establish whether the data table includes a factor of safety. Drawing the wrong conclusion can have serious consequences. As a rule, it is best to include factors of safety and avoid calculations when preparing reference tables for field use. The simplest tables are those that organize loading conditions and allow users to simply compare the actual situation or load to that in the table without making additional calculations or adjusting for various conditions. Assumptions about factors of safety or other conditions can be included within tables or in footnotes.

Other properties of materials and structures are important in mining. For example, pressurized fluid streams are used to cut rock. Failing or leaking hydraulic lines can produce fine streams of fluid at high pressure. The fluid stream can cause injury because human tissue is relatively weak compared to other materials.

Columns and their load capacities are important. Columns are normally divided into long and short columns based on the ratio of length to cross-section. Long columns under compression loads will fail by bowing or buckling when a load reaches a certain level. Short columns are less likely to buckle and can carry greater loads for the same cross-section compared to a long column.

A property of loose materials important in mining safety is called the angle of repose. When loose materials form a pile, the pile will have sloped sides. The angle formed naturally by the side of a pile is called the angle of repose. Different materials will form a different slope because the tension, compression, and shear properties of the materials vary. During excavations, soils and other loose materials may initially stay vertical. Eventually, the wall will collapse to form the angle of repose. The likelihood of collapse can be affected by the type of material or soil, moisture content, and nearby vibration from equipment or blasting. Collapse is more likely also when equipment or piled up; material increases the compressive load near the remaining excavation wall.

Some soils and loose materials can change properties quickly. Some materials can carry a large load if it is well distributed or if the material is compressed to just the right density. Some soils that carry loads in normal conditions will quickly change properties and act like fluids when vibrated in an earthquake or from some other source. Fluids have little (there may be a little shear capacity depending on viscosity) or no load bearing capacity. To ensure safety of structures of various kinds, it is essential to know:

- The material involved
- The load-bearing properties of the materials
- The loads that will be encountered from operations
- The weather conditions, such as snow, rain, floods, and ice
- Any other sources, such as vehicles
- How to analyze the different modes of failure.

The loading must be analyzed in terms of the modes of failure of structural components. Consider roof bolts, which are used to anchor structures that keep ceilings from collapsing in tunnels and mine shafts. When a roof bolt is in place vertically, it may be carrying a load in tension. The bolt itself could fail in tension. The interface between the bolt and the surrounding material (rock or soil) is in shear. The bolt may be more likely to pull out as the surrounding material fails in shear before the bolt fails in tension. If the bolt were placed at an angle, there may also be a bending load on the exposed part of the bolt. Then, bending failure must be considered. Analysis will determine which mode of failure will occur first.

Mechanical Systems

Machines are used to cut, bore, transfer, haul, and load mined materials or materials used in mining. There are machines and tools for maintenance and repair. Each contains hazards of various kinds. This discussion will be limited to three major considerations with machines and tools: energy and energy sources, machine actions and protecting people from them, and man-machine interfaces.

Energy and Energy Sources   Each machine and tool relies on some energy source for its power. There are engines that run on gasoline or natural gas. There are electric motors. There is steam, compressed air, and pneumatic power. Some tools use explosive charges for their energy. Some machines store energy in springs or flywheels. Some rely on falling mass or mass in motion to achieve their function.

The kinds of energy hazards vary with the energy source. Petrochemical fuels have fire and explosive hazards. They produce products of potentially hazardous combustion. They may generate heat. Steam has thermal hazards. Electrically powered equipment hazards vary with the frequency for alternating current, the current flow, the charge stored, and other characteristics.

One must also consider the form of energy. Is there potential, kinetic, or internal energy? Mass that could fall is an example of potential energy. Kinetic energy involves mass in motion. Stored energy can include the internal heat value of combustible fuels, or the energy stored in a spring, pressurized steam, or compressed air line.

What is important is recognizing the various kinds and quantities of energy involved in equipment, machines, and tools and managing the energy safely for those operating, maintaining, cleaning, or servicing them or working close to them. Haddon's energy management strategies help to identify possible solutions to energy release hazards. Very often, lock out and tag out procedures are used to help protect those working on machines, equipment, and tools from energy releases. Depending on the kind of energy, various design features may be required to provide protection.

For example, the hydraulic system in an off-highway haul truck may contain 50 or more gallons of hydraulic fluid that may burn, particularly when atomized during a rupture of a line or connector. Having that amount of combustibles available to be released from the system requires analysis of potential effects of a failure and the need for controls. Haddon's strategies would suggest reducing the volume of hydraulic fluid used, find a nonflammable fluid to eliminate energy release through combustion, separating heat sources from hydraulic lines using shields, or increasing the barriers to potential release by using solid hydraulic lines near heat sources rather than flexible lines.

Machine Actions and Protecting People from Them   Machines create hazards. The hazards and options for controlling them are related to the kind of actions contained in the machines. Most literature classifies machine actions into five categories: rotation, transverse, in-running nip points, cutting and punching, and shearing and bending. Most often, power transmission and point-of-operation guards, guard devices, and various other controls protect operators from machine hazards. Distance can also be a control for machine hazards. Government publications[1] and national standards[2] identify a wide range of controls to protect people from machine actions. Most manufacturers provide detailed literature for safe operation of machines and equipment. Failure to install or maintain protective devices on machines is likely to result in injury or damage. Training of those operating or maintaining equipment is essential.

A particular problem is protecting those who clean, service, or maintain machines and equipment. Often they must get at components that are within zones protected during normal operations. Accidents and injuries often occur because there is no low-speed, low energy, or manual mode for machines, only an operational, full-speed mode. The full-speed mode is often very dangerous for cleaning, servicing, and maintenance procedures (refer to Haddon's energy strategies). Many manufacturers provide detailed procedures for safe cleaning, maintenance, and servicing.

Man-Machine Interfaces   Another important consideration in machines and equipment is the interface with users. Ergonomics or human factors engineering principles are often critical in the design of machines and equipment. There are many opportunities to improve productivity and reduce errors in operations that may result in accidents by understanding the visual, auditory, tactile, physical, and mental processing capabilities and limitations of people. One must also recognize that many variables in people can affect performance of machines and equipment.

---

1. One example is *Concepts and Techniques of Machine Safeguarding*. 1980. OSHA 3067. U.S. Government Printing Office.
2. The American National Standards Institute publishes standards on many kinds of machines and the safeguarding of machine hazards. They are updated periodically. One example is the ANSI B11 series on presses of various types.

Consider these questions. Are emergency shut-off switches within reach of every operator in case something goes wrong? Is information that is presented in displays easy to read and interpret? Are the forces required to operate hand, finger, or foot controls within the strength range for all operators? Are the functions of the machine logically related to controls and displays? These and many other questions may be critical to the safe operation or maintenance of machines and equipment.

Other Kinds of Hazards

There are many other kinds of hazards that safety engineering must recognize, evaluate, and control. Included are electrical, low and high pressure, thermal, chemical, fire, explosion, waste, vibration, noise, ionizing and non-ionizing radiation, visual, biological, materials handling, transportation, and others. Many of these are addressed elsewhere in this book.

DESIGNING FOR PEOPLE AND THEIR SAFETY AND HEALTH

A primary focus of safety engineering is eliminating or reducing hazards and unsafe conditions through engineering controls (refer to Figure 6.1). Administrative controls require teaching people to recognize remaining hazards and how to protect themselves. Safety engineering can also affect human behavior that may be required for protection. Through effective design, many opportunities for unsafe behavior can be eliminated or reduced. Processes and tasks can be simplified and made easier and more productive for workers, operators, and others. Many high-risk tasks can be transferred to equipment and machines. Instructions can be clearly written for performing tasks properly and safely or using equipment, machines, and tools safely. Designers can also create safety features for those times when systems and equipment fail. Fail-safe designs, which ensure safe modes or conditions when failure occurs, can minimize danger. Fail-safe designs can reduce the need to observe and perceive that something is going wrong. Fail-safe designs can minimize the need to complete corrective actions that would otherwise lead to injury when a failure occurs.

Ergonomics

Ergonomics is the science of work. Some prefer the terms human factors engineering or human engineering. In general, this field can be partitioned into two main areas. One area deals with the physiological aspects of work and the physical capabilities and limitations of people. The other area deals mainly with the cognitive aspects of human interfaces with process and equipment. Ergonomics is applied through design. Ergonomics references will provide many of the details expanded upon in the summary.

Ergonomics involves relationships between people and things. Ergonomics requires an understanding of the characteristics of people, derived from anthropometrics, physiology, biomechanics, psychology, and sociology. Ergonomics requires an understanding of the characteristics of things, such as machines, vehicles, environments, buildings, processes, tasks, publications, and physical, chemical, social, and managerial environments.

In ergonomics, there are three general classes of relationships with overlaps among them. One kind of relationship focuses on performance and productivity. Safety and health forms the second. The third is satisfaction and involves such concepts as comfort, convenience, and being attractive and pleasant.

Some Basics

This section covers only a few aspects of ergonomics. Included are some basic concepts and a few examples. In the last few years, ergonomics has become an integral part of safety and health. The primary focus has been on cumulative trauma disorders resulting from repeated and continuous activity. For many years, safety has been concerned with lifting and materials handing and associated back injuries. Those concerns are now part of the ergonomics focus. But ergonomics goes well beyond those issues when preventing accidents and injuries, whether singular or continuous events.

TABLE 6.1   A comparison of some capabilities of people and machines[*]

People are better at:	Machines are better at:
Detecting information (visual, auditory) from among background conditions	Quick response (human reaction time and response time is greater)
	Sensitivity to stimuli (humans have limited ranges of sensitivity)
Handling unexpected occurrences	Precise, repeated operations
Reasoning inductively	Deductive reasoning
Learning from experience	Storing and processing large amounts of data
Creativity and originality	Exerting force and power
Flexibility and adjusting to change	Monitoring functions

*Derived from Meister, D., and G.F. Rabideau. 1965. *Human Factors Evaluation in System Development.* New York: John Wiley & Sons.

Effective Allocation of Functions   In designing work, it is essential to know the capability and limitations of humans and how those contrast with machines and equipment. The capability of machines and equipment has increased rapidly with the infusion of microcomputer technology. Some machines and equipment may now be better at some functions for which humans were better in the past. Table 6.1 lists some of the differences between people and machines.

Design the Job to Fit the Person   Because people are not alike and have many different characteristics, it is important to allow for such variability in design. People are not all the same size. They do not all have the same strength. They do not all have the same knowledge or skills. As a result, it is important to fit the job or task to the person, rather than having each person adjust. Here are a few guiding principles in designing for people.

1. *Know the population you are designing for.* Will workers be young or old or any age? What previous experience do they have? What skills do they have? Will both genders be involved? Can the work be performed by people with disabilities? What size, strength, or range of motion will people have?

2. *Design so machines and equipment are adjustable.* One size does not fit all. Today, one can often find adjustable features for controls, seating, furniture, fixtures, and other equipment, particularly in consumer products, vehicles, and manufacturing equipment. Similar features may be needed for workstations and equipment in various mining settings.

3. *Design for the 95th percentile male to fit and the 5th percentile female to reach.* In general, the U.S. population is getting taller and larger. Populations in other parts of the world may be much different. Usually, there are anthropometric tables listing various body dimensions and strength data. One must be careful in the use of such tables. The information in the tables may be derived from a population of subjects who are significantly different from the population for which a solution is sought. For example, the data in a table may be from unclothed or lightly clothed people and inappropriate when designing for workers who wear heavy protective or winter gear. However, assuming that some valid data sources are available, the principle stated here suggests that the upper end of the male population is the concern when people or their limbs must be able to fit into a space or through an opening. The lower end of the scale for women is the main concern when reaching.

Understand the People–Machine Interface   Another important ergonomics concept is the interface between people and machines, illustrated in Figure 6.4. The complexities of the interface go beyond the physical characteristics and extend to cognitive and performance factors. The two must work together effectively to minimize errors that may lead to accidents. The concept assists in evaluating conditions for potential hazards.

Functions of people are above the horizontal line and machine functions are below the line. As a machine performs some function, the operator must know what the machine is doing or how well it is doing in order to guide its operation. Information about the machine and its performance are presented in some form of display. Displays may be dials, gauges, images, audio signals, etc. For the operator to understand what the displays are reporting, the operator must sense the information through visual, auditory, tactile, or other senses. The operator must then process the information to

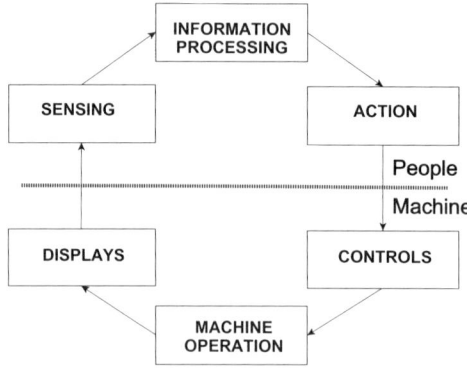

FIGURE 6.4   Information flow between people and machines affects systems design solutions

decide if the action of the machine should be changed from its present state. The operator transfers actions to the machine through controls. The controls then change the machine function. Some elements of this model are often ignored when designing work and the equipment used to accomplish it.

On the person side, the information from sensors must be within the range of sensation. For example, people cannot see in the infrared or ultraviolet regions. One may need to evaluate a workstation to ensure that sufficient light is required to see a display. One may need to recognize the fact that some workers are older and less likely to hear higher frequencies within the range of hearing. One may need to analyze the rate at which information occurs during an emergency and is within a rate that can be interpreted by workers and not confused with competing information.

Even if information is sensed, it has to be meaningful, perceived, and processed. One may have to compare the information to previously learned conditions or differentiate it from other information of a similar nature. An example is the difference in meaning between a fire alarm that says get out of a building and a tornado alarm that means take cover within the building. The receiver must know what sounds are to be converted to specific actions. The wrong action could be disastrous. Some situations may not occur often. The person may not recall from memory that a dangerous situation exists with a particular set of signals.

The action taken must be timely and of the right magnitude or duration to affect the machine's function. The person may not have enough strength to operate a control. A person may not be capable of the proper action or have the ability, knowledge, or skill to operate the control. For example, a person may not know the correct command to operate a speech-activated control. Or the action of a control may not be consistent with conventions learned for similar controls in other settings.

The desired response from the machine may not be within its range of responses. For example, a vehicle has a limited turning radius and may be unable to turn sharp enough to avoid some situations.

One can use this people–machine interface model to analyze machines, equipment, processes, and other situations to determine what can go wrong and whether the entire system is capable of responding to a given set of circumstances. While this model may seem elementary, the events at Three Mile Island and the design of control room equipment provided many examples of failures in the interface between systems and operators.

Material Handling

Mining involves moving materials. Most material handling is handled by equipment, usually large equipment. Some mining activities involve manual material handling. Manual material handling is a leading cause of accidents, injuries, and cumulative trauma disorders. The revised National Institute of Occupational Safety and Health (NIOSH) lifting equation provides an analytical tool for evaluating lifting activities of various types (Waters et al. 1993; Waters, Putz-Anderson, and Garg 1994). The new version of the equation includes factors for asymmetry and hand holds. In general the lifting equation involves the following structure:

$$RWL = LC \times HM \times VM \times DM \times AM \times FM \times CM \qquad \text{(EQ 6.2)}$$

where:

RWL	=	recommended weight limit (lower than that acceptable to at least 90% of females)
LC	=	load constant (an RWL for ideal conditions at the standard lifting location)
HM	=	horizontal multiplier (position of hands forward from the body)
VM	=	vertical multiplier (distance of hands from the floor)
DM	=	distance multiplier (vertical travel distance from origin to destination of the lift)
AM	=	asymmetric multiplier (involving angular position from the sagittal plane; essentially the amount of twisting involved in the lift)
FM	=	frequency multiplier (measured in lifts per minute)
XCM	=	coupling multiplier (effectiveness of handles or hand holds).

Based on many studies, NIOSH provides the following information to apply Equation 6.2 in calculating the RWL.

Component		Metric System	US Customary System
LC = load constant	=	23 kg	51 lb
HM = horizontal multiplier	=	(25/H)	(10/H)
VM = vertical multiplier	=	$(1-(0.003 \mid V-75 \mid))$	$(1-(0.0075 \mid V-30 \mid))$
DM = distance multiplier	=	$(0.82 + (4.5/D))$	$(0.82 + (1.8/D))$
AM = asymmetric multiplier	=	$(1-(0.0032A))$	$(1-(0.0032A))$
FM = frequency multiplier (from Table 6.2)			
CM = coupling multiplier (from Table 6.3)			

where:

H	=	horizontal distance of hands from midpoint between the ankles—measure at the origin and the destination of the lift (cm or in, depending on measurement system)
V	=	vertical distance of the hands from the floor—measure at the origin and destination of the lift (cm or in, depending on measurement system)
D	=	vertical travel distance between the origin and destination of the lift (cm or in, depending on measurement system)
A	=	angle of asymmetry: angular displacement of the load from the sagittal plane—measure at the origin and destination of the lift (degrees)
F	=	average frequency rate of lifting measured in lifts/min—duration is defined to be: ≤ 1 hr; ≤ 2 hr; or ≤ 8 hr assuming appropriate recovery allowances (see Table 6.2).

Procedures, Warnings, and Instructions

The writing of instructions, warnings, and procedures for safety operations also involves expertise from ergonomics. College writing classes seldom cover how to write instructions. The legal system considers failure to warn just as important in product liability cases as design and manufacturing defects. Litigation has forced major improvement in the art of writing warnings about hazards that remain in a product and instructions for protecting the product user from injury or illness. The lessons from product liability can carry over to writing safe procedures. Well-written procedures, warnings, and instructions are essential for safe operations. However, they are not always sufficient to protect people, because they must be learned, understood, remembered, followed, and implemented in a timely manner when situations call for their use.

MANAGEMENT SYSTEMS

In a particular process, operation, or equipment item, there may be many hazards. Once they are identified, one has the problem of sorting them out and deciding what controls should be put in place and how much money to spend doing so. Hazards need to be evaluated along with control options. The purpose of this section is to comment on approaches to handling these important safety engineering activities.

TABLE 6.2   Frequency multiplier, FM, for Equation 6.2

Frequency, lifts/min*	Work duration					
	≤ 1 hr		≤ 2 hr		≤ 8 hr	
	V < 75	V ≥ 75	V < 75	V ≥ 75	V < 75	V ≥ 75
0.2	1.00	1.00	0.95	0.95	0.85	0.85
0.5	0.97	0.97	0.92	0.92	0.81	0.81
1	0.94	0.94	0.88	0.88	0.75	0.75
2	0.91	0.91	0.84	0.84	0.65	0.65
3	0.88	0.88	0.79	0.79	0.55	0.55
4	0.84	0.84	0.72	0.72	0.45	0.45
5	0.80	0.80	0.60	0.60	0.35	0.35
6	0.75	0.75	0.50	0.50	0.27	0.27
7	0.70	0.70	0.42	0.42	0.22	0.22
8	0.60	0.60	0.35	0.35	0.18	0.18
9	0.52	0.52	0.30	0.30	0.00	0.15
10	0.45	0.45	0.26	0.26	0.00	0.13
11	0.41	0.41	0.00	0.23	0.00	0.00
12	0.37	0.37	0.00	0.21	0.00	0.00
13	0.00	0.34	0.00	0.00	0.00	0.00
14	0.00	0.31	0.00	0.00	0.00	0.00
15	0.00	0.28	0.00	0.00	0.00	0.00
>15	0.00	0.00	0.00	0.00	0.00	0.00

* Note: Values of V are in cm; 75 cm = 30 in.

TABLE 6.3   Coupling multiplier, CM, for Equation 6.2

Couplings	Coupling multipliers	
	V < 75 cm (30 in.)	V > 75 cm (30 in.)
Good	1.00	1.00
Fair	0.95	1.00
Poor	0.90	0.90

Risk Analysis

Risk involves the combination of frequency and severity. Frequency considers the likelihood that a hazard will lead to an undesired event, incident, or accident. Severity deals with the extent of damage, injury, or harm. Both qualitative and quantitative approaches may be used in risk analysis. The topic of risk is covered in more detail elsewhere in this book. In general, the goal is to decide which hazards are most in need of controls. Clearly, those hazards that have both high frequency and high severity require the greatest attention. Ideally, all hazards should be eliminated or reduced, but that is not always practical or financially feasible. Risk analysis techniques have been expanded over time for particular classes of hazards and particular methods may be called for in certain cases. Risk analysis is a very important part of the process of hazard recognition, evaluation, and control.

System Safety

System safety involves a family of methods for deciding how to design equipment, systems, and processes. These methods have emerged from aerospace settings and are now applied to many different kinds of complex equipment, plants, and operations. Today, system safety methodologies are an integral part of safety engineering. Often the application of system safety techniques requires a team of specialists from various disciplines.

Frequency of Occurrence	HAZARD CATEGORY			
	1 Catastrophic	2 Critical	3 Marginal	4 Negligible
A. Frequent	1A	2A	3A	4A
B. Probable	1B	2B	3B	4B
C. Occasional	1C	2C	3C	4C
D. Remote	1D	2D	3D	4D
E. Improbable	1E	2E	3E	4E

Hazard Risk Index	Suggested Criteria
1A, 1B, 1C, 2A, 2B, 3A	Unacceptable (corrections required)
1D, 2C, 2D, 3B, 3C	Undesirable (management decision required)
1E, 2E, 3D, 3E, 4A, 4B	Acceptable with review by management
4C, 4D, 4E	Acceptable without review

FIGURE 6.5   Schematic risk decision table

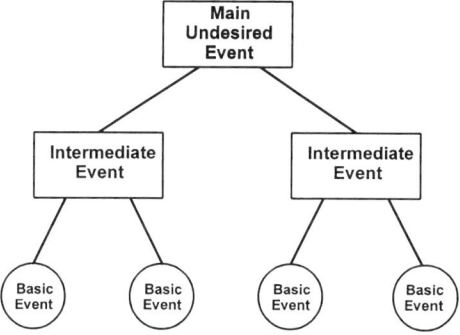

FIGURE 6.6   A fault tree helps to analyze causes of failures

Hazard Analysis   A foundation for system safety activities is hazard analysis. It may involve charting all components in a system and the hazards associated with them. The analysis may include hardware, equipment, software, human operators, and other elements. Various forms of hazard analysis may be required, depending on the complexity of the system being analyzed.

Risk Analysis   Another group of methods used in system safety involve risk analysis. In many cases, the hazards are charted into a risk decision table or risk assessment matrix (see Figure 6.5). The severity of hazards is rated and charted on one axis of the chart. The probability of occurrence is on the other axis. Then severity-probability cells are marked for the kind of action required, such as risk reduction required, management approval, or that the operation is permissible.

A classic case involves the space shuttle *Challenger* (McConnell 1987). Conditions encountered on the day of the fatal launch placed the flight into a mission-critical category. System safety analysis indicating that it was likely that a seal problem would result in loss of the mission and space shuttle. Management decided to change the risk category and fly.

Fault Tree Analysis   A well-known safety technique is fault tree analysis. It is often applied to complex systems with the goal of identifying factors that contribute to the top event. When various factors contributing to the top event are evaluated, the top event branches out into a sequence of conditions that individually or in combination contribute to the likelihood of the top event or intermediate ones. A conceptual version of a fault tree appears in Figure 6.6. Actual fault diagrams can become very complex. One can assign quantitative values to each basic event and then use Boolean algebra to compute the probability of intermediate events and the final event. One can also use qualitative analysis to analyze a fault tree and identify high-risk branches of the tree.

In mining for example, a top event might be the collapse of a mineshaft or an explosion. Use of the technique would seek to uncover all contributing factors. Once the fault tree has been developed, it can be analyzed qualitatively and quantitatively to establish the probability of the top event based on the probability that lower events will occur. Then designers can select the corrective action for the most likely causes for the top event.

Failure Mode and Effects Analysis   Another method is failure mode and effects analysis. It considers what may go wrong and what the consequences will be. Most people are familiar with this method through diagnostic charts that aid in trouble shooting automobiles or other equipment. By locating the failure or symptom in the chart, one can locate possible causes and solutions for the problem. In failure mode and effects analysis for safety, one is trying to identify what controls will prevent or reduce the danger of some hazard.

Other Methods   There are many other techniques and components of system safety or derived from system safety. Some analysis includes the cost to implement controls for hazards, the effectiveness of the controls, and the degree of risk reduction. Overall, the techniques allow one to make recommendations or decisions about which hazards have the greatest risk and which controls will be most cost effective.

SUMMARY

Safety engineering is an important part in the process of recognizing, evaluating, and controlling hazards. Safety engineering emphasizes the use of engineering controls for eliminating or reducing hazards through design of work, equipment, machines, vehicles, and facilities. Other important approaches give attention to administrative controls and overall management of the safety enterprise. All elements affect the bottom line of the organization and its productivity while decreasing the risk for employees, contractors, and the public.

REFERENCES

Brauer, R.L. 1994. *Safety and Health for Engineers*. New York: John Wiley & Sons.

——. 1980. *Concepts and Techniques of Machine Safeguarding*. OSHA 3067. U.S. Department of Labor, Occupational Health and Safety Administration (OSHA).

Chaffin, D.B., and G. Andersson. 1991. *Occupational Biomechanics*. 2nd ed. New York: John Wiley & Sons.

Christensen, W.C., and F.A. Manuele, editors. 1999. *Safety Through Design*. Itasca, IL: National Safety Council.

——. 1983. *Guidelines for Controlling Hazardous Energy During Maintenance and Servicing*. DHHS (NIOSH) Publication No. 83-125. Morgantown, WV: NIOSH Division of Safety Research.

Deming, W.E. 1986. *Out of the Crisis*. Cambridge: Massachusetts Institute of Technology Center for Advanced Engineering Study.

Haddon, W., Jr. 1970. On the escape of tigers: an ecological note. *Technology Review* (May).

Hammer, M., and J. Champy. 1993. *Reengineering the Corporation*. New York: HarperBusiness.

Juran, J.M. 1992. *Juran on Quality by Design: The New Steps for Planning Quality into Goods and Services*. New York: The Free Press.

Manuele, F.A. 1997. *On the Practice of Safety*. 2nd ed. New York: Van Nostrand Reinhold.

McConnell, M. 1987. *Challenger: A Major Malfunction*. New York: Doubleday & Company.

Meister, D., and G.F. Rabideau. 1965. *Human Factors Evaluation in System Development*. New York: John Wiley & Sons.

Salvendy, G. 1997. *Handbook of Human Factors and Ergonomics*. 2nd ed. New York: John Wiley & Sons.

Sanders, M.S., and E.J. McCormick. 1993. *Human Factors in Engineering and Design*. 7th ed. New York: McGraw-Hill.

Schoff, G.H., and P.A. Robinson. 1991. *Writing and Designing Manuals*. 2nd ed. Chelsea, MI: Lewis Publishers.

Spellman, F.R., and N.E. Whiting. 1999. *Machine Guarding Handbook: A Practical Guide to OSHA Compliance and Injury Prevention*. Rockville, MD: Government Institutes Division, ABS Group.

Waters, T.R., V. Putz-Anderson, A. Garg, and L.J. Fine. 1993. Revised NIOSH equation for the design and evaluation of manual lifting tasks. *Ergonomics* 36(7) 749–776.

Waters, T.R., V. Putz-Anderson, and A. Garg. 1994. *Applications Manual for the Revised NIOSH Lifting Equation*. DHHS (NIOSH) Publication No. 94-110. Morgantown, WV: U.S. Department of Health and Human Services, Public Health Service, Centers for Disease Control, NIOSH.

CHAPTER 7

Federal Regulation of Mine Safety and Health

Michael T. Heenan
Partner, Heenan, Althen & Roles, Washington, D.C.

INTRODUCTION

Catastrophic explosions and mine fires are the reasons that the U.S. government originally became involved in mine safety and health. Thousands of people died in mines and risks to miners were enormous at the beginning of the twentieth century. The year 1907 was the worst in history with 3,242 deaths in the coal mining industry alone. The Bureau of Mines was created within the U.S. Department of the Interior in 1910, but the bureau was not given authority to actually enter and inspect mines until 1941. Following catastrophic explosions in the 1960s and 1970s, government inspection and control of mines was substantially expanded.

Today, the safety and health of all mine personnel is regulated by the United States Department of Labor. This responsibility was assigned to the Secretary of Labor by the Federal Mine Safety and Health Act of 1977 (Mine Act).[1] The designated agency for mine oversight and enforcement within the Labor Department is the Mine Safety and Health Administration (MSHA). MSHA administers a comprehensive regulatory program aimed specifically at ensuring safe and healthy working conditions at mines.

With industry modernization and government regulations, the risk of catastrophic explosions and fires has been substantially reduced. In 1998, the mining industry experienced its safest year of the twentieth century with an all time low of 80 fatalities in all types of mining. One fatality is one too many, but the industry and MSHA continue to strive for "zero fatalities." The record to date shows enormous success of safety and health enhancements over time. The contrast between the early 1900s and the present is extraordinary. Throughout the United States, mine operators are diligently complying with the law.

Most mines in the United States are surface mines that do not pose risks of catastrophic explosions or fires. Virtually all mines, however, present some risks that are unique to mining. At the same time, they pose a wide variety of risks akin to those in other heavy industries. All of these risks come within the purview of MSHA.

OVERVIEW OF THE REGULATORY PROGRAM

Delegation of Authority

Regulatory agencies such as MSHA are primarily an outgrowth of modern economic development, industrialization and mechanization and their attendant complexities. Although traditionally the three branches of government under the U.S. Constitution—legislative, executive, and judicial—are separate, the specialized aspects of complex topics such as mine safety and health have caused Congress to delegate powers to executive agencies. While Congress is the traditional body that creates new legislation, the detail-intensive task of making and periodically updating specialized safety and health requirements for mines is not a practical ongoing function for Congress. Thus, the function of developing safety and health standards for mines has been delegated by Congress to the Executive Branch of government, and specifically to the Department of Labor.

Administrative Rulemaking

While Congress has developed some safety and health standards for mines in the past, today it is the Labor Department, through MSHA, that typically promulgates new standards and regulations pursuant to executive authority. The rulemaking process for development of mine safety and health standards and regulations by an administrative agency, in this case MSHA, is subject to two principal safeguards. First, the Labor Department must give advance notice of proposed new rules or proposed changes to existing rules, so that interested persons, including labor and management representatives, can comment on the proposed rules. Second, if concerns or objections of interested persons are not resolved, objectionable aspects of the new rules can be challenged in federal court, provided it can be demonstrated that issues were raised during the notice and comment period of the rulemaking procedure.

Administrative Litigation

Were it not for federal mining legislation, the federal courts would have to conduct numerous trials regarding the validity of enforcement actions by MSHA. Parties subject to government sanctions in the form of mine closure orders or civil penalties are entitled to their day in court. However, Congress has provided in the Mine Act that legal review proceedings are to be heard and decided initially by a specialized, independent agency called the Federal Mine Safety and Health Review Commission. This agency is not part of the Labor Department. Rather, it was established by Congress specifically to consider and independently decide disputes arising under the Mine Act.[2]

Mine Act proceedings that are fully litigated begin with a trial before an Administrative Law Judge (ALJ) under the commission. If even one party objects to the ALJ decision, review by the full five-member commission panel may be sought. Thus, the commission oversees both trial and appellate proceedings. Because these proceedings are conducted by an administrative agency, they are deemed administrative, rather than judicial, in nature. Parties are required to exhaust their administrative remedies before they may seek judicial review. Consequently, only after such administrative review is completed does the Act permit appeal to a federal court.

Operators Under the Act

While other industries are regulated by programs administered by other various agencies, few programs could claim to be more intensive or more vigorous than the mining industry program enforced by MSHA under the Mine Act. For example, Mine Act requirements apply to everyone who goes onto mine property to do work. Even though an independent contractor may be engaged by a mining company to do specialized non-mining work (roofing for example), that contractor will be deemed an "operator" at a mine and will have to meet all of the Mine Act's requirements while present on the property.[3] In this connection, direct enforcement by MSHA against any operator on mine property is authorized. Moreover, in any case where an independent contractor operator is found at fault, the mine owner may also be charged for the violation. This raises complicated issues that are dealt with elsewhere in this book.

Safety and Health Rules and Regulations

The focus of mine safety and health regulation is always the safety and health of persons at mines. Thus, compliance with mandatory standards developed pursuant to the Mine Act is the central responsibility of mine operators and miners. Mandatory standards are the dos and don'ts of mine safety and health. The standards are published in the *Code of Federal Regulations* (CFR). Also published in this same volume are various administrative regulations associated with enforcement.

The mandatory standards include requirements specific to mines such as those pertaining to roof support, ventilation, permissible electrical equipment, ground control, hazardous dust control, and other standards that would be pertinent to any heavy industry. The mandatory standards also impose duties on operators to perform pre-shift or on-shift examinations of work areas and equipment to eliminate hazards.[4] They also require that operators provide paid training of miners, including comprehensive training for new miners—40 hours of training for underground miners and 24 hours of training for surface miners. Independent contractors at mines are also to be trained, but not always to the same extent as mine employees of mine operators. Short-term contractors, who are not exposed to mine production hazards, may not need full-scale training. MSHA regulations and policy must be consulted in every case.[5]

The foregoing is simply an overview of the types of regulations promulgated under the Mine Act. This chapter will not provide more details on regulations as the purpose of this chapter is not to review specific mandatory standards or administrative rules, but rather to explain the scheme developed in the Mine Act and how standards and regulations are enforced, as well as how enforcement and other administrative actions are subject to legal challenge and review.

ORIGINS OF THE MINE ACT

The very forceful penalties prescribed for violation of the Mine Act did not, for the most part, originate with that law in 1977. Rather, they were introduced under a predecessor statute, the Federal Coal Mine Health and Safety Act of 1969.[6] A large portion of the Labor Department's existing Mine Act interpretations grew out of the 1969 Coal Act. That Act was enforced by the United States Department of the Interior, and specifically by the Bureau of Mines (later the Mining Enforcement and Safety Administration [MESA]) within the Interior Department.

The 1969 Coal Act had a significant effect not only on the coal industry, but also on industry in general. It introduced the concept of rigorous civil monetary penalties to enforce safety and health in the workplace. Within one year of the 1969 Coal Act, Congress passed the Occupational Safety and Health Act of 1970 (the OSHA statute), which was to be administered by the Occupational Safety and Health Administration (OSHA).[7] The OSHA statute prescribed a somewhat similar, but generally less intrusive program, to regulate the safety and health of all workers in the United States not covered by the 1969 Coal Act or any other specific safety and health legislation.[8]

OSHA Jurisdiction Distinguished

OSHA was not given jurisdiction over coal mines or noncoal mines. That is because, as indicated above, there already were specialized laws for mines and these laws were enforced by the Secretary of the Interior. The law for noncoal mines was called the Federal Metal and Nonmetallic Mine Safety Act of 1966 (1966 Metal/Nonmetal Act).[9] This law did not have the same degree of formidable enforcement mechanisms as were introduced in the 1969 Coal Act, but it did provide for comprehensive rulemaking and inspections by the Interior Department. Standards promulgated under the 1966 Metal/Nonmetal Act were, in many cases, advisory rather than mandatory, and the law did not provide for civil penalties.

Effects of the Mine Act

Today, and ever since enactment of the Mine Act in 1977, all mines are under a single statute administered by MSHA. The regulations promulgated for coal mines are aimed at preventing the same kinds of hazards as have been addressed in regulations for metal/nonmetal mines. However, because of differences in the evolution of standards for coal and noncoal mines, two sets of rules exist in the CFR today, one specifically addressing coal and one addressing metal ore and also nonmetallic materials such as stone, sand, shells, and clay.[10] Each set of rules is fully divided depending on whether they pertain to surface or underground operations. Organizationally, MSHA maintains two divisions to separately administer coal mines and metal/nonmetal mines. However, all types of mines are subject to identical enforcement procedures and all have the same obligations, rights, and duties.

SCOPE OF REGULATION

By enacting the Mine Act, Congress declared that the first priority of the mining industry must be the health and safety of the miner and that there is an urgent need to provide more effective means to improve working conditions to prevent death and serious bodily harm, and prevent occupational diseases, such as pneumoconiosis and silicosis.

Responsibilities of Operators and Miners

Congress stated that the operators of mines, with the assistance of the miners, have the primary responsibility to prevent unsafe and unhealthy conditions in mines. The term "operator" is defined in the Mine Act as "any owner, lessee, or other person who operates, controls or supervises a coal or other mine or any independent contractor performing services or construction at such mine."[11]

Unlike OSHA, which regulates employers, MSHA regulates land and all of the work that takes place on such land. MSHA jurisdiction attaches at the functional borders of a mine and any milling or preparation facilities. A mine operator could own a large tract of land, on which various activities aside from what is traditionally considered to be mining may be conducted (ranching, asphalt, or ready-mix concrete production, for example), and MSHA's jurisdiction would be limited to those parts of the property that fall within the definition of "mine" as set forth in the Mine Act.

Definition of Mine

The Mine Act defines "mine" as:

(A) An area of land from which minerals are extracted in nonliquid form (the Act does not cover oil or gas operations but would extend to such operations if conducted with workers underground).

(B) Private ways and roads appurtenant to such land—if a mine relies on a public road to access its property, that road is not subject to MSHA jurisdiction, because it is not a private road or way.

(C) Lands, excavations, underground passageways, shafts, slopes, tunnels and workings, structures, facilities, equipment, machines, tools, or other property including impounds, retention dams, and tailings ponds, on the surface or underground, *used in, or to be used in, or resulting from, the work of extracting such minerals* from their natural deposits in nonliquid form, or if in liquid form, with workers underground, *or used in, or to be used in, the milling of such minerals, or the work of preparing coal or other minerals*, and includes custom coal preparation facilities.[12]

As the foregoing indicates, mining includes not just extraction, but all mineral milling and coal preparation activities as well. Moreover, land on which such mineral milling and coal preparation activities are conducted qualifies as a mine subject to regulation by MSHA. This broad definition applies notwithstanding that mineral milling or coal preparation facilities miles away from any extraction site at a location where mined materials must be transported by rail, truck, or barge. The fact that a cement plant does not have its own quarry, for example, does not alter MSHA's jurisdiction over the plant as a "mine" facility.

Everything that is "used in, or to be used in, or resulting from, the work of extracting minerals from their natural deposits ... or used in, or to be used in, the milling of such minerals or the work of preparing coal or other minerals" is included within MSHA's jurisdiction.[13] Various legal case decisions challenge MSHA's assertion of jurisdiction in specific cases. Frequently, it is argued that a certain facility is not a mine and should be regulated by OSHA instead of MSHA.

MSHA and OSHA Interagency Agreement

Pursuant to statutory authority, MSHA and OSHA entered into an interagency agreement regarding a variety of jurisdictional questions and this agreement is indispensable in connection with any review of MSHA's or OSHA's authority to regulate a specific site.[14] The main effect of the interagency agreement is to address instances where a question may exist as to the point at which it can be said that mined materials have finally left the mining and mineral milling processes and are no longer part of MSHA jurisdiction. For example, there is a big difference between milling clinker from limestone that has been fired in a kiln and mixing finished cement into other materials, such as sand, gravel, and water, to prepare ready-mix concrete. In the first instance, the process of making cement is considered to be "mineral milling" and it is subject to MSHA jurisdiction. In the second instance, ready-mix concrete preparation is deemed a "post-milling" process and is not considered part of mining. This process is subject to OSHA jurisdiction.

Jurisdictional questions are not always as easily resolved, however. There are as many jurisdictional issues as there are types of materials mined and processed. From clay extraction for cat litter to mineral mining for chemical components, innumerable permutations often arise when determining whether MSHA jurisdiction applies to all or part of an operation.

REGULATORY SCHEME

The question of when MSHA jurisdiction applies is an important one, because as soon as it is determined that a particular property falls within the definition of a "mine" under the Mine Act, a variety of affirmative obligations must be fulfilled by the mine operator.

Operator Identification

First and foremost, all mine operators must identify themselves to MSHA. Under rules promulgated by MSHA, all mine operators must complete a standard form with basic information, including whether the company is a corporation, partnership, sole proprietorship, or some other business entity, such as a joint venture.[15] From this information, MSHA determines what actions are required from a new operator in connection with the new mining operation as well as subsequent operations.

MSHA also uses information on this identity report to determine the total size of the business for purposes of evaluating the size of civil money penalties that the operator will be subject to if the mine is cited for violations. Given the vigorous and comprehensive nature of Mine Act administration citations are a virtual certainty. Corporations must declare whether they are subsidiaries, and if so, they must name the parent company. By linking a subsidiary with all other mining subsidiaries of the corporate parent, MSHA establishes what it calls the "size of the controlling entity." This size is a factor used in assessing civil penalties for all MSHA violations.[16]

Information on the MSHA legal identity form also informs MSHA as to whether special enforcement mechanisms pertinent to corporate agents might apply. Under the Mine Act, corporate agents are subject to being personally prosecuted. (However, this is not true for agents of a partnership or sole proprietorship.) Under the Mine Act, an agent is defined as "any person charged with responsibility for the operation of all or a part of a coal or other mine or the supervision of the miners in a coal or other mine."[17] The personal liability of agents will be discussed in connection with civil and criminal penalties.

Failure to File Identity Report   Any mine that does not identify itself to MSHA is at risk for criminal prosecution. MSHA has brought numerous legal actions against such companies and their principals. Such cases are not subject to the administrative procedures of the Mine Act. Rather, they are a matter of criminal law and prosecuted by the United States Attorney in the federal district court for the jurisdiction where the offense is committed.[18]

Heavy fines and jail sentences have been imposed for failure to file an identity report. Unidentified mines are considered outlaws and are subject to the most severe type of enforcement. If need be, the Labor Department can seek an injunction, and obtain the assistance of federal marshals to gain entry to a mine that is trying to keep agency officials away. MSHA may also seek daily civil penalties from the operator for every day that the operator persists in refusing admittance.

MSHA INSPECTIONS

Inspections are conducted for a variety of reasons. Besides regular inspections—two times a year for surface mines and four times a year for underground mines—there are any number of special occasions for particular inspections such as what are commonly called "spot" inspections.[19] Inspections may be conducted to evaluate the entire operation, monitor dust control, evaluate electrical compliance, or inquire into any other compliance issue. Inspections are always conducted without prior notice. Indeed, as a matter of criminal law under the Mine Act, any person who gives advance notice of an inspection stands to be criminally prosecuted.[20]

Miners' Right to Accompany Inspector

Notwithstanding the foregoing, the law allows opportunity for a representative of the operator and a representative authorized by the miners at the mine to accompany the inspector for purposes of aiding in the inspection and participating in any pre- or post-inspection conferences at the mine. Moreover, a representative of the miners is entitled to "suffer no loss of pay during such participation."[21] If there is no miners' representative, the inspector proceeds with a representative of the operator, but if the operator delays excessively in providing a representative the inspector proceeds alone. In either case, the inspector may talk to miners on the job about safety and health issues.

Special Hazard Complaint Inspections

Representatives of miners are entitled to ask MSHA to inspect a mine with alleged safety problems. Where the employees are represented by a union, the union generally provides the representation, but other individuals at the mine can be active as well and, as a practical matter, MSHA tends to conduct an inspection in response to any safety or health complaint filed with the agency. The complaint is supposed to be in writing and the operator is to be given a copy by MSHA, with the names of persons lodging the complaint removed.[22] This anonymity is designed to encourage miners to take action with regard to unsafe conditions or practices at a mine without fear of reprisals.

ENFORCEMENT

The two main vehicles for initiating sanctions under the Mine Act are *citations* and *orders*. Citations notify the operator that something is unlawful, but do not close any part of the operation. Orders of Withdrawal (Orders) close all or part of an operation.

Citations and Correction of Conditions

Any time that an inspector forms a belief that an operator has violated the Mine Act or any mandatory health or safety standard or regulation promulgated pursuant to the Act, it is the inspector's duty to charge the operator with the violation. In most instances the charge is set out in what is referred to as a citation. Apart from notifying the operator of the charge, the most immediate consequence of a citation is that the operator is given a specified period to correct the alleged violation.[23]

Citations and Civil Penalties

After correction of a cited condition or practice, the citation will, in due course, be sent to MSHA's Office of Civil Penalty Assessments. The level of a proposed penalty will generally be based on various findings made by the inspector on the face of the citation, including the level of negligence of the operator, the seriousness of the condition or practice, and whether the condition or practice is "significant and substantial" (commonly called S&S). Since the Mine Act is a "strict liability statute," a mine operator must pay penalties for all violations even if the operator is not negligent at all. However, negligence is a critical factor in determining how high a penalty should be assessed.

Significant and Substantial (S&S) Findings

Apart from negligence, possibly the most significant finding on a citation has to do with whether the condition cited was "of such a nature as could significantly and substantially contribute to the cause and effect of a mine health or safety standard."[24] As the Mine Act is enforced, there are three principal ways in which the S&S or non-S&S designation may have a significant impact:

(1) Unless the mine is determined by the Assessment Office to have an excessive history of violations (more than 2.1 violations per inspection day), non-S&S citations are eligible for nominal penalties (originally $50, but adjusted for inflation over time).

(2) An S&S finding fulfills a prerequisite for a citation to be evaluated under one of MSHA's sternest enforcement mechanisms—the "Unwarrantable Failure" citation, which will be discussed in detail under the section on Orders of Withdrawal below.

(3) Under the Mine Act and regulations promulgated by the Secretary of Labor, special elevated enforcement mechanisms are prescribed for any operator who is determined to have a pattern of S&S violations. MSHA regulations provide details as to how this type of enforcement is to be implemented.

Orders of Withdrawal

There are a number of instances where an inspector is authorized to close (order miners to be withdrawn from) all or part of a mine.[25] When an inspector issues such an order, the cited equipment or practice must be taken out of operation and work discontinued immediately, except work to correct the cited condition. No one is allowed to enter the area except those needed to correct the condition, government officials, and under certain circumstances, representatives of the miners.

Orders of Withdrawal are very disruptive to mine operations and often result in a complete cessation of work, causing a related loss of production. Getting an order is expensive for an operator in more ways than one. Days of production may be lost until the condition is fully corrected. In addition, orders are subject to very high civil penalties. They also often carry allegations of high danger or high negligence that can have added repercussions with respect to the operator's history of compliance and can make subsequent enforcement actions more severe. The specific effects of any given order will depend in part on whether a violation was charged and what findings were associated with the charged violation.

Types of Orders

Not all orders are issued for violations; orders may be issued without charges of violation. Whether or not a violation is associated with an order is of great importance. Orders with violations are typically subject to high money penalties. Moreover, miners idled by any order, regardless whether a violation is charged, are protected to a degree from loss of pay—remainder of the shift on which the order is issued and four hours of the oncoming shift. If they are idled by an order related to a violation, however, they have a much greater entitlement, up to one week of lost wages. The miners are also entitled to bring a legal action against the operator to collect such pay.[26]

Discussed below are two basic types of orders that may be issued without regard to whether a violation exists.

Imminent Danger—The "A Order"   The Mine Act provides that if an inspector finds an Imminent Danger in a mine, the inspector shall determine the extent of the area involved. The inspector issues an order to require the mine operator to withdraw everyone who could potentially be affected "until the conditions or practices which caused such imminent danger no longer exist." Under the Mine Act, "imminent danger" means "the existence of any condition or practice ... which could reasonably be expected to cause death or serious physical harm before such condition or practice can be abated."[27] Such orders are sometimes referred to as "A orders," referring to section 107(a) of the Mine Act.

As indicated, there does not have to be a violation of law for an inspector to issue this type of order, but in practice, a citation is often associated with the issuance of such an order. High civil penalties may result from a citation issued with such an order. Typically, such a citation will be referred for an elevated civil penalty assessment under MSHA's "Special Assessment" procedures, particularly if the operator is charged with high negligence.

Control—The "K Order"   MSHA has authority to take varying degrees of control in the event of a mine accident. Typically, at the start of an accident investigation, MSHA issues a Control Order—or K Order, referring to section 103(k) of the Mine Act—to prohibit any unauthorized entry to the accident scene.[28] (Although rarely used, there is also a "J" Order in which MSHA may assume direct control of rescue and recovery operations following a mine accident.) Control Orders do not cite violations at all and they are not subject to civil penalties. They are simply a vehicle for MSHA to control an accident site pending investigation and other official actions.

Some orders ARE based on charges related to cited violations.

Failure to Abate—The "B Order"   According to the Mine Act, an inspector should issue an order withdrawing the miners (also called a Closure Order) if on any follow-up inspection it is found that a previously cited condition or practice "has not been totally abated," and it is further found that the original period prescribed for abatement "should not be further extended." In this situation, the inspector is to issue a Closure Order under section 104(b) of the Mine Act that remains in effect until the cited condition is fully abated.[29] These B orders are usually given high civil penalty assessments under MSHA's special assessment procedures.

Unwarrantable Failure—The "D Order"   Earlier it was mentioned that any S&S violation may be evaluated as to whether it involves an "unwarrantable failure of the operator to comply." In practice, charges of unwarrantable failure are reserved for more serious conduct on the part of the operator or the operator's agents. Unwarrantable failure has been defined as "aggravated conduct, constituting more than ordinary negligence by a mine operator in relation to a violation of the Act … Unwarrantable failure is characterized by such conduct as 'reckless disregard,' 'intentional misconduct,' 'indifference,' or a 'serious lack of reasonable care.'"[30]

If an inspector concludes that a particular S&S violation resulted from an unwarrantable failure of the operator to comply, the inspector will issue a citation that states that an unwarrantable failure exists. That citation is referred to as an unwarrantable failure citation or a "D citation" (referring to section 104(d) of the Act).[31]

In practice, there are three principal effects of the unwarrantable designation in any citation. First, the operator is essentially put on probation. If any further unwarrantable failures are found in the next 90 days—even if the violations are not S&S—an order (not a citation) will be issued. Once an order is issued under these circumstances, every unwarrantable failure results in an order unless and until the mine undergoes a complete inspection and no further unwarrantable failures are found.[32] Multiple unwarrantable failures result in what is sometimes referred to as a "sequence" or "chain." As a practical matter, it seems that very often after one unwarrantable failure is issued, others tend to follow.

The second effect of the unwarrantable designation is that any citations or orders with this designation are assessed elevated civil penalties under MSHA's special assessment procedures. (The differences between special and regular assessments are discussed in connection with civil penalties below.)

The third effect of the unwarrantable failure designation is that any citation or order having this designation may be referred for "special investigation." A very substantial portion of unwarrantable citations and orders are specially investigated. A special investigation is a very serious event and is fraught with potential legal problems for individual managers and supervisors, as well as the company.

Pattern Orders   The Mine Act and regulations provide for very heavy sanctions in the form of multiple orders at any mine deemed to have a "pattern of violations." The prerequisite procedures for pattern orders are complex. Because the procedures have not been invoked often, they are not being covered in depth here. If a mine is ever deemed to have a pattern of violations, that mine will be issued an order (not a citation) for every S&S violation found by any inspector, unless and until an inspection of the entire mine reveals no S&S violations.[33]

INFORMAL REVIEW OF CITATIONS AND ORDERS

MSHA regulations provide that all parties at a mine may review any citation or order with their MSHA district manager, or a delegate of the district manager.[34] These conferences, as they are called, can present valuable informal review opportunities for ensuring inspection results are fair and consistent with the goals of the Mine Act. They may include discussion regarding any or all findings.

Conferences should be requested within ten days of the time the citation is issued. Once a conference is scheduled, it does not have to be conducted within ten days or any other set period. However, it is critical to understand that the pendency of a conference (or of conference results) does not affect any of the very important time limits for *formal* review discussed below.

Seeking review of a citation or order by MSHA in a conference is not the same as contesting a citation in court. Rather, a conference simply provides an opportunity for MSHA to reconsider a citation or order.

A citation or order could be made more severe as a result of information MSHA receives in a conference. This does not happen with great frequency, but it does happen. At a minimum, parties should be thoroughly prepared and should understand clearly whether the evidence they are relying upon helps or hurts them. In some cases, parties may wish to submit a written explanation as to why a citation should be vacated or reduced because of mitigating circumstances. This is permitted and in certain cases can be more effective than an actual conference.

One reason in particular that operators might seek informal review of a citation or order is to try to avoid the possibility of a special investigation. Such investigations are time consuming, expensive, and can lead to serious legal liability. Again, because such cases frequently become the subject of formal proceedings—and admissions made during a conference *may* be introduced as evidence in formal proceedings—a conference participant must have a very clear understanding of the evidence, arguments, and implications of all that is communicated to MSHA in the conference. In any event, if an operator is successful at the conference in convincing MSHA to eliminate findings such as unwarrantable failure or imminent danger, this will go a long way toward preventing a special investigation from occurring. However, when MSHA continues to believe that the charges in a citation or order are justified, a special investigation may be inevitable.

As indicated previously, special investigations are one of the various types of investigations that MSHA regularly conducts. Consequences of any investigation may be quite serious depending on what findings are made by MSHA after review of the investigation record.

INVESTIGATIONS

The most serious legal events to occur with respect to mines generally arise out of investigations. In practice, investigations and inspections are reasonably distinct from one another. The primary difference is that in an inspection, an inspector ordinarily gathers evidence based on what the inspector personally *observes* at a mine. An investigator, for the most part, gains evidence based on what persons interviewed *say* and what is reported in any documents provided to the investigator. Each type of investigation has its own purpose. The initiation of one type of investigation does not preclude another on the same matter. In addition, there may be crossover allegations as well as evidence that the different investigations share. For example, evidence gained by MSHA in an Accident Investigation may be shared in connection with a later special investigation.

There are three basic types of investigations.

Accident Investigations

Under the Mine Act and regulations, operators at mines must immediately report all accidents to MSHA so that it can be determined whether an immediate accident investigation will be conducted.[35] Such investigations contain elements of an inspection where the investigators go and look at the scene and the equipment involved, along with other relevant factors. MSHA always investigates fatal accidents and may choose to investigate any of the other types of accidents subject to immediate reporting by the operator. These are:

- Any death on mine property
- Any injury with a reasonable potential to cause death
- Any entrapment of an individual for more than 30 minutes
- Any unplanned flood of liquid or gas
- Any unplanned ignition of gas or dust
- Any unplanned fire not extinguished in 30 minutes
- Any unplanned ignition of blasting materials
- Any unplanned roof fall above the anchorage zone
- Any coal or rock outburst that causes withdrawal of miners or disrupts activity for more than 1 hour
- Any unstable impoundment
- Any damage to hoisting equipment in a shaft interfering with equipment for 30 minutes
- Any event at a mine that caused death or bodily injury to persons off mine property.[36]

During an accident investigation, the mine operator and miners are usually permitted to participate as representatives on a panel of inquiry convened at the time of the investigation. Sometimes, however, MSHA proceeds in a confidential rather than public manner. In either event, parties with knowledge, including the operator, agents of the operator, and the miners, will be interviewed. As a matter of law—unless the investigation is performed in connection with a properly convened public hearing—statements are voluntary and no person is compelled to submit to an interview. In most cases, however, there is cooperation with MSHA and the investigation proceeds unimpeded.

As described with respect to control orders, MSHA may prohibit all entry to an accident site pending completion of the investigation. The purpose of such is twofold: first, MSHA wants to make sure all relevant evidence is gathered before it is destroyed by resumed operations or otherwise, and second, MSHA wants to make sure that any hazard is completely resolved before legal control is returned to the operator. Typically, before being able to resume operations, the operator must advise MSHA specifically what will be done to protect the miners and prevent another accident. This may call for exceeding the minimum requirements of law in certain circumstances.

After an accident investigation, MSHA will notify the operator of any citations or orders that will be issued for any violations identified during the investigation.[37] Penalties will eventually be assessed and they can be quite high—up to the statutory maximum (more than $50,000) for each violation cited. An official Accident Investigation Report will be issued and this will be referred to the MSHA Civil Penalty Assessment Office for consideration in determining the amount of penalty to be assessed under MSHA's Special Assessment program. Final resolution of civil penalty assessments against the operator does not necessarily bring matters related to the investigation to a conclusion. Both the operator—and the operator's agents, if the operator is a corporation—are subject to further criminal or civil penalties for any offenses that may be the subject of a later special investigation or other investigation into possible criminal conduct.

Special Investigations

As has been stressed, special investigations can be monumental events. They always involve serious violations and always raise the possibility that one or more individuals, including directors, officers, managers, or supervisors (agents) of corporate operators, will be prosecuted civilly or criminally as a result of alleged personal culpability with respect to the violation or violations under investigation.[38] The triggers for special investigations may include unwarrantable failure charges, imminent danger charges with high negligence findings, citations, or orders that point blame at a particular person by name or position, and findings from other types of investigations. Such other types of investigations may include investigations into alleged unlawful discrimination by the mine operator against a miner in a protected status under the Act, and investigations into hazard complaints filed by miners.

Every MSHA district office has special investigators. Organizationally, they report to MSHA headquarters, but they also are under the direction of the district manager of their particular district. At MSHA headquarters, reports of special investigators are reviewed by the Chief of the Technical Compliance and Investigation Division for the particular type of mining at issue (coal or metal/nonmetal). Determinations are made, with the assistance of attorneys from the Department of Labor (Office of the Solicitor), whether and to what extent alleged violations of individuals will be prosecuted civilly by the Labor Department or referred to the U.S. Department of Justice for criminal prosecution by the appropriate U.S. Attorney.

The time limit for completing a special investigation and filing a criminal case against an individual is 5 years.[39] Sometimes MSHA will notify a person that its investigation is being closed, but generally it will not. MSHA is reluctant to make such notifications because there may be later discovered evidence.

As with other types of investigations, providing a statement to MSHA is a completely voluntary matter. However, giving a statement is everyone's right and no person may interfere with that right or direct a person to not give a statement to MSHA investigators.

Discrimination Investigations

Section 105(c) of the Mine Act provides:

> No person shall discharge or in any manner discriminate against ... or otherwise interfere with the exercise of the statutory rights of any miner, representative of miners or applicant for employment ...[40]

The Mine Act, in section 105(c), provides detailed procedures to address discrimination against miners, miners' representatives, and applicants for employment because any such person has a protected status or has engaged in protected safety activity. The following are specifically protected:

- Persons who exercise any rights provided by the act
- Persons who complain about an alleged danger or safety or health violation

- Persons who refuse to work in the face of a hazardous condition
- Persons who are the subject of medical evaluation and job transfer under law
- Persons who institute any proceedings under the act
- Persons who testify, or who are about to testify, in any proceeding under the act.[41]

In practice, investigations into possible unlawful discrimination begin when an individual files a written complaint with MSHA identifying the alleged discriminatory actions. Assuming that the complainant has stated facts that constitute unlawful discrimination under the Mine Act, MSHA will promptly investigate with the intention of producing a determination on the case within ninety days. If the investigation is deemed to establish a violation by the operator, the Secretary of Labor will represent the miner in legal proceedings to redress the violation. Even before such a case is tried, however, MSHA can seek temporary reinstatement of a discharged miner, and this is done routinely. The temporary reinstatement normally keeps the complainant at work unless and until a decision is rendered in the legal case finding that there was no actionable discrimination.[42]

Where a violation of the section 105(c) discrimination provisions of the act is found, the operator will be ordered to reinstate the complainant, make up back pay and benefits, take such other actions as may be ordered to put the miner in the position he or she would have been in had the discrimination not occurred.[43] The operator will also be assessed a civil penalty under MSHA's Special Assessment Program.

Hazard Investigations

There is one other event at mines that sometimes proceeds in the manner of an investigation. Special inspections done to inquire into complaints of hazardous conditions by miners or their representatives may only focus on current conditions and, therefore, are much like any other inspection. However, in many cases allegations may pertain to past events or conditions. In such cases, the special inspection may take on the character of an investigation.

Inspectors ask probing questions of persons at the mine and may even seek to record interviews by using tape recorders or making detailed notes. If an inquiry takes this tack, it essentially becomes an investigation with all of the serious legal implications attached. Moreover, it may possibly produce evidence that will lead to a special investigation later.

If an inspector conducting this inquiry concludes that violations or dangers exist, that inspector is required to issue appropriate citations or orders. (They may, and often do, issue such citations or orders based solely on information provided by witnesses.) If no hazards or violations are uncovered, the inspector is required to issue a "notice of negative finding." Such findings are subject to informal review by MSHA at the request of the party that made the complaint in the first place. Such requests for informal review must be filed with MSHA within ten days.[44] As with all violations, citations and orders issued during a Hazard Investigation are subject to mandatory civil penalty assessments, and occasionally they may be subject to criminal penalties.

PENALTIES FOR VIOLATIONS

Civil Penalties

As the Mine Act has been interpreted, civil penalties are mandatory for every violation cited by an inspector.[45] By law MSHA can only *propose* civil penalties. They are not final or collectible unless and until they become a final order of the Federal Mine Safety and Health Review Commission. However, the program is set up so that if an operator or other person fails to challenge a proposed penalty within thirty days, then the penalty will become a final order of the commission by operation of law.[46]

Operators are the primary parties subject to civil penalty assessments, but they are not the only ones. A miner who violates rules prohibiting smoking or having smoking materials may be personally assessed a civil penalty. Also, as previously indicated, directors, officers, and agents (managers and supervisors) may be subject to personal civil penalties for violations that such persons "knowingly authorized, ordered or carried out." The various types of civil penalties applicable to operators, and sometimes individuals, are described on the following page.

Nominal–Non-S&S Penalty Assessments   Some violations are technical and do not really involve risk to persons. They are not of such a nature as could significantly and substantially contribute to the cause and effect of a mine hazard. In such cases, unless MSHA makes a determination that a higher penalty is warranted, the non-S&S violation will be assessed a nominal penalty of a relatively low fixed amount. The major exceptions are violations deemed unwarrantable or resulting in imminent danger and the like. Such violations, even if they do not carry an S&S designation, will be assessed under MSHA's special assessment procedures. In addition, if the operator is deemed to have an excessive history of violations, the operator will be ineligible for a nominal assessment.[47] In cases of excess history, there is no nominal penalty; rather, the regular assessment calculation is done, but a factor is added to substantially inflate the penalties.

Regular (Computer Calculated) Assessments   Under MSHA's regulations, a formula is provided for calculation of proposed civil penalties based on points assigned for each finding made by an inspector with respect to a cited condition.[48] For all civil penalty assessments, MSHA is to take into account six specific criteria established by Congress for determining final assessments by the commission. The six criteria are:

- Operator's history of previous violations
- Size of the business of the operator
- Whether the operator was negligent
- The effect of the penalty on the operator's business
- The gravity of the violation
- The operator's good faith in correcting the cited condition.[49]

Daily Penalty Assessments   Under the Mine Act, MSHA has authority to propose daily civil penalties for every day that an operator fails to correct a violation.[50] In practice, daily civil penalties are rarely used. Operators are not inclined to engage in a course of conduct that would unlawfully defy MSHA, even if they think the agency is completely wrong about something because MSHA has so many enforcement tools at its disposal. In any event, daily penalties are one more way for MSHA to enforce the Mine Act.

Special Assessments   By regulation, MSHA may elect to waive the normal computer formula for assessing penalties if "conditions surrounding the violation warrant special assessment." MSHA regulations state in essence that some types of violations may be of such a nature or seriousness that the computer formula will not be appropriate. In other words, the MSHA Assessment Office must make a specific determination with respect to the penalty.[51] Invariably, special assessments are much higher than regular assessments. The maximum penalty of $50,000 per violation is periodically adjusted upward for inflation.

The list of cases that call for a special assessment is essentially as follows:

- Fatalities and serious injuries
- Unwarrantable failures
- Defiance of a MSHA Closure Order
- Refusal of entry to an inspector
- Violations for which individuals are liable
  - Imminent danger
  - Discrimination violations
  - Violations due to extraordinarily high negligence or aggravating factors.[52]

Individual Civil Penalty Assessments   Generally speaking, individuals are subject to civil penalties if they are agents of a corporate operator and they knowingly authorize, order, or carry out a violation.[53] In practice, before such assessments are proposed, a special investigation is conducted to gather evidence—or evidence is gathered from some other investigation record, such as an accident or discrimination investigation.

Before a proposed assessment is finally decided upon, the individual in question is given an opportunity to have a conference with the MSHA district manager or delegate. Thereafter, if the case proceeds it will be referred to MSHA's Assessment Office. After an assessment is proposed, the individual has 30 days from the date of service of the papers to contest the violation. Failure to timely contest will typically result in the proposed assessment's becoming final and not subject to further review.

Criminal Penalties

Willful Violations   Individuals as well as companies can be prosecuted for violations of law that they willfully authorize, order, or carry out. Individuals may be sentenced to prison, house detention, work release, or probation. There have been numerous instances in which these various aspects of criminal sentencing have been invoked. Among the most frequent reasons for prosecution are illegal mining and fraudulent activity related to MSHA compliance obligations.

The Mine Act (like so many other federal laws) makes reference to certain maximum penalty amounts that are no longer applicable. Today, criminal penalties are set in conformity with mandatory sentencing guidelines that were subsequently enacted by Congress. Fines for criminal violations by a company, generally speaking, can be as high as $500,000 for any violation associated with a fatality and $250,000 for other criminal violations.[54] One company paid a total of $500,000 for two misdemeanor violations under a plea agreement in a case that did not involve any injury.

Advance Notice of Inspection   Because of an expressed concern among certain members of Congress that the effectiveness of MSHA inspections was perhaps being compromised under prior legislation, the Mine Act includes criminal penalties, including imprisonment, for any person who gives advance notice of any inspection to be conducted under the Act.[55] Again, the penalties specified in the act as enacted are now greatly magnified.

False Statements   The Mine Act provides for criminal fines against anyone who knowingly makes a false statement or certification in any application, record, report, or other document filed or required to be maintained under the Act.[56] Again, sentencing guidelines, not the Mine Act, will control the sentence imposed.

Misrepresented Equipment   Under the Mine Act, certain types of equipment must be certified as approved or permissible. In acquiring such equipment from manufacturers, distributors, or prior owners, companies naturally rely on representations as to the equipment's suitability under the law. Thus, the Mine Act makes it a crime, subject to fine and imprisonment, to knowingly distribute or sell any equipment represented as suitable for use in a mine, if the equipment or component does not fully comply with legal requirements.[57]

LEGAL PROCEEDINGS

Federal Mine Safety and Health Review Commission

The Mine Act created an independent agency that hears and decides cases arising under the act. The commission is a panel of five commissioners appointed by the president and confirmed by the Senate. The normal term for each commissioner is six years. Terms are staggered so they do not expire at the same time. New appointments or reappointments occur every two years.[58]

The main types of cases that the commission hears are:

- Operator contests of citations or orders
- Contests of proposed penalties by operators or individuals
- Complaints for compensation by miners idled by an order
- Complaints of discrimination related to safety.[59]

In practice, each type of case is initiated within a prescribed time period by the interested party, with service of documents on all other parties. Most proceedings are initiated by the Secretary of Labor (MSHA) and operators. Miners and their representatives participate in cases as they deem appropriate. Cases are initially assigned to an ALJ for a trial and a decision based on application of pertinent law. If any party objects to the outcome then the commission will act as an appellate tribunal and review the ALJ's decision.[60]

Labor Department—Petitions for Modification

One type of case has not been assigned to the commission. Petitions for Modification are proceedings in which operators (or miners) seek to have MSHA modify the application of a particular safety standard at a particular mine. To obtain a modification, an applicant or petitioner must prove either that applying the standard as it exists would cause a "diminution of safety" or that there is another way that the goals of the regulation can be accomplished in a better or equally safe manner.[61] If a resolution is not worked out with MSHA after a preliminary inquiry by the agency, the case will be referred to an ALJ who works, not for the commission, but rather directly for the Labor Department. The ALJ is required to follow the usual administrative procedures aimed at securing an independent and impartial decision supported by findings of fact and conclusions of law.[62]

Federal District Court

Under the Mine Act, federal district courts have a specialized role. Primarily, they hear criminal cases involving violations of the Mine Act or other provisions of criminal law. District courts also hear government requests for injunctions in cases where operators refuse entry to inspectors or resist enforcement in other ways that may require some force, such as federal marshals, to correct. Finally, federal district courts also hear collection proceedings in cases where persons have not paid final civil penalties.[63]

U.S. Courts of Appeals

The U.S. Courts of Appeals hear all petitions from final agency actions including cases arising out of challenged rulemaking and promulgation of safety and health standards. Courts of Appeals also hear all appeals from final actions of the commission.[64]

CONCLUSION

The Mine Act has established a comprehensive and intense regulatory program for mines. Meeting the requirements of the Mine Act is a continual challenge for operators and miners. Moreover, MSHA inspectors and investigators are always monitoring performance and if operators do not comply, they will be subject to serious civil and criminal penalties. The most important thing, however, is for every mine to be safe. It takes mine operators and miners working together to make good compliance a reality.

Citations are to the *U.S. Code* (USC), the *Code of Federal Regulation* (CFR), the Federal Mine Safety and Health Review Commission (FMSHRC) cases, the *MSHA Program Policy Manual*, and the *Federal Register* (Fed. Reg.).

1. Federal Mine Safety and Health Act of 1977, 30 USC §§ 801–962 (1999).
2. 30 USC § 823.
3. 30 USC § 802(d); 30 CFR Part 45.
4. *See* 30 CFR Parts 56, 57, 70, 71, 75, 77.
5. 30 USC § 825; 30 CFR Part 48; *MSHA Program Policy Manual,* Vol. III, Release III-3 (1990).
6. 30 USC § 961.
7. Occupational Safety and Health Act of 1970, 29 USC § 651, *et seq.*
8. The National Institute for Occupational Safety and Health (NIOSH), within the Department of Health and Human Services (HHS), was created by the OSHA statute and serves to research safety and health standards in the workplace and to make recommendations to the Department of Labor based on its research. 29 USC § 671. Under the Mine Act, NIOSH, as part of HHS, has authority to inspect and investigate a mine in order to gather information for its research. 30 USC § 813(a).
9. 30 USC § 961.
10. 30 CFR Parts 56, 57 (Metal and Nonmetal Mine Safety and Health); 30 CFR Parts 70–72 (Coal Mine Health); 30 CFR Parts 75, 77 (Coal Mine Safety).
11. 30 USC § 802(d).
12. 30 USC § 802(h)(1).
13. *Id.*
14. MSHA–OSHA Interagency Agreement, 44 Fed. Reg. 22827 (1979), *amended by* 48 Fed. Reg. 7521 (1983).

15. 30 USC § 819(d); 30 CFR Part 41.
16. 30 CFR § 100.3.
17. 30 USC § 802(e).
18. 30 USC § 820; 30 CFR § 41.13.
19. 30 USC § 813(a),(i).
20. 30 USC § 820(e).
21. 30 USC § 813(f).
22. 30 USC § 813(g).
23. 30 USC § 814(a).
24. 30 USC § 814(d)(1), (e)(1). A violation will be Significant and Substantial "if, based upon the particular facts surrounding that violation, there exists a reasonable likelihood that the hazard contributed to will result in an injury or illness of a reasonably serious nature." *Secretary of Labor v. Cement Div., National Gypsum Co.*, 2 MSHC (BNA) 1201 (FMSHRC 1981).
25. 30 USC §§ 813(j), (k), 814(b), (d), (e), (f), (g), 817(a).
26. 30 USC § 821.
27. 30 USC §§ 802(j) (definition of imminent danger), 817(a) (imminent danger order).
28. 30 USC § 813(k).
29. 30 USC § 814(b).
30. *Emery Mining Corp. v. Secretary of Labor*, 4 MSHC (BNA) 1585 (FMSHRC 1987).
31. 30 USC § 814(d).
32. *Id.*
33. 30 USC § 814(e).
34. 30 CFR § 100.6.
35. 30 USC § 813(j).
36. 30 CFR § 50.2(h).
37. 30 USC § 815(a).
38. 30 USC § 820.
39. 18 USC § 3282.
40. 30 USC § 815(c).
41. 30 USC § 815(c); *see also Robinette v. United Castle Coal Company*, 2 MSHC (BNA) 1213 (FMSHRC 1981) (holding that the Mine Act protects a worker who refuses to work because of a good faith, reasonable belief that a hazardous condition exists).
42. 30 USC § 815(c)(2), (c)(3); 29 CFR § 2700.45.
43. 30 USC § 815(c)(2).
44. 30 CFR Part 43.
45. 30 USC § 820(a).
46. 30 USC § 815(a).
47. 30 CFR § 100.4.
48. 30 CFR § 100.3; *see also* 30 CFR § 100.4.
49. 30 CFR § 100.3; *see* 30 USC § 820(i).
50. 30 USC § 820(b).
51. 30 CFR § 100.5.
52. *Id.*
53. 30 USC § 820(c).
54. *See* 18 USC § 3571.
55. 30 USC § 820(e).
56. 30 USC § 820(f).
57. 30 USC § 820(h).
58. 30 USC § 823.
59. *See* 29 CFR Part 2700.
60. 30 USC § 823(d).
61. 30 USC § 811(c).
62. 30 CFR Part 44, Subpart C, § 44.15.
63. 30 USC §§ 818, 820.
64. 30 USC §§ 811(d), 816.

CHAPTER 8

Other Regulatory Requirements Impacting Mining

Mark N. Savit, Esq.
Patton Boggs LLP, Washington, D.C.[1]

Adele L. Abrams, Esq.
Law Office of Adele L. Abrams, Calverton, Maryland

JURISDICTION: WHO ARE THE REGULATORS?

Aside from the Mine Safety and Health Administration (MSHA), there are myriad federal, state, and local agencies that can affect health and safety at mining operations. Perhaps because of their greater variety, the intervention of many of these agencies appears to be more prevalent at metal and non-metal mining operations than at coal mines. Nevertheless, as shown below, intervention of any federal agency described in this chapter could occur at virtually any mining operation at any time. Often, their intervention follows a major accident at which not only MSHA but also several other agencies may appear. In fact, in the authors' experience, it is common for four or more federal and state agencies to appear on site in the immediate aftermath of a major accident.[2]

The fact that multiple agency intervention is most likely to occur following a major accident makes it all the more important for prudent mine operators or health and safety officers to familiarize themselves, to the extent appropriate, with each of the agencies that could play a role in the regulation of the mines operations. This chapter discusses the most significant of these federal agencies:

- Occupational Safety and Health Administration (OSHA)
- Federal Railroad Administration (FRA)
- Environmental Protection Agency (EPA)[3]
- National Institute for Occupational Safety and Health (NIOSH)
- National Transportation Safety Board (NTSB)
- Chemical Safety and Hazard Investigation Board (CSB)
- U.S. Coast Guard
- Bureau of Alcohol, Tobacco and Firearms (ATF), in the most general sense.

1. The authors acknowledge the contributions of Patton Boggs' associates Michael D. Bloomquist, Amy B. Chasanov, and Michael T. Palmer to this project.
2. This chapter does not discuss any state or local enforcement or regulatory agencies. However, sometimes state health and safety agencies will play a pivotal role in the investigation of an accident, the enforcement of health and safety related regulations, and the institution of enforcement actions, if any.
3. Because EPA regulations deal with environmental quality, the discussion in this chapter is limited to the rules regarding hazardous waste operations (HAZWOPER).

An attempt is made to discuss the extent, as well as the limits, of each agency's jurisdiction, as well as its most salient regulatory authority. Anyone who may interact with the agencies discussed in this chapter should consult additional sources before engaging in any activity that could result in liability.

AGENCIES REGULATING HEALTH AND SAFETY AT MINING OPERATIONS

Occupational Safety and Health Administration

OSHA was created pursuant to the Occupational Safety and Health Act of 1970 (the OSH Act), 29 USC § 651 *et seq.*, and is a separate agency within the U.S. Department of Labor. Like the Mine Act, the OSH Act gave authority to the Secretary of Labor to promulgate standards for regulating health and safety in the workplace.

OSHA standards cover four main categories: General Industry Standards, 29 *Code of Federal Regulations* (CFR) Part 1910; Construction Standards, 29 CFR Part 1926; Maritime and Longshoring Standards, 29 CFR Parts 1915, 1918; and Agricultural Standards, 29 CFR Part 1928. The relevant specific industry standard is cited with respect to workplace conditions found in violation of the OSH Act. However, where a specific standard is not applicable, OSHA may cite employers for violating its General Duty Clause.[4]

The OSH Act covers employment in all 50 states, the District of Columbia, Puerto Rico, the Virgin Islands, and most remaining U.S. territories and possessions.[5] However, there are certain jurisdictional limits under the OSH Act. Operators of mines, as that term is defined in the Mine Act, are exempt under Section 4(b)(1) of the OSH Act because MSHA has primary jurisdiction. As mentioned above, MSHA is a separate agency within the Department of Labor, which regulates mining workplace and exercises authority to promulgate and enforce standards over such facilities, and its activities and powers are discussed in detail elsewhere in this book.

To delineate certain areas of authority and provide a procedure for resolving general jurisdictional questions, MSHA and OSHA entered into an interagency agreement (IA).[6] Not surprisingly, one of the guiding principles between the two entities is that, with respect to unsafe working conditions on mine sites and at milling operations, MSHA is charged with enforcement. However, the IA provides that where the provisions of the Mine Act do not otherwise cover health and safety conditions at a mine or mill (e.g., hospitals at mine sites), then the Secretary of Labor may apply provisions of the OSH Act. Additional principles in the agreement provide that a worksite, which would normally fall under the jurisdiction of the Mine Act, shall be regulated under the OSH Act where no existing MSHA standards apply to the site.[7]

The IA provides a list of certain industries—and operations within certain industries—that have been deemed to fall within the jurisdictional sweep of either MSHA or OSHA. In addition to the facilities commonly thought of as mines (e.g., stone quarries, strip mines, and underground coal and metal mines), MSHA jurisdiction includes salt processing facilities on mine property, electrolytic plants where the plants are an integral part of milling operations, stone cutting and stone sawing operations on mine property where such operations do not occur in a stone polishing or finishing plant, and alumina and cement plants.[8]

OSHA jurisdiction includes the following, whether or not they are located on mine property: brick, clay pipe, and refractory plants; ceramic plants; fertilizer product operations; concrete batch,

---

4. The General Duty Clause is found in Section 5(a) of the OSH Act and provides that covered employees shall provide a workplace that is free from acknowledged hazards causing, or likely to cause, death or serious physical harm or illness. To prove a General Duty Clause violation, the Secretary of Labor must demonstrate: (1) a condition or activity in the employer's workplace presented a hazard or could potentially prove to be hazardous for employees; (2) the employer or the employer's industry had full or partial knowledge of the hazard; (3) the hazard could potentially have caused or was likely to cause death or serious physical harm; and (4) reasonable means existed to eliminate or reduce the threat posed by the hazard.

5. In recent years the OSH Act's jurisdiction has been expanded to cover certain additional employees in the public sector, including the U.S. Postal Service. In addition, states and territories may enforce their own health and safety standards if they have a state plan approved by the Secretary of Labor.

6. 44 Fed. Reg. 22827 (April 17, 1979), *amended by* 48 Fed. Reg. 7521 (February 22, 1983).

7. IA at A(3).

8. IA at B(6)(a).

asphalt batch, and hot mix plants; smelters and refineries.[9] In addition, OSHA jurisdiction extends to salt distribution terminals, cement distribution terminals, and milling operations associated with gypsum board plants, provided those facilities are not located on mine property.[10] Finally, the IA specifies that borrow pits are subject to OSHA jurisdiction unless the pits are located on mine property or are related to mining.[11]

The courts have generally granted MSHA broad jurisdiction over both primary and ancillary activities conducted at the mine site,[12] although the text of the Mine Act defines MSHA's jurisdiction as extending only to mines and then, only if the products of the mine enter or affect commerce.[13] The term mine is defined, in pertinent part, as:

> *an area of land from which minerals are extracted in nonliquid form ... private ways and roads appurtenant to such area, and ... lands, excavations, underground passageways, shafts, slopes, tunnels and workings, structures,* facilities, equipment, machines, tools, or other property *including impoundments, retention dams, and tailings ponds, on the surface or underground, used in, or to be used in, or resulting from, the work of extracting such minerals from their natural deposits ... or used in, or to be used in, the milling of such minerals, or the work of preparing coal or other minerals .... In making a determination of what constitutes mineral milling for purposes of this Act, the Secretary shall give due consideration to the convenience of administration resulting from the delegation to one Assistant Secretary of all authority with respect to the health and safety of miners employed at one physical establishment ...*[14]

In recent legal challenges to MSHA's authority, MSHA was found to have jurisdiction over demolition contractors at a site where coal was handled for processing at a cogeneration plant,[15] but not at a coal-fired electric power plant,[16] an electric utility,[17] or an abandoned coal silo.[18] MSHA has long resisted any attempt to split off functions so as to avoid its jurisdiction. In *Mineral Coal Sales, Inc.*,[19] the Federal Mine Safety and Health Review Commission affirmed MSHA jurisdiction, noting:

> *[I]nherent in the determination of whether an operation properly is classified as 'mining' is an inquiry not only into whether the operation performs one or more of the ... activities [listed in § 3(i) of the Mine Act], but also into the* nature *of the operation performing such activities....*

Otherwise, facilities could avoid Mine Act coverage simply by adopting separate business identities along functional lines, with each performing only some part of what, in reality, is one operation.[20]

---

9. IA at B(6)(b).

10. *Id.*

11. A "borrow pit" is an area of land where the overburden is extracted from the surface. Extraction occurs on a one-time-only basis or only intermittently as the need occurs, for use as fill materials by the extracting party in the form in which it is extracted. If milling is needed, other than for removal of large rocks, wood, and trash, the operation likely would constitute mining and be subject to MSHA jurisdiction. See IA at B(7).

12. The Senate Report on the 1977 Act stated:

   > *... it is the Committee's intention that what is considered to be a mine and to be regulated under this Act be given the broadest possibl[e] interpretation, and it is the intent of this Committee that doubts be resolved in favor of inclusion of a facility within the coverage of the Act.*

   S. Rep. No. 181, 95th Cong., 1st Sess. 14 (1977).

13. *See* 30 USC § 804.

14. Section 3(h)(1) of the Mine Act, 30 USC § 802(h)(1) (emphasis added).

15. *RNS Services, Inc.* v. *Secretary of Labor,* 115 F.3d 182 (3d Cir. 1997).

16. *Herman* v. *Associated Electric Cooperative, Inc.*, 172 F.3d 1078 (8th Cir. 1999). *But see United Energy Services, Inc.* v. *FMSHRC,* 35 F.3d 971 (4th Cir. 1994) (affirming MSHA jurisdiction over contractors at electric cogeneration power plant).

17. *Old Dominion Power Co.* v. *Donovan,* 772 F.2d 92 (4th Cir. 1985).

18. *Lancashire Coal Co.* v. *Secretary of Labor,* 968 F.2d 388 (3d Cir. 1992).

19. *Mineral Coal Sales, Inc.,* 7 FMSHRC 615 (Commission, 1985).

20. *Id.* Judicial interpretation of the Mine Act holds that a company is not required to extract minerals before being subject to MSHA jurisdiction, nor is a connection with the extractor required for a facility to be regulated by MSHA. *See Donovan* v. *Carolina Stalite Co.,* 734 F.2d 1547 (D.C. Cir. 1984); *Alexander Brothers, Inc.,* 4 FMSHRC 541, 543-44, n. 8 & 9 (Commission, 1982).

MSHA jurisdiction has also been conferred on what might otherwise be an OSHA operation when some equipment (i.e., conveyors and electric motors) is used at both mining and nonmining facilities. The commission looks at "the integrated nature of the operation" and whether exposure of workers to mine hazards is sufficient to confer jurisdiction upon MSHA.

When a question of MSHA/OSHA jurisdiction arises, the IA directs the appropriate MSHA district manager and OSHA regional administrator or OSHA state designee to attempt to resolve the matter at the local level. If unsuccessful, they are to refer the matter to their respective national offices. In the absence of litigation, the Secretary of Labor makes the final decision.

Federal Railroad Administration

Congress enacted the Federal Railroad Safety Act in 1970 "to promote safety in all areas of railroad operations and to reduce railroad-related accidents, and to reduce deaths and injuries to persons and to reduce damage to property caused by accidents involving any carriers of hazardous materials" (45 USC § 421). The Secretary of Transportation established the FRA **pursuant** to this legislation. As part of its mandate, the FRA has established regulations regarding railroad safety standards and operating rules as well as railroad installation, maintenance, inspection, and repair. It enforces its rules through civil and criminal penalties that may be levied against railroad owners or operators who fail to adhere to FRA rules.

Because many mines have railroad tracks and/or rail yards on their property to convey materials to and from their mines, potential jurisdictional conflicts between MSHA and the FRA do arise. A common example is MSHA's attempt to impose its training requirements on railroad employees because MSHA interprets the employees' conduct as a mining function. By contrast, the FRA may interpret the same employees' conduct as a railroad function that does not require mine-specific training. Despite the relative frequency of such debates, there are no formal memoranda between MSHA and the FRA regarding issues of overlapping jurisdiction, nor are there established processes to resolve jurisdictional disputes. When conflicts do arise, they are generally worked out between the FRA's Office of Chief Counsel and the Department of Labor's Office of the Solicitor. However, this is not always the case, and any mine operator who may have to contend with potential conflicts between the FRA and MSHA should be prepared before they arise.

Although the FRA has broad authority to regulate railroads, the FRA does not currently exercise its jurisdiction to the full extent possible. Instead, the FRA regulates only railroads operating on the general railroad system (i.e., the network of standard gauge railroads over which passengers travel and goods are transported; 49 CFR Part 209, Appendix A). FRA's regulations do not extend to "plant railroads," where the entire operation of the railroad is confined to the boundaries of the industrial installation. Thus, to the extent a mine operates a completely internal railroad system, MSHA is likely to have jurisdiction over that railroad's operations, rather than the FRA. In fact, MSHA has promulgated regulations relating to such railcar activities.[21]

There are instances when a major railroad operating as part of the general railroad system enters a mine or industrial plant. If that major railroad enters the mine property for a limited period of time, its activities remain subject to FRA regulations while on mine property. Similarly, a mine railroad may find itself subject to FRA regulations when it operates on the general railroad system. Given the FRA's broad authority, it is important to remember that the FRA could decide in the future to amend its regulations to include railroads that are currently excluded from its jurisdiction.

In some instances, MSHA may assert jurisdiction over railroad workers or the owners and operators of a railroad. As noted above, Congress intended a broad definition of a "mine" under MSHA. As such, the Mine Act defines a "coal or other mine" to include "private ways and roads appurtenant to such area [from which minerals are extracted]" and "facilities, equipment ... or other property ... used in ... the work of preparing coal or other minerals" [30 USC § 802(h)(1)]. The work of preparing coal includes storing and loading coal [30 USC § 802(i)]. Given this focus on preparation, activities relating to the delivery of raw coal to a processing facility are covered under the Mine Act, but those relating to the delivery of processed coal to the ultimate consumer are unlikely to be covered by the

---

21. See, e.g., 30 CFR § 57.14214 (train warnings) and § 77.1607 (v)-(aa) (loading and haulage equipment-operation).

Act.[22] Further, mine operators may be held liable for MSHA violations of their independent contractors, such as companies providing rail-switching services, or owners of tracks used for loading coal at a mine.[23] In addition, railroad owners themselves may be considered an operator under MSHA, since MSHA has asserted broad jurisdiction over independent contractors that perform services at a mine.[24]

Additionally, individuals employed by railroad companies or whose jobs are rail-related may be considered miners if the tasks are performed at an MSHA-regulated site. A number of decisions have found that railroad employees who work at mines (e.g., shoveling and cleaning coal out of railroad cars before cars taken to coal preparation plant for loading) should be considered miners who are eligible for blacklung benefits under the Black Lung Benefits Act.[25]

In short, to the extent that railroad or railway companies are considered operators, or rail employees are considered miners, such companies may be subject to MSHA safety and health standards and the statutory provisions of the Mine Act.

Hazardous Waste Operations and Emergency Response Standard

OSHA mandates that in some instances emergency response operations undertaken to respond to releases of hazardous substances must meet particular standards. There are two applications of this standard that could potentially apply to mines [29 CFR Part 1910.120(a)(1)]:

> *(1) Operations involving hazardous wastes that are conducted as treatment, storage, and disposal (TSD) facilities regulated by 40 CFR parts 264 and 265 pursuant to RCRA* (Resource Conservation and Recovery Act)*; or by agencies under agreement with U.S.E.P.A. to implement RCRA regulations and*

> *(2) Emergency response operations for releases of, or substantial threats of releases of, hazardous substances without regard to the location of the hazard.*

For facilities under (1) above, OSHA requires an emergency response plan and training. There are more exacting requirements for facilities under (2) above; these include a safety and health program, site control procedures before cleanup begins, medical surveillance of employees, monitoring of exposure, and informational programs, among others.

The MSHA/OSHA IA, discussed previously, confirms the relationship between the two agencies.[26] When MSHA does not have enforceable standards, the agency refers matters to OSHA for appropriate action. However, MSHA has promulgated regulations governing mine rescue teams, which detail the requirements for training mine rescue teams (30 CFR § 49.8) and mine emergency notification plans (30 CFR § 49.9). MSHA also provides for hazard training of mine workers under 30 CFR § 48.11 (underground mining) and § 48.31 (surface mining). Given the existing regulations promulgated by MSHA, it does not appear that EPA or OSHA may impose the 29 CFR § 1910.120 standards on mines.

Nevertheless, situations have arisen in areas of disputed or confused jurisdiction where either EPA and OSHA have insisted that the hazardous waste operations (HAZWOPER) rules must be followed. In such situations, operators must understand the limits of each agency's jurisdiction and be prepared to support the position that is legally correct and most advantageous to the operation in question.

---

22. See *Pennsylvania Electric Co.* v. *FMSHRC*, 969 F.2d 1501 (3d Cir. 1992) (affirming MSHA jurisdiction over electric company's conveyors that were used to transport coal from mine to processing station).

23. See, e.g., *Harman Mining Corp.* v. *FMSHRC*, 671 F.2d 794 (4th Cir. 1981).

24. *See* 30 USC §802(d) (operator definition includes "any independent contractor performing services or construction at such mine); *Otis Elevator Co.* v. *Secretary of Labor*, 921 F.2d 1285 (D.C. Cir. 1991) (all independent contractors performing services at a mine are operators).

25. For example, in *Mitchell v. Director, Office of Worker's Compensation Programs*, 855 F.2d 485 (7th Cir. 1988), the court found that a railroad employee who worked under the direction of coal mine employees at the mine site and who helped prepare coal for delivery should be considered a miner. Additionally, a railroad brakeman/conductor was a coal miner under the Black Lung Benefits Act because he hauled raw coal from mines to a preparation plant and spent a significant amount of time in or around the mine. *Norfolk & Western Railway Co.* v. *Roberson*, 918 F.2d 1144 (4th Cir.), *cert. denied*, 500 U.S. 916.

26. 44 Fed. Reg. 22827 (April 17, 1979), amended by 48 Fed. Reg. 7521 (February 22, 1983).

National Institute for Occupational Safety and Health

NIOSH is part of the Centers for Disease Control and Prevention (CDC) within the Department of Health and Human Services (HHS). NIOSH is the federal agency responsible for research and prevention of workplace hazards. It is headquartered in Washington, D.C., and has facilities in Anchorage, Alaska; Atlanta, Georgia; Cincinnati, Ohio; Morgantown, West Virginia; Pittsburgh, Pennsylvania; and Spokane, Washington. HHS is responsible for implementing the Mine Act[27] 30 USC § 801 *et seq*.

Sec. 101(a) (6) (B) of the Mine Act provides, in relevant part:

> *The Secretary [of HEW] ... on a continuing basis ... shall, for each toxic material or harmful physical agent which is used or found in a mine, determine whether such material or agent is potentially toxic at the concentrations in which it is used or found in a mine [and] submit such determinations with respect to such toxic substances or harmful physical agents to the Secretary [of Labor].... Within 60 days after receiving any criteria ... relating to a toxic material or harmful physical agent which is not adequately covered by a mandatory health or safety standard promulgated under this section, the Secretary [of Labor] shall either appoint an advisory committee to make recommendations with respect to a mandatory health or safety standard covering such material or agent ... or publish a proposed rule promulgating such a mandatory health or safety standard ... or shall publish his determination not to do so.*

In recent years, NIOSH has fulfilled this obligation by issuing criteria documents, reports, and comments, and conducting research on such "materials" and "agents" as coal dust, silica, and diesel particulate matter, as well as on health issues such as noise and ergonomics. In fiscal year 1997, NIOSH completed the assimilation of the former Bureau of Mines, creating a new Office for Mine Safety & Health Research. NIOSH's mine research is conducted through two laboratories, located in Pittsburgh and Spokane. These facilities conduct surveillance of occupational fatalities, injuries, and diseases; carry out research into control of toxic substances to which miners may be exposed; develop control technology and protective equipment; conduct field investigations and laboratory studies; and develop and recommend criteria for new standards.

The Mine Act also directs NIOSH to coordinate the activities of a Mine Safety and Health Research Advisory Committee (MSHRAC).[28] The committee was formed in 1984 and has been active in advising MSHA and NIOSH on various mining-related health issues and potential research areas. NIOSH's findings frequently form the basis for rulemaking or increased enforced emphasis by MSHA.

Under section 103 (a) of the Mine Act, authorized representatives of NIOSH, like MSHA inspectors, have the right to enter the mine site for the purpose of carrying out investigations, inspections, and other authorized activities, including health research, review of records required by statute, and sampling. The warrantless search authority provided to MSHA under the Mine Act extends equally to NIOSH activities.[29] Thus, as part of its research and investigative functions, NIOSH is authorized to visit mine sites for investigations and to conduct medical examinations and tests.[30] NIOSH also can require mine operators to "establish and maintain such records [and] reports, and provide such information as [NIOSH] may reasonably require" [30 USC § 813 (h)].

Interference with NIOSH's exercise of its statutory powers may result in civil actions against the mine operator. Remedies for violations include permanent or temporary injunctions, restraining orders or other appropriate relief ordered by the U.S. District Court. 30 USC § 818 (a) (1). Civil penalties[31] can also be issued against anyone who is found to have impeded an inspection or investigation conducted by MSHA or NIOSH pursuant to Section 103 (a) of the Mine Act, 30 USC § 813 (a).

---

27. Pub.L. 95-164.
28. 30 USC § 812 (b). It is subject to the requirements of the Federal Advisory Committee Act, 5 USC App. 2.
29. 30 USC § 813(a).
30. Sec. 101 (a) (7) states: "... In the event ... medical examinations are in the nature of research, as determined by the Secretary [of HEW], such examinations may be furnished at the expense of the Secretary [of HEW]. The results of examinations or tests made pursuant to the preceding sentence shall be furnished only to the Secretary [of Labor] or the Secretary [of HEW], and, at the request of the miner, to his designated physician."
31. Citations are issued pursuant to 30 USC § 814 (a) or 30 USC § 814 (d), and the maximum civil penalty per violation is currently $55,000, subject to future increases indexed to inflation.

Any records that the mine operator must prepare and retain under the Mine Act or pursuant to standards promulgated by MSHA—such as injury/illness/fatality reports and inspection and equipment examination records—must be made available to NIOSH representatives for examination at the mine site. The Mine Act does not specifically provide NIOSH with statutory authority to review records and/or results of medical examinations provided to workers by mine operators, either voluntarily or pursuant to regulatory mandates. Subpoena power under the Mine Act does not extend to health research investigations or inspections carried out by NIOSH.[32] Mine operators and their employees may have a privacy interest in the documents, which do not have to be compiled or maintained by law (e.g., medical surveillance and exposure monitoring records, personnel files, and business records). Although NIOSH may be granted legal access to such materials where they are related to mine safety and health research, the agency cannot inspect or copy such documents without legal authorization. Therefore, NIOSH may be required to obtain an administrative warrant to gain access to materials that are not required by statute.

In summary, NIOSH possesses extremely broad powers, virtually the same as those granted to MSHA. The agency has become increasingly active at mine sites over the past several years. Although a visit by NIOSH may not be a common occurrence, all mine operators should be fully prepared to deal with the possibility at all times.

National Transportation Safety Board

The NTSB was created in 1967 to investigate all civil aviation accidents and certain highway accidents, railroad accidents, pipeline accidents, and marine accidents to determine the cause or probable cause of the accident. Consequently, the NTSB may be involved in mine site accident investigations involving rail transportation facilities on mine property or, more rarely, involving over-the-road trucking. Its role is purely investigative and while it has no regulatory authority, attendant to its investigative duties, the NTSB also issues recommendations to other federal, state, and local agencies and private organizations about transportation accidents. On its own initiative it also conducts investigations and studies to determine the adequacy of current safeguards and safety in transportation. To ensure its autonomous status, the NTSB is independently funded and has had no ties to the Department of Transportation or its satellite agencies since 1975.

The NTSB has delegated its investigative duties to its directors and their employees. Under certain circumstances, the directors of the Office of Aviation Safety and the Office of Surface Transportation Safety may order an investigation into any accident or incident involving transportation safety. Once an investigation is initiated, the actual investigation is conducted by the designated investigator in charge. The investigator in charge has extraordinarily broad powers over the conduct of the field investigation, including determining who obtains "party" status and participates in the investigation through that status. The investigator in charge also exerts some influence over the eventual findings of fact and probable cause determination adopted by the NTSB.

The investigator is charged with the responsibility for determining the facts and conditions that led to the accident and making a probable cause determination. The NTSB's investigations are ostensibly nonadversarial fact-finding missions with no formal issues in contest. In practice, however, these investigations can become quite contentious. Ultimately, however, neither the board's factual analysis nor its probable cause determination with respect to an accident are admissible as evidence in court.

At the NTSB's discretion, its investigation will take priority over all other accident investigations conducted by other federal agencies under NTSB jurisdiction. Criminal investigations are the only exception to this broad mandate. Under those circumstances, the Federal Bureau of Investigation (FBI) normally takes charge. This is not to say that other federal agencies are required to place a moratorium over their investigations. This simply means that the other agency's investigation may not interfere with the NTSB investigation.[33]

With the NTSB's limited resources, the investigator in charge usually names parties to an investigation to assist with the investigation. The designated parties are limited to those federal agencies,

---

32. Section 103 (b), 30 USC § 813 (b).

33. In practice, the other federal agencies involved in the accident investigation normally abstain from continuing their investigations until the NTSB has concluded its investigation.

persons, companies, and associations that can provide personnel and technical assistance to the investigation. Insurance company representatives, claimants, and legal representatives are specifically excluded from obtaining party status. Those entities that obtain party status respond to the NTSB and lose party status if they do not comply with their assigned duties or act in a manner prejudicial to the investigation.

The NTSB investigator in charge also has broad discretionary authority with respect to gaining access to property and obtaining evidence of the accident wreckage. In addition, the investigator is provided with express statutory authority to obtain copies of relevant documents and records in the course of the investigation. To assist the investigator in carrying out the statutory duties, the NTSB may issue subpoenas, enforceable in Federal District Court, to obtain evidence or testimony. The investigator is charged with the responsibility of preserving the evidence to the "maximum extent feasible," however, there are no assurances that the evidence will not be lost, destroyed, or irrevocably altered.

Investigations may take several months to complete depending on the nature of the accident and whether any fatalities are involved. In the course of its investigation of major accidents, the NTSB may also hold a public hearing. These hearings are usually held within 6 months of the accident and provide an opportunity to elicit testimony about the accident and investigation. The hearing may also provide an opportunity to provide information to the public about the course of the investigation.

Before making its final report with respect to an accident investigation, any person, federal agency, company, or association whose employees, functions, or products were involved in an accident that is the subject of NTSB investigation may submit to the NTSB written proposed findings, a proposed probable cause, and proposed safety recommendations with respect to the accident.

Although not admissible in court, it is easy to understand how the agency's findings can influence both enforcement actions and actions for damages by or against the entity at which the accident occurred. Care must be taken to ensure that, to the maximum extent practicable, the NTSB is not permitted to reduce the evidentiary value of key components involved in an accident and to ensure that important legal rights are not compromised as a result of NTSB investigative actions.

Chemical Safety and Hazard Investigation Board

The CSB is an independent federal agency that investigates chemical incidents at commercial and industrial facilities, including mines. The CSB's mission is to ensure the safety of workers and the public by determining incident causation,[34] issuing public reports and safety recommendations, and evaluating the effectiveness of other governmental agencies involved with chemical safety. These include MSHA, OSHA, and the EPA.[35]

The CSB is not an enforcement or regulatory body, but functions as a scientific investigatory organization. It is a five-member board modeled after the NTSB. The CSB was established under Section 112 (r)(6)(G) of the Clean Air Amendments of 1990 42 USC § 7412, but it did not begin operations until January 1998. Incidents meeting CSB investigation criteria are those where:

- A chemical release is involved.
- The incident occurred at a fixed facility or in transportation within the United States.
- The incident resulted in one or more of the following:
  - At least one fatality
  - Hospital treatment of at least one person
  - Property damage greater than $250,000
  - Workplace or community evacuation
  - Closure of major transportation arteries
  - Spill cleanup lasting longer than one day.

---

34. The CSB is statutorily required to take an "all cause" approach in investigating accidents, so as to identify all contributory circumstances and not merely the "single, necessary or sufficient cause ...." Pub.L. 101-549, 42 USC § 7412(r) 6 (C).
35. Currently, the CSB has signed Memoranda of Understanding with OSHA and EPA but it has not formalized its relationship with MSHA.

The CSB takes a leadership role in coordinating investigation activities among federal, state, and local agencies and company personnel. As with the NTSB, CSB's conclusions or recommendations may not be used as evidence in any litigation arising from any matter mentioned in a CSB report.[36] Again, as with the NTSB, the mere fact that CSB findings cannot, themselves, be used as evidence, does not mean that these findings cannot form the basis for extremely damaging civil suits or civil or criminal enforcement actions. Between the startup of operations in 1998 and the date of this publication, the CSB has engaged in a limited number of investigations, and it is, therefore, difficult to predict how it will act in a mining-related scenario. For this reason, mine operators should be particularly cautious when CSB is involved with an incident investigation at their operations.

U.S. Coast Guard

The Coast Guard is the principal federal entity responsible for maritime safety, security, and environmental protection. Accordingly, the Coast Guard plays a limited role in the regulation of mining operations involving vessels and commercial mining dredges.

To reduce possible confusion, MSHA and the Coast Guard agreed to cooperate with each other with regard to mining vessels and dredging operations shortly following passage of the Mine Act.[37] Even though the Coast Guard acknowledged that few areas of overlapping jurisdiction and responsibility exist, Coast Guard representatives agreed that MSHA will, in general, regulate vessels that are uninspected under Coast Guard regulations. The Coast Guard continues to inspect and certify vessels engaged in mining. Where there is overlapping regulatory jurisdiction between MSHA and the Coast Guard, the two entities take a mutually appropriate course of action. The agencies apparently still believe that, because of the good working relationship between the MSHA and Coast Guard field offices, there is no need to develop formal agreements. Thus, although each agency regulates different aspects of vessel operations, mining vessels and mining dredges are under the joint jurisdiction of the Coast Guard and MSHA.

Because the agencies regulate such different aspects of vessels operations, it is essential that any operator engaged in marine mining operations on navigable waterways possesses detailed familiarity with the regulations of both agencies. To the extent that compliance with the requirements of any single agency might conflict with those imposed by another, that conflict should be brought to the attention of each agency immediately to eliminate any liability that might result from the conflict.

Bureau of Alcohol, Tobacco, and Firearms

The presence and use of explosives is regular occurrence at most mine sites. Commonly known as the ATF, the bureau is the entity of the federal government that generally regulates and enforces federal laws and regulations relating to the storage and use of explosives. In the context of mine sites, however, ATF's jurisdiction is coextensive with that of MSHA. In addition to setting forth its own standards for the use, handling, and storage of explosives, MSHA's regulations specifically reference and incorporate ATF and U.S. Department of Transportation (DOT) regulations and standards regarding explosives, as well as the voluntary standards of the Institute of Makers of Explosives (IME). [38]

The applicable MSHA metal/nonmetal explosives standards set forth detailed requirements for the storage,[39] transportation,[40] and use of explosives.[41] In many cases, these regulations specifically reference ATF, DOT, or IME requirements.[42] For instance, 30 CFR § 56/57.6000 requires that a "magazine" be a "[B]ATF Type 1 or Type 2 facility" and that a "storage facility used to store blasting agents correspond to an [B]ATF Type 4 or 5 storage facility." Additionally, the MSHA regulations reference

---

36. See Pub.L. 101-549, 42 USC § 7412 (r) 6 (G).
37. Letter from United States Coast Guard to Mine Safety and Health Administration, November 29, 1978.
38. The IME requirements are available at MSHA headquarters, at all MSHA district offices, and at the Office of the Federal Register in Washington, D.C.
39. 30 CFR § 56/57.6100. Facilities, bins, or tanks must also post so visible the appropriate DOT placards or other appropriate warning signs that indicate the contents.
40. 30 CFR § 56/57.6200.
41. 30 CFR § 56/57.6300.
42. The IME requirements for what constitutes a laminated partition are referenced in the MSHA's definitions, storage section, transportation section, and use section of 30 CFR Parts 56/57.

the DOT regulations as to what constitutes a blasting agent, a detonator, or an explosive.[43] Finally, the regulations direct operators to the ATF regulations (tables) affecting storage facilities containing explosive material.[44]

MSHA regulations addressing the use of explosives in coal mining operations stand in sharp contrast to 30 CFR Parts 56/57, in that they do not reference any other agency's regulations. Underground coal blasting regulations are found at 30 CFR §§ 75.1300–1328; surface coal blasting standards are published at 30 CFR §§ 77.1300–1304.

Because MSHA references ATF regulations and standards, the two entities agreed that it was more efficient for mine site inspections to be performed by a single agency. Therefore, the ATF and MSHA executed an IA to define jurisdiction and ensure that industry complied with all applicable regulations.[45] Under the IA, MSHA "agrees to perform on behalf of [B]ATF inspections of storage facilities and records required at the storage site (under 18 USC 841 et seq and applicable regulations in 27 CFR [Part 55]) of all mines subject to MSHA jurisdiction."[46] Further, MSHA will conduct these inspections on behalf of ATF at the same time MSHA performs its regular mine inspection. In the event of a conflict between MSHA and ATF standards, the provision providing for the greater safety or security of persons in and around the mine shall govern. Therefore, the IA makes MSHA responsible for ensuring that mine operators under its jurisdiction comply with ATF and MSHA regulations regarding explosives.

CONCLUSION

The discussion above illustrates the variety of mine activities that may be subject to multiple or competing jurisdictional claims by federal and state agencies. To determine whether a facility may be subject to dual or conflicting jurisdiction, mine operators should contact the individual regulatory agencies or counsel for additional information.

---

43. 49 CFR § 173.114a(a) (blasting agent); §§ 173.53 and 173.100 (Class A and Class C detonators); §§ 173.53, 173.88, and 173.100 (explosive).
44. 30 CFR § 56.6131 cites to 27 CFR §§ 55.218 and 55.220.
45. See 45 Fed. Reg. 25564 (1980).
46. 45 Fed. Reg. at 25565.

CHAPTER 9

Management Strategy and System for Education and Training

George L. Germain
GL&M Associates, Flowery Branch, Georgia

Robert Arnold, Jr.
Newmont Gold, Indonesia

DEFINING THE DISCIPLINE

Many people emphasize the difference between education and training, saying that education focuses on *knowledge* and training focuses on *skills*. Our view is that more emphasis should be given to the similarities, rather than the differences, between them (Germain et al. 1997). Whether we call it education, training, or development, the primary focus should be on *learning*. And, for practical purposes, learning involves the affective, cognitive, and behavioral domains, in other words, attitudes, knowledge, and skills.

Attitudes

Psychologists often call this the *affective* domain. It relates to vital factors such as feelings, emotions, beliefs, convictions, and values. Existing attitudes have a huge impact on the learning process. Conversely, the learning process helps to shape or change attitudes.

Knowledge

Psychologists often label this the *cognitive* domain. It relates to factors such as information, concepts, perception, principles, reasoning, creativity, and the intellect. In the learning process, there are many things that learners need to know in order to be able to do.

Skills

This is within the *behavioral* domain, including factors such as actions, words, demeanor, dexterity, motor coordination, and physical capabilities. Skills are a major consideration in the training/learning process, where the major goal is to prepare people to do something, to perform specific tasks.

Figure 9.1 (modified from Bird and Davies 1996) depicts the relationship of holistic education and training to safety success.

DEVELOPING ALEARNING ORGANIZATION CULTURE

In his book *The Fifth Discipline: The Art and Practice of the Learning Organization*, Peter M. Senge (1990) pictures the learning organization as one

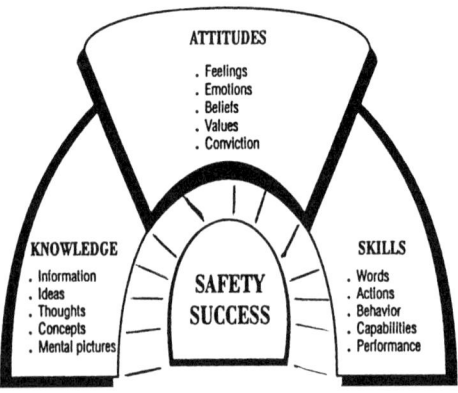

FIGURE 9.1   Holistic education and training

... where people continually expand their capacity to create the results they truly desire, where new and expansive patterns of thinking are nurtured, where collective aspiration is set free, and where people are continually learning how to learn together.

Simply stated, the learning organization puts major emphasis on education, training, and learning.

A company's culture reflects its values, beliefs, practices, and goals throughout its communication system. For instance, super-successful Southwest Airlines initiates its learning culture in its mission statement: "We are committed to provide our employees a stable work environment with equal *opportunity for learning and personal growth*" (emphasis added).

Culture is communicated by what leaders say and do. Mining managers and supervisors should show through word and action that they are MINERS for knowledge and skills and MINERS for safety education and training. Their mining operations include:

M—*Motivating* every person in the organization to continuously learn, grow, develop, and progress.

I—*Integrating* safety education and training into the overall operational process.

N—*Nurturing* the right (safe, efficient, and productive) way of performing each and every task.

E—*Encouraging* and empowering every person, every day, toward lifelong learning.

R—*Reinforcing* with abundant rewards and recognition, the behaviors that show that people are learning, and applying the learned knowledge and skills.

S—*Showing* the way. Setting the example. Supporting what you say by what you do.

Education, training, and learning should become a natural part of everyday life in the organization, or "the way we operate around here." This must be reflected in the mission statement, policies, procedures, goals, objectives, responsibility statements, management information system, and leadership actions. Day by day, people must "walk the talk" regarding education, training, learning, and doing for safety, along with quality, production, and cost control.

Figure 9.2 (based on the system described by Bird and Germain 1996) shows vital aspects of a safety system that ought to be included in the education, training, and learning process throughout the organization.

FACILITATING ADULT LEARNING (Reprinted from Germain et al. 1997)

Many of us have memories of being school kids; sitting in one of a long row of desks; facing the back of someone's head; constrained by a host of rules regarding dress, demeanor, talking, raising our hand, or getting permission to go to the bathroom; and confronted with the potential of punishment and being sent to the Principal's Office! These kinds of memories of the teaching/learning situation

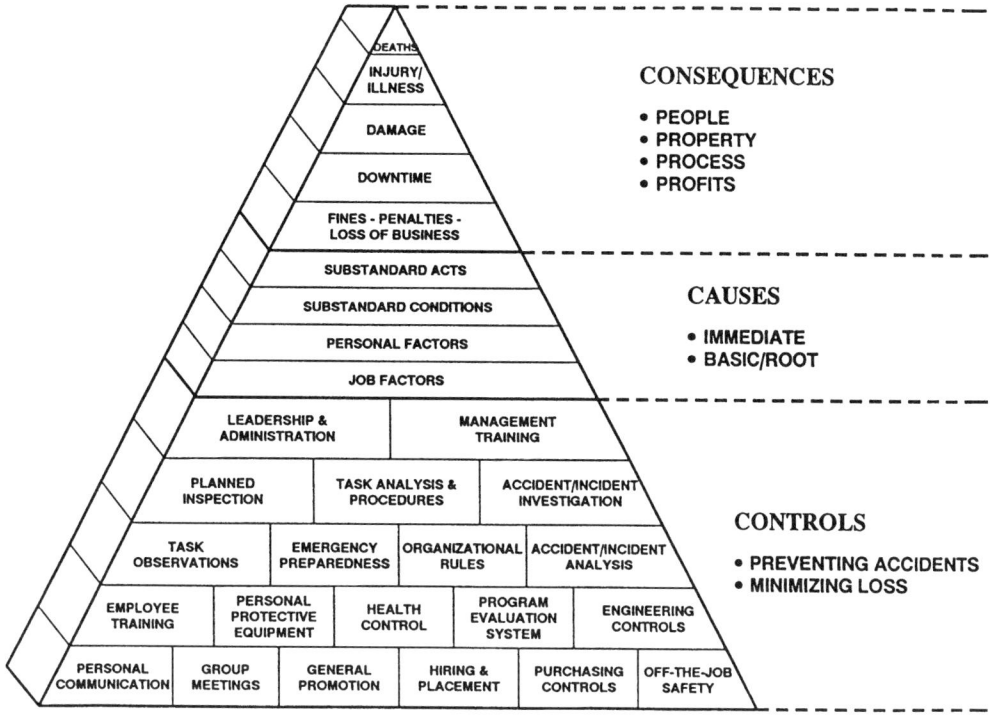

FIGURE 9.2   **Vital aspects of education and training for safety action and accomplishment**

all tend to be negative. These mental pictures may be what comes to mind when adults are asked (worse yet, told) to attend "a training program."

Whether or not the environment and methods for teaching children work, adults are not just bigger children. Adults have characteristics which call for adult-oriented learning environments and methods. Following are some of these characteristics.

Adults have a significant variety of life experiences stored in their personal data bank. They have an abundance of attitudes, knowledge, and skills to draw on and build on. They want to use their past experiences as the foundation for new learning. They are used to choosing and deciding. They can help each other learn.

Adults have significant concerns which may compete with the learning process. They have jobs that demand time, thought, and effort. They have family responsibilities. They may be busily involved in community, club, and volunteer activities. They tend to have many things on their minds.

Adults have progressed from total dependence (as infants), to independence (as youths), to interdependence. They recognize the need and values of working together, of teamwork, of learning from one another. But they also want to be self-directing and self-respecting. Adults may be a bit rusty regarding sustained study habits. They may feel somewhat apprehensive about appearing to be slow; being able to keep up with the group and learning requirements; or having to "pass the test."

All adult learners are tuned in to the same radio station—WIIFM. They want to know What's In It For Me? They tend to be problem-centered rather than fact-centered.

They seek and appreciate practical application of the knowledge and skills involved in the training/ learning activity. Some adults have needs related to visual acuity, hearing loss, arthritis, back problems, and other physical concerns. They appreciate a learning environment which accommodates such special needs. Adults are not sponges or tabula rasa. They want more than "transmittal and absorption" in the training/learning situation; they want an experiential learning process.

BEYOND COMPLIANCE TO EXCELLENCE

Compliance is critical. Miners and managers must obey the laws of the land and meet generally accepted standards for safety, health, and environmental control. This is not easy because laws and regulations have become so numerous and complex that it seems almost impossible to keep up with them.

As just one example, here are the 20 subparts of the 216-page *Federal Metal and Nonmetallic Mine Safety and Health Standards* (30 CFR [*Code of Federal Regulations*] 56/57/58, 9th ed.):

A	General		K	Electricity
B	Ground Control		L	Compressed Air and Boilers
C	Fire Prevention and Control		M	Machinery and Equipment
D	Air Quality, Radiation, and Physical Agents		N	Personal Protection
E	Explosives		O	Materials Storage and Handling
F	Drilling and Rotary Jet Piercing		P	Illumination
G	Ventilation		Q	Safety Programs
H	Loading, Hauling, and Dumping		R	Personnel Hoisting
I	Aerial Tramways		S	Miscellaneous
J	Travel Ways and Escape Ways		T	Gassy Mines

Gaining commitment and compliance to such codes and standards requires a great deal of motivation, communication, education, and training. Effective plans and actions are necessary throughout the mining operation, including at least these aspects:

1. Obtain all applicable codes and regulations.

2. Train appropriate employees on how to read and interpret the codes and regulations and keep up to date with changes.

3. Determine where and how these codes and regulations affect your site.

4. Modify facilities and processes to minimize impacts.

5. Implement action plans to control accidental loss.

6. Monitor, audit, and evaluate the compliance process.

7. Maintain continuous compliance.

Document, Document, Document

Although compliance is critical, it is not enough. It does build a solid foundation for your safety management system. But *excellence* requires much more, such as the following strategies to strengthen support for and success with the process of safety and health education, training, learning, and *doing*:

- Tying needs assessment and training/learning activities to the company's strategic plan

- Ensuring support from decision makers and strengthening their commitment by seeking and using their involvement in decisions and activities

- Forming and using an internal steering/advisory committee or, perhaps better, team

- Considering perceived needs as well as underlying needs in training design, delivery, and evaluation

- Prioritizing needs in terms of relevance and importance

- Setting clear goals, measurable objectives, and realistic expectations, and fulfilling them

- Meeting people's desire to "be in on" what's going on, by sharing information and reports generously

- Evaluating training at all feasible levels: reaction, learning, behavior, results, and return on investment

- Maximizing motivation through recognition, rewards, and reinforcement

- Doing meaningful cost-benefit analyses to show that the training/learning process is not an expense, but an investment

- Promoting transfer of training into performance through the actions of managers, participants, and trainers/facilitators before, during, and after the training/learning activity
- Publicizing and celebrating success
- Repeating the process. Repeating the process. Repeating the process.

Figure 9.2 reflects the types of safety training/learning topics used at thousands of worldwide locations in their journeys toward excellence. Leading organizations realize that people need to know the consequences of mistakes and accidents, not only on people, but also on property, the operational process, and profits.

People need education and training on the causes of loss-producing events; not just the substandard acts and conditions, but also the personal and job factors that are the root causes. There are never-ending needs for education and training on the 20 vital topics shown in Figure 9.2 as the controls for preventing accidents and minimizing loss.

THE ESSENCE: WHY—WHO—WHEN—WHERE—WHAT—HOW

WHY Educate and Train?

First and foremost, every organization should ensure the education and training to continuously improve the knowledge and skills of its most important asset–human capital.

Change is never-ending. Tools and technology change; policies, procedures, and practices change; laws and standards change; society's culture changes; the workforce changes; and so forth. Change creates a continuing need for education, training, and learning.

Regulatory requirements are an important reason for education and training. Many safety, health, and environmental laws and standards relate to the need for training. For instance, looking back at the list of the 20 subparts for 30 CFR 56/57/58, it is easy to see the tremendous need for knowledge and skills in mining operations.

Safety, health, and environmental acronyms abound, as we can see from this partial list:

- ACGIH–American Conference of Governmental Industrial Hygienists
- ANSI–American National Standards Institute
- CFR–Code of Federal Regulations
- DOT–Department of Transportation
- EPA–Environmental Protection Agency
- ISO–International Standards Organization
- MSHA–Mine Safety and Health Administration
- NFPA–National Fire Protection Agency
- NIOSH–National Institute for Occupational Safety and Health
- OSHA–Occupational Safety and Health Administration.

And there are many other related acronyms, all of which reflect the vast need for a variety of knowledge and skills, for ongoing education and training.

Here are some of the benefits of effective safety and health education, training, and learning:

- Reduced accidents, personal harm, property damage, and related losses
- Increased awareness of the value of tools, materials, equipment, supplies, and facilities
- Decreased downtime and delays
- Improved morale and motivation
- Reduced mistakes and waste
- Optimum performance, productivity, and profitability.

If you think education and training are expensive, try ignorance and inefficiency.

The WHO of Education and Training

Two basic concerns here are (1) Who needs education and training? and (2) Who should facilitate the education and training? Basically, the answer to the first question is "everyone."

Associates (workers, employees) must have the education and training to perform proficiently, meaning safely, efficiently, and productively. In this information era, they must learn how to function in new and demanding organization structures and handle team membership and empowerment, computer and communication technology, statistical techniques, problem-solving systems, and so much more.

Front line supervisors must learn how to bridge the huge gap from "boss" to team leader–mentor–support provider–facilitator.

For instance, executives must learn totally new strategies such as how to:

- Both compete and collaborate locally and globally
- Develop and implement missions, values, paradigms, and ethical principles
- Change and communicate the company culture.

Staff professionals for safety, health, environmental, and training functions must also be lifelong learners. As internal consultants, they need to know:

- What's on the leading edge of developments in their fields
- Changes in related regulations and standards
- How to attain and maintain their professional qualification, certification, or licensing status
- How to tie their special functional interest in with the organization's mission, strategic plan, and operational processes.

Education and training are also vital aspects of contractor management. Here, for example, is a summary of a *Professional Safety* article (Roughton 1995) on contractor safety:

Contractors should be able to complete prequalification forms detailing past safety performance. Their formal written safety programs should be up-to-date and fully implemented. Training records on topics such as HAZWOPER, lockout/tagout, confined space entry, respiratory protection, blood-borne pathogens, confined spaces, and hot work should be complete and readily available. Contractors should be able to demonstrate how they have evaluated employee understanding and retention of training. Once hired, contractors must work with facility owners to define how much additional training is needed.

And, of course, visitors should have an orientation that includes adequate safety considerations. As we said earlier, "Who needs education and training?" Everyone.

Who Should Facilitate the Training?   We used to think that safety and/or training professionals had to do most of the training themselves. We thought it was easier to prepare staff professionals to instruct for a great variety of subject matters than it would be to prepare the subject matter experts (SMEs) in how to instruct in their own fields of expertise. Not so now. While safety and training staff professionals may still do some of the formal education and training, they are just as likely to stimulate, coordinate, and facilitate education and training systems and activities conducted by SMEs. SMEs are the people who know the subject and the system; do the work; and have the operational responsibility, accountability, and experience. They are people such as miners, mechanics, and managers; technicians, engineers, analysts; and suppliers, consultants, and computer specialists. These people have the necessary knowledge, experience, and credibility for helping others to learn. Experience shows that a bit of train-the-trainer activity can prepare them to instruct very effectively.

The WHEN of Education and Training

Education, training, and learning are not simply a number of periodic programs, but a continuous process. This process spans the entire period, from orientation to separation.

However, precise timing to meet certain specific needs is also important. The training should not be conducted too long before it is needed or can be applied. Unapplied knowledge and skills tend to wither and be forgotten. This is the Disuse (use-it-or-lose-it) Principle of Learning.

Also, it can be disastrous not to provide the training until after it is needed. This is an open invitation to inefficiency, mistakes, waste, and accidental loss in terms of people, property, productivity, and profitability.

The WHERE of Education and Training

Learning can take place anywhere and training can occur everywhere: in the meeting room, at the computer, on the job, at home, at a college/university, association, or institute.

Most training tends to occur either on the job or in some sort of classroom. Following are four aspects of comparison for these locations:

Classroom training tends to ...	On-the-job training tends to ...
Be for groups	Be for individuals
Occur in an artificial environment	Occur in the real work environment
Have relatively few learning distractions	Have many learning distractions (other equipment and materials, people trying to meet the production push, etc.)
Involve quite a variety of teaching/learning techniques	Emphasize the hands-on teaching/learning technique

Analysis shows that good classroom training and on-the-job training share some significant features. For example, both

- Are designed to satisfy pinpointed needs
- Are focused on specific objectives
- Are learner-centered
- Benefit from proper preparation
- Depend on good communications
- Apply basic principles of learning, such as readiness, association, involvement, repetition, and reinforcement
- Include meaningful implementation, evaluation, and follow-up
- Produce measurable results.

The WHAT of Education and Training

The overall strategy should be Total Accident Control Training, or TACT. People at all organizational levels, in all functional areas, need to learn what the system is, how it operates, what their responsibilities and accountabilities are, and how they fit into the system. This encompasses a great variety of education and training topics.

Here is one way of categorizing the vast number of aspects within TACT:

- Safety orientation training and education
- Specific technical safety and health training and education
- Leadership/management education and training.

Safety Orientation Training and Education   Orientations typically include two types of information: general and worksite or job-specific. They may be covered together or in separate sessions. They may be conducted by the same or different people.

In large sites, representatives from departments such as Human Resources Development, Personnel, and/or Safety, Health, and Environment conduct orientation. In smaller sites, the site manager or a supervisor may present orientation material. Regardless of who does it, the orientation should acquaint the person with:

- General or site-wide safety
- Health and environmental issues, such as policy and procedures
- Hazard awareness rules and regulations
- General personal protective equipment (PPE) requirements
- Emergency procedures.

Figure 9.3 shows the types of topics covered by many organizations.

ORIENTATION CHECKLIST FOR EMPLOYEES
(for all new employees - regular and temporary)
An Equal Opportunity Employer

DATE	EMPLOYEE'S NAME	NAME HE/SHE GOES BY

PRE-HIRE:
- ☐ Update Job Description and Critical Job Procedures if necessary
- ☐ Use up-to-date application form
- ☐ Conduct reference checks consistent with location practice

UPON OFFER OF EMPLOYMENT:
- ☐ Verify Identity and Employment Eligibility, Complete 1-9 Form (where applicable)
- ☐ Drug Screening Consent Form
- ☐ Parts B and C of the Medical Examination Form
- ☐ Medical Examination
- ☐ Drug and Alcohol Test

ON FIRST DAY:
- ☐ Explain Any Benefits
- ☐ Health, Life, Dental Insurance
- ☐ Vacation
- ☐ Holidays
- ☐ Others

MISCELLANEOUS Hire Forms
- ☐ Employment Record Form
- ☐ W-4 Form (Federal and also state if required)
- ☐ Employee Confidential Information/Invention Agreement
- ☐ Other

MISCELLANEOUS Hire Procedures, Advise Employee of:
- ☐ Direct Deposit
- ☐ Payroll Deductions
- ☐ Credit Union
- ☐ Other

EXPLAIN BASIC POLICIES AND PROCEDURES
- ☐ Wages
- ☐ Formal Probationary Period - length, expected performance
- ☐ Performance Review (if applicable)
- ☐ Disciplinary Policy
- ☐ Drug and Alcohol Policy
- ☐ Attendance Policy
- ☐ Call-In Procedure-Absenteeism/Tardiness
- ☐ Hours Worked
- ☐ Overtime
- ☐ Breaks/Lunch

FIGURE 9.3   Orientation checklist for employees

Job-specific orientation should be conducted or coordinated by the new employee's immediate supervisor or team leader. Here are the types of topics often covered in this portion of the orientation process:

- Getting acquainted with the people, the work environment, and how the person's job fits in
- Specific worksite safety, health, and environmental rules and PPE requirements
- Personnel policies relating to attendance, reporting-off, overtime, discipline, employee assistance services, training, and career development
- Work schedules and performance standards
- Reporting accidents, injuries, damage, illnesses, spills, and harmful releases
- First aid and medical matters
- Drug testing and special medical tests

❑ Housekeeping
❑ Other
EXPLAIN EEO POLICY
    ❑ Company's Commitment to Equal Employment Opportunity
    ❑ EEO Representative, EEO Facility Coordinator and Corporate EEO Department
    ❑ Policy Against Harassment
    ❑ EEO Compliant Resolution Procedure
SHOW EMPLOYEE AROUND
    ❑ Parking Lot/Employee's Entrance
    ❑ Restroom/Locker Room/Lunch Room
    ❑ Shop/Supply Storage Room
    ❑ Introduce to Other Employees and to Immediate Supervisory Group
EXPLAIN WHAT WE DO AT OUR LOCATION
    ❑ Outline the Organization of the Division/Department and its relationship to the rest of the Company
    ❑ The Work Flow and How Employee's Jobs Fits into the Total Operation
JOB INSTRUCTION
    ❑ Review and Provide Copy of Plant Rules and/or Employee Handbook
    ❑ Discuss Employee's Primary Duties and Responsibilities
    ❑ Identify the Standard of Performance Expected
    ❑ Review and Provide Copy of Job Procedure, Critical Task Procedure, etc.
    ❑ Encourage Employee to Ask Questions At Any Time
    ❑ Find Out What the Employee Already Knows
    ❑ Train Employee (Tell/Show/Watch/Follow-up)
    ❑ Check Back Several Times to See How Employee Is Progressing
    ❑ Other
SAFETY HEALTH AND ENVIRONMENTAL INSTRUCTION
    ❑ Provide Copy of SHE Rules
    ❑ Explain SHE Policies, Procedures and Practices
    ❑ Tell Where to Get First Aid and Medical Treatment
    ❑ Explain P.E.O. Programs
    ❑ Required Safety Equipment
    ❑ Reporting Injuries/Illnesses, environmental spills and Unsafe Practices/Conditions
    ❑ Other

I have reviewed and/or received all items contained in this checklist and understand the information provided.

EMPLOYEE SIGNATURE	DATE	SUPERVISOR

FIGURE 9.3 Orientation checklist for employees (continued)

- Specific hazards and special work permit procedures
- Reporting unsafe/at risk conditions and practices
- Housekeeping and personal hygiene
- Emergency procedures
- Mutual expectations.

Follow-up is a vital but sadly neglected part of the ongoing orientation process. There is an awful lot of information for people to understand, remember, and apply. They cannot do it instantaneously. Also, it may not have been presented perfectly. There is a great need to check back, review, supplement, reinforce, and continue to show interest. Some organizations find the 1-1-1 approach helpful (i.e., a planned, formal follow-up of the orientation is conducted at least one week, one month, and one quarter after the original session). These follow-up sessions are checkpoints regarding comprehension, retention, questions, suggestions, and opportunity for positive reinforcement.

Specific Technical Safety and Health Training and Education   Here is a sampling of the types of topics that are part of TACT in many organizations:

- Behavioral observation and discussion
- Confined space
- Critical task analysis
- Critical task procedures
- Damage control
- Electrical safety
- Emergency preparedness
- Ergonomics
- Explosives
- Fire prevention and control
- First aid and medical services
- Hazard communication
- Hot or special work permits
- Housekeeping
- Incident/accident investigation
- Inspection
- Job/task instruction technique
- Lock out or tag out
- Machine guarding
- Materials handling and storage
- Methane control
- Personal protective equipment
- Personnel hoisting
- Rules and regulations
- Safety meetings
- Self-rescue devices
- Shafts
- Signaling
- Ventilation.

Consider the items on this list and answer these three questions for each item:

- Does this apply to our organization?
- How well are we educating and training our people regarding this aspect of health and safety?
- What should we do for both short-term and long-term improvement?

To get an idea of a specific program, here is a list of courses offered for Georgia Mine Safety and Health Training by the Mine Safety Department of the Appalachian Technical Institute in Jasper, Georgia:

Part 48 Training
- Forty-hour underground miner training
- Twenty-four-hour surface new miner training
- Eight-hour annual refresher training.

Part 49 Training
- Underground mine rescue training.

Equipment Operator Safety Training
- Forklift operator
- Front-end loader operator

- Haul truck operator
- Motor grader operator
- Drill operator
- Track dozer operator
- Crane training (32 hours, including introduction to basic crane operation, rigging, inspections, and operator proficiency)
- Train the trainer for operators (haul truck, front-end loader, and plant operator helper).

Supervisory Training Programs

- Role of the supervisor
- Motivation
- Communication
- Holding safety meetings
- Accident investigation
- Safety observation
- Safety inspections
- Safety orientation and training
- Job safety analysis
- Enforcing rules and regulations
- MSHA and the supervisor.

Other

- First aid—8-hour medic first aid (includes basic first aid and CPR)—MSHA and OSHA accepted
- MSHA instructor training course
- DuPont "Take-Two" safety meetings
- Additional short topic presentations for safety meetings or short training sessions on virtually any aspect of mining
- National Safety Council (NSC) Defensive Driving Course (6 or 8 hours).

Leadership/Management Education and Training   You cannot have TACT without leadership/management education and training. You cannot have an effective safety system without effective leadership, without effective management of the system.

Turn back to Figure 9.2 and study the 20 elements in the "controls" area. These 20 elements form the foundation of a safety and health management system included in education and training programs all around the world. This system is detailed in books such as Bird and Germain 1996 and Germain et al. 1997. Figure 9.4 is an example of an introductory training program agenda for supervisors using the 20-element management system.

Another leading system is the one promulgated by the NSC. It is built around the following 14 elements (covered in detail in the NSC's *14 Elements of a Successful Safety & Health Program*).

- Hazard recognition, evaluation, and control:
  - Inspections
  - Incident/accident investigations
  - Industrial hygiene exposure assessments
  - Systems safety reviews
  - Industrial hygiene monitoring
  - Job safety analysis
  - Preventive maintenance
  - PPE standards
  - Redesign.

Total Accident Control Training

- Three-Day Supervisory Program -

First Day

1. INTRODUCTION - getting acquainted; program explanation; small group discussion exercise to spotlight key areas of concern for participants.

2. PEOPLE, PROPERTY & PROFITS - business and social reasons for a more professional job of supervisory management than ever before; basic concepts of risk management and Total Accident Control (TAC).

3. PROFESSIONAL SUPERVISORY MANAGEMENT - marks of a "pro"; "management/leadership work" vs. "operating work"; guiding principles; benefits.

4. PROBLEM CAUSES, EFFECTS & CONTROLS - supervisory management as a key to control; difference between "symptoms" and basic causes; three stages in a managing control; twenty elements for successful accident control.

5. SUPERVISORY INVESTIGATION - a practical, professional approach to accident/incident investigation; how effective investigation saves time and reduces losses; how to measure the quality of investigation; tips on interviewing, analyzing, documenting and following-up.

Second Day

6. EFFECTIVE SUPERVISORY INSPECTIONS - kinds of inspections; why and how to inventory "critical parts;" the importance of housekeeping; an effective hazard classification system; tips on using inspection reports to get more employee involvement and management action.

7. GROUP COMMUNICATION SKILLS - why supervisors should have group TAC meetings with workers; how to give a good talk (the 5P formula); when meetings should be held and how to make them most effective.

8. MEASUREMENT AS A MANAGEMENT TOOL - three key types of measurement (consequences - causes - controls); how to make best use of TAC measurements; values and benefits.

9. PERSONAL SUPERVISORY COMMUNICATION SKILLS - the supervisor's role in pre-job orientation; how to give key point tips for efficiency, safety and productivity; the "Motivate - Tell & Show - Test - Check" technique for proper job instruction; effective coaching guidelines.

10. THE SUPERVISOR'S ROLE IN DAMAGE CONTROL - bridging the gap between injury control and TAC; uncovering and reducing huge hidden costs; protecting people, preserving property and promoting profits.

Third Day

11. MAINTAINING EFFECTIVE DISCIPLINE - tips on obtaining proper use of personal protective equipment, compliance with rules and regulations and better handling of "problem cases"; comparing punitive and positive discipline.

12. CRITICAL TASK PROCEDURES - how to use the three-column (steps - potential problems - controls) analysis worksheet; how to save time, effort and money with the "improvement check"; how to write the procedure from the worksheet; eight ways to put procedures to work.

13. EMERGENCY PREPAREDNESS - doing a needs analysis; developing, implementing and monitoring a system; the use of emergency teams; key point tips on emergency response and emergency care.

14. GENERAL PROMOTION - variety is the spice of promotion; how to get the most benefit for the least expenditure; the place of "gimmicks"; double-barreled contests; employee involvement and supervisory leadership example.

15. MOTIVATING TAC PERFORMANCE - five basic guidelines for understanding motivation; six practical principles for managing motivation; basic aspects of a performance management and motivation system for supervisors.

The length of the program, the number of topics covered, what they are and the amount of time devoted to each can be changed in many ways…to meet the needs of the sponsor and the participants.

FIGURE 9.4   Total accident control training—3-day supervisory program

- Workplace design and engineering
  - Preoperational design and start-up review
  - Ergonomic controls
  - Codes and standards
  - Facilities, workstations, and machine safeguarding
  - Material handling
  - Life safety and fire protection
  - Automated processes, including cellular manufacturing and robotics.

- Safety performance management
  - Performance standards/guidelines
  - Conformance to standards
  - Performance reviews and appraisals
  - Communicating results.
- Regulatory compliance management
  - Assessing compliance
  - Standards identification, review, and application.
- Occupational health
  - Employee health services
  - First aid
  - Medical records
  - Individual hygiene services
  - Worker disabilities
  - Worksite monitoring
  - Periodic medical examinations
  - Medical surveillance.
- Information collection
  - Cost analysis
  - Incident management controls
  - Workplace conditions
  - Trend analysis
  - Injury and illness case analysis
  - OSHA logs
  - Off-the-job injury data.
- Employee involvement
  - Joint participation
  - Team concepts.
- Motivation, behavior, and attitudes
  - Positive recognition and reinforcement plans
  - Job safety observation
  - Behavior and attitude assessment.
- Training and orientation
  - Safety management training
  - Safety technique training
  - Task training
  - Orientation
  - Compliance/regulation training
  - Training standards/controls
  - Follow-up observation and retraining
  - Periodic observations/contacts.
- Organizational communications
  - Communication of goals and results
  - Publicizing, promoting, and campaigns
  - Public relations/media management
  - Senior management involvement, policy statement, commitment, and accountability.

- Management and control of external exposures
  - Contractor control programs
  - Vendor assessment of liability exposure
  - Product safety control
  - Public liability exposures
  - Natural disaster preparedness
  - Fleet management
  - Environmental management.
- Workplace planning and staffing
  - Hiring and job placement
  - Safety work rules
  - Employee assistance programs
  - Office safety
  - Americans with Disabilities Act requirements program.
- Assessments, audits, and evaluations
  - Self-assessments
  - Third-party assessments
  - Voluntary regulatory assessments.

So far in this section, we have considered the why, who, when, where, and what of safety and health education and training. Now let's look at how it's done.

The HOW of Education and Training

Perhaps the most important point is to treat training, not simply as programs, but as a continuous process, a system that facilitates education, learning, application, and results. OSHA's seven-step training guidelines model (U.S. Department of Labor 1992) reflects the widely accepted steps in this process.

1. Determine if training is needed. Training is not always the best solution to performance problems. A lot of time, effort, and other resources are wasted because training is conducted for non-training problems. It pays to have a thorough and systematic process for identifying and specifying what the real needs are, rather than rushing headlong into an extensive, expensive training activity.

Many performance problems should be solved by nontraining tools and techniques such as:

- Better hiring, selection, and placement of employees
- Improved design, layout, and maintenance of the workplace
- Ergonomically improved tools, facilities, and processes
- Job aids such as task procedures, flow charts, checklists, diagrams, decision tables, reference manuals, and troubleshooting guides or hotline
- More efficient and effective organization and communication
- A better performance management system.

Education and training are appropriate solutions when the problems are lack of the knowledge and/or skills required for the desired performance.

2. Identify training needs. Three major considerations here are (a) regulatory requirements, (b) work requirements, and (c) performance improvement potentials.

A basic starting point is to ensure that the training/learning system meets all regulatory requirements. A helpful publication for this purpose is *Training Requirements in OSHA Standards and Training Guidelines* (see References at the end of this chapter). For mining operations, see this chapter's *Appendix*, "OSHA and MSHA Training Requirements," an especially helpful selection of information from the actual regulations.

The second major consideration in identifying training needs is the work requirements. The basic question is "What knowledge and skills does the work require?" The answer tells what the focus of the training/learning system should be, i.e., what the employees need to *know* and what they must *do*.

Useful tools for this purpose include job analyses and descriptions, task analyses and procedures, work practices, performance observations, tests, and surveys.

The third consideration is performance improvement potentials. This boils down to comparing what people presently know and can do, with what they should know and be able to do, and analyze the gap between the two.

3. Identify goals and objectives.   Goals are the general end results desired of the training. For example, "To integrate damage control as a vital aspect in the control of accidental loss." Objectives are the specific, measurable results sought. For example, "To reduce accidental loss by 20% within 6 months."

Learning objectives reflect what the learners are to *know* and/or be *able to do* upon completion of the training/learning process. For example, "given all needed equipment, paramedic learners can demonstrate the proper lift-and-carry method of an occupied emergency stretcher, as determined by the facilitator's completion of an evaluation checklist." Objectives of this sort serve as guides to instruction, learning, and evaluation.

In his book *Developing Attitude Toward Learning* (Second Edition, 1984), Robert Mager expressed the importance of objectives in a memorable fashion:

There once was a teacher
Whose principal feature
Was hidden in quite an odd way.
Students by millions
Or possibly zillions
Surrounded him all of the day.
When finally seen
By his scholarly dean
And asked how he managed the deed,
He lifted three fingers
And said, "All you swingers
Need only to follow my lead.
"To rise from a zero
To Big Campus Hero,
To answer these questions you'll strive:
Where am I going,
How shall I get there, and
How will I know I've arrived?"

4. Develop learning activities.   When you have done the prior three steps well, you will have a good picture of what is needed to do the training/learning job well:

- Lesson plans
- Visual and/or audio aids
- Hand-outs and study materials
- Facilities
- Tools, machines, and equipment
- Electronic support system.

In some cases, you may be able to purchase a program and/or training services from outside your organization. Your decision regarding do-it-yourself vs. purchasing from outside should be based on feasibility, potential learning effectiveness, and cost effectiveness.

5. Conduct the training.   Schedule the facilities, the facilitators, and the participants. Conduct or coordinate the training/learning activities. Use knowledge and proficiency tests to determine the degree to which the objectives are met. Issue certificates to those who meet the standards for successful completion. Where appropriate, issue a company permit or license.

Good training results in better performance. But good training is much more than having good classroom sessions. It depends on the learning culture of the company; on what managers do before,

HOW WELL DO I (OR, OUR MANAGERS) FACILITATE TRANSFER OF KNOWLEDGE AND SKILLS FROM THE TRAINING/LEARNING SITE TO THE WORK SITE?				
0 = Not at all 1 = Somewhat 2 = Well 3 = Very Well				
Before The Training/Learning Activity				
1.	Involve trainees in the planning process.	0	1	2	3
2.	Brief the potential participants on the importance of the activity, the objectives, content, process, and application to the job.	0	1	2	3
3.	Build responsibility for transfer of training/learning into supervisory performance standards.	0	1	2	3
4.	Review instructional content and materials.	0	1	2	3
5.	Provide time for completing precourse assignments.	0	1	2	3
6.	Offer rewards and promotional preferences to learners who demonstrate the new behaviors.	0	1	2	3
7.	Select participants carefully and let them know the basis of selection.	0	1	2	3
8.	Encourage trainee attendance at all sessions.	0	1	2	3
9.	Use supervisor/trainee contracts which summarize what each will do regarding the training/learning process.	0	1	2	3
During The Training/Learning Activity				
10.	Prevent interruptions.	0	1	2	3
11.	Communicate and demonstrate real support for the activity.	0	1	2	3
12.	Monitor attendance, participation and accomplishment.	0	1	2	3
13.	Give recognition for attendance, participation and accomplishment.	0	1	2	3
14.	Work with participants in planning transfer actions.	0	1	2	3
15.	Plan for assessing transfer of new skills to the job.	0	1	2	3
After The Training/Learning Activity				
16.	Provide opportunities for practicing new skills.	0	1	2	3
17.	Monitor the transfer of new knowledge and skills to the job.	0	1	2	3
18.	Provide role models for the desired behaviors.	0	1	2	3
19.	Schedule trainee briefings for co-workers on the activity's objectives, content, method and results.	0	1	2	3
20.	Set mutual expectations for improvement.	0	1	2	3
21.	Give positive reinforcement for application of new skills.	0	1	2	3
22.	Give promotional preference to those who successfully apply the learned knowledge and skills to the job.	0	1	2	3
23.	Publicize and celebrate success.	0	1	2	3

FIGURE 9.5   Sample employee questionnaire

during, and after the training activity. Figure 9.5 is a useful tool for profiling management behavior in this area. It can be used to profile either a specific person or the whole management system.

6. Evaluate program effectiveness.   The classic model for training evaluation was developed by Donald L. Kirkpatrick. It is built around four levels:

- REACTION—What do the participants think of and feel about the training/learning activity?
- LEARNING—Considering knowledge, skills, and attitudes, what did the participants learn?
- BEHAVIOR—What changes in job behavior (e.g., more of, less of, different than) occurred as a result of the training/learning activity?
- RESULTS—What difference did the training/learning process make regarding factors such as:
  - Safety
  - Quality

- Production
- Cost
- Absenteeism
- Turnover
- Grievances
- Customer complaints
- Tons produced
- Equipment failures
- Downtime
- Injuries
- Spills
- Toxic emissions
- Repair costs
- Waste
- Morale.

The model was published more than 40 years ago, has persisted, and was updated in Kirkpatrick's 1994 book *Evaluating Training Programs: The Four Levels.*

7. Follow-up. Apply steps such as shown here for better training/learning application and follow-up:

- Have the trainees brief their coworkers on the training's objectives, content, method, and results.
- Use supervisor/trainee contracts that summarize what each will do regarding application of what was learned.
- Provide opportunities for application of the new knowledge and skills.
- Show empathy and tolerance for the trainees' difficulty in perfecting new behaviors, skills, and ways of doing the work.
- Model the desired behaviors.
- Give positive reinforcement for the application of the new skills.
- In personal contacts and performance reviews, give credit to applications and accomplishments related to the new knowledge and skills.
- Have periodic alumni days, in which graduates share how they have used their new knowledge and skills; discuss their application failures and successes.
- Use a newsletter to spread the word about the payoff from the training/learning process.
- Develop, implement, and monitor continuing action plans.
- Celebrate application success!
- Conduct periodic refresher and update training/learning activities.

The next section includes more "how" ideas, in terms of specific tools and techniques.

METHODS, MEDIA, AND MATERIALS

Thinking first of the overall approach, you should decide how much emphasis to give to:

- Individual instruction
- Group/classroom instruction
- Instructor-centered training
- On-the-job training and/or independent study.

Then you can make decisions about the use of specific methods, media, and materials such as shown in Figure 9.6.

Training/Learning
Methods - Media - Materials

• Apprenticeships	• Models
• Audio aids	• Multimedia
• Brainstorming	• On-the-job training
• Buzz groups	• Overhead transparencies
• Case studies	• Panel presentations
• Computer assisted instruction	• Problem-solving scenarios
• Critical incidents	• Programmed instruction
• Debates	• Projects
• Demonstrations	• Questionnaires
• Discussions	• Questions and answers
• Exhibits	• Quizzes
• Field trips	• Reading assignments
• Field work assignments	• Recitation
• Flip pads/charts	• Reports (verbal and/or written)
• Flow charts	• Role-plays and modeling
• Guest speakers	• Simulations
• Guided experience	• Skill practice
• Handbooks	• Slides
• Handouts	• Small group exercises
• Hands-on practice	• Team tasks
• Home study materials	• Tests and feedback
• Instructional games	• Videos
• Job aids	• Visual aids
• Lectures	• Workbooks
• Mind-mapping	• Worksheets
• Mockups	• Workshops

FIGURE 9.6   Training/learning: Methods—media—materials

Especially for skill training and on-the-job instruction, the best method happens to be an old method. It goes by many names, such as Proper Job/Task Instruction, Effective Job/Task Instruction, the Four-Step Method of Instruction, and Job Instruction Training (or JIT, as it was known when it was systematized at the time of World War II). The four steps are practical and easy to remember:

1. Motivate	2. Tell and Show	3. Test	4. Check
Put learner at ease	Demonstrate the operation	Have learner show and tell	Tell learner who to go to for help
Find out what learner knows about the job	Use step-by-step approach	Have learner explain key points	Put learner on his/her own
Position learner properly	Stress key points	Ask questions and correct or prevent errors	Follow up often, answer questions, review key points
Build learner's interest	Instruct clearly and completely	Continue until you know the learner knows	Taper off to normal amount of supervision
		Reinforce positive parts of performance	

8. Job aids. Job aids deserve a special note. Many people tend to underrate and underuse them. Job aids are prompters or guides for doing a job, for jogging the memory. They reduce the need to rely on fallible memory and can significantly reduce the need for additional training. They include learning facilitation tools such as:

- Checklists, diagrams, and flow charts
- Templates, patterns, forms, and worksheets
- Job placards and postings
- Troubleshooting guides and written step-by-step job/task guides
- Decision guides—charts and tables with options and criteria listed to guide choices
- Reference manuals and technical documentation
- Electronic performance support systems.

Most job aids can be kept where the work is performed, to be readily available when the user needs them. Sometimes they are used in conjunction with or in place of other training/learning activities.

Briefly, you should choose the methods, media, and materials that are both appropriate and practical. They should meet the training/learning needs and objectives; should satisfy as many principles as possible; and should be as functional and economical as feasible. In each instance, the best ones are the simplest and most cost-effective.

RETURN ON INVESTMENT: THE FIFTH LEVEL IN EVALUATING RESULTS

Earlier, we presented the classic model for training evaluations: reaction, learning, behavior, and results. Recently, considerable attention has been given to a fifth level: return on investment (ROI). This compares the training/learning activity's monetary costs and the monetary benefits. The basic question is, "Did the monetary value of the results exceed the cost of the process?" This requires careful calculation of:

- Total (direct and indirect) training costs
- Monetary measurement of results attributed to the training/learning activity
- The difference between the two.

Although it's difficult, it's being done. Showing payoff is a powerful management motivator.

The payoff from education and training is not limited to measurable monetary payoff. ROI includes many psychosocial benefits for which it may be difficult to assign a specific monetary value. For example:

- A safer, healthier work environment
- Improved commitment, cooperation, and collaboration
- More applied creativity and innovation
- Broader, faster employee development and career growth
- Reduced waste, absenteeism, turnover, and lost time
- Better, more widespread understanding of economic principles and the business process
- More efficient and effective attainment of business goals
- Decreased groaning, gripes, and grievances
- Increased motivation and morale.

Whether or not benefits such as these can be measured on a monetary scale, there should be no doubt of their tremendous value, and their ROI. As we pointed out earlier, "If you think education and training are expensive, try ignorance and inefficiency!"

REFERENCES

Bird, F.E., Jr., and R.J. Davies. 1996. *Safety and the Bottom Line*. Loganville, GA: Institute Publishing.
Bird, F.E., Jr., and G.L. Germain. 1996. *Practical Loss Control Leadership*. Loganville, GA: Det Norske Veritas (U.S.).
——. 1997. *The Property Damage Accident*. Loganville, GA: FEBCO.

CFR. 1997. *Federal Metal and Nonmetallic Mine Safety and Health Standards* (30 CFR, 56/57/58). 9th ed. Washington, DC: Mine Safety Associates.

Germain, G.L., R.M. Arnold, Jr., J.R. Rowan, and J.R. Roane. 1998. *Safety, Health, and Environmental Management*. Washington, DC: International Risk Management Institute.

Kirkpatrick, D.L. 1994. *Evaluating Training Programs—The Four Levels*. San Francisco: Berrett-Koehler Publishers.

Mager, R.F. 1985. *Developing Attitude Toward Learning.* Belmont, CA: Lake Publishing Company.

NSC. 1994. *14 Elements of a Successful Safety and Health Program*. Chicago, IL: NSC.

——. 1997. *Accident Prevention Manual for Business and Industry.* Administration & Programs, 11th ed. Chicago, IL: NSC.

OSHA. 1992. *Training Requirements in OSHA Standards and Training Guidelines.* U.S. Department of Labor.

Roughton, J. 1995. "Contractor Safety." *Professional Safety* 40(1): 31–34.

Senge, P.M. 1990. *The Fifth Discipline: The Art and Practice of the Learning Organization.* New York: Doubleday/Currency.

APPENDIX: OSHA AND MSHA TRAINING REQUIREMENTS

The continued importance of training is evidenced by the requirements of both the Occupational Safety and health Administration (OSHA) and the Mine Safety and Health Administration (MSHA).

OSHA REQUIREMENTS
Listed next are the major parts of the OSHA regulations (Title 29—Labor, *Code of Federal Regulations*) covering training requirements. (Table 23–A gives a convenient index of the types of hazards and the parts of the regulations requiring training to protect against the hazards.)

- Part 1910, Safety and Health Training Requirements for General Industry
- Part 1915-18, Safety and Health Training Requirements for Maritime Employment
- Part 1926, Safety and Health Training Requirements for Construction
- Part 1928, Occupational Safety and Health Requirements for Agriculture

MSHA REGULATIONS
The following is a summary of the training requirements under the MSHA Regulations, 30 *CFR*, PART 48—TRAINING AND RETRAINING OF MINERS (See §48.2 and §48.22 for definitions of terms used in Part 48)

Subpart A—Training and Retraining of Underground Miners

§48.1 Scope
The provisions of this subpart A set forth the mandatory requirements for submitting and obtaining approval of programs for training and retraining miners working in underground mines. Requirements regarding compensation for training and retraining are also included.

§48.3 Training Plans; Time of Submission; Where Filed; Information Required; Time for Approval; Method for Disapproval; Commencement of Training; Approval of Instructors
(a) Each operator of an underground mine shall have an MSHA approved plan containing programs for training new miners, training newly-employed experienced miners, training miners for new tasks, annual refresher training, and hazard training for miners.
(b) The training plan shall be filed with the District Manager for the area in which the mine is located.
(d) The operator shall furnish to the representative of the miners a copy of the training plan two weeks prior to its submission to the District Manager. Where a miners' representative is not designated, a copy of the plan shall be posted on the mine bulletin board 2 weeks prior to its submission to the District Manager. Written comments received by the operator from miners or their representatives shall be submitted to the District Manager. Miners or their representatives may submit written comments directly to the District Manager.
(e) All training required by the training plan submitted to and approved by the District Manager as required by this sub

part A shall be subject to evaluation by the District Manager to determine the effectiveness of the training programs. If it is deemed necessary, the District Manager may require changes in, or additions to, programs. Upon request from the District Manager the operator shall make available for evaluation the instructional materials, handouts, visual aids and other teaching accessories used or to be used in the training programs. Upon request from the District Manager the operator shall provide information concerning the schedules of upcoming training.
(f) The operator shall make a copy of the MSHA approved training plan available at the mine site for MSHA inspection and for examination by the miners and their representatives.
(g) Except as provided in §48.7 (New task training of miners) and §48.11 (Hazard training) of this subpart A, all courses shall be conducted by MSHA approved instructors.
(h) Instructors shall be approved by the District Manager.
(i) Instructors may have their approval revoked by MSHA for good cause which may include not teaching a course at least once every 24 months. A decision by the District Manager to revoke an instructor's approval may be appealed by the instructor. . . . Such an appeal shall be submitted to the Administrator within 5 days of notification of the District Manager's decision. Upon revocation of an instructor's approval, the District Manager shall immediately notify operators who use the instructor for training.
(j) The District Manager for the area in which the mine is located shall notify the operator and the miners' representative, in writing, within 60 days from the date on which the training plan is filed, of the approval or status of the approval of the training programs.
(k) Except as provided under §48.8(c) (Annual refresher training of miners) of this subpart A, the operator shall commence training of miners within 60 days after approval of the training plan, or approved programs of the training plan.
(l) The operator shall notify the District Manager of the area in which the mine is located, and the miners' representative of any changes or modifications the operator proposes to make in the approved training plan. The operator shall obtain the approval of the District Manager for such changes or modifications.
(m) In the event the District Manager disapproves a training plan or a proposed modification of a training plan or requires changes in a training plan or modification, the District Manager shall notify the operator and the miners' representative in writing.
(n) The operator shall post on the mine bulletin board, and provide to the miners' representative, a copy of all MSHA revisions and decisions which concern the training plan at the mine and which are issued by the District Manager.

§48.4 Cooperative Training Program
(a) An operator of a mine may conduct his own training programs, or may participate in training programs conducted by MSHA, or may participate in MSHA approved training programs conducted by State or other Federal agencies, or associations of mine operators, miners' representatives, other mine operators, private associations, or educational institutions.
(b) Each program and course of instruction shall be given by instructors who have been approved by MSHA to instruct

in the courses which are given, and such courses and the training programs shall be adapted to the mining operations and practices existing at the mine and shall be approved by the District Manager for the area in which the mine is located.

§48.5 Training of New Miners; Minimum Courses of Instruction; Hours of Instruction

(a) Each new miner shall receive no less than 40 hours of training as prescribed in this section before such miner is assigned to work duties. Such training shall be conducted in conditions which as closely as practicable duplicate actual underground conditions, and approximately 8 hours of training shall be given at the minesite.

(b) The training program for new miners shall include the following courses:
    (1) Instruction in the statutory rights of miners and their representatives under the Act; authority and responsibility of supervisors.
    (2) Self-rescue and respiratory devices.
    (3) Entering and leaving the mine; transportation; communications.
    (4) Introduction to the work environment.
    (5) Mine map; escapeways; emergency evacuation; barricading.
    (6) Roof or ground control and ventilation plans.
    (7) Health.
    (8) Cleanup; rock dusting.
    (9) Hazard recognition.
    (10) Electrical hazards.
    (11) First aid.
    (12) Mine gases.
    (13) Health and safety aspects of the tasks to which the new miner will be assigned.
    (14) Such other courses as may be required by the District Manager based on circumstances and conditions at the mine.

(c) Methods, including oral, written, or practical demonstration, to determine successful completion of the training shall be included in the training plan.

(d) Upon proof by an operator that a newly employed miner has received the courses and hours of instruction set forth in paragraphs (a) and (b) of this section within 12 months preceding initial employment at a mine, such miner need not repeat the training, but the operator shall give and the miner shall receive and complete the instruction and program of training set forth in paragraph (b) of §48.6 (Training of newly employed experienced miners), and §48.7 (New task training of miners), if applicable, before commencing work.

§48.6 Training of Newly Employed Experienced Miners; Minimum Courses of Instruction

(a) A newly employed experienced miner shall receive and complete training in the program of instruction prescribed in this section before such miner is assigned to work duties.

(b) The training program for newly employed experienced miners shall include the following:
    (1) Introduction to work environment.
    (2) Mandatory health and safety standards.
    (3) Authority and responsibility of supervisors and miners' representatives.
    (4) Entering and leaving the mine; transportation; communications.

(5) Mine map; escapeways; emergency evacuation; barricading.
(6) Roof or ground control and ventilation plans.
(7) Hazard recognition.
(8) Self-rescue and respiratory devices.
(9) Such other courses as may be required by the District Manager based on circumstances and conditions at the mine.

§48.7 Training of Miners Assigned to a Task in Which They Have Had No Previous Experience; Minimum Courses of Instruction

(a) Miners assigned to new work tasks as mobile equipment operators, drilling machine operators, haulage and conveyor systems operators, roof and ground control machine operators, and those in blasting operations shall not perform new work tasks in these categories until training prescribed in this paragraph and paragraph (b) of this section has been completed. This training shall not be required for miners who have been trained and who have demonstrated safe operating procedures for such new work tasks within 12 months preceding assignment. This training shall also not be required for miners who have performed the new work tasks and who have demonstrated safe operating procedures for such new work tasks within 12 months preceding assignment. The training program shall include the following:
    (1) Health and safety aspects and safe operating procedures for work tasks, equipment, and machinery.
    (2) (i) Supervised practice during nonproduction.
        (ii) Supervised operation during production.
    (3) New or modified machines and equipment.
    (4) Such other courses as may be required by the District Manager based on circumstances and conditions at the mine.

(b) Miners under paragraph (a) of this section shall not operate the equipment or machine or engage in blasting operations without direction and immediate supervision until such miners have demonstrated safe operating procedures for the equipment or machine or blasting operation to the operator or the operator's agent.

(c) Miners assigned a new task not covered in paragraph (a) of this section shall be instructed in the safety and health aspects and safe work procedures of the task, prior to performing such task.

(d) Any person who controls or directs haulage operations at a mine shall receive and complete training courses in safe haulage procedures related to the haulage system, ventilation system, firefighting procedures, and emergency evacuation procedures in effect at the mine before assignment to such duties.

(e) All training and supervised practice and operation required by this section shall be given by a qualified trainer, or a supervisor experienced in the assigned tasks, or other person experienced in the assigned tasks.

§48.8 Annual Refresher Training of Miners; Minimum Courses of Instruction; Hours of Instruction

(a) Each miner shall receive a minimum of 8 hours of annual refresher training as prescribed in this section.

(b) The annual refresher training program for all miners shall include the following courses of instruction:
    (1) Mandatory health and safety standards.
    (2) Transportation controls and communication systems.

(3) Barricading.
(4) Roof or ground control and ventilation plans.
(5) First aid.
(6) Electrical hazards.
(7) Prevention of accidents.
(8) Self-rescue and respiratory devices.
(9) Explosives.
(10) Mine gases.
(11) Health.
(12) Such other courses as may be required by the District Manager based on circumstances and conditions at the mine.

(d) Where annual refresher training is conducted periodically, such sessions shall not be less than 30 minutes of actual instruction time and the miners shall be notified that the session is part of annual refresher training.

§48.9 Records of Training

(a) Upon a miner's completion of each MSHA approved training program, the operator shall record and certify on MSHA form 5000-23 that the miner has received the specified training. A copy of the training certificate shall be given to the miner at the completion of the training. The training certificates for each miner shall be available at the minesite for inspection by MSHA and for examination by the miners, the miners' representative, and State inspection agencies. When a miner leaves the operator's employ, the miner shall be entitled to a copy of his training certificates.

(b) False certification that training was given shall be punishable under section 110 (a) and (f) of the Act.

(c) Copies of training certificates for currently employed miners shall be kept at the minesite for 2 years, or for 60 days after termination of employment.

§48.10 Compensation for Training

(a) Training shall be conducted during normal working hours; miners attending such training shall receive the rate of pay as provided in §48.2(d) (Definition of normal working hours) of this subpart A.

(b) If such training shall be given at a location other than the normal place of work, miners shall be compensated for the additional cost, such as mileage, meals, and lodging, they may incur in attending such training sessions.

§48.11 Hazard Training

(a) Operators shall provide to those miners, as defined in §48.2(a)(2) (Definition of miner) of this subpart A, a training program before such miners commence their work duties. This training program shall include the following instruction, which is applicable to the duties of such miners:
(1) Hazard recognition and avoidance;
(2) Emergency and evacuation procedures;
(3) Health and safety standards, safety rules, and safe working procedures;
(4) Use of self-rescue and respiratory devices
(5) Such other instruction as may be required by the District Manager based on circumstances and conditions at the mine.

(b) Miners shall receive the instruction required by this section at least once every 12 months.

(c) The training program required by this section shall be submitted with the training plan required by §48.3(a) (Training plans: Submission and approval) of this subpart A and shall include a statement on the methods of instruction to be used.

(d) The operator shall maintain and make available for inspection certificates that miners have received the hazard training required by this section.

(e) Miners subject to hazard training shall be accompanied at all times while underground by an experienced miner, as defined in §48.2(b) (Definition of miner) of this subpart A.

§48.12 Appeals procedures

The operator, miner, and miners' representative shall have the right of appeal from a decision of the District Manager.

Subpart B—Training and Retraining of Miners Working at Surface Mines and Surface Areas of Underground Mines

The provisions of this subpart B set forth the mandatory requirements for submitting and obtaining approval of programs for training and retraining miners working at surface mines and surface areas of underground mines. Requirements regarding compensation for training and retraining are also included.

§48.23 Training Plans; Time of Submission; Where Filed; Information Required; Time for Approval; Method for Disapproval; Commencement of Training; Approval of Instructors

(a) Each operator of a mine shall have an MSHA approved plan containing programs for training new miners, training newly-employed experienced miners, training miners for new tasks, annual refresher training, and hazard training for miners.
(2) Within 60 days after the operator submits the plan for approval, unless extended by MSHA, the operator shall have an approved plan for the mine.
(3) In the case of a new mine which is to be opened or a mine which is to be reopened or reactivated after the effective date of this subpart B, the operator shall have an approved plan prior to opening the new mine, or reopening or reactivating the mine unless the mine is reopened or reactivated periodically using portable equipment and mobile teams of miners as a normal method of operation by the operator. The operator to be so excepted shall maintain an approved plan for training covering all mine locations which are operated with portable equipment and mobile teams of miners.

(b) The training plan shall be filed with the District Manager for the area in which the mine is located.

(d) The operator shall furnish to the representative of the miners a copy of the training plan 2 weeks prior to its submission to the District Manager. Where a miners' representative is not designated, a copy of the plan shall be posted on the mine bulletin board 2 weeks prior to its submission to the District Manager. Written comments received by the operator from miners or their representatives shall be submitted to the District Manager. Miners or their representatives may submit written comments directly to the District Manager.

(e) All training required by the training plan submitted to and approved by the District Manager as required by this subpart B shall be subject to evaluation by the District Manager to determine the effectiveness of the training programs. If it is deemed necessary, the District Manager may require changes in, or additions to, programs. Upon request from the District Manager the operator shall make available for evaluation the instructional materials, hand-outs, visual aids, and other teaching accessories used or to be used in the training programs. Upon request from the District Manager the operator shall provide information concerning schedules of upcoming training.

(f) The operator shall make a copy of the MSHA approved training plan available at the mine site for MSHA inspection and examination by the miners and their representatives.

(g) Except as provided in §48.27 (New task training of miners) and §48.31 (Hazard training) of this subpart B, all courses shall be conducted by MSHA approved instructors.

(h) Instructors shall be approved by the District Manager

(i) Instructors may have their approval revoked by MSHA for good cause which may include not teaching a course at least once every 24 months. A decision by the District Manager to revoke an instructor's approval may be appealed by the instructor. Such an appeal shall be submitted to the Administrator within 5 days of notification of the District Manager's decision. Upon revocation of an instructor's approval, the District Manager shall immediately notify operators who use the instructor for training.

(j) The District Manager for the area in which the mine is located shall notify the operator and the miners' representative, in writing, within 60 days from the date on which the training plan is filed, of the approval or status of the approval of the training programs.

(k) Except as provided under §48.28(c) (Annual refresher training of miners) of this subpart B, the operator shall commence training of miners within 60 days after approval of the training plan, or approved programs of the training plan.

(l) The operator shall notify the District Manager of the area in which the mine is located and the miners' representative of any changes or modifications which the operator proposes to make in the approved training plan. The operator shall obtain the approval of the District Manager for such changes or modifications.

(m) In the event the District Manager disapproves a training plan or a proposed modification of a training plan or requires changes in a training plan or modification, the District Manager shall notify the operator and the miners' representative in writing.

(n) The operator shall post on the mine bulletin board, and provide to the miners' representative, a copy of all MSHA revisions and decisions which concern the training plan at the mine and which are issued by the District Manager.

§48.24 Cooperative Training Program

(a) An operator of a mine may conduct his own training programs, or may participate in training programs conducted by MSHA, or may participate in MSHA approved training programs conducted by State or other Federal agencies, or associations of mine operators, miners' representatives, other mine operators, private associations, or educational institutions.

(b) Each program and course of instruction shall be given by instructors who have been approved by MSHA to instruct in the courses which are given, and such courses and the training programs shall be adapted to the mining operations and practices existing at the mine and shall be approved by the District Manager for the area in which the mine is located.

§48.25 Training of New Miners; Minimum Courses of Instruction; Hours of Instruction

(a) Each new miner shall receive no less than 24 hours of training as prescribed in this section. Except as otherwise provided in this paragraph, new miners shall receive this training before they are assigned to work duties. At the discretion of the District Manager, new miners may receive a portion of this training after assignment to work duties: Provided, That no less than 8 hours of training shall in all cases be given to new miners before they are assigned to work duties. The following courses shall be included in the 8 hours of training: Introduction to work environment, hazard recognition, and health and safety aspects of the tasks to which the new miners will be assigned. Following the completion of this preassignment training, new miners shall then receive the remainder of the required 24 hours of training, or up to 16 hours, within 60 days. Operators shall indicate in the training plans submitted for approval whether they want to train new miners after assignment to duties and for how many hours. In determining whether new miners may be given this training after they are assigned duties, the District Manager shall consider such factors as the mine safety record, rate of employee turnover and mine size. Miners who have not received the full 24 hours of new miner training shall be required to work under the close supervision of an experienced miner.

(b) The training program for new miners shall include the following courses:

(1) Instruction in the statutory rights of miners and their representatives under the Act; authority and responsibility of supervisors.

(2) Self-rescue and respiratory devices.

(3) Transportation controls and communication systems.

(4) Introduction to work environment.

(5) Escape and emergency evacuation plans; firewarning and firefighting.

(6) Ground control; working in areas of highwalls, water hazards, pits and spoil banks; illumination and night work.

(7) Health.

(8) Hazard recognition.

(9) Electrical hazards.

(10) First aid.

(11) Explosives.

(12) Health and safety aspects of the tasks to which the new miner will be assigned.

(13) Such other courses as may be required by the District Manager based on circumstances and conditions at the mine.

(c) Methods, including oral, written or practical demonstration, to determine successful completion of the training shall be included in the training plan.

(d) Upon proof by an operator that a newly employed miner has received the courses and hours of instruction set forth in paragraphs (a) and (b) of this section within 12 months preceding initial employment at a mine, such miner need not repeat the training, but the operator shall give and the miner shall receive and complete the instruction and program of training set forth in paragraph (b) of §48.26 (Training of newly employed experienced miners) and

§48.27 (New task training of miners), if applicable, before commencing work.

§48.26 Training of Newly Employed Experienced Miners; Minimum Courses of Instruction
(a) A newly employed experienced miner shall receive and complete training in the program of instruction prescribed in this section before such miner is assigned to work duties.
(b) The training program for newly employed experienced miners shall include the following:
   (1) Introduction to work environment.
   (2) Mandatory health and safety standards.
   (3) Authority and responsibility of supervisors and miners' representatives.
   (4) Transportation controls and communication systems.
   (5) Escape and emergency evacuation plans; firewarning and firefighting.
   (6) Ground controls; working in areas of highwalls, water hazards, pits, and spoil banks; illumination and night work.
   (7) Hazard recognition.
   (8) Such other courses as may be required by the District Manager based on circumstances and conditions at the mine.

§48.27 Training of Miners Assigned to a Task in Which They Have Had No Previous Experience; Minimum Courses of Instruction
(a) Miners assigned to new work tasks as mobile equipment operators, drilling machine operators, haulage and conveyor systems operators, ground control machine operators, and those in blasting operations shall not perform new work tasks in these categories until training prescribed in this paragraph and paragraph (b) of this section has been completed. This training shall not be required for miners who have been trained and who have demonstrated safe operating procedures for such new work tasks within 12 months preceding assignment. This training shall also not be required for miners who have performed the new work tasks and who have demonstrated safe operating procedures for such new work tasks within 12 months preceding assignment. The training program shall include the following:
   (1) Health and safety aspects and safe operating procedures for work tasks, equipment, or machinery.
   (2) (i) Supervised practice during nonproduction.
      (ii) Supervised operation during production.
   (3) New or modified machines and equipment.
   (4) Such other courses as may be required by the District Manager based on circumstances and conditions at the mine.
(b) Miners under paragraph (a) of this section shall not operate the equipment or machine or engage in blasting operations without direction and immediate supervision until such miners have demonstrated safe operating procedures for the equipment or machine or blasting operation to the operator or the operator's agent.
(c) Miners assigned a new task not covered in paragraph (a) of this section shall be instructed in the safety and health aspects and safe work procedures of the task, prior to performing such task.
(d) All training and supervised practice and operation required by this section shall be given by a qualified trainer, or a supervisor experienced in the assigned tasks, or other person experienced in the assigned tasks.

§48.28 Annual Refresher Training of Miners; Minimum Courses of Instruction; Hours of Instruction
(a) Each miner shall receive a minimum of 8 hours of annual refresher training as prescribed in this section.
(b) The annual refresher training program for all miners shall include the following courses of instruction:
   (1) Mandatory health and safety standards. The course shall include mandatory health and safety standard requirements which are related to the miner's tasks.
   (2) Transportation controls and communication systems.
   (3) Escape and emergency evacuation plans; firewarning and firefighting.
   (4) Ground control; working in areas of highwalls, water hazards, pits, and spoil banks; illumination and night work.
   (5) First aid.
   (6) Electrical hazards.
   (7) Prevention of accidents.
   (8) Health.
  (10) Self-rescue and respiratory devices.
  (11) Such other courses as may be required by the District Manager based on circumstances and conditions at the mine.
(d) Where annual refresher training is conducted periodically, such sessions shall not be less than 30 minutes of actual instruction time and the miners shall be notified that the session is part of annual refresher training.

§48.29 Records of Training
(a) Upon a miner's completion of each MSHA approved training program, the operator shall record and certify on MSHA form 5000-23 that the miner has received the specified training. A copy of the training certificate shall be given to the miner at the completion of the training. The training certificates for each miner shall be available at the mine site for inspection by MSHA and for examination by the miners, the miners' representative and State inspection agencies. When a miner leaves the operator's employ, the miner shall be entitled to a copy of his training certificates.
(b) False certification that training was given shall be punishable under section 110 (a) and (f) of the Act.
(c) Copies of training certificates for currently employed miners shall be kept at the mine site for 2 years, or for 60 days after termination of employment.

§48.30 Compensation for Training
(a) Training shall be conducted during normal working hours; miners attending such training shall receive the rate of pay as provided in §48.22(d)
(b) If such training shall be given at a location other than the normal place of work, miners shall be compensated for the additional costs, such a mileage, meals, and lodging, they may incur in attending such training sessions.

§48.31 Hazard Training
(a) Operators shall provide to those miners, as defined in §48.22(a) (2) (Definition of miner) of this subpart B, a training program before such miners commence their work duties. This training program shall include the following instruction, which is applicable to the duties of such miners:
   (1) Hazard recognition and avoidance;
   (2) Emergency and evacuation procedures;
   (3) Health and safety standards, safety rules and safe working procedures;

(4) Self-rescue and respiratory devices; and,

(5) Such other instruction as may be required by the District Manager based on circumstances and conditions at the mine.

(b) Miners shall receive the instruction required by this section at least once every 12 months.

(c) The training program required by this section shall be submitted with the training plan required by §48.23(a) (Training plans: Submission and approval) of this subpart B and shall include a statement on the methods of instruction to be used.

(d) In accordance with §48.29 (Records of training) of this subpart B, the operator shall maintain and make available for inspection, certificates that miners have received the instruction required by this section.

§48.32 Appeals Procedures

The operator, miner, and miners' representative shall have the right of appeal from a decision of the District Manager.

CHAPTER 10

Mine Safety in the Twenty-First Century: The Application of Computer Graphics and Virtual Reality

Damian Schofield, Robin Hollands, and Bryan Denby
AIMS Research Unit, University of Nottingham School of Chemical, Environmental and Mining Engineering Nottingham, United Kingdom

INTRODUCTION

Inevitably, the future will be digital—digital cameras and videos, electronic document storage, network commerce, Internet business, intelligent search agents, computer animations, and virtual simulators are already in use. The minerals industry is no exception, even though it can be slow to accept new technology. The modern mine is, however, a high-technology environment, often with millions of dollars invested in digital equipment.

Computer technology in the mining industry has altered the fundamental way in which certain parts of the mining operation are performed. As computers become more powerful, minerals industry users redefine their problems to use the capabilities of the technology. The future of computing in the minerals industry is not always led by the demands of the mining engineer, but sometimes by the academics and commercial software developers who devise new techniques and products that may change the way certain traditional operations are carried out (Denby and Schofield 1999).

These technological developments have often improved the safety of the mining environment. We will discuss some of the areas where this technology can be applied and introduce the technologies that are likely to continue to improve safety in the future. This chapter will focus on the application of computer graphics (CG) and virtual reality (VR) as technologies that have significant potential to improve the safety of mining personnel.

The ability to visualize complex and dynamic systems involving personnel and equipment within the mine layout is a potential advantage of applying the CG and VR technology. In this chapter, we will introduce the use of CG and VR systems and the ways in which they can be used to improve the safety of a variety of mining situations.

SAFETY IN THE MINING INDUSTRY

Work in the minerals sector is still among the most hazardous of all occupations. Inherent risks exist because of the potential for rockfalls, explosions, and fires, the often-confined nature of the workplace, and the proximity of dangerous equipment and personnel. Some of these risks can be managed at a system level, but much still depends on the performance of individual miners.

In the past, western mining industries had a very traditional attitude toward safety. Safety was seen as costly and counterproductive, concerned more with complying with industrial law rather than ensuring the health and well-being of those who worked in the industry (Staley 1992). Worldwide attitudes toward industrial safety have advanced significantly in recent years. Various new techniques have been introduced to try to raise the safety awareness of the workforce.

There can be no doubt that accident rates have been progressively reduced in the mining industry. Changes in the frequency of different accident types have also occurred over the years. As greater understanding of the technical risks has developed and regulatory regimes have changed, major disasters have become less common. This has, however, exposed the smaller scale events to greater scrutiny. Hence, the highlight has shifted toward trying to improve the safety of individual, unit operations through improved ergonomic design and placing greater emphasis on risk assessment and enhanced training of individuals.

Evidence from everyday life shows that well trained and careful workers may avoid injury on a dangerous job, while untrained and careless workers may be injured under the safest possible conditions. Before any employee can work safely, they must be shown safe procedures for completing their tasks. Safety training should be designed to improve safety awareness in employees and to show them how to perform their jobs without endangering themselves and their fellow employees.

In general, successful training helps mining personnel to acquire the skills, knowledge, and attitudes to make them competent and safe in all aspects of their work—whatever their position on the mine. Training often includes formal off-the-job training; instructions to individuals and groups; and on-the-job coaching, practical sessions, and counseling (Allison 1992; Cole and Staff 1988). Initial work done at the University of Nottingham on traditional miner training methods identified a number of problems (Churchill and Snowden 1996):

- A large amount of training is carried out through media that are very hard to transfer (e.g., paper and pencil, verbal games).

- Instructions for rote learning of information is the most common technique used by trainers with the same sets of training media being used from year to year. Many teaching methods present too much material, too rapidly, with little or no opportunity for worker involvement.

- Trainees frequently fail to attend to the problem at hand, often dividing their attention between what is going on at the front of the classroom and interpersonal interactions with those around them.

- When verbal games are used, they usually focus on low-level factual recall of information. In addition, the mechanics of the games tend to compete for trainee and instructor attention and detract from the content.

- Because the training has a limited number of scenarios, the trainees learn to use the surface features of their training. Trainees really need to be learning about the more general underlying features of safe behavior.

- Skill degradation is an important issue. When the hazards of a mine environment are combined with the issue of skill degradation, the need for realistic training becomes paramount. There are legal requirements in the mining industry to ensure that regular formal retraining is undertaken.

- There is a general feeling that training should be better. One of the most important factors in effective training is motivation. The more involved trainee and trainer are in the teaching process the more effective the learning will be.

The University of Nottingham report also stated that instructional and training materials that have good potential for engineering training often fail to achieve that potential (Churchill and Snowden 1996). Many studies have shown that it is far more effective to focus on one or two issues that have direct relevance for the learners and to encourage active involvement in these issues (Cole and Staff 1988; Halpern 1984).

Large mineral organizations must continually look for ways to improve their safety performance and training. Any new technology that may help to reduce accident statistics needs to be explored. The rapid advances in CG and VR provide a very real way in which complex ideas and information can be transmitted to a workforce. These new techniques allow videos, simulators, and planning systems to be developed quickly and efficiently. The capacity to remember safety information from a three-dimensional computer world is far greater than the ability to translate information from a printed page into a "real" three-dimensional environment (Rheingold 1991; Krueger 1991).

COMPUTER GRAPHICS AND VIRTUAL REALITY TECHNOLOGY

Major mining software companies have kept pace with computer technology advances, developing software that utilizes the hardware available. Many people are now familiar with three-dimensional computer-aided design (CAD) systems and engineers use them routinely in their workplaces. Mining CAD software now incorporates advanced visualization tools that allow engineers to view their three-dimensional designs.

CG refers to a set of computer applications that can be used to produce images and animations. CG uses numerical models of real-world objects to create artificially created views. Each object is reduced to a representation consisting of points, edges, and flat sides. Once the object is in this form, the computer modeler can use numerical models of lighting sources and reflection characteristics and can apply realistic textures over the artificial objects to make them more closely resemble their real counterparts. However, since it can take time to generate an image, these images can be stored off-line. The computer can then build an animation frame by frame. This is how commercial computer-based movies such as *Toy Story* and *A Bug's Life* are made (Hollands et al. 1999).

However, computer animations like these are passive and always show the same sequence regardless of any user action. VR, on the other hand, is interactive in nature and must respond to user actions, such as moving around the virtual world and turning on equipment.

VR can be described as the science of integrating humans with information. It consists of three-dimensional, interactive, computer-generated environments. These environments can be models of real or imaginary worlds. The key to many people's definition of VR lies in the underlying processes, the simulations, the reactions, and the behavior of the objects or people within the virtual environment (VE). A VR user can, for example, sit in a vehicle and drive it. The vehicle will have responsive behavior associated with it, and other vehicles in the world may have predefined actions and responses.

For the virtual world to appear to respond "instantly" to such actions, the computer must generate a new view of the world at least 20 or so times per second. This requirement to generate virtual worlds in real time often means that the visual quality of VR worlds is not as realistic as the impressive computer animations on the same computer platform; however, it is currently essential for the interactivity that makes VR worlds engaging and useful as a training medium.

The way a virtual world is experienced can vary widely. "Immersive" VR uses output devices designed to map as directly as possible onto the user's perceptual organs. A head-mounted display (HMD) encases the audio and visual perception of the user in the virtual environment and cuts out all outside information. Many HMDs present an image directly in front of each eye and magnify it so that it fills a wide field of view, creating the impression of actually being in a place, rather than looking at a screen. Head, body, and hand sensor tracking may move users around the world and allow them to interact with objects. However, HMDs often support relatively low resolutions, which are compounded by being spread over a wide field of view, and may have a number of disadvantages including encumbrance, isolating experience, and occasional simulator sickness.

Many VR systems opt instead to use a standard computer screen as an interface into the virtual world. Using this system, standard computer peripherals such as the joystick and the mouse can be used to navigate around the world and interact with it. Larger monitors make the experience more immersive, and the use of projectors to display very large images allows a number of people to be involved at the same time. This has been found to be an attractive compromise to many end users, made more appealing by the ready availability of existing personal computers and peripheral devices.

These systems comprise hardware and software components as shown in the schematic in Figure 10.1. The major hardware features can be classified as follows:

- Input devices—These allow the user to interact with and control the actions in a VR system. They can range from simple keyboard input (the least preferred option), through mouse or joystick control to more advanced specialist controls such as spaceballs, control simulators, or body tracking devices.

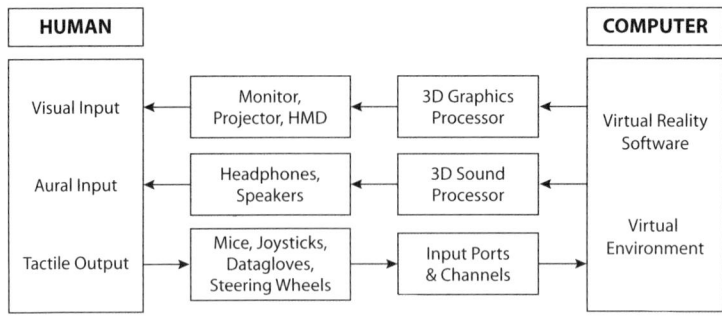

FIGURE 10.1 **A generic VR system**

- Processors—Here the input signals are processed, specific calculations underlying the simulation are carried out, and output signals are generated.

- Memory and disk storage—As most VR systems generate images in real time, they require relatively little memory and are usually highly efficient in terms of disk storage.

- Output devices—These range from monitors, through projection systems to fully immersive HMDs.

The rapid developments in PC technology in recent years and the huge potential market for desktop VR in a wide range of sectors means that this area is seeing some of the fastest developments. Multinational corporations are investing hundreds of millions of dollars in ensuring that VR system performance increases. Even though the technology drive has largely been focused on the home computer games market, the spin-offs into engineering have resulted in high-quality systems becoming available for serious applications (Aukstakalnis and Blatner 1992; Earnshaw et al. 1995; Wilson et al. 1996).

At the same time that hardware costs and performance have reached sensible levels, there is a growing market for VR software. This demand is resulting in continuous reductions in software development costs. As the market for VR applications in mining increases, major reductions in unit costs of complete training systems should be realized. Hence the argument that VR is an expensive technology no longer holds, and the opportunity for mass training using VR opens up as unit costs drop dramatically.

Examples of VR-based training exist in a number of other sectors that can be used to indicate a future path for the mining industry. Anyone who has recently flown in a large passenger aircraft has trusted his or her life to someone who has been trained with the assistance of a VR flight simulator (Stewart 1994). The techniques that have been developed over a number of decades in this area are now available on desktop PCs and have been adapted into a whole range of other training applications including such diverse areas as military, nuclear, and even surgical training (British Nuclear Fuels Limited 1999; Bentowitz 1997; Halff et al. 1986; and Thurman 1992). Figure 10.2 shows an example from a military helicopter flight-simulator application developed by Evans and Sutherland. These types of systems offer major potential training advantages in terms of the increased retention caused by the visual nature of the medium and the role-playing nature of the interactivity.

A common theme of these examples is training for hazardous environments in a manner that minimizes the exposure of the trainee to real risk. Although some of these advanced training environments also help to develop tactile skills, the key developmental aspects revolve around procedural or knowledge-based training. VR training is an accepted and effective approach in these industries.

The extensive research literature about these simulations provides much information about the effectiveness of these types of simulators when teaching and assessing proficiency in fields where critical judgment and decision making are required (Halff et al. 1986; Imanche et al. 1995). The possibility of embedding many different scenarios and many different events into the training simulator allows the trainee to gain experience of many different types of situations that they may encounter (Theasby 1992). Trainees have so much new and dynamic information that they are less likely to learn just the surface features of a few training scenarios. This makes it easier for them to move their knowledge from the training situation to the real world (Thurman 1992).

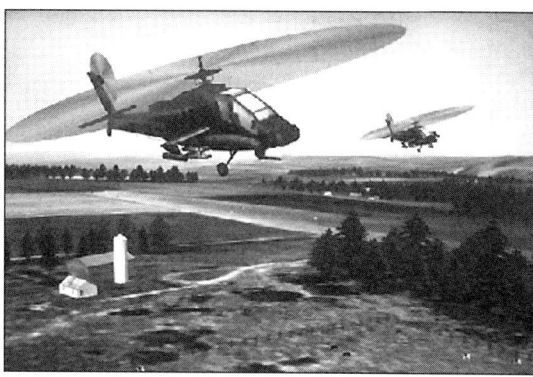

FIGURE 10.2   A military training application (Evans and Sutherland 1999)

A number of academic groups, companies, and government institutions around the world have been developing VR systems for the mining industry. It is interesting to note that the large government research institutions listed below are currently developing VR applications for the mining industry in the following areas (Denby and Schofield 1999):

- The Council for Scientific and Industrial Research (CSIR) in South Africa has developed a training system for the gold mine stope environment.
- The Commonwealth Scientific and Industrial Research Organisation (CSIRO) in Australia has a number of VR projects under way, including a large mine data visualization project.
- The National Institute of Occupational Safety and Health (NIOSH) in the United States is developing a hazard awareness system for underground coal environments.

The AIMS Research Unit at the University of Nottingham in the United Kingdom (UK) is a leading researcher into VR-based systems for the mining industry. AIMS has taken advantage of the advances in hardware and software to research and develop a variety of graphical based systems for safety and training in the minerals industry. The unit has found that systems developed using PC technology are more easily ported into industry because of the reduced costs, the existing user base, and the familiarity of PC technology (Schofield et al. 1994). In particular it now appears that the technologies have developed sufficiently and costs reduced to levels that allow even the smallest companies to consider them seriously.

A number of CG and VR applications have been developed at Nottingham, including environmental visualization, safety awareness training systems, accident reconstruction, data visualization, ergonomic design, simulation systems, driving simulators, training systems, and hazard awareness systems (Schofield 1997).

VR training systems can provide a far more varied learning experience for the trainee. Systems can be configured so that each time the trainee enters the VR world the scenario changes. Sometimes these changes are minor and sometimes they are more obvious. The fact that the training experience is potentially different, however, means that the trainee must concentrate on each occasion. Reinforced learning can be structured in this approach and the immersive nature of the experience again tends to improve knowledge retention (Denby et al. 1998).

In addition, VR-based simulation allows consistent training scenarios. This consistency results in improved quality control, both of subjects and training, because it can be more readily quantified (Halpern 1984). The grading of the performance and the comparison between trainees is facilitated. The improved assessment techniques allow the teaching to become contingent on the performance of the individual or group, and the next training scenario can emphasize the skills that still require the most development. This can also be achieved by adjusting the pace of learning and providing context-sensitive help for particular learners. In addition, the consistent nature of the training means that the scenarios themselves can be assessed and modified over time to make them more effective.

Different information and different controls may also lead to trainees learning information that will be accessed differently. Implicit knowledge is knowledge that can be used without conscious thought and is robust under stress (Svendson 1991). An intuitive interface that is highly immersive may allow this learning to take place (Egsegian et al. 1993). This difference is important when considering who is going to be trained. Novice trainees may need explicit instruction to help them acquire necessary skills, whereas a trainee on refresher courses may respond best to implicit information. The interface could be manipulated subtly to adjust for each situation (Berry and Dienes 1993).

CG- and VR-based training systems will form an important element of the mine training systems of the future. It is only a matter of time before low-cost VR training develops to reach its full potential. However, it is apparent that in order for VR training to become an established methodology for the mining industry, careful consideration must be given to the introduction and integration of this technology. Few people with a thorough understanding of training needs and VR technology suggest that VR systems will completely replace conventional training methods. Classroom training and work experience are still vital in many respects. A sensible implementation strategy must therefore look closely at the integration of this new technology into a carefully planned approach that will include conventional classroom teaching, on-the-job training, and supervised work experience. Examples of AIMS' applications of CG and VR technology will be described in the following sections.

IMPROVING SAFETY AWARENESS WITH GRAPHICS AND VIDEO TRAINING

A good knowledge and a sound commitment to safety give a manager or supervisor the confidence to go out and "sell" safety to the workforce. Many techniques are used by mining companies to make employees more aware of safety and health issues. This includes safety awards, primary and refresher training, competitions, and publicity. However, the most effective way to influence people about safety is communicating effectively. The best type of communication about the workplace occurs when it is done either in the workplace or by using representations of the workplace.

Employees who have experienced training courses, videos, computer animations, or virtual environments can be reminded of that experience through poster campaigns, leaflets, and other more traditional safety communication media.

CG images and animations can be used to express symbolic or abstract concepts that can help to reinforce safety awareness to a workforce. An example of this is shown in Figure 10.3. This is taken from a British Coal safety awareness campaign. In the figure a free-steered vehicle (FSV) is shown carrying a powered support that grows teeth, a concept that suggests that these vehicles are comparable to wild animals roaming underground and should be avoided at all costs. This type of message, abstract but simple, gets a safety message across clearly and quickly, and reinforces current company safety campaigns. The repetitive use of this image in posters and leaflets reminds employees of the safety information seen in videos and training programs.

Although modern lecture-based training makes use of a variety of media, one of the most engaging forms of the traditional media is film or video presentations. Unlike text summaries or slide shows, the moving image captures the dynamic nature of the workplace, and a well-produced, up-to-date presentation will usually keep the audience interested long enough to get its message across.

Unfortunately, professionally produced videos can be prohibitively expensive to create. A number of skilled technicians are required to create the material, and in addition to filming time, scripting, storyboarding, and final editing must all be figured into the final presentation budget.

The production of filmed media can have another financial implication where real equipment or personnel are involved. The disruption caused by location filming is often significant and where production is lost, this secondary cost implication can far outweigh the primary cost of the production. Even where access to real equipment can be provided, the scenarios that can be presented are limited to normal working practices and only to those hazardous situations that can be safely simulated (Hollands et al. 1999).

CG animation allows entire video clips to be created using artificially created worlds and models only. As the plant and equipment have been created within the computer model, no access to or downtime of the real process is required. Because there is no risk associated with synthetic props, any hazardous situation can be demonstrated. CG animation is also comparatively cheap, and professional quality results can be generated using PC software, including video postproduction and editing.

AIMS has also produced a number of "toolbox" training videos. One example is an FSV awareness video produced for British Coal. This was aimed at educating pedestrians who work in free-steered

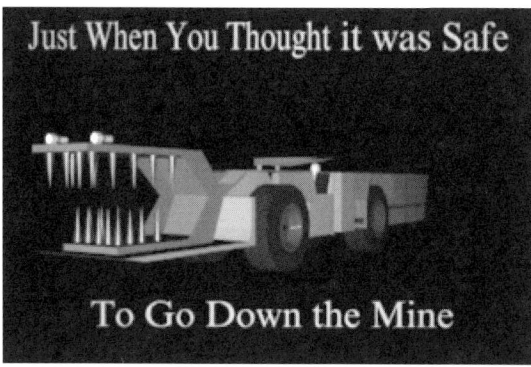

FIGURE 10.3   A computer-generated image from a safety awareness campaign

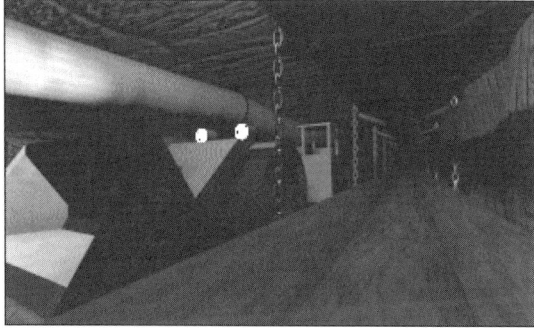

FIGURE 10.4   A scene from a computer-generated mining safety video

vehicle roadways of the dangers associated with the vehicles. A still from this animation is shown in Figure 10.4. CG was used exclusively to produce this video in which:

- Dangerous situations and accidents were recreated.
- Accidents were viewed from various viewpoints (e.g., the driver's cab, or from a pedestrian's view).
- The driver's lines of sight were shown as graphical three-dimensional objects, marking the danger zones.
- A range of analogies from everyday life was used to reinforce the safety message.
- The ability of good safety techniques to prevent accidents was shown and proved.

The still shown in Figure 10.5 is from a training video for a major UK civil engineering firm. It teaches the importance of safety procedures for pedestrian personnel around a mobile plant. In the image shown, a pedestrian steps out from behind parked vehicles into the path of an oncoming mobile site plant.

If safety is to be sold to a workforce, management needs to use the tools of the salesperson. Safety can be sold using videos, posters, brochures, and safety campaigns. CG animations are already used extensively by the advertising industry, and these animations are ideal tools for getting a message across to a workforce. Abstract and symbolic ideas can be used to place an impression and scenario into the minds of mine personnel.

SAFETY THROUGH ERGONOMIC DESIGN

Mining equipment has traditionally suffered from poor ergonomic design. Although this situation is changing, the industry is still equipped with large amounts of machinery that could be improved through better ergonomic analysis and a stronger commitment to the operator's safety. One key problem of design and planning is the need to visualize the often-complex interaction of layout, equipment, and personnel.

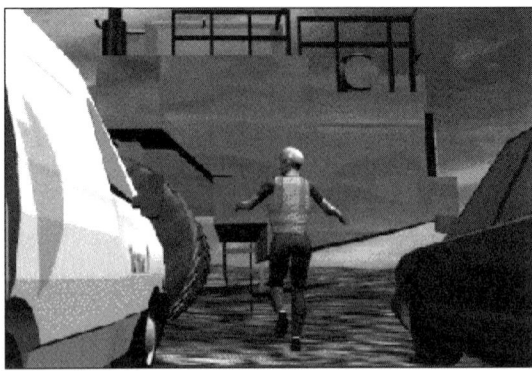

FIGURE 10.5   A scene from a computer-generated construction safety video

In 1991, the HM Inspectorate of Mines investigated the safety of FSVs in British Coal Mines (*Health and Safety Executive* [HSE] 1992). The resulting report highlighted the visibility limitations inherent in FSV design by referring to roadway plans and sections that showed where a seated driver was unable to see objects at less than a given height in the vicinity of the machine. HSE has subsequently developed two-dimensional computer-based methods for producing such visibility plots (Boocock et al. 1994). Mason and Simpson (1990) also undertook work in this area, generating visibility charts for FSVs using a CAD design package called SAMMIE.

Even though these techniques are useful and identify potential improvements to equipment design, it is important to reevaluate techniques as computer technology advances and use this technology to extend the assessment into three dimensions (Schofield 1997). AIMS has recently undertaken research work funded by SIMRAC (Safety in Mines Research Advisory Council), which is investigating the ergonomic problems associated with FSVs (Denby and Schofield 1998b).

Working with health, safety, and engineering consultants, AIMS has developed a system for investigating visibility problems associated with FSVs. The VR system developed indicates dynamic risk zones (areas of low visibility) as vehicles move around within three-dimensional environments.

The application generates "view bars" that indicate, per frame of animation, the height above which the driver of the vehicle can see. Thus, in the image shown in Figure 10.6, the driver can see only about half of the mineworker. The view bars are color-coded:

- Green indicates that the driver can see the floor, or close to the floor.
- Yellow indicates that the driver cannot see the bottom half of the roadway.
- Red shows the areas where the driver cannot see anything in the roadway.

The VR simulator can also generate a minimum-height three-dimensional representational *graph, or a two-dimensional plan*, over the specified time period, showing those regions that the driver can never see below the specified height.

MAJOR INCIDENTS AND HAZARDS

The importance of planning for major hazards and training staff in how to cope in the event of such a hazard has become increasingly recognized. Most of this planning and training can be carried out with CG and VR tools (Lyons 1993).

As part of a European Coal and Steel Community (ECSC) project, AIMS is investigating the use of VR to simulate the hazardous environments that result from underground fires and explosions. It has been reported that 85% of fires are detected by mine personnel (Pomroy and Carigiet 1995), so the need for concise, relevant training in the detection of mine fires seems to be of paramount importance.

Fundamentally, the VR system acts as a front end to a dynamic, environmental simulator in which various hazardous situations can be examined and interacted with. As users navigate around the virtual mine, they are given feedback on ventilation direction and speed. At some point in the mine layout a fire or explosion situation can be simulated and the accompanying changes in environmental parameters begin. A still from the VR system developed is shown in Figure 10.7.

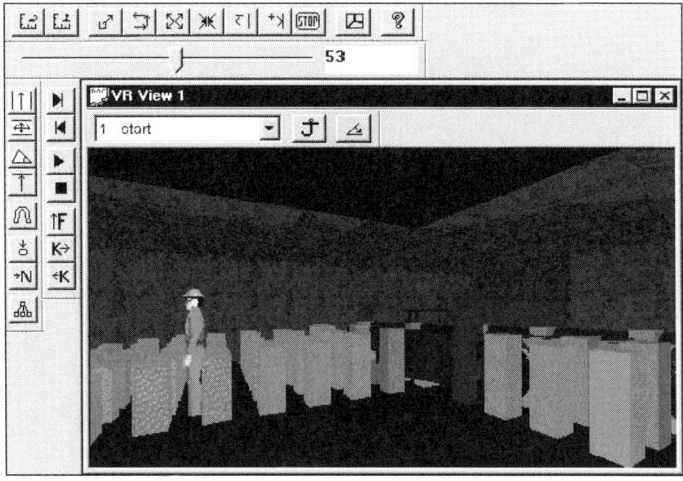

FIGURE 10.6   Three-dimensional visibility simulator showing restricted area of vision

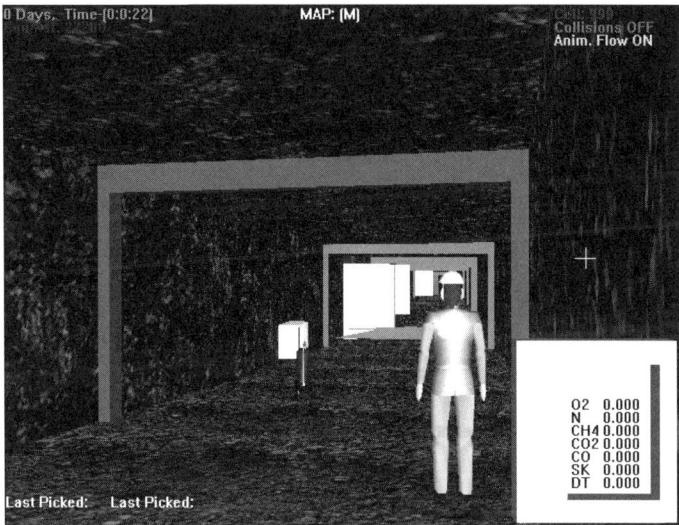

FIGURE 10.7   Visualization of environmental conditions in an underground environment

Users can take the role of a mine worker or supervisor, in which egress from the mine might be the primary concern, or they can take the role of a rescue team member, in which the objective is to travel safely into the mine to rescue trapped workers. If atmospheric conditions start to deteriorate, the likely physiological effects can be fed back to the user to simulate differing levels of stress. The monitoring of hazardous situations and reaction to those hazards can be logged for later assessment.

It must be noted that this work is still at the preliminary stages of development and more work is necessary to develop it to the stage where it could be used to enhance training of mine workers or mine rescue teams. The potential for using VR in these types of situations, however, is significant.

An earlier example of the way VR can be applied as a major hazard planning tool is an oil rig evacuation scenario. Figure 10.8 shows images from the oil rig VR system.

A user in this scenario begins within an accommodation block of the simulated oil rig and can then move out onto the deck and either to a helipad or down to the sea. A helicopter that has been incorporated into the virtual world flies in and lands on the helipad. Two cranes on the rig can be operated by the user and used to move containers on the central section of the rig. The user can also enter one of the production modules. Within this world, various escape routes may be blocked by fire

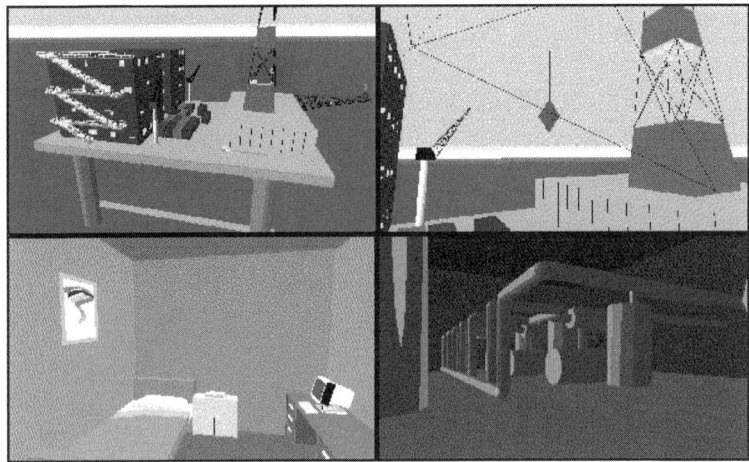

FIGURE 10.8 Images from an offshore oil rig evacuation simulator

or falling debris, meaning that the user has to use some initiative and their knowledge of the oil rig layout to escape. The user's progress through this environment is monitored and can be reported and assessed at the end of a simulation.

Increased media publicity of major incidents means that the public no longer regards industrial processes as perhaps they once did—something remote from them, run by engineers with an incomprehensible language of their own. Today, hazardous industries are seen as being capable of giving rise to events that may affect ordinary people directly and perhaps disastrously. This increase in public awareness means that mining companies, now more than ever, have to use all the facilities at their disposal to plan against major hazards. CG and VR systems are additional tools that can be used and may help to provide training and increase awareness among the workforce (Schofield 1997).

INFREQUENT PROCESS PLANNING

In cases where infrequent or "one off" (one of a kind) operations are to be considered, management needs to devote attention to a number of health and safety implications. Failure to do so can result in a number of unacceptable conditions (HSE 1991). It is inevitable that in these cases, where the task to be performed is not routine, the safety of the operation is, at least in part, dictated by the specific technology involved and the specific hazards/risks to which the operations are prone. However, although there may be safety implications from these specific, technical aspects, we should also look for common training/safety elements that will, by definition, be beyond the detailed technical issues.

Examples of the need for infrequent process planning in the mining industry can range from the need to maneuver large pieces of unusual equipment from the shaft bottom to the workplace through to major salvage and reinstallation of longwall face equipment. These processes involve the manipulation of large items of equipment, in confined three-dimensional spaces. Often these operations are critical to the production environment and failure to plan them effectively can reduce the mine's profitability.

CG and VR techniques are ideal for evaluating design criteria, testing tolerances and clearances, and training personnel. The training aspect is particularly important because a range of high-risk, high-cost situations, such as underground longwall face salvages, can be recreated within the computer model (Denby and Schofield 1998b).

The operation of a longwall face salvage has been simulated and assessed. Virtual objects representing the equipment were manipulated to examine whether they will fit through narrow roadways, or whether they needed to be dismantled. An image from the face salvage VR planning system is shown in Figure 10.9. Personnel can be shown animations of the face salvage and how it is to be performed or trained using a VR simulator to recreate the movement of the equipment in the constrained virtual roadways.

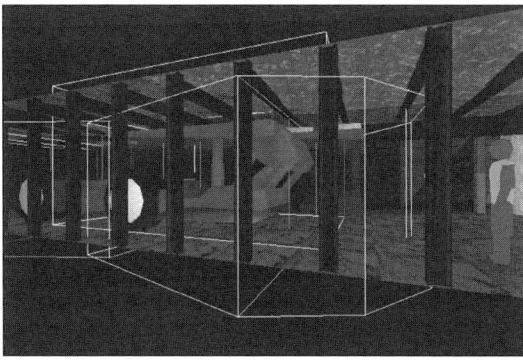

FIGURE 10.9   An image from the VR longwall face salvage planning system

A number of general conclusions can be drawn from infrequent activity incidents. On many mines, infrequent tasks such as underground face salvages, or the movement of large items of equipment, are left to contractors. The increasing pressure on the minerals industry to improve safety in all aspects of the job means that low-cost configurable training tools are needed to train both contract and regular employees (Schofield 1997).

EQUIPMENT SIMULATION

Equipment simulators offer a number of advantages over other testing environments (Alicandri 1994). CG imagery allows tremendous flexibility; any required equipment and surrounding environment can be developed.

Many surface mines are in operation throughout the world; all require the safe transfer of material around the site. In many cases this is achieved by haulage trucks. These large vehicles, often the size of a small house, have many associated safety issues. Their huge size, together with the difficult environmental conditions in which they must operate, introduces handling and visibility problems. There is a high level of risk associated with each truck, as the consequences of an accident can be extremely severe. In the United States, the Occupational Safety and Health Administration (OSHA) found, on average, 107 fatalities and 38,330 injuries associated with these trucks occurred annually in the workplace. OSHA also found present training standards to be ineffective in reducing the number of accidents involving powered industrial trucks (OSHA 1995).

AIMS has been involved in research to develop fixed-base simulators for a number of mining applications. One of these applications is a truck-driving simulator for surface mining and quarrying operations. Using the VR system shown in Figure 10.10, a trainee can navigate a truck into a mine and experience many of the hazards that this entails. The truck is controlled using a specially designed interface that replicates some of the controls found in the truck driver's cab. The simulation uses the inputs to update the vehicle's position, speed, and orientation.

The VR truck driving system includes:

- Realistic truck behavior based on rimpull and retarder curves
- Intelligent loading and queuing operations
- Customizable site layouts that can be imported from mine CAD models
- Variable atmospheric and texture conditions
- Introduction of hazards into the simulation
- The ability to handle multiple exit junctions on the haul roads.

As mining progresses from phase to phase, haul road networks and truck routes must adapt as the landform changes. To create more relevant training scenarios, it was important that the trainers were able to accurately recreate their own workplaces and conditions. The virtual world geometry can be imported from mining industry standard modeling packages such as Vulcan or Surpac. Road layouts, truck movements and loading points, and lighting and fogging conditions can also be configured (Williams et al. 1998).

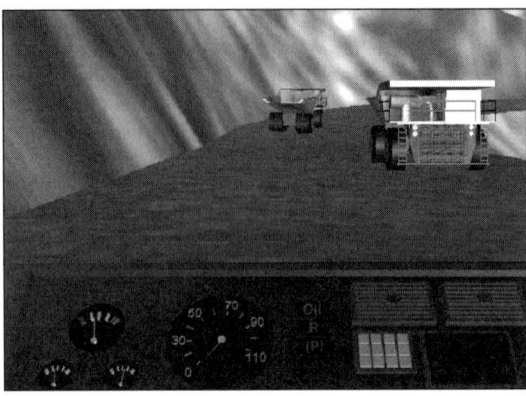

FIGURE 10.10   An image from the surface mine truck simulation system

Code from the VR truck simulator developed by AIMS has been incorporated into a commercial product called VROOM (Earthworks 1999). This is used to create realistic virtual models and allows users to visualize their mine sites and drive around their site layout.

An example of an underground application is shown in Figure 10.11. This is used for the simulation of underground room and pillar operations. The user can configure the number of entries and the size of the pillars. The software then automatically recreates the mine layout. The user then selects which equipment is to operate within the mine layout. The system is preprogrammed with the intelligence and behavior of the different pieces of equipment.

Figure 10.11 shows the system being used with multiple windows: the upper left window shows a map of the room and pillar operation with the locations of all the items of equipment in the mine. This map is dynamically updated. The upper right window is a floating viewpoint that allows the user to walk\travel around the mine. The lower two windows are anchored to items of equipment. This VR environment operates in both a desktop mode and in an immersive mode. In the immersive mode, the user views the world using a HMD and gains a true three-dimensional perspective of the world.

The increasing use of teleremote systems in mining operations provides an ideal activity for the application of VR simulation for training. The user watches a computer screen instead of a video screen and can be trained without the possibility of sustaining damage to expensive equipment. Most of these simulation systems are controlled using joysticks; these are a natural control device, as most mine personnel are familiar with how they work from experience with computer games. They are also easy for new users to master. Joysticks are also the preferred method of teleremote control for mineral operations, giving them an added advantage (Kosuge et al. 1995).

ACCIDENT RECONSTRUCTION

Traditionally management effort has been directed at preventing repetitions of accidents that have already occurred. This is done largely on the basis of information derived from detailed accident investigations (Bird and Germain 1986). Investigation is a small part of safety and health program administration, yet it is essential if management is to profit from the errors and omissions that have resulted in any unintended loss of resources.

The highly technical nature of accident reports makes them inappropriate as a means of mass communication. A summary of the information is usually used to distribute the findings throughout the company or industry, but can often fail to sufficiently convey the situation (Ferry 1988).

The use of CG animation to reconstruct the events leading up to and occurring during the accident in question can provide a powerful means of presentation. The intuitive visual nature of the results can be easily understood without any semantic problems associated with a textual summary. The ability to observe a version of the simulated accident from any time and at any position can demonstrate or resolve any potential conflicts in witness reports (Hollands et al. 1999).

AIMS has been involved with UK police force accident investigation units, providing forensic animations of traffic accidents. Initial experience in courtrooms has demonstrated the overwhelming

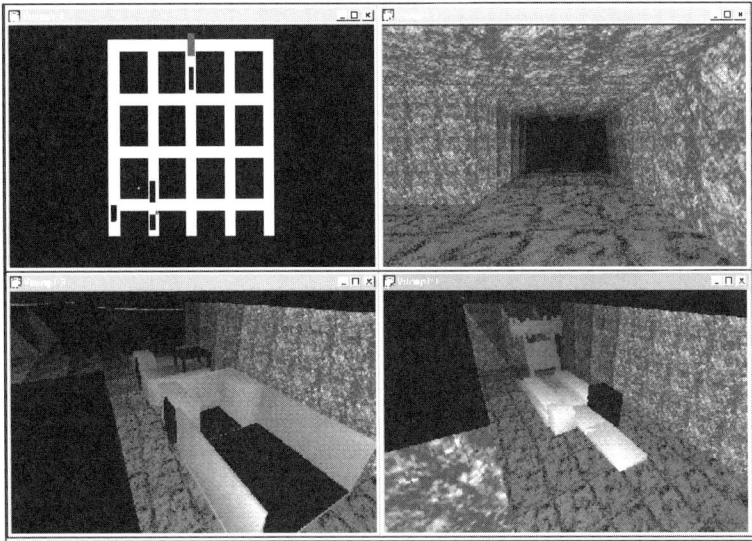

FIGURE 10.11   Image from a room and pillar training system

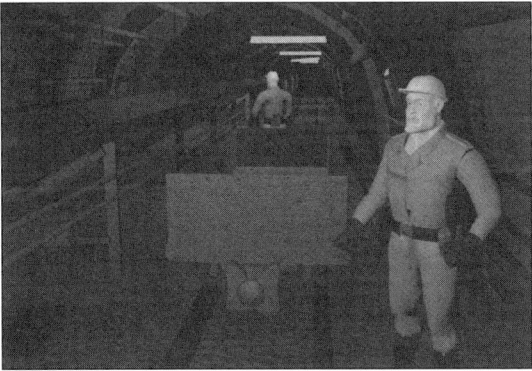

FIGURE 10.12   A computer-generated reconstruction of a mine accident

advantage of using CG evidence to aid understanding among all people involved in an accident inquiry (Schofield and Noond 1999).

This experience has been applied to a number of mining accidents. Figure 10.12 shows a still from an animation of an accident in an underground coal mine. This accident involved a runaway mine car, which traveled down an intake roadway and killed two mine workers. Figure 10.12 shows two miners working around the mine car before the accident. In this particular scenario, the accident was rerun from a variety of viewpoints showing errors in the behavior of various people involved in this particular accident. The scenario was also repeated under various altered conditions to show how the accident could have been avoided.

Figure 10.13 shows a second example of an accident reconstruction. This is a still from a reconstruction created for a major civil engineering firm and demonstrates the importance of safety procedures for pedestrian personnel around a mobile plant. In the image shown, the confusion caused by identical vehicle reversing alarms led to the death of a complacent linesman.

Investigation is a critical element of safety, and without the adequate and detailed knowledge required for such an investigation, management has no true knowledge of the reasons why accidents occur or how to prevent their recurrence. With technology developing so fast the need to model accidents and simulate dangerous occurrences has never been greater. CG and VR systems provide the

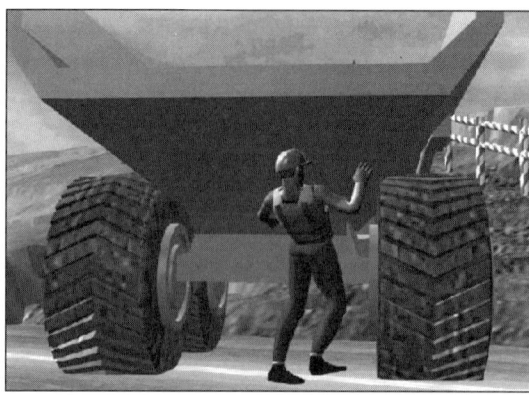

FIGURE 10.13   A computer-generated reconstruction of a construction site accident

speed and flexibility necessary to model such accidents and provide tools to consider many "what if" scenarios rapidly and effectively.

ASSESSING THE RISK

The tasks of hazard identification and risk assessment are closely linked— both require the assessors to visualize the operation (Cooper and Chapman 1985). In a complex situation, particularly one that does not yet exist in reality, it may be difficult to visualize all the factors that affect the risk, which leads to a greater likelihood of human error. Therefore, staff must be trained in how to perform a risk assessment. The skills needed will often be fully developed only after some considerable period of working in the real environment. Training is obviously extremely important, but the conventional classroom-based training is often ineffective (Bransford et al. 1986) and training in the real environment will inevitably expose inexperienced personnel to the very risks that companies are aiming to minimize.

CG and VR can be used to visualize more than real-world objects. Visual indicators of abstract data provide a powerful medium for learning about concepts or ideas. Where these ideas relate to measurement of risk, the visualization tools can be instrumental in assessing risk within the workplace (Hollands et al. 1999). One of the most difficult parts of objective risk assessment is obtaining a numerical measure for risk. AIMS has experimented with a number of different methods for assessing risk in mining environments (McClarnon et al. 1995).

The method shown in Figure 10.14 uses the concept of risk regions around a mobile plant. The wireframe shapes indicate the boundaries of a volume around the object within which there is a significant measure of risk. The VR system can be used to automatically perform risk analysis on any operation. The risk is measured at specific points where "risk markers" are placed. These markers are colored boxes that change from green (low risk) to yellow to red (high risk). The risk regions around equipment are dynamic (i.e., they change over time, dependent on the state of the virtual world at that time). Risk markers can be placed anywhere within the virtual world and can even be attached to mobile objects. This means that risk markers can be assigned to people, or to the user, and the risk to either or both monitored over a period of time.

The specific shapes of the risk regions are particular to the risks associated with that individual object and change dynamically as the risk changes. For example, while a truck is moving, the risk region extends forward in its direction of travel to represent the increased risk of collision resulting from braking time. If the vehicle is already carrying a load, or traveling on treacherous terrain, the risk region will also increase. Combining risk regions with a simulation of a typical process allows an indication of the spatial distribution of risk. Where one or more risk regions intersect, the total risk within that volume is increased.

Another study of risk around a mobile plant combines a number of spatial factors to determine the total risk at any one point. Figure 10.15 shows an image from a shuttle car training system funded by SIMRAC. This work illustrates the risks to pedestrian miners from shuttle cars moving around the mine.

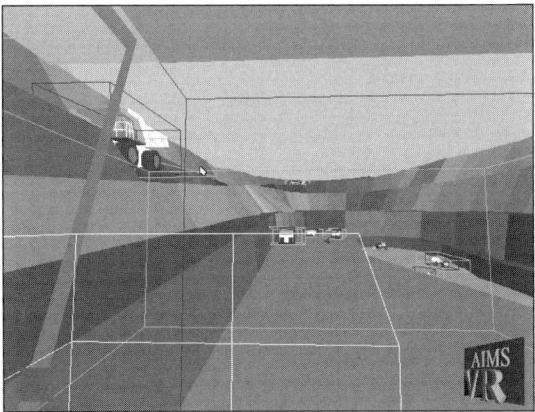

FIGURE 10.14   Using VR for open-cast risk assessment

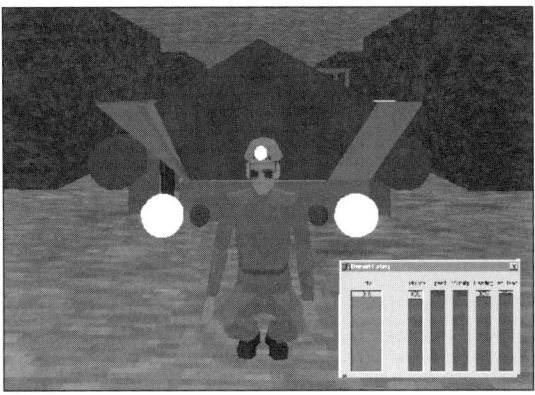

FIGURE 10.15   Combining risk components for a mobile plant

The VR system allows the user to be any one of the participants within the scene, whether the shuttle car driver, the pedestrian, or a remote observer. As the user walks around the world or drives the shuttle car, a number of risk indicators illustrate the risk that the vehicle poses to the pedestrian. Some of the risk components are intuitively simple—if the shuttle car is closer to the pedestrian the proximity risk is higher; if the shuttle car is heading away from the pedestrian, the risk is lower than if it is heading directly toward him. Finally, the faster the shuttle car, the greater the risk.

However, the two other risk components may not be as obvious. Because the pedestrian worker may well be wearing ear defenders and may work in areas of high ambient noise, a risk component determines whether the pedestrian is facing the approaching vehicle. Similarly, the areas that are visible to the shuttle car driver are also stored within the computer model. If the pedestrian is hidden from view by the load on the vehicle, or obscured by struts or paneling, the associated risk is higher than if the driver has an unobstructed view of the pedestrian (Hollands et al. 1999).

As risk assessment becomes an everyday part of many mineral operations, new and efficient ways of performing that assessment need to be considered. Because these techniques take into account many of the diverse factors involved, CG and VR are ideal for risk assessment.

IMPROVING HAZARD AWARENESS

Mining production personnel frequently and unnecessarily expose themselves to hazardous situations during routine work. Identifying potential hazards requires knowledge, skill, awareness, and aptitude. Assessing the likely severity of the hazard depends on an understanding of the hazard itself and the possible injury that may occur if things go wrong. Assessing the likely chance of the hazard leading to an incident is again based on an understanding of the environment, equipment, and processes. Although this can be taught, it is fundamentally based on the experience of the person making the assessment. VR systems developed to address this problem utilize a methodology based on the key concepts of hazard identification and risk assessment (Denby and Schofield 1998a).

Many of the VR systems developed can be used in two similar but differing modes (i.e., training and testing). In training mode a VR system can be triggered to highlight potential hazards as a trainee navigates around the world. In testing mode a trainee is presented with a similar, but different, world in which a variety of hazards exist. Instead of the hazards being highlighted as they are approached, the user must positively identify hazards by clicking a mouse, or touching a joystick button or a screen. The user must then select from a series of options to identify the hazards, to rate their potential severity, and to predict their probability of occurrence.

One of the benefits of using a VR system for hazard spotting is the ability to customize scenarios and apply random hazards. This is important because it means that trainees cannot necessarily learn to pass the test by repeated trial and error. Because each test can be unique, knowledge retention is assessed.

Competency-based testing is also possible using this approach. In certain areas of the world, there are particular problems with drug and alcohol abuse by mine operatives. Domestic problems can compound these abuses and lead to mine workers arriving for duties in an unfit state to do their jobs effectively and safely.

One of the primary groups that can benefit from VR-based training are those who may have problems with existing training programs because of limitations of language or literacy. Since it is highly unlikely that these users would be significantly computer-literate, the user interface must be kept simple, so that its operation does not form a barrier to learning from the training package.

VR technology has been investigated for application in the South African mining industry to provide improved hazard identification training for underground workers, primarily, but not exclusively, in relation to rock-related hazards. This work was conducted as a jointly funded 2-year project of SIMRAC and the Mining Technology division of the CSIR. The developer of this project recently completed a Ph.D. in VR in the AIMS Research Unit at the University of Nottingham (Squelch 1999).

Hazards represented in the South African stope model currently include falling rocks and moving machinery. An image from the system developed is shown in Figure 10.16. Each hazard is triggered by the trainee "walking" into its region of influence if no prior corrective action has been performed. In each case the implication of incorrectly responding to or recognizing the hazard is depicted to the trainee through sound and visual effects, which includes video clips where appropriate (Squelch 1996). The success or failure of a trainee is recorded for each hazard during his or her session in the virtual world, and can be subsequently rated for evaluation purposes and future comparison.

This stope model has been developed and tested with the aid of field trials at gold mine training centers in South Africa. These trials have indicated an encouraging level of relevance, understanding, and acceptance of the VR-generated mine environment among the trainee target group of underground workers. Current indications that VR technology can be successfully applied to mine safety training are very favorable (Squelch 1999).

AIMS has 10 years experience in creating a variety of VR training systems. Recently, it became apparent that a large number of the VR training applications developed shared a common set of requirements:

- Generate a three-dimensional representation of a working environment.
- Place representations of hazardous objects or situations within the world.
- Allow the user to find, identify, and categorize any hazards present.
- Simulate the operation and dynamics of objects and equipment within the virtual world.
- Allow the user to carry out actions within the virtual world.
- Tag or report any actions that result in a hazardous situation.

In order to be able to develop such applications without the programming skills normally required, AIMS has developed SAFE-VR, a graphical user interface (GUI) application development tool. Using SAFE-VR, virtual worlds can be created and populated with hazards simply by using the mouse and a simple point and click interface.

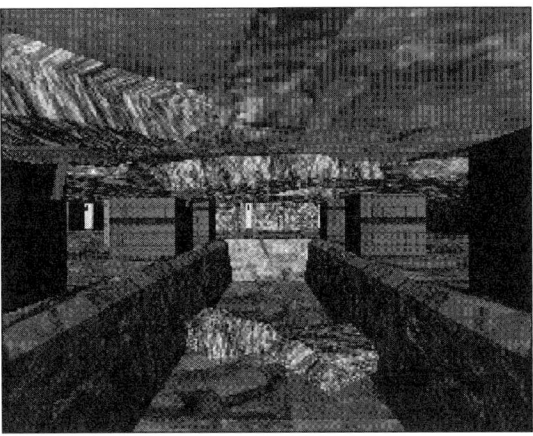

FIGURE 10.16   CSIR's gold stope training system

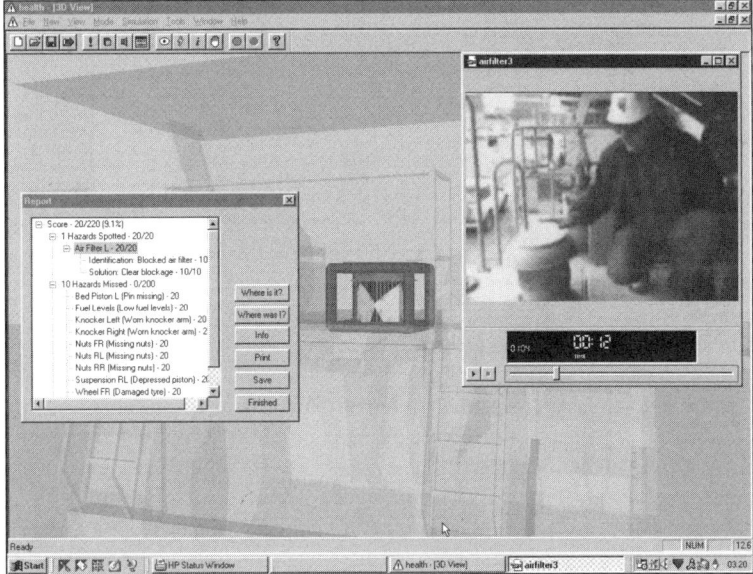

FIGURE 10.17   Example session report from a SAFE-VR preshift truck inspection, showing hazard location and multimedia video clip

In a typical SAFE-VR hazard spotting application, the user moves through the virtual world and must seek out and identify any hazards present. Once a hazardous object has been spotted, the user is presented with multiple-choice lists from which they must choose the appropriate identification and solution. Where existing training material exists within an organization, this can be incorporated into a SAFE-VR training application. The existing material then acts as a context-sensitive revision aid, as shown in Figure 10.17.

In addition to simple hazard spotting applications, SAFE-VR also has a method for creating simulations of dynamics, procedural operations, as well as fault tree diagnosis. Any object can have a number of possible actions associated with it, actions that can initiate events within the SAFE-VR simulation (Hollands et al. 1999).

As an example of a SAFE-VR scenario, Figure 10.18 shows an image from a hazard-spotting system that involves a preshift inspection of a surface mine haulage truck. This world consists of a single truck with about 25 different hazards associated with different components of the truck. The hazards themselves vary in apparent severity from missing securing pins to litter around the air filter. The system

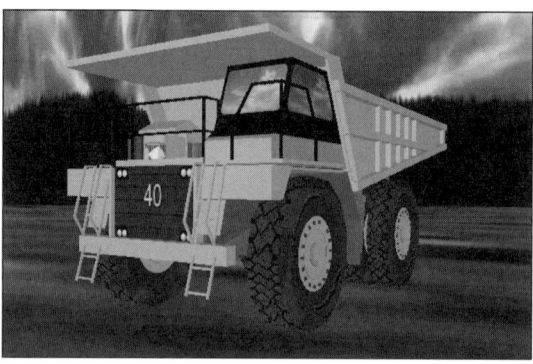

FIGURE 10.18   Image from a SAFE-VR preshift truck inspection

makes use of samples from existing training videos to explain the repercussions of overlooking any hazards. Missing securing pins may cause the entire load bed to drop from the truck, and the litter around the air intake could cause the vehicle to stall, either causing the driver to lose control, or to be stuck at a particularly dangerous point on the haul road.

Figure 10.19 is a shot from a SAFE-VR simulation of a Universal MkII 650 drill rig. These rigs can be complex to operate and extremely hazardous if handled incorrectly. This simulation combines hazard spotting with the operational simulation of the rig. In addition to the plant itself, this simulation also includes the personnel involved in the activity, who may be acting dangerously, such as the worker in the picture failing to wear protective headgear.

In addition to hazard spotting, the functions of the controls are simulated. This allows trainees to familiarize themselves with control location and function before they are allowed to operate real equipment. In addition, the trainees may operate the controls to take the rig through a standard drilling procedure. When controls are operated in the wrong sequence, the simulation logs the error and informs the user. Similarly, should the user forget any safety-related procedures, such as applying locking bars, the omission is logged, and the trainee's score is penalized.

The ability to include a functional simulation of the equipment operation also allows the inclusion of equipment fault trees. Where an item of equipment has failed, and has not been spotted during the preoperation inspection, the repercussions will be passed on to the equipment operation until the fault has been rectified. A simple example of this in the rig context is the failure to spot low fluid levels in a poorly maintained battery, which results in insufficient power to start the equipment compressors.

Figure 10.20 shows an underground roof support application developed using SAFE-VR. This application allows the user to inspect a section of roadway in an underground coal environment. The trainee is expected to spot a range of hazards such as unsupported areas, water seepage, sidewall shearing, badly installed roof bolts, and other irregularities. The trainee is also expected to identify deviations from the mines support regulations in both the roadway and at junctions. These are displayed and explained to the trainee when the application begins.

Within the underground roof support application, the trainee may be called upon to perform definite actions to create a safe situation, such as withdrawing all personnel from a dangerous, unsupported area. Although this application was developed for a coal mining environment, the methodology could be adopted for a range of mining environments.

The systems described above have demonstrated how VR-based hazard walkthroughs can train and test workers and supervisors in how to spot hazards. The advantages of this approach include:

- Real workplaces can be created, making training more relevant.
- A variety of potentially hazardous situations can be entered into the world.
- In training mode, the system can highlight hazards as the trainee navigates through the virtual workplace.
- In testing mode, the trainee must carry out an inspection of the workplace, identifying hazards, assessing risk, and identifying the correct procedures to reduce risk.

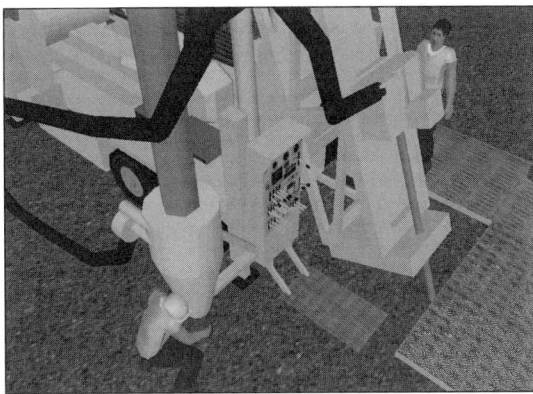

FIGURE 10.19   Image from a SAFE-VR drill rig application

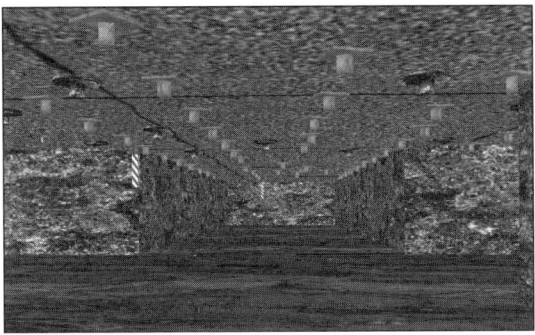

FIGURE 10.20   Image from a SAFE-VR underground roof support application

- Computerized logging of the inspection allows training procedures to be assessed.
- Hazard assessment can be considered as the first step in a quantitative risk assessment procedure.

CONCLUSIONS

Most people would agree that much of the progress made in improving the safety record of the mining industry is in large part attributable to technological advances. Improvements in engineering will no longer sustain past rates of improvement—the industry must now look at other methods of securing further improvements. Recognizing the importance of human factors in the overall safety of an organization is the first step on the path toward improved safety performance. The use of a wide range of innovative tools, simulators, and training aids will move an organization's workforce into the new century with a commitment to and motivation for an active safety culture.

Introducing CG and VR into areas associated with mine safety can be done in a number of ways, some of which have been discussed briefly in this chapter. Experience from other industries suggests that the application of these techniques can improve safety if carefully developed and integrated sensibly into a planned training program. Every organization has its own safety requirements and objectives and must decide how these tools can be used within its own workplace.

CG and VR technology is now well developed and has reduced costs to levels that allow even small mining organizations to consider its use. The flexibility of these systems means that they can be configured quickly and produced relatively cheaply. Most of the CG and VR examples highlighted in this chapter were produced in less than a month. In addition, most will run on standard, currently available desktop PCs.

VR-based simulator systems will form an increasingly important element of the training systems of the future. The ability of computers to create synthetic representations of the real world, whether in CG or VR, offers a number of opportunities to enhance current training methods. Using computer models of real equipment is free of risk and allows endless experimentation without ever taking the real equipment off-line and risking production. Allowing users to learn within computer-generated environments gives them the opportunity to make mistakes and suffer the consequences without necessarily putting themselves at risk.

The computer-based nature of the simulations often provides much-needed novelty value to the training process, resulting in users paying more attention and learning more efficiently. However, great care has to be taken to ensure that both the visual nature and simulation dynamics accurately reflect the real world to prevent the simulation from losing credibility in the eyes of cynical trainees.

The rapid developments in the computer technologies we have discussed must be matched by willingness by the industry and regulators to make use of them. There is still much that needs to be done before routine VR-based training is accepted within the mining industry. In particular there is perhaps a shift in culture that must take place amongst management and employees. Universities and government bodies and industry-based research groups may advise on the capabilities of the technology, but without support and guidance from industry the technology will fail to realize its true potential.

This technology exists now and can be embraced cost effectively by any forward-looking engineering organization on a cost effective basis. The next step is for the industry to recognize the potential and seriously invest in the development of training packages that meet various organizational needs exactly. As understanding of the techniques grows and further systems and examples develop, acceptance will continue to grow. It is only a matter of time before CG and VR applications in the mining industry reach their full potential.

REFERENCES

AIMS. 1999. AIMS Solutions. URL: www.aims-solutions.com (version current October 12, 1999).

Alicandri, E. 1994. The Next Best Thing to Being on the Road, URL: www.tfhrc.gov/pubrds/winter94/p94wi19.htm (version current October 14, 1999).

Allison, R.S. 1992. Safety in high hazard industries. *Proceedings of the Safety, Hygiene and Health in Mining Conference*. Harrogate, UK 1: 231–243.

Bentowitz, S. 1997. Computers add new twists to medical school training. *Scientists* 11:1.

Berry, D., and Z. Dienes. 1993. *Implicit Learning: Theoretical and Empirical Issues*. New York: Hillsdale.

Bird, F.E., and G.L. Germain. 1986. *Practical Loss Control Leadership*. Loganville, GA: International Loss Control Institute.

Boocock, M.G., T.C. Corlett, and J. Naylor. 1994. Visibility from free steered vehicles: a case study. *The Mining Engineer* 154(396): 81–84.

Bransford, J., R. Sherwood, N. Vye, and J. Reiser. 1986. Teaching, thinking and problem solving: research foundations. *American Psychology* 41(10): 1078–1089.

British Nuclear Fuels Limited (BNFL). 1999. BNFL–Where Science Never Sleeps. URL: www.bnfl.com (version current March 3, 1999).

Churchill, E., and D. Snowden. 1996. *Mine Training, Internal Project Report*. Nottingham, UK: University of Nottingham.

Cole, H.P. et al. 1988. *Miner and Trainer Responses to Simulated Mine Emergency Problems, Information Circular*. U.S. Bureau of Mines.

Cooper, D.F., and C.B. Chapman. 1985. An overview of risk analysis for underground projects. *Underground Space* 9: 35–40.

Denby, B., R. Hollands, and D. Schofield. 1999. Virtual reality based safety training technology for the mining industry. *Proceedings of the 28th International Conference on Safety in Mines Research Institutes*. June 7–10. Sinaia, Romania.

Denby, B., and D. Schofield. 1998a. The role of virtual reality in the safety training of mine personnel. *Proceedings of SME Annual Meeting and Exhibit*. March 9–11. Orlando, FL.

——. 1998b. Virtual reality as an aid to safety design. *Proceedings of Developments in Underground Transport Symposium*. March 26. Nottingham, UK.

——. 1999. Advanced computer techniques: developments for the minerals industry towards the new millennium. *Proceedings of the International Symposium on Mining Science and Technology*. August. Beijing, China.

Denby, B., D. Schofield, and D. McClarnon. 1995. *The Use of Virtual Reality and Computer Graphics in Mining Engineering, Information Bulletin*, Community Ergonomics Action, European Coal and Steel Community 32: 1–6.

Denby, B., D. Schofield, D.J. McClarnon, M. Williams, and T. Walsha. 1998. Hazard awareness training for mining situations using virtual reality. *Proceedings of the XXVII APCOM Symposium*. April 19–23. London, UK.

Earnshaw, R.A., M.A. Gigante, and H. Jones. 1995. *Virtual Reality Systems*. London: Academic Press.

Earthworks. 1999. Virtual Mining. URL: /www.earthworks.com.au/vrnews.htm. (version current October 14, 1999).

Egsegian, R., K. Pittman, K. Farmer, and R. Zobel. 1993. Practical applications of virtual reality to firefighter training. *Proceedings of the 1993 Simulation Multiconference of the International Emergency Management and Engineering Conference, Tenth Anniversary, Research and Applications*. April. San Diego, CA.

Evans and Sutherland Corporate Site. URL: www.es.com. (version current March 3, 1999).

Ferry, T. 1988. *Modern Accident Investigation and Analysis*. Canada: John Wiley and Sons.

Halff, H.M., J.D. Holan, and E.L. Hutchins. 1986. Cognitive science and military training. *American Psychology* 41(10): 1131–1139.

Halpern, D.F. 1984. *Thought and Knowledge: An Introduction to Critical Thinking*. Hillsdale, NJ: Erlbaum.

Health and Safety Commission. 1992. *Management of Health and Safety at Work Regulations 1992. Approved Codes of Practice*. London: HSMO.

HSE. 1991. *Successful Health and Safety Management*. London: HSMO.

——. 1992. *The Safety of Free Steered Vehicle Operations Below Ground in British Coal Mines*. London: HSMO.

Hollands, R., B. Denby, D. Schofield, G. Brooks, and A. Burton. 1999. Use of virtual reality in improving safety awareness and performance. *Proceedings of the National Oil and Gas Offshore Safety Conference*. May 26–27. Perth, Australia.

Imache, R., B. Mezhoud, and M. Maaoui. 1995. Computer aided medical training systems. *Modelling, Measurement & Control Part C: Energetics, Chemistry, Earth, Environmental & Biomedical Problems*. 48(3–4): 51–63.

Kobitec. 1999. Modelling and Simulation. URL: www.kobitec.co.za/simulate.htm. (version current October 14, 1999).

Kosuge, K., K. Takeo, and T. Fukuda. 1995. Unified approach for teleoperation of virtual and real environments–manipulation based on reference dynamics. *Proceedings of IEEE International Conference on Robotics and Automation*. Japan: IEEE. 1: 938–943.

Krueger, M.W. 1991. *Artificial Reality*. New York: Addison Wesley.

Lyons, M. 1993. *What Can Virtual Reality Offer the Building Services Industry?* Publicity Information, Colt Technology Ltd.

Mason, S. and G.C. Simpson. 1990. *Ergonomics Principles for the Design of Free Steered Vehicles*. Report No. SSL/90/173. Bretby, UK: British Coal Corporation, Scientific Services – Ergonomics Technical Department.

McClarnon, D.J., B. Denby, and D. Schofield. 1995. The use of virtual reality to aid risk assessment in underground situations. *Mining Technology* 77(892): 377–388.

Mueller, E.R. 1979. Simplified dispatching board boosts truck productivity at Cyprus Pima. *Mining Engineering* 68(4): 72–76.

OSHA. 1995. Powered Industrial Truck Operator Training. URL: gabby.osha-slc.gov/FedReg_osha_data/FED_19950314.html (version current January 22, 1997).

Pomroy, W.H., and A.M. Carigiet. 1995. *Analysis of Under-Ground Coal Mine Fire Incidents in the United States from 1978 through 1992*. Pittsburgh, PA: U.S. Department of the Interior, Bureau of Mines, IC 9426.

Rheingold, H. 1991. *Virtual Reality*. London: Secker and Warburg.

Schofield, D. 1997. Virtual reality associated with FSVs, quarries and open cast vehicles—Training, risk assessment and practical improvements. Workshop on Risks Associated with Free Steered Vehicles, Safety and Health Commission for the Mining and Other Extractive Industries, European Commission, Luxembourg.

Schofield, D., and J. Noond. 1999. Accident reconstruction: possible futures. Paper presented at Senior Accident Investigators Conference. April 24–25, Essex Police Training School, Chelmsford, Essex.

Squelch, A. 1996. Hazard recognition using artificial intelligence and virtual reality techniques. *Proceedings of the SIMRAC Symposium*. September 5. Mintek, Johannesburg.

——. 1999. Ph.D. Thesis. University of Nottingham. Application of virtual reality for hazard awareness training in South African gold mines.

Staley, B.G. 1992. Culture shock—changing attitudes to safety in mines. *Proceedings of the Safety, Hygiene and Health in Mining Conference*. Harrogate, UK. 1: 263–273.

Stewart, J.E.I. 1994. Using the backward transfer paradigm to validate the AH-64 simulator training research advanced test bed for aviation. *Human Factors and Ergonomics Society* 2: 1238–1241.

Svendsen, G.B. 1991. Influences of interface style on problem solving. *International Journal of Man-Machine Studies* 35: 379–397.

Theasby, P.J. 1992. Virtues of virtual reality. *GEC Review*, Marconi Simulation 7(3): 131–145.

Thurman, R. 1992. Simulation and training based technology. *Proceedings of the 1992 EFDPMA Conference on Virtual Reality*. December 1–2. Washington, D.C.

Williams, M., D. Schofield, and B. Denby. 1998. The development of an intelligent truck simulator. *Proceedings of Virtual Worlds 98, First International Conference on Virtual Worlds*. July 1–3. International Institute of Multimedia. Paris, France.

Wilson, J.R., M. D'Cruz, S. Cobb, and R. Eastgate. 1996. *Virtual Reality for Industrial Applications*. Nottingham, UK: Nottingham University Press.

CHAPTER 11

Inspections and Auditing

Douglas K. Martin, C.M.S.P.
Arizona State Mine Inspector, Phoenix, Arizona

H.L. Boling, C.M.S.P.
President, H.L. Boling & Associates, Inc., Pima, Arizona

INTRODUCTION

When an organization provides a safe, clean, and hazard-free work environment, a productive work environment is engendered as well. Auditing furnishes the check-and-balance system necessary for successful safety management. Actual observations in the workplace allow for real comparisons between work performances and established standards. An effective audit can be a valuable tool for all levels in a company to use for identifying potential problem areas and people who are not functioning at expected levels, and for evaluating the various processes. If used to their maximum potential, audits offer a thorough, effective assessment of existing safety management systems.

The overall objectives of auditing are to:

- Prevent injuries and property loss
- Reinforce positive safety behavior
- Elevate safety awareness
- Establish safety standards
- Test understanding of standards
- Test compliance with standards
- Identify weaknesses within the safety system
- Correct unsafe situations
- Motivate people.

SAFETY AUDIT

Training, in reality, is a positive investment in the future of employees and the company. Failure to train employees on how to properly audit specific work areas may set up a situation ripe for possible incidents or worse. The success of any audit depends on the thoroughness of training.

Guidelines to Successful Safety Audits

A standard audit form should be developed and used by all divisions or departments. This form must be clearly understood by all auditing teams and strictly adhered to as the standard tool. An example of such an audit form is shown in Figure 11.1.

The purpose of safety audits must be instilled in all management, from the front-line supervisors to the chief executive officer. Every person in the company must make a commitment to safety auditing. Auditing should also become a part of performance evaluations for hourly and supervisory personnel.

STATE CAPITOL MINING COMPANY

Safety Audit

Date: _____   Audit Team: _____

Areas Audited: _____   _____

_____   _____

Time: _____   _____

_____

OBSERVATIONS	CLASS	RESPONSIBILITY	COMPLETION

Copies to: _____   _____   _____

Positive recognition (complimenting employees on doing things right) ......PR _____

Safety improvement (employee with an idea to improve safety .... SI _____

Health (dust, noise, fumes, solvents)..H _____

Safety rule violation (actual observation, or the evidence that a rule
has been violated)... SRV _____

Environmental (spills, storage, disposal) .... E _____

Unsafe condition (a condition, obviously unsafe) .... UC _____

Unsafe act (an act obviously unsafe, not covered by a written rule
or practice) ....UA _____

FIGURE 11.1   Example of a possible audit form

Internal audits must be conducted with a positive attitude, the importance of which should be stressed to all audit team members. Training should be provided to audit team members on how to correct safety violations; deal with employee complaints, comments, and suggestions; and positively recognize and reinforce safe acts observed.

Audits must result in immediate corrective action when unsafe acts are observed. Such actions will show employees the seriousness of working safely and help to promote the safety audit process. Prompt follow-up is mandatory to demonstrate the quality of the process and the company's commitment to safety.

Audit results should be posted and discussed with all employees. Audits need to be performed on a continual basis, so that they become second nature and standard practice.

Internal audit teams should include employees ranging from top management to hourly employees. The teams should rotate members and incorporate teams from other crews, departments, or divisions. This ensures that new perspectives are constantly added to the assessment.

Auditing Criteria

Establishing a commitment and then developing audit schedules are the first steps of a sound safety program. Observe people in the workplace and communicate with employees about safe behavior. Point out observations of unsafe acts or conditions and discuss avenues to accomplish the job safely. Thanking the employees for their time, which puts the audit in a positive light, is very important.

Document the audit and file it in a centralized place for reference. Once all factors are reviewed, develop an action plan based on the observations and apply that plan.

The Audit Process

Make a commitment to spend a predetermined amount of time auditing. Although auditing does not require a great amount of time, it does require dedication.

When auditing, sample conditions in one or more small areas, rather than attempting to cover the entire area. By varying the location of the audits, all areas of audit responsibility can be assessed on a regular basis. Appropriate action during audits sets the safety climate within each department. Never let a safety violation pass without taking immediate corrective action. This reaction, or failure to react, shows employees what is acceptable and unacceptable to a supervisor.

Make it a point to recognize and mention positive behaviors and conditions during each audit. Use subsequent audits to build awareness for improvement. As work groups meet one set of goals, increase that positive motivational pressure for improved work areas.

Each auditor must make a formal list of all observations. Use these lists when discussing audit results with each group and for establishing a follow-up system. Each auditor should maintain a tickler file or notebook and follow up on audit items personally. This personal involvement is a vital step in establishing recognition, trust, and respect. Employees will not usually be motivated enough to correct unsafe practices or conditions unless they are convinced that you will be back to check. Personal follow-up maintains the positive pressure of the auditing process.

The approach to conducting audits may vary. Generally, employees should be notified when their work practices will be observed. Audit teams should discuss with employees the nature of their jobs and any hazards they are likely to encounter. To obtain a more realistic sample of work behaviors, however, the audit team may occasionally make unannounced audits and enter work areas by different routes. Before announcing that an audit will be conducted, note that the audit may simply determine an approach for a future audit.

Team size and frequency will depend on the size of the property. At the beginning of every shift, employees should inspect their work areas and equipment *before* starting work to ensure that all defects are noted and corrected. Figure 11.2 is a sample daily audit form. The safety reminder checklist is not a complete list of safety topics and should be structured for your work area or facility. Note that the items listed in Figure 11.2 are not only positive work practices, but also government requirements.

Here are some sample audit team assignments. They can be adjusted to the size of your operation and its culture.

- Team One—top management, area supervision, and at least two hourly employees
  - Frequency: one to four times a month, depending on size of the area
- Team Two—area supervisor, the front-line supervisor, and at least two hourly employees
  - Frequency: one to four times each month, depending on the size of the area
- Team Three—front-line supervisor and at least two hourly employees
  - Frequency: three to five times each week
- Team Four—safety professional (part of the checks and balances in the process)
  - Frequency: three to five times each week.

Training in Audit Methods

The most effective audit training method couples classroom instruction with actual work area walk-throughs. All employees conducting audits must understand that an effective audit program serves two purposes. Because all injuries result from unsafe behavior and/or conditions, a training system must be in place to teach employees to identify these situations and allow them to be corrected before they result in injury. Training ensures that audits are done properly, and that people are motivated, empowered, and involved. All of these contribute to establishing safety as a personal value.

It is imperative that we train people on proper auditing techniques, elements to look for, the importance of using good communication skills, and ways to always make audits a positive experience. We must never assume that because a person is a long-time employee, he or she automatically knows what to do and how to do it. We must ensure that *everyone* is properly trained.

```
DAILY WORK AREA AUDIT EXAMPLE
SAFETY REMINDER CHECKLIST

❑  Safety glasses
❑  Face shield
❑  Grinding shields
❑  Hearing protection
❑  Hard hat
❑  Steel-toed shoes
❑  Gloves
❑  Respirator
❑  Work clothing in good condition
❑  Hair containment
❑  Area housekeeping
❑  Equipment guarding
❑  Barricades
❑  Eyewash station
❑  Emergency showers
❑  Fire protection inspected
❑  Seat belts
❑  Vehicle inspection checklist
❑  Fall protection
❑  Tag-out procedure followed
❑  Berms-roadway/dumps
❑  Ladder inspection
❑  Power tools inspected
❑  Electrical cords inspected
❑  Overhead hazards
❑  Scaffolds inspected
❑  Tie-off protection
❑  Hazard communication
❑  Confined space permits
❑  Other: _____

The safety reminder checklist is not a complete list of safety topics and should be
structured for your work area or facility.
```

FIGURE 11.2 Example of a possible safety reminder checklist

Objectives and Benefits of Audits

Audits should promote safe behaviors, in addition to motivating and empowering employees. Hazardous acts and conditions must be identified and eliminated. Building safety awareness is an important part of the process. The audit should locate and correct defects in the safety system.

Focus on certain factors at the time of audit, such as safe behavior, physical hazards, and personal protective equipment. Other concerns are work processes, body mechanics, unsafe acts or procedures, equipment use, and the pace of work.

Behavior and Physical Audits

A successful audit incorporates both behavior and physical audits, properly blended into a safety system that provides a safe and healthy work environment for the employee.

Behavior audits survey employees as they carry out their tasks, looking for unsafe behavior. First, determine whom to audit, and obtain their permission. Next, observe them at work. Remember that most unsafe behaviors are caused by time constraints, attempts for convenience or comfort, and an "it can't happen to me" attitude. Provide feedback to the employee or employees at the conclusion of the audit (keep the feedback both positive and constructive). As always, document audit results and develop a follow-up plan that includes corrective actions.

Physical audits evaluate the safety of working conditions and identify workplace hazards. First, determine where to conduct the audit. Always communicate with employees working in the area. List items of concern when documenting the audit results. Again, develop a follow-up or corrective action plan and implement it.

Audit Observation Techniques

The key to successful auditing is making precise observations. Getting an overview of the audit area or "the big picture" and deciding where attention should be focused can enhance observation efficiency. Attempt to catch the evaporating act—the one that ceases before you notice it.

Specific questions in different categories can be asked during observation:

Positions and actions of people—Is anyone in danger of injury by pulling or lifting heavy objects? Is anyone in a position to fall or be trapped, hit by, or collide with anything?

Proper use of personal protective equipment—Does the employee always use the proper personal protective equipment (PPE)? Does the PPE provide adequate protection against exposure to hazards? Has the employee been trained in how to properly use and wear the PPE? Is the PPE inconvenient to wear, or hampering in any way?

Tools and equipment—Does the employee know how to use them properly and safely? Are they in a safe condition? Are they being inspected regularly? Are homemade tools that are against company policy being used?

Adherence to procedures—Are the procedures adequate to perform the job in an efficient and safe manner? Do they address and prevent risk? Are they followed at all times? If not, why not?

Neatness and organization—Is the workplace neat and in order? Are tools and items being returned to their proper place? Do employees clean up workstations before leaving for breaks, lunch, or the end of their shift?

AUDIT CHECKLIST

An audit checklist can vary depending on the type of work performed at a company or organization. Here is an example of a suggested checklist, intended to give you an idea of what they are and possibly how they should be structured. (Note: this audit checklist is not all-inclusive.)

- Personal protective equipment. Is it adequate? Used properly? In good condition? Does it protect the:
  - Ears
  - Head
  - Arms and hands
  - Legs and feet
  - Respiratory system
  - Torso.
- Positions of personnel (injury causes)
  - Striking against, struck by
  - Caught between
  - Falling
  - Temperature extremes
  - Electric current
  - Inhaling, absorbing, swallowing
  - Overexertion
  - Miscellaneous: explanation: _____
- Actions of employees
  - Adjusting protective equipment
  - Changing position
  - Rearranging job

- – Stopping job
- – Attaching grounds or locks
- – Miscellaneous: explanation: _____
- ▪ Tools and equipment
  - – Correct for the job
  - – Used correctly
  - – In safe condition.
- ▪ Procedures and orderliness
  - – Adequate, reviewed, and upgraded
  - – Established and understood
  - – Maintained.

Always take time to develop and continuously upgrade the audit checklist as technology changes or improves.

AUDIT QUALITY

As a supervisor or leader, you need to ensure that the audits conducted in your area are effective and of a consistent standard. When we properly train our people (both hourly and management) to audit, and work with them to increase their awareness of what auditing is all about, we raise the standard of audits in our area and provide a safe, clean, hazard-free, productive work environment.

We should also frequently observe audits conducted by people in other areas to compare the results and ensure that we have a consistent process. The comparison will also serve as a check and balance system and point out areas where further training is needed to ensure a common standard of excellence.

PROPRIETORSHIP

The single concept that will make a positive, well-thought-out audit work is the idea of proprietorship. We must all understand that we "own" the auditing process, which is a very important component of a safety system designed to protect all of us—employees, contractors, and visitors alike. All managers and supervisors, from the top through first-line supervisors, are responsible for everything that happens in their areas. If we are to have buy-in and expect people to take proprietorship of the audit, we must ensure that they are provided with proper training, tools, time, and support to complete the job correctly.

Jobs and work areas are only as safe or unsafe as we choose to make them. Taking proprietorship ensures that we follow the correct direction.

ANNOUNCED AND UNANNOUNCED SAFETY AUDITS

Safety audits can be conducted using several different methods, and feedback can take both written and verbal forms. Choose the method that aligns with your company's culture and size.

To capture a broad area, general audits encompass large physical areas and behaviors. Specific audits focus on specific areas, such as looking only at electrical defects, auditing specific behavior, or looking for unsafe acts, such as improper lifting.

You may audit as a team or individually. It is not the number of auditors that counts, but the thoroughness of the audit. Differing methods carry equal value, depending on your need.

Announced Audits

Announced and scheduled audits held each week can be effective in getting neglected areas cleaned up and ensuring that employees focus on behaviors and practice safe work habits. Announced audits promote buy-in from employees, which builds trust. Employees normally like to know when they will be audited so they can prepare and look good on the audit report.

Unannounced Audits

Unannounced audits are a good tool to determine how a work area and the employees are functioning or following safe work habits without prior knowledge of being observed. These types of audits measure how well the safety assessment program is working. Additionally, unannounced audits are a good way to inspect contractor work areas.

REPORTING AND POSTING AUDIT RESULTS

Reporting audit results can create a positive and open auditing process. It lets all employees know that audits are being conducted and removes the common stigma that says that "management does not want to know about defects and improper acts." It emphasizes the importance of audits by publicizing who is part of the audit team. The names of employees audited should not be reported to maintain positive reactions to audits.

Internal audit results should be posted in the division office on the safety bulletin board and on bulletin boards in the area being inspected. Results should be posted immediately upon completion, with action items noted on the form. Positive recognition should be listed first, indicating items that were noted during the review as safe and in compliance with company policy.

Results of each audit should also be regularly reviewed during safety meetings. Trend analysis, such as bar or line graphs, can be used to demonstrate progress being made in safe work behaviors. Such charts should not only be used to show trends on types of defects, but on the completion of audits, themselves. To show commitment to eliminate all accidents, there must be follow-up on unsafe acts and conditions, giving employees a general feeling for the status of safety in that area.

AUDIT FOLLOW-UP

Develop a system that ensures follow-up or effective action. Obvious hazards *must* be followed up on *immediately*! Without delay, a copy of the report must be filed with routing instructions so it can be tracked through the system. Follow-up evaluations on audit items should be done before the next scheduled audit, then documented and filed appropriately.

Items discovered during an audit that present obvious hazards must be acted upon and remedied immediately. Less serious issues should be put in order of priority and a schedule developed to correct each item in a timely fashion.

All such remedies must be completed before the next scheduled audit. Audits, no matter how detailed, are of little or no value when we fail to consistently follow up with corrective action. Failure to follow up sends a clear message to the employees that the company is not concerned about their safety and health.

CONCLUSION

An audit's success depends on the understanding, caring, motivation, and skill of all involved. A program that ensures regular audits covering all areas and involving every employee will encourage total participation. Consistent follow-up is the key to correcting issues revealed through both physical and behavioral audits.

Auditing is an essential tool for identifying current and potential problems. This enables management to evaluate problem-solving options and provide a safe and productive work environment.

Auditing results measure the safe working environment on the entire property and zero in on specific areas. Employee commitment is the key to safety.

Positive, consistent audits give us a clear picture on how well we manage the safety process. They will prove to be invaluable to ensure that our people are properly trained, follow-up actions are carried out consistently, and a positive attitude is maintained toward both the process and the employees.

Please keep the following reasons in mind when employees question the need to audit: Auditing prepares safe work areas for people. Failure to properly audit places people at risk. In a nutshell, audits are the right thing to do.

Hazards are blind, they do not discriminate against gender, skin color, physical characteristics, or company affiliation.

CHAPTER 12

Incident Reporting and Analysis

Douglas K. Martin, C.M.S.P.
Arizona State Mine Inspector, Phoenix, Arizona

H.L. Boling, C.M.S.P.
President, H.L. Boling & Associates, Inc., Pima, Arizona

INTRODUCTION

Incident reporting and analysis determines what happened during an incident, allowing the causes to then be eliminated. The overall goal is to prevent injuries and property damage by learning from our mistakes.

Specifically, the purposes of incident analysis are to:

- Learn from mistakes
- Prevent recurrences
- Increase the level of safety awareness
- Demonstrate commitment to continuous improvement.

Established procedures for evaluating causes of incidents should be in place at all companies and organizations. Incident analysis should be followed by the implementation of controls to prevent future similar occurrences. Comprehensive procedures should also include the analysis of near incidents. Potential causes can be controlled before an incident occurs. All incidents that result in fatalities or serious injuries to more than one person should have the analysis conducted under the direction of corporate safety and with legal advice.

Incident analysis should always be conducted as a fact-finding mission, not a fault-finding one. Good, positive communication is the key ingredient to success. It is understood that incidents do not just happen, they are caused. The cause is often not readily apparent, but it is always the crux of the problem. The cause may be a wide variety of events, or a single episode initiated by the affected employee. Effective analysis will result in a positive attitude toward the job, employment, supervisor, company, and safety procedures. The single most effective way to determine an incident cause is through direct communication between the employee involved in the incident and the analysis team.

Avoid finger pointing and fixing blame. Even though a company safety rule may clearly have been violated and discipline may be warranted, the analysis should be allowed to unfold and bring to light the causes and responsible parties. Discipline, should always be done in private, away from the incident analysis team. This is a one-to-one meeting between the supervisor and employee involved. A detailed explanation about why discipline is warranted should be given. Discipline should always aim to correct, never to punish. This forum will provide an opportunity to stress the importance of the employee to the company and the care and concern that the supervisor, management, and the company has for his or her safety and well-being. Incident prevention goes hand-in-hand with a thorough incident analysis, which should include a caring, consistent discipline policy.

The incident area is first made safe by eliminating immediate causes. All incidents are to be reported immediately with an individual form completed for each employee involved. All incidents are to be analyzed immediately by the supervisor and affected employee. If the employee is not available because of trauma, an employee who performs the same type of work should be called upon.

The initial team (employee/supervisor) shall determine if a full team is required. This decision is based on the depth, severity, and complexity of the incident. If a full team is not needed, the supervisor and employee will complete the analysis immediately and carry out a corrective action plan.

If a full team is formed, it continues the analysis, starting by collecting incident data. The immediate causes and root causes of the incident are based on known facts and an action plan for eliminating the root causes is formulated.

Completion dates and responsible individuals are then assigned to implement the action plan. The incident analysis team shall then prepare and distribute a report to all supervisors for discussion with their employees. The Health and Safety Department collects the results of the analysis, compares this incident with previous records, and determines if a trend exists.

Points to Remember

- Always keep your attitude toward the analysis and the employee positive.
- Never rush an analysis. Give everyone a chance to talk. Listen to each person's explanation and his or her perception of what happened.
- The only way similar types of incidents can be prevented from recurring is if every incident is thoroughly analyzed and its true cause determined.
- Communicate! Communicate! Communicate!

RESPONSIBILITIES AND TRAINING

In the preplanning stage of the process, the persons responsible for analyzing the incident must be clearly designated. The first level of supervision is most often assigned as coordinator. This person is the management representative closest to the day-to-day activities that resulted in the mishap. It is not meant to imply the front-line supervisors should have total responsibility. In most instances, other members of the analysis team should share the responsibility and assist the supervisor. Other responsibilities may include:

- **Employees** advise the supervisor of facts associated with the incident and immediately report all occupational or property incidents, near incidents, and illness.
- **Safety professional(s)** assist the analysis team in fact finding, causal analysis, and the development of conclusions and recommendations.
- **Engineering** supplies detailed process information and assists in developing effective engineering solutions to any problems identified.
- **Maintenance** assists in determining if the lack of preventive maintenance, or any maintenance procedure, contributed to the incident.
- **Corporate Safety Department** directs analysis in the event of fatalities, or of serious injuries to more than one person, and assigns members to the investigation team. Corporate safety staff assists in developing reports to regulatory authorities, final in-house reports, and news releases.
- **Legal Department** assists in advising accuracy in reporting, circulation of reports, remedial actions, and potential liability.
- **Management** reviews incident reports, assists in developing recommendations, and assigns personnel to oversee corrective action.

Everyone who is given responsibility to conduct incident analysis must be trained in the proper procedure for gathering facts, analyzing causes, developing corrective actions, and reporting results. In particular, the training program should emphasize the properties of causal analysis, resulting from effective analysis. A thorough investigation produces meaningful conclusions and corrective recommendations.

Usually the facility safety department is charged with the initial training of all individuals who are promoted into supervision and those assigned to the analysis team. Emphasis is placed on how to conduct an effective and positive incident analysis. Annual refresher training is suggested for all supervisors and analysis team members to enhance and sharpen skills.

INCIDENT ANALYSIS AND REPORTING FORMS

Training employees to properly fill out incident analysis report completely is essential. Depending on the incident's severity, reports may be narrative or documented on the incident analysis forms or checklists. A narrative report contains detailed answers to the following questions (see Figure 12.1):

- **What was the employee doing?** Explain in detail the activity of the employees at the time of the incident.

- **What happened?** Indicate in detail what took place. Describe the incident, type of injury, parts of the body affected, and whether the employee was wearing appropriate safety equipment properly.

- **What caused the incident?** Explain in detail the condition, act, or malfunction that caused the incident. Remember, it is common to have more than one reason or cause for an incident. Carelessness is not a cause. Example: An employee is moving along a walkway next to a conveyor carrying rock. He steps on a stone and twists his ankle. The initial team must visualize the total picture of where the rock came from and how it ended up on the walkway. Blaming the employee for not watching where he or she was walking will lose credibility with the employee and not arrive at the root cause.

- **What can be done to prevent a similar incident?** Identifying root causes, performing corrective procedures, and communicating this information to all employees will prevent similar incidents in the future.

An incident analysis form or checklist should contain, as a minimum, employee identification, dates, time, department, shift, location of the incident, a thorough description of the event, and an analysis of the causal factors. As the investigation continues, the checklist should list action items completed or pending to correct the problem (see Figure 12.2).

Signatures of the incident analysis team members are necessary to indicate review and approval. It is important that the report is submitted to management before leaving the facility on the day the incident occurred. Incomplete or inadequate reports should be returned to the supervisor for additional attention.

DEFINITIONS

Incidents

An occurrence or event that interrupts normal procedure or precipitates a crisis is an incident. Include all events that could have resulted in injury or damage to facilities. This includes what is typically thought of as near incidents. The potential consequences are the same in a near incident as in a serious injury. Types of incidents requiring analysis are:

- Near incidents
- Property damage
- Illness
- First aid injuries
- Medical treatment injuries
- Lost-time injuries
- Fatalities.

The difference between a near incident and a fatality is pure luck. It is essential that all incidents are viewed equally and analysis performed with the same intensity. Some definitions follow:

- **Property damage**—impairment of the usefulness or value of equipment, tools, or facility. Include all incidents that result in property damage, no matter how minor.

- **Injury incidents**—damage to a person. Include all incidents that result in injury, no matter how minor. Include near incidents.

Incident and Reporting Form

Near Incident: _____   First Aid: _____

Property Damage: _____   No Time Lost: _____

Illness: _____   Lost Time: _____

Employee Name: _____   PR: _____

SSN: _____   Regular Job Title: _____   Dept./Crew: _____

Job Title at Time of Incident: _____

Date of Incident: _____   Time of Incident: _____   (a.m./p.m.)

Date of Shift Rotation: _____   Day of Week: _____

Location of Incident: _____

Supervisor Name: _____

Description of Incident: _____

_____

_____

_____

Was there an injury?:   Yes   No   If yes, describe: _____

_____

_____

FIGURE 12.1   Incident and reporting form

- **Analysis**—separation of the substantial whole into its constituent parts for individual study. A thorough analysis should be conducted on every incident.

REPORTING RESPONSIBILITY

All employees, regardless of position, are responsible for immediately reporting all types of incidents to their supervisor. When an injury incident is not reported promptly, it may become more serious through lack of medical attention. Additionally, another employee caught in the same circumstance may be critically hurt if no action has been taken to eliminate the original causes.

Recognizing and removing a potential hazard before an incident occurs is the responsibility of all employees. It is the responsibility of management, including front-line supervision, to maintain an atmosphere where all incidents can be analyzed thoroughly and objectively. Therefore, reporting, analysis, and implementation of the action plan should be a shared responsibility of all employees.

The reporting and analysis of all types of incidents is a responsibility of employees and management. The Health and Safety Department can assist in managing safety in several ways. These professionals have special training and expertise in the area of root cause analysis. Their services are very valuable in identifying potential hazards and contributing causes, which you may not recognize.

After an occurrence, the department can classify and accurately report the incident for precise record keeping. The department receives the Incident Report and the Incident Analysis Team Report, then calculates data trends. These results are then distributed to the appropriate internal divisions and other companies.

The Health and Safety Department professionals' knowledge can be essential in building a safety program and audit system that complies with laws and regulations.

```
                        Years   Months    Incident happened during:

Total Mining Experience:        _____   _____     Regular time: _____

Experience at this Mine:        _____   _____     Overtime: _____

Experience at this job title:   _____   _____

Employee Recommendation to Prevent Recurrence: _____

_____

_____

Immediate Action Taken to Prevent Recurrence: _____

_____

Action Taken by: _____      Date Completed: _____

Supervisor Signature:                     Employee Signature:

_____              _____

Note:  Use attachment if more space is needed for descriptions or recurrence
information.

   A copy of this form must be given to the Safety Department on date of incident

                    Routing of Original Report

                       (Review and initial)

Gen Supervisor: _____          Superintendent: _____

      Manager: _____           Safety: _____
```

FIGURE 12.1   Incident and reporting form (continued)

THE ANALYSIS TEAM

An incident analysis team prevents the recurrence of similar incidents. The team should always be thoroughly trained on what to do and what not to do. They must understand the importance of this tool that helps eliminate all incidents. Attitude plays a large role in the ability to reach the root cause. For example, if our reaction is to get angry and point a finger, the employees will not volunteer information freely. Under these circumstances, the root cause may elude the analysis team. Any lost time in eliminating a hazard places workers at risk.

The start of every analysis should be an explanation by the supervisor as to the direction, purpose, and importance of the analysis. Every member of the team must understand failure to arrive at a root cause could jeopardize others working in similar conditions. Knowing how to and eliminating causes properly protects workers and companies.

Establishing a Team

The front-line supervisor, hourly employees, management, and safety department comprise the team as follows:

- The analysis team is established as soon as possible after the incident.
- Management supports and participates.
- Team size is based on needs of the analysis.
- Peers of the involved employee should be included if at all possible, especially individuals who perform similar work.

Incident Analysis Checklist

The following (example) checklist is intended to serve only as a guide to possible causes of an incident. The list is not complete, but should function as a starting point to help guide the analysis team toward finding both the immediate, and most importantly, the root cause.

Equipment or Facility
Unrecognized hazard
Recognized hazard, inadequate action
Design factor
Installation factor
Improper use of equipment/facility
Inadequate equipment/facility
Insufficient equipment/facility

People Indirectly Involved
Unsafe work procedures
Unsafe acts
Lack of safety awareness
Lack of proper training
Lack of experience
Lack of judgment
Not following procedure/practice
Acceptance of unsafe practice or condition
Lack of supervision
Lack of adequate personnel

Operating Conditions
Normal, repetitive operations
Normal, nonrepetitive operations
Abnormal situation
Employee-created unsafe conditions
Work environment unsafe condition
Environmental issues

People Directly Involved

Unsafe work procedures
Unsafe acts
Lack of safety awareness
Lack of proper training
Lack of experience
Lack of judgment
Acceptance of unsafe practice or condition
Lack of supervision
Not following procedure/practice
Lack of adequate personnel

Procedure
Inadequate for the job
Outdated because new equipment is available
Not understood by employees

FIGURE 12.2   Incident analysis checklist

- Whenever possible, always include subject matter experts.
- Involve safety and health professionals.
- Deploy additional resources that enable the team to reach the root cause.

When we are committed, we will find a solution. When we are not committed, we place people at risk. If we are willing to accept risk, then we must be willing to accept tragic consequences to friends and coworkers.

The role of the team leader is to establish the analysis team, obtain consensus on the objective, and build trust and consistency in the analysis process. All type of fault finding must be eliminated and no fingers must be pointed. Copies of the standard operating procedures should be read before a team member investigating an incident. All results and recommendations must be based on facts, not opinions.

The team is charged with collecting all the pertinent information. From this data, a determination of the immediate and root causes is made. The action plan is then formulated and responsibility for implementation taken.

To prevent recurrence, the team must begin the analysis as soon as possible. All circumstances and events that immediately led up to the incident must be discovered and the root cause or causes identified. An action plan based on previously found facts must be written, approved, and acted on. Communicate the results of the analysis to all employees. An incident affecting a fellow worker is meaningful. Allowing the analysis team to function for the betterment of safety will make a lasting impression, boost moral, and improve safe production.

The benefits of a successful analysis can be realized by identifying potential hazards that can be corrected before an injury occurs. Areas in need of safety emphasis will be recognized. Existing procedures, practices, and safety training will be modified to prevent incidents. The collection and assimilation of incident reports indicate trends that can be averted by responding with appropriate safety management.

The *initial team* is the affected employee and supervisor. A *full team* comprises the employee, a peer employee, the front-line supervisor, a management representative, and a safety professional.

The *peer employee* is one who performs similar work with a background or experience in the work process. Peer contribution is important for two reasons:

1. Knowledge of the work environment or job procedures helps to uncover the underlying root cause and their involvement ensures the action plan is pertinent and acceptable to other employees doing similar work.

2. The incident analysis team may also include other departments, divisions, or individuals at any organizational level depending on the need.

EMPLOYEE PERCEPTIONS

Conducting an incident analysis is precipitated by care about employee health and safety. The analysis is not a means to find fault, punish anyone, or cover up information. By reacting quickly to incidents and taking time to ensure they are analyzed thoroughly and objectively, the importance of safety is shown. It is important to use good interpersonal skills to eliminate negative perceptions.

An employee must always be treated with dignity and respect. All actions should accentuate the positive. Information should be gathered in a factual manner, eliminating hearsay and opinions. Persons who have acted properly or responded well to the situation must be praised. Those who need improvement should be given additional training. Always show compassion for anyone injured or traumatized by the incident. An incident of serious nature will affect many people throughout the job site and off the property.

TIMING

All types of incidents should be analyzed immediately. The circumstances surrounding the incident may change as a result of operations, weather, or personnel, among other factors. People involved in the incident may have a problem remembering details and may unknowingly substitute conjecture or opinion for fact. Witnesses may discuss the incident and influence each other's version of the details.

Injured employees may be in pain, emotionally upset, or in need of medical attention. In these cases, the supervisor may have to take their statements later. If employees are willing, the supervisor may interview the injured employee at the hospital or home in order to determine the cause of the incident.

GUIDELINES FOR COLLECTING FACTS

It is important that factual information be carefully recorded. The individual collecting data must take detailed notes to accurately record the employee's account. Verify the data with the employee to ensure accuracy and to confirm that the impact is fully understood. Employees should not be interrupted with questions when describing the incident. Ask questions after the employee has finished. Do not attempt to explore the incident causes at this point. The focus should be exclusively on understanding what happened.

Collection of facts

- All information possible from the injured, ill, or affected employee
- List of witnesses and their statements
- Physical data at the scene

- All records, including training and personnel
- Workplace auditing reports
- Equipment maintenance records
- Description of equipment loss
- Photos and videos
- Planned safe reenactment
- Training and standard operating procedures
- Any other documentation that will assist in determining the root cause.

When gathering facts, care should be given so blame is not placed or perceived. The supervisor should explain the purpose of incident analysis. It is important that everyone feels relaxed and a good relationship exists between the supervisor, the employee, and any witnesses.

The following questions do not establish facts and may hinder the analysis:

"Didn't you know you had to wear goggles?"

"Why didn't you get another ladder?"

"Why didn't you slow down when you realized the road was slick?"

Fact-finding questions do not accuse, blame, or threaten, but allow witnesses to speak freely and unhampered.

"What were you doing at the time of the incident?"

"How were you doing the task?"

"How do you think the incident occurred?"

"What do you believe could have prevented this incident?"

If possible, the interview should be conducted at the scene of the incident to make it easier for the employee to demonstrate the exact location or body position. The number of people at the scene should be minimized to avoid putting the employee on the defensive or becoming embarrassed or uncomfortable.

Interview all witnesses. Witnesses may hesitate to say anything that places a coworker in a bad light. You should help them understand this is not a fault-finding mission, and the main purpose of the analysis is to prevent future injuries. If possible, witnesses should be interviewed separately to prevent influencing each other's accounts or being subjected to peer pressure. They should be interviewed in a similar manner as the procedure used with the injured employee. Do not forget compassion.

The analysis team should accomplish the following steps:

- Visit the scene of the incident and examine the equipment involved to gain perspective.
- Review all applicable work procedures to ensure they contain specific instructions on the safety hazards of the job.
- Ascertain if the employee received proper task training.

Determining the cause of an incident is the most important responsibility of the incident analysis team. The *immediate cause* is the act or condition that directly resulted in a near incident, injury, or property damage. The *root cause* is the underlying system, actions, or conditions that allow the immediate cause to occur.

For example, an individual cuts his finger when handling a recently purchased machine part. The immediate cause may be not wearing appropriate gloves. The root cause may be that the tool room was not open and the employee could not obtain gloves, or the employee was not trained to recognize the need for gloves in this type of situation. The immediate cause relates specifically to the incident, whereas the root cause is more general and can be applied to a variety of situations.

To find the root cause, continue to ask "why" until a solution is found or until "why" cannot be answered. Why was the employee's finger cut? Simple, no gloves. Why were gloves not available in the work area? The tool room was closed or the employee did not take time to walk to the locker for his gloves.

Improper procedures, and lack of training, should always be addressed or eliminated as a potential root cause. Environmental and long-term health issues should be included. Personal factors may have contributed to the incident and should be considered. Personal factors play an important part when determining root causes. Sometimes they may seem more subjective than objective, but must be made part of the analysis. Questions such as: Were they attempting to save time or effort? Was there emotional stress? Were safety rules violated? Was the employee fatigued?

No greater amount of importance can be placed on ensuring that the analysis is fact finding, not fault finding. You must look at all possible contributing cause or causes, and continue to ask why.

All the time and effort put into an incident analysis will be wasted if there is no action plan or incomplete follow up. The action plan must attack root causes. Once root causes have been identified and agreed on by the analysis team, an action plan should be made to prevent the occurrence of similar incidents. This may apply to a particular situation, job, area, branch, or to the entire operation. If you fail to arrive at the root cause, you are destined to repeat the incident again. What we invest in people and the process is what we get out of it. Everyone must be properly trained in incident analysis.

Each action plan should contain items that supervision, management, and the individual will do to correct each cause and prevent recurrence. The individual responsible for implementation of each item must be identified. All action plan items should have a target date with a leader assigned the responsibility to follow items through to completion. As implied before, incidents should not be kept secret. Records need to be kept, compared, and the results shared throughout the operation. Awareness instigates thought.

A written incident analysis team report must be completed as a means of organizing findings and recording conclusions for future reference and follow-up. Keep the report factual and positive.

REPORTS

The following information should be included in the detailed report of the incident analysis team:

Employee Information

- Occupation
- Age
- Payroll number
- Total experience in job classification
- Training
- Length of service with the company
- Service at this particular task.

Injury Information

- Date of incident, injury, or illness
- Time occurred
- Time reported by employee or other
- Time employee reported for medical attention
- Location of the incident
- Nature of injury or illness
  - Part of body affected
  - Simple diagnosis.

Physical Damage

List the equipment involved, including:

- Purpose
- Serial number
- Make
- Model
- Age
- Maintenance records
- Condition.

Incident Analysis Process

Purpose
Improve workplace safety
Determine root cause
Uncover defects in safety management systems
Demonstrate commitment for continuous improvement

The Analysis Process
Establishing a team
       Front-line supervisor
       Hourly employee
       Management
       Safety department

Collecting pertinent information
       Interviews
       Observations

Validating root causes
       Fact finding (not fault finding)

Determining corrective/preventive actions
       Using all available resources
       Closing the loop

Management Responsibilities
Direct participation
Oversight
Final approval
Evaluation of analysis performance
Case studies

Follow-up
Evaluating incident reports
       Thoroughness and accuracy
       Timeliness
       Specific causes listed
       Remedies suggested
       Responsibilities established

Corrective/preventive actions
       Eliminate root causes
       Eliminate underlying causes
       Eliminate the hazard
       Construct a barrier
       Institute new procedures
       Train employees

FIGURE 12.3   Incident analysis process

Physical Conditions
- Location
- Weather
- Temperature
- Position of sun
- Flooring—wet or dry, asphalt, concrete, dirt, stone, sand.

Incident History
- Background information relevant to the incident description
- Body position when incident occurred
- Activity at the time of incident
- List of tools and equipment in use at the time
- Description of any unsafe conditions or acts that led to the incident.

Incident Description

Describe the unexpected event.

Security Actions

Immediate action taken for the protection or rescue of employees.

- **Analysis**—interview of affected people, list of witnesses with statements including activities and physical location when incident occurred
- **Determination**—root cause of the incident with validation, appropriate corrective and preventive actions
- **Assignment**—individual to oversee and take responsibility for completion of entire action plan, team members, dates of team meetings
- **Action plan**—elimination of the root causes, dates for completion of each item, person responsible for each item
- **Trends**—compare incident information
- **Team report**—detailed report for selected distribution
- **Distribution report**—summary of the team report for general distribution (this distribution report must protect the privacy of the individuals involved; do not include personal information)
- **Approvals**—management, legal, safety and health, supervisor
- **Communication**—discuss distribution report with all employees.

When we fail to conduct an incident analysis properly, we place people and property at risk. Jobs, procedures, and work areas are only as safe or unsafe as we choose to make them. If we properly conduct incident analyses, we can, and will, eliminate chance and risk in the process. Figure 12.3 summarizes the incident analysis process.

CHAPTER 13

Safety Communications[1]

George L. Germain
GL&M Associates, Flowery Branch, Georgia

INTRODUCTION

This chapter focuses on selected aspects of a fascinating, often frustrating, process related to most of our problems and progress—the vital process of communication. Other than thinking, virtually everything we do includes some aspect of communication. As an anonymous sage once said: *You cannot not communicate*. The renowned Stephen Covey expressed it even more broadly and strongly: *Communication is the most important skill in life* (1989, p. 237). In operations such as mining, communication often is, in fact, an injury prevention and life-saving tool.

No attempt is made here to cover all, or even most, aspects of communication. Rather, the focus is on a practical definition, a few principles and tips, key listening skills, group/team communications, and an introduction to personal (one-on-one) communication tools such as orientation, job instruction, key point tipping, and planned personal contacts.

PRACTICAL DEFINITION

Communication is a two-way process that involves sending and receiving symbols, signs, or signals, in the form of words, pictures, things, and actions. It is speaking and listening, writing and reading, behaving and observing behavior. Its goal is to achieve understanding. Here is a simple, practical definition used around the world:

> *Communication is what we do to send and receive understanding. Expressed another way, the communication process is ... interaction resulting in meaning and understanding. The interaction may be between two people; among a group of people; or between people and written words, pictures, sounds, smells, tastes, objects, or animals.*

It can be quite challenging to interact in such a way that *mutual* meaning and understanding occur. Two big reasons for this are "personal mind filters" and "selective perception." As depicted in Figure 13.1 all of the inputs—words, pictures, sounds, smells, tastes, and behaviors—go through the receiver's mind filter—cultural background, past experiences, values, attitudes, biases, feelings, needs, desires, and roles. What comes through the filter, the output, is the receiver's interpretations, meanings, and reactions.

The second reason why good communication can be so challenging is selective perception; that is, what we see is determined by what we look for. We tend to see what we have seen before, what we

---

1. Adapted, with permission, from related chapters in (1) Bird, F.E., Jr., and G.L. Germain. 1996. *Practical Loss Control Leadership*. Loganville, GA: Det Norske Veritas (USA.), Inc.; (2) Bird, F.E., Jr., and G.L. Germain. 1997. *The Property Damage Accident*. Loganville, GA: FEBCO, Inc.; (3) Germain, G.L., R.M. Arnold, Jr., R.J. Rowan, and J.R. Roane. 1998. *Safety, Health and Environmental Management*. Dallas, TX: International Risk Management Institute.

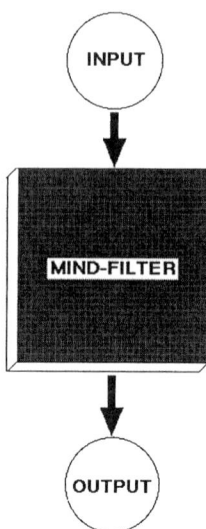

FIGURE 13.1   Communication or confusion?

expect to see, what we want to see, what we are tuned in to. We pay attention to specific aspects of our environment and don't notice others. How we interpret what happens around us depends, in large measure, on whether we are male or female, conservative or liberal, rich or poor, majority or minority, miner or manager, and so on. Diversity increases the communication challenge.

As shown in Figure 13.2, communication can be the bridge from one mind to another. Good communication bridges the gaps of confusion and misunderstanding and results in mutual meaning and understanding. It is a wonderful way to reduce mistakes, wastes, accidents, injuries, damage, and harm to the environment.

GUIDING PRINCIPLES AND IMPROVEMENT TIPS

Several tested and proven management principles emphasize the importance of good communication. Here are four of them:

- **The Information Principle: Effective communication increases motivation.** When people understand clearly the results they try to accomplish and how they contribute to those results, they are more highly motivated. In addition, the person who makes a sincere effort to keep people informed, and to truly listen to them, is telling them, "I think you are important. I want to be sure you and I both know what's going on."

- **The Distortion Principle: The more levels a communication goes through, the more distorted it becomes.** The more people involved in the line of communication, the greater the probability of distortion, delay, and loss of meaning. When a message is communicated from one person to another, each human brain and tongue that relays the message tends to change it. Unintended meaning may be added, information may be omitted, or the original intent may be altered. Each person through whom the communication is transmitted tends to hedge the message with safeguards as he/she passes it on, and to add CYA (Cover Your Anatomy) thoughts.

- **The Psychological Appeal Principle: Communication that appeals to feelings and attitudes tends to be more motivational than that which appeals only to reason.** We tend to think with our emotions. If you want a person to grasp your meaning, find an emotional peg upon which to anchor that understanding. Even if your message is factual and impersonal, people listen

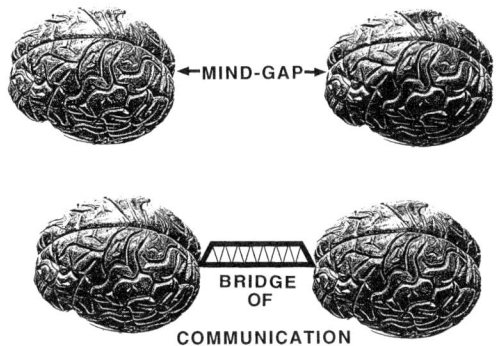

FIGURE 13.2   Interaction resulting in meaning and understanding

and understand better when you introduce the idea by relating it to their personal interests, jobs, families, desires, and value system. A sincere emotional appeal can produce understanding and action most quickly and effectively.

- **The Utilization Principle: The sooner and more often an idea or skill is put to work, the better it is learned and remembered.** If we hear something and understand it, our possession of the information tends to be temporary, unless we do something to reinforce it. Once the new thought is applied, it starts to become our own, to become a permanent part of us. To make a communication your own, use it. To help other people understand and remember your ideas, help them put those ideas to work. Application converts ideas into action and gets results.

Before we get into specific safety and health communication techniques, here are some practical tips for communication in general:

- Seek first to understand, then to be understood.
- Respect the other person's uniqueness.
- Communicate in the receiver's world and demonstrate empathy.
- Practice the art of asking questions.
- Use the "enlightening rod"—reflection, open questions, and directive questions.
- Practice active listening; learn to listen; and listen to learn.
- Create clear mental pictures; help people to see what you mean.
- Replace or supplement abstract ideas with concrete, down-to-earth explanations.
- Notice behavioral cues, like stance, facial expression, eye contact, and body language.
- Focus more on the sender's substance than his or her style.
- Control your emotional reactions. Count to 10, at least.
- Accentuate the positives.
- Give credit where credit is due.

Learn to Listen; Listen to Learn

A survey of successful leaders determined which activities provided the biggest return on investment of time. Of 20 identified activities, many focused on various aspects of communication, such as communicating decisions, speaking effectively, explaining work, using feedback, and writing effectively. The second most important one was "Give clear, effective instructions." The one that topped the whole list was "Listen actively."

There is a big difference between hearing and listening. Hearing is a physical process involving sound waves, ears, and the nervous system. Listening is more of a psychological process involving meanings, mind, and heart—feelings, emotions, attitudes, beliefs, and values.

Just as a quick check, take a pen or pencil and mark "yes" or "no" for each item on the following checklist. Give the answers that truthfully apply to your typical listening pattern. It should take only about three minutes. It's best if you do it right now.

1.	Are you waiting impatiently for the other person to shut up so you can talk?	Yes	No
2.	Are you in such a hurry to suggest a solution that you don't wait to hear the real problem?	Yes	No
3.	Are you listening primarily for what you want to hear, or expect to hear?	Yes	No
4.	Do feelings, attitudes, or emotions interfere with your listening?	Yes	No
5.	Do biases and prejudices significantly influence your listening?	Yes	No
6.	Do your thoughts take side excursions while the other person is talking?	Yes	No
7.	Are you so wrapped up in your own view of the situation that you fail to see things from the other person's viewpoint, i.e., to have empathy?	Yes	No
8.	Do you quit listening when the subject matter gets difficult?	Yes	No
9.	Do you have a negative attitude during the communication process?	Yes	No
10.	Do you just pretend to listen?	Yes	No
	Totals	____	____

Interpretation of Results

If you answered no to nine or ten of them, your ears are open and your mind is positively at work. No to seven or eight shows better than average listening skills. Five or six no answers indicate an in-and-out listener who is trying to improve. If you answered no to four or fewer, you can profit significantly from working to improve your listening skills.

Tips for Better Listening

Listening is learnable. It may not be easy, but it can be improved. Below, for example, are 18 tips for better listening.

- **Show your interest.** Use eye contact. Maintain an alert posture. Let your actions—such as a smile, a nod, a leaning toward the speaker—reflect your interest. Verbally acknowledge what you hear, with comments such as "I see," "That seems like a significant part of the picture," "That's a big decision," or "How did that make you feel?"

- **Concentrate on communication cues.** Pay close attention to the speaker's verbal, vocal, and visual cues. In other words, concentrate on what they say, how they say it, and what they do as they speak.

- **Control distractions.** Try to eliminate or minimize external distractions such as radio, TV, competing conversations, machinery noises, interruptions, ringing phones, or competing activities. Try to control internal distractions such as your aching back, thoughts about your own problems, all the work you have to do, and so forth.

- **Listen for main ideas.** Zero in on key concepts, the common threads woven through the conversation, the critical issues.

- **Wait your turn.** Control your impatience. Let the other person finish his or her own sentences. Try to avoid interrupting, arguing, or debating. Keep quiet until the other person has finished the train of thought. Be sure you understand before you seek to be understood.

- **Clarify and verify.** Listen for answers to questions. Serve as a psychological mirror by reflecting back to the speaker how you think they feel, as well as what you think they said or meant. Determine areas of agreement and disagreement between what you have perceived and what the other person intended.

- **Ask questions appropriately.** Make it an inquiry, not an interrogation. Try to avoid complex, multiple questions; keep questions clear and concise. Don't answer your own question before letting the other person answer. Try not to embarrass the person. Keep questions relevant to the topic.

- **Understand before you challenge or question.** Remember, the other person really wants to be understood.

- **Evaluate evidence.** Mentally differentiate between facts and feelings, opinions, or assumptions. Consider the implications of what you perceive. Identify stereotypes that are indicated.

- **Attend to psychological factors.** Pay special attention to feelings, attitudes, emotions, beliefs, and values.

- **Serve as a sounding board.** Reflect back to the other person what they seem to be saying and feeling. Do this not as a judge or preacher, but simply as an interested listener. Show that you really are trying to understand and be helpful.

- **Control "I" trouble.** Try to avoid being self-centered and wrapped-up in your own situation. Don't overdo the "I," "I," "I" bit. Focus on the other party and their situation.

- **Stay on the subject.** Show that you really are listening and interested by avoiding tangents, keeping the communication focused on the main track.

- **Avoid selective listening.** We all have a tendency toward "wishful twisting." We tend to listen for what we want to hear or expect to hear, believe what we want to believe, and twist what we hear to suit ourselves. Guard against this.

- **Control negative emotional reactions.** What you hear may make you upset, fearful, angry, disgusted, and so on. Try to keep from letting that color everything you say and do during the communication. The old reliable "count to 10" idea comes in very handy here. Typically, loud, explosive, emotional responses tend to interfere with effective communication. Controlled, considerate conversation is more effective.

- **Show empathy.** Listen empathetically, not pathetically. Show that you are tuned in to where the other person is coming from; that you are trying to see things from their viewpoint; that, though you may not condone their ideas and behavior, you can understand why they think and feel as they do. This nonjudgmental listening promotes more and better communication.

- **Respect periods of silence.** Try to avoid filling every little pause with sound. Sometimes the person needs some time to gather their thoughts or to summon the courage to say what they want to say. Even though 30 seconds of silence may seem more like 30 minutes, respect that silence. It may be golden.

- **Summarize.** Reinforce the key issues, main concepts, and common thread of the communication. If action steps are involved, ensure understanding of who is to do what, when. Give credit where credit is due for communicating effectively.

A deaf ear is the first symptom of a closed mind. You can learn a lot by listening. Active listening may well be your most important communication skill for learning things such as:

- Where others are coming from, how they view their environment, how they feel about what's going on, and why they feel that way
- Why people take risks and behave unsafely
- Why people exercise caution and behave safely
- What miners and others see as significant hazards and accident causes
- What people have to offer as possible solutions to safety and health problems.
- A good listener is not only popular everywhere, but after a while she/he knows a lot.

Learn to listen. Listen to learn.

PERSONAL COMMUNICATIONS

Let's take a look at five vital applications of one-on-one communication skills:

1. Orientation
2. Job instruction
3. Key point tipping
4. Planned personal contacts
5. Job performance coaching.

Orientation

Employees new to the job and work environment are at an especially dangerous point. Accomplished leaders use effective orientation to help new or transferred workers get safely through that critical period.

Orientations typically include two types of information: general and job-specific. They may be covered together or in separate sessions. They may be conducted by the same or by different people.

General Orientation   In larger organizations, staff specialists such as those in Human Resources Development, Personnel, and/or Safety, Health, and Environment (SHE) oversee general orientation. In smaller facilities, the site manager or the trainee's supervisor may be in charge. Regardless of who does it, orientation should acquaint the person with general or site-wide SHE issues such as policy and procedures, hazard awareness, rules and regulations, general personal protective equipment (PPE) requirements, and emergency preparedness. (For a checklist of items to be included in orientation, refer back to Figure 9.3 in Chapter 9.)

Here are some key questions you can answer in assessing the general orientation process in your facility:

1.	Is there a process to ensure that all employees new to the location receive a general orientation to the site's SHE program?	Yes	No
2.	Do employees receive the orientation before they actually begin doing their assigned work?	Yes	No
3.	Are checklists and/or other written guides used to ensure consistent coverage in general orientations?	Yes	No
4.	Are records of those receiving general orientation maintained?	Yes	No
5.	Are records kept which document a systematic follow-up of each person's orientation?	Yes	No
6.	Is there documentation showing that the orientation content is changed when significant organizational and/or process changes occur?	Yes	No

Job-Specific Orientation   Whenever possible, this should be conducted or coordinated by the trainee's immediate supervisor or team leader. It is the only chance these people have to make a good first impression regarding care and concern about the employee's safety, health, and general well being. Remember, "First impressions are lasting impressions" and "You never get a second chance to make a good first impression."

The orientation should be a process, not just an event. The process can be considered in terms of the preparation, welcome, essentials, and follow-up.

To prepare, take action to ensure a smooth and effective orientation. Bear in mind that this is one of the most important days in the new employee's work life. When the person sees that you also consider it important, it will go a long way toward establishing a good relationship. Several little things can make a big difference, such as:

- Be sure you know the person's name, experience, education, and general background.
- Alert others in the department. Have them primed and ready to meet and greet their new associate.
- Arrange your schedule to avoid or minimize interruptions.
- Schedule and communicate a definite time and place. Try to make it a place that is relatively free of distractions and permits good communication.
- See that the person's workstation, desk, or office is properly equipped and ready for operation.
- Anticipate the kinds of questions the person is likely to ask, and try to have answers in mind.
- If remaining paperwork must be done, be sure that the required forms are handy, and that you know exactly how they are to be completed and processed.
- Be sure that all required PPE, visual aids, tools, equipment, and handout materials are readily available.

To welcome the trainee, do those important little things that help make the person feel really welcome. A warm personal greeting helps. So does showing interest in them as a person, not just an instrument of production. Include non-work aspects of life in your questions and comments. Topics such as these are **FOR** putting people at ease: **F**amily, **O**ccupation, and **R**ecreation.

Another important part is to introduce the person to others in the area. Also, let them know that you really are open to questions; that the only dumb questions are those they have in mind, but do not ask.

The essentials refer to actually presenting information, touring the area, explaining the work process, and highlighting key procedures and practices. The following list shows topics to cover. Of course, yours depend on the specific nature of your work processes and environment. The topics are:

- Getting acquainted with the people and the work environment, and understanding how the person's job fits in
- Specific safety and health rules and PPE requirements
- Personnel policies relating to factors such as attendance, reporting off, overtime, discipline, employee assistance services, training and development
- Work schedules and performance standards
- Reporting accidents, injuries, damage, illnesses, and spills
- First aid and medical matters
- Drug testing and special medical tests
- Special work permit procedures
- Special hazards
- Reporting unsafe conditions and practices
- Housekeeping and personal hygiene
- Emergency procedures
- Mutual expectations.

As you probably already know, the follow-up is a vital, but sadly neglected part of orientation. Effective orientation is not an event, it's an ongoing process.

There is an awful lot of information for people to understand, remember, and apply. They cannot do it instantaneously. In addition, it may not have been presented perfectly. There is a great need to check back, review, supplement, reinforce, and show continuing interest. Some worksites find the 1–1–1 approach helpful (i.e., a planned, formal follow-up of the orientation is conducted at least one week, one month, and one quarter after the original session.). These follow-up sessions are checkpoints regarding comprehension, retention, questions, suggestions, and opportunity for positive reinforcement. Figure 13.3 illustrates a type of tool that can be helpful in the follow-up process.

Here are some key questions you could answer in assessing the job-specific orientation in your company:

1.	Is there a process to ensure that specific orientations are given to newly placed employees?	Yes	No
2.	Is the work-specific orientation conducted before the employee actually does the work?	Yes	No
3.	Are checklists, or other guides, used to ensure consistency of the orientations?	Yes	No
4.	Are these topics addressed:		
	a. SHE work rules?	Yes	No
	b. Emergency procedures?	Yes	No
	c. Work-specific SHE procedures?	Yes	No
	d. Accident/incident reporting?	Yes	No
	e. Employee SHE roles and responsibilities?	Yes	No
	f. Site-specific hazards?	Yes	No
	g. Legislative compliance requirements?	Yes	No
	h. PPE requirements?	Yes	No
	i. SHE management/leadership roles and responsibilities?	Yes	No

---

OPINION SURVEY

Last week you completed our Employee Orientation Training Course. By now, we're sure you have formed an opinion of the course. We rely on your opinion to make our training as effective as possible. Would you please answer the following questions to help us evaluate the orientation course?

1.   Rate the Orientor/Instructor

    a.   Circle one: POOR   FAIR   GOOD   EXCELLENT

    b.   Circle one: Talked Clearly   Generally Understandable   Couldn't understand

2.   Presentation

    a.   Was the material: (Circle one)   Difficult   Moderate   Easy to Understand

    b.   Was the information presented: (Circle one or more)

        Interesting   Dull   Just what I needed
            Not detailed enough   Too detailed

    c.   Was the method of presentation: (Circle one or more)

        Dull   Just so-so   Enthusiastic

3.   What did you like most about the orientation?

    _____

    _____

4.   What did you like least about the orientation?

    _____

    _____

5.   What are your suggestions to improve the orientation?

    _____

    _____

6.   Add here additional comments or questions you may have.

    _____

    _____

    _____

FIGURE 13.3   Sample opinion survey

5.	Are records kept on who was oriented, and when?	Yes	No
6.	Is there an orientation for contractors?	Yes	No
7.	Are orientation programs reevaluated whenever processes, facilities, equipment, and procedures change?	Yes	No
8.	Do programs link SHE with quality, production, and cost control?	Yes	No

Job Instruction

It is hard to think of any work-related skill that is more important than giving good job instruction. It helps a person learn how to perform a task correctly, quickly, conscientiously, and safely. Instruction also systematically substitutes for trial-and-error learning and is a reliable replacement for hit-or-miss instruction. Think of how wonderful it would be if we helped every person perform every task correctly, quickly, conscientiously, and safely! The great thing is that a proven technique exists for effective instruction, especially for, though not limited to, manual tasks.

Originally called JIT (Job Instruction Training), its four steps were described as:

1. Preparation
2. Presentation
3. Performance
4. Follow-up.

	Explanations were clearly understood	I would like more information
DO YOU KNOW		
1. HOW TO REPORT FOR WORK		
How to record your time?		
How you should dress for work?		
Where to leave personal property?		
2. HOW YOU ARE PAID		
Your rate of pay?		
When & how paid?		
Days & hours of work?		
3. HOW TO REPORT		
An absence, accident, your problems?		
Change of address, marital status, number of dependents?		
4. DO YOU UNDERSTAND		
Smoking, safety, fire protection and env. rules?		
Security regulations?		
Rules of conduct?		
Clean area regulations?		
Attendance rules?		
5. YOUR BENEFITS?		
Group insurance?		
Retirement plan?		
Holidays?		
Vacation?		
Worker's Compensation?		
Social Security?		
6. NAMES		
Your supervisor's name?		
Your fellow employee's name?		

LIST BELOW ANY FURTHER QUESTIONS YOU MAY HAVE CONCERNING THE COMPANY, YOUR JOB, ETC.:

_____

_____

_____

EMPLOYEE SIGNATURE	DATE

FIGURE 13.3   Sample opinion survey (continued)

A modification that has been used around the world for about 30 years is summarized as follows:

Motivate

- Put the learner at ease.
- Find out what the learner knows about the job.
- Position the learner properly, with the same vantage point as the instructor's.
- Build the learner's interest.

Tell and Show

- Demonstrate the operation.
- Use a step-by-step approach.
- Stress key points.
- Instruct clearly and completely.

Test

- Have the learner tell and show.
- Have the learner explain key points.
- Ask questions and correct or prevent errors.
- Continue until you know the learner knows.

Check

- Tell the learner who to go to for help.
- Put the learner on his or her own.
- Follow-up often, answer questions, and review key points.

- Taper off to a normal amount of supervision/leadership.
- Reinforce positive parts of performance.

Here is how you can prepare to give effective job instruction:

Have a Plan

- Know about the job to be taught.
- Consider how much skill you expect the learner to have, and how soon.

Break Down the Job

- List the important steps.
- Highlight key points.

Have Things Ready and Orderly

- Furnish the proper equipment, materials, supplies, and environment.
- Arrange these as the learner will be expected to keep them arranged.

Practice

- Check the effectiveness of your instruction technique.
- Review and refresh your knowledge and skills periodically.

This technique has survived for half a century because it works. Moreover, it brings many benefits, which can be summarized as ESP:

- **E**fficiency (fewer mistakes, less turnover, reduced waste, and better quality)
- **S**afety (fewer accidents, less property damage, reduced injuries, fewer environmental degradations, and safer work habits)
- **P**roductivity (improved knowledge and skill, higher morale and motivation, less downtime and lost time, better cost control and profitability).

Here are some key questions you could answer in assessing job/task instruction.

1.	Are those who give job/task instruction required to use a defined technique for such instruction?	Yes	No
2.	Have those who are required to use the defined job/task instruction technique been adequately trained to do so?	Yes	No
3.	Is the defined instruction technique typically used?	Yes	No
4.	Are appropriate people selected to do effective job/task instruction?	Yes	No
5.	Are records kept regarding the initial and refresher training of job/task instructors?	Yes	No
6.	Is there a follow-up system to assess how well the learners apply their instruction?	Yes	No

Key Point Tipping

"Tip" means just what it does in everyday life—a piece of information given in an attempt to be helpful, or a small gift, hint, or suggestion. So key point tipping is the organized process of giving employees helpful hints, suggestions, reminders or tips about key quality, efficiency, cost, or safety points.

Key points are those vital bits of information that

- Make or break the job
- Show special tricks of the trade that make the task more efficient and effective
- Demonstrate the feel or knack that is the mark of a pro
- Illustrate critical points of quality, productivity, cost control, and safety.

Both people and jobs have individual differences. Every person is unique. Every job has its own special hazards, circumstances, and problems. You can take maximum preventive action only if you zero in on each specific hazard or problem, face-to-face with the person doing the job—at the job scene, as the job is about to be done. Ask yourself the question, "If this particular person could have a serious problem on this particular job or task, what is it most likely to be?" Reach down into the well of your experience with this job and your knowledge of this person, his or her work habits and experience.

Think of the *specific* person, the *specific* task, the *specific* most probable problem, and the most important *specific* preventive action. Give that employee the benefit of your knowledge and experience; give a key point tip.

The best tips are short tips. And they should always be given as reminders rather than formal instruction. A safety tip, for example, could be as simple as: "Jake, when you go into that posted area, be sure to use hearing protection; I don't want you to damage your hearing."

Simple, isn't it? But it can have a tremendous impact if it is done by *every* supervisor, with *every* worker, on *every* critical task. Not only is it another avenue to improved safety, production, cost control, and quality, but it's also an excellent human relations tool. As the above example illustrates, each tip should reflect a genuine interest in the well-being of the employee.

Key point tipping is a specific, specialized contact technique that:

- Is easy to learn
- Takes hardly any time
- Costs practically nothing
- Contributes significantly to safe, high quality, injury-free, damage-free production.

It gives you another top-notch tool of personal communication. It makes full use of the motivational power of repetition, reminders, and reinforcement. It is not a substitute for training or for any other part of the leadership job. Rather, it is an added tool in your leadership kit. It can help you get efficiency, safety, and productivity while improving employee morale. So make it a spontaneous habit—give a key point tip with every critical task.

Here are some key questions you could answer in assessing the key point tipping process at your location:

1. Do written procedures for SHE activities include key point tipping, or its equivalent?	Yes	No
2. Have supervisors been trained to do key point tipping?	Yes	No
3. Do we have records of the training?	Yes	No
4. Do we have a system for periodic monitoring of the key point tipping process, in terms of		
a. The leader's responsibility?	Yes	No
b. The worker's behavior regarding the tips?	Yes	No

Planned Personal Contacts

Whether or not you have planned *group* contacts such as safety meetings, you should have planned *individual* contacts with each employee. These are an excellent supplement to group meetings, and they are especially critical when conditions do not permit getting people together for group meetings.

Many personal contacts are spontaneous. They just happen in the normal course of events. These informal contacts provide hundreds of chances to give key point tips and reinforce desired attitudes and behavior. However, these chance contacts should be supplemented with planned personal contacts, which give you opportunities for:

- Personalizing critical aspects of safety, quality, productivity, and cost control for each worker
- Building better safety awareness and attitudes
- Showing each worker your personal concern for his or her well-being
- Improving your leader-team member relationships
- Enabling you to make best use of the time you invest in direct contact with each worker.

These contacts should be frequent enough to influence the person's attitude, knowledge, and/or skills. The specific number will vary with the number of employees involved, the size of the work area, and similar factors. A planned contact with each person each week would be good. A minimum standard should be at least one per person per month.

Five key steps in conducting a planned personal contact are:

- Pick a critical topic—one that is important in the employee's work and promotes proactive safety and health.

- Prepare the contact. Note the main thought you want to stress. Decide what facts, figures, forms, or aids you want to use.
- Make the contact. Tell why the topic is important and facilitate a two-way discussion. Agree on an action step.
- Record the contact. Keep a simple record to document what you have covered in planned personal contacts with each person, and when.
- Follow up; ensure that both you and the employee do what you agreed to do. Continue communication, coaching and positive reinforcement. (See Figure 13.4 for additional points.)

Here are some questions you could answer in assessing the planned personal contacts process at your worksite:

1.	Do our SHE policies, procedures or practices include planned personal contacts or an equivalent?	Yes	No
2.	Have supervisors/team leaders been trained to conduct contacts?	Yes	No
3.	Is the planned personal contact training documented?	Yes	No
4.	Is there a written requirement regarding the minimum standard for frequency of planned personal contacts?	Yes	No
5.	Are we using a system to monitor the continuing use of planned personal contacts?	Yes	No
6.	Are we accumulating evidence of the effectiveness of planned personal contacts?	Yes	No

GROUP/TEAM COMMUNICATIONS

Challenges and Benefits

Group/team communications may be even more complex and challenging than the personal communications discussed above. As mentioned before, one definition of communication is "interaction resulting in mutual meaning and understanding." As depicted in Figure 13.5, the interaction potential in groups is infinitely greater than in one-to-one relationships. Likewise, the difficulty of gaining mutual meaning and understanding is significantly greater.

But there are some important advantages and benefits of team meetings, safety meetings, and other group communications. For example:

- They can provide quick communication with many people at once.
- They give everyone involved the same exposure to the messages.
- They enable sharing of viewpoints, experiences, and expertise.
- They can aid innovation, creativity, and problem solving.
- They can facilitate group consensus and acceptance of action steps.
- They can help to build the facilitator's image as a leader.
- They can create a cooperative climate through effective participation and interaction.

"Izzle" Factors

Feedback from thousands of people has pinpointed the sorts of things that make the difference between meetings that *fizzle* and those that *sizzle*. The feedback says that fizzle factors include:

- Unprepared leadership
- Disorganization
- Irrelevancies
- Impracticalities
- Too much lecture, sometimes uncontrolled and boring
- Domination by one or two people
- "Too-ness"—Too hot, too cold, too noisy, too dark, too crowded, and especially, too long.

PLANNED PERSONAL CONTACTS		
DEPARTMENT: SUPERVISOR: SIGNATURE:		
DATE	PERSON	TOPIC

(Front)

- PLANNED PERSONAL CONTACTS -

1. PICK A CRITICAL TOPIC
- Important to the specific person on the specific job
- A source of actual or potential loss
- A target for improved efficiency - safety - productivity

2. PREPARE THE CONTACT
- Note key facts and figures
- Pinpoint the main message
- Decide how to personalize it
- Prepare to show as well as tell
- Develop a prescription

3. MAKE THE CONTACT
- Introduce: explain what the topic is and why it is important
- Discuss: tell - show - ask - listen
- Summarize: re-emphasize main point and give prescription for action

4. RECORD THE CONTACT
- Keep track of what you have covered, with whom and when
- Use as evidence of accomplishment
- Use in planning additional communications

5. FOLLOW-UP
- Get promised information for the person
- Contact others if necessary to relay information, suggestions or requests
- Tie additional communications in with the contact topic

(Back)

FIGURE 13.4   Planned personal contact log sheet

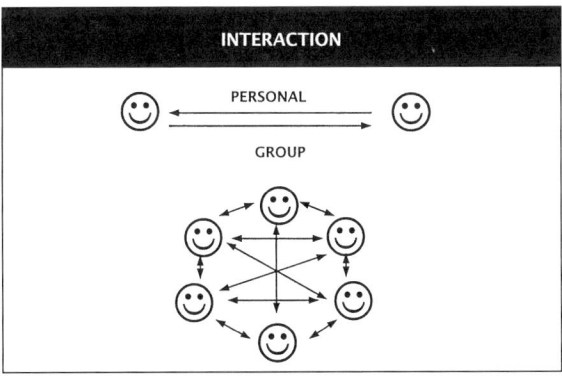

FIGURE 13.5   Interaction flow chart

Things that make meetings sizzle include:
- A meaningful agenda
- Effective leadership
- Effective membership
- Positive participation
- Relevance
- Practicality

IS EVERYBODY READY?

Preparing Yourself

1.	Are the objectives of the meeting, what you want to accomplish, clearly fixed in your mind?	No	Yes
2.	Have you figured out a clear, concise, effective way of presenting the problem and/or information?	No	Yes
3.	Have you done your "homework"? Do you know the background material thoroughly?	No	Yes
4.	Do you have the facts and figures you need to make things meaningful to others?	No	Yes
5.	Are you prepared to adjust to personalities and communication styles of the meeting members?	No	Yes
6.	Have you checked to make sure you have invited everyone that you should, and no one that you shouldn't?	No	Yes
7.	Have your prepared some questions and/or provocative statements to use in case the session seems to bog down a bit?	No	Yes
8.	Do you have a sufficient supply of any material you plan to distribute?	No	Yes
9.	Have you developed or obtained appropriate diagrams, flip charts, pictures, videos, recordings, models or other aids which will make a clearer and/or stronger impressions on members' minds?	No	Yes

Preparing The Meeting Members

10.	Have you let meeting members known in advance what the meeting will be about?	No	Yes
11.	Have you offered suggestions regarding what the members can do to be well prepared?	No	Yes
12.	Have you informed them of the specific time and place?	No	Yes
13.	Have you let them know what, if anything, they should bring to the meeting?	No	Yes
14.	Have you given them enough advance notice so that they can schedule and prepare adequately?	No	Yes

FIGURE 13.6   Meeting preparation checklist

- Proper physical environment
- Enthusiasm
- Timing—meet at the right day and time; start on time; allot time segments properly; end on time!

Making Meetings Effective

If you want a "meeting of the minds" rather than just a meeting, consider these five aspects of effective meetings:

- Preparation
- Presentation
- Visualization
- Participation
- Evaluation.

Preparation   A well-led meeting gets under way long before the members assemble in their seats. The way you set the stage has a lot to do with how smoothly things go when the curtain goes up. As a facilitator or leader, you should be concerned with preparing yourself, the meeting members, and physical surroundings. Figure 13.6 is a checklist that can help you prepare for better meetings.

<table>
<tr><td colspan="4" align="center">**Preparing The Physical Surroundings**</td></tr>
<tr><td>15.</td><td>As far as possible, have you ensured an environment that enables an efficient, effective, reasonably comfortable meeting?</td><td>No</td><td>Yes</td></tr>
<tr><td>16.</td><td>Have you checked, or has someone checked, the adequacy of</td><td></td><td></td></tr>
<tr><td></td><td>• ventilation?</td><td>No</td><td>Yes</td></tr>
<tr><td></td><td>• heating/air conditioning?</td><td>No</td><td>Yes</td></tr>
<tr><td></td><td>• lighting?</td><td>No</td><td>Yes</td></tr>
<tr><td></td><td>• seating (accommodations and arrangement)?</td><td>No</td><td>Yes</td></tr>
<tr><td></td><td>• pencils or pens, paper and writing surfaces?</td><td>No</td><td>Yes</td></tr>
<tr><td></td><td>• flip pad, screen, projector and/or other aids?</td><td>No</td><td>Yes</td></tr>
<tr><td>17.</td><td>If you are going to use mechanical equipment (such as tape recorder, projector, or video monitor), have you:</td><td></td><td></td></tr>
<tr><td></td><td>• made sure its available?</td><td>No</td><td>Yes</td></tr>
<tr><td></td><td>• ensured proper outlets, extension cords, spare bulbs, etc. ?</td><td>No</td><td>Yes</td></tr>
<tr><td></td><td>• checked your skill in operating it properly (or arranged for a skilled operator)?</td><td>No</td><td>Yes</td></tr>
<tr><td></td><td>• secured the proper films, tapes, slides or transparencies ?</td><td>No</td><td>Yes</td></tr>
<tr><td></td><td>• determined the location of power panels and switches?</td><td>No</td><td>Yes</td></tr>
<tr><td>18.</td><td>Have you checked the availability of the meeting room for the day and time you need it?</td><td>No</td><td>Yes</td></tr>
<tr><td>19.</td><td>Have you ensured, as far as possible, minimal "sound pollution" from other meeting and activities?</td><td>No</td><td>Yes</td></tr>
<tr><td>20.</td><td>Have you determined the adequacy of items such as refreshments (if appropriate) and rest rooms?</td><td>No</td><td>Yes</td></tr>
<tr><td colspan="4" align="center">**Special Preparations**</td></tr>
<tr><td>21.</td><td>Are you psychologically prepared for the inevitable occurrences often attributed to "Murphy's Law?" (You might list some of the possibilities below.)</td><td>No</td><td>Yes</td></tr>
</table>

FIGURE 13.6   Meeting preparation checklist (continued)

Presentation   Here are some key considerations to keep in mind for a good presentation:

- Start on time.
- State the purpose.
- Capture their interest.
- Speak plainly and loudly enough to be heard in the back of the room.
- Maintain eye contact.
- Follow the agenda.
- Facilitate discussion.
- Ask questions.
- Encourage others to ask questions.
- Listen actively.
- Monitor the time factor.
- Properly introduce other presenters, if any, and their role or topic.
- Give positive reinforcement to people for their good questions, contributions, and ideas.
- Summarize.
- Verify action steps (who, what, when).
- End on time.

Visualization   Have you noticed what people tend to say when they really get the message? "I see what you mean," or "I get the picture." A vital part of any speech or presentation is to paint clear mental pictures in people's minds; to help them understand and remember.

Sometimes you can do this with word devices or memory aids such as acronyms, alliteration, rhymes, analogies, and contrasts. An acronym is formed from the initial letters or groups of letters in a phrase. For example: PLUS (Positive Leadership Upgrades Safety) or SHARE (Safety Helps And Recognizes Everyone). Alliteration is using the same letter or word in a series of words—for example, conceive, believe, and achieve; or people, property, process, and profit. Rhymes have endings that sound the same. For example: "Don't be a fool, when using this tool." An analogy compares two different things and stresses their similarities like the human heart and a mechanical pump, or the human eye and a camera. Contrast compares two items or situations and stresses their differences. For example, "Let's see how today's workplace safety differs from the time of our parents or grandparents."

Visual (and audiovisual) aids are the most commonly used tools for helping to create clear mental pictures; they cause people to pay *attention* to the message, help them to *understand* the message, and improve their capacity to *remember* the message. Good aids make people use both their ears and eyes, help them to both hear and "see what you mean." The key point of presentation is to:

- Use both sound and sight.
- Make the presentation both verbal and visual.
- Paint vivid mental pictures for the listeners.
- Use some combination of:
  - Demonstrations
  - Graphs
  - Discussions
  - Samples
  - Displays
  - Questions
  - Quizzes
  - Posters
  - Charts
  - Models
  - Mockups
  - Videos
  - Computer-assisted learning
  - Newspaper items
  - Photographs
  - Illustrations
  - Tools
  - Transparencies
  - Paintings
  - Drawings
  - Diagrams
  - Slides
  - Actual equipment.

Remember that visual aids are supposed to aid the vision. To be effective, they must be clearly visible to every member of the audience; each one should make a key point in a simple, clear way. They should be something more than just words; they should create clear, memorable mental pictures.

Participation   Medical science has not yet found a cure for snoring, but meeting specialists have. It is participation. In fact, active involvement not only prevents snoring, it also improves interest, motivation, sharing, learning, and remembering.

Questions can be a tremendous tool for stimulating participation. As a leader or facilitator, you can both ask questions and motivate others to ask questions. The following nine types of questions can be used:

1. **Open questions**—invite a true expression of opinion and feelings; show that you are interested and want to understand and cannot be answered "yes" or "no." *Example:* "How should discipline apply to those involved in accidents?"

2. **Factual questions**—seek data, information, facts, and figures. *Example:* "How many property damage accidents were reported in your area last period?"

3. **Leading questions**—introduce a thought of your own and suggest the desired answer. *Example:* "Don't you agree that this is excess absenteeism?" (Leading questions should be used sparingly).

4. **Provocative questions**—stimulate new thoughts and challenge traditional concepts. *Example:* "What's your reaction to the idea that something is safe when its risks are judged to be acceptable?"

5. **Probing questions**—get additional information or to broaden discussion. *Example:* "How could we go about implementing that suggestion?"

6. **Decision questions**—agree on a course of discussion or action. *Example:* "Which of these two proposed investigation forms will be best for us?"

7. **Justification questions**—challenge a statement or get more substantiation. *Example:* "Can you tell us where those figures came from?"

8. **Hypothetical questions**—explore assumptions or suppositions. *Example:* "What might happen if downsizing eliminates the Safety Coordinator position?"

9. **Directive questions**—direct discussion toward positive factors. *Example:* "*How much* time do you think this corrective action will save in your department?"

Other tools and techniques for stimulating participation include scenarios, role plays, case studies, brainstorming, problem solving, "buzz groups," team exercises, or getting participants to help with the presentation.

Many authors, managers, and staff professionals emphasize the importance of meeting leaders in stimulating participation and making meetings successful. The importance of the meeting *members* should also be emphasized. Figure 13.7 is a self-evaluation checklist for meeting participants.

Evaluation   Although there are many excellent meetings, there is no perfect one. Continuous improvement is the goal. Systematic and continuing improvement requires evaluation of performance (self-evaluation and/or evaluation by others), and application of what's learned from the evaluation. What are the negatives to overcome? The positives to build on? Items such as those shown in Figure 13.8 can be helpful for this type of evaluation.

SAFETY PROMOTION GUIDELINES

What the mind attends to ... it considers.
What the mind does not attend to ... it dismisses.
What the mind attends to regularly ... it believes.
What the mind believes ... it eventually does.

Ensure that safety, health, and environmental protection permeate your whole communication system, including policies, procedures, goals, objectives, standards, rules, job descriptions, task procedures, budgets, publications, meetings, training programs, performance appraisals and reviews, and recognition and awards.

Use effective general promotion tools and techniques. Take your pick from a host of possibilities such as those shown in Figure 13.9.

Apply the following 10 guidelines for effective safety promotion:

1. **Set specific promotion targets.** For example, your general promotion activities can be designed to:

   ▪ Increase *awareness* of specific SHE aspects

   ▪ Improve *attitudes* about specific SHE factors.

- Add to *knowledge* of specific SHE concerns.
- Motivate specific SHE *behaviors.*

2. **Focus on critical problems.** Select materials to address specific critical problems, based on historical need and/or the potential for major loss. Try to both identify the problem and offer a solution for it. Problems requiring engineering or administrative controls are not likely to be solved by a promotional campaign. Promotion efforts should be directed at problems for which there is a high probability that awareness and attitudes have preventive power.

3. **Relate the messages to specific accident causes and preventive actions.** General messages such as "Be Safe," "Drive Safely," or "Be More Careful" are quite vague and of limited value. Specific messages such as "Bend Your Knees to Save Your Back" are of much greater value.

4. **Practice point-of-control promotion.** Studies show that posters, for instance, are most effective when used at the point of need. As an example, posters reminding people to "Use the Handrails for Safety on the Stairs" should be posted where people are about to ascend or descend the stairs. Similarly, job aids such as critical task checklists and procedures can be most effective when posted where the work is performed.

HOW GOOD A GROUP PARTICIPANT AM I?

Circle either Plus or minus

#	Question	+	-
1.	Do I propose new ideas, activities or procedures? (+) Or do I just sit and listen? (-)	+	-
2.	Do I ask questions to increase understanding? (+) Or do I fail to admit that I do not understand? (-)	+	-
3.	Do I share my knowledge and experience when they might be helpful? (+) Or do I keep things to myself? (-)	+	-
5.	Do I try to synthesize (bring together) and summarize our ideas and activities? (+) Or do I focus only on details and ignore the big picture? (-)	+	-
6.	Do I try to understand the group's goals and keep discussion directed toward them? (+) Or do I tend to get off track too often? (-)	+	-
7.	Do I properly question the practicality of projects and the logic of the ideas? (+) Or do I simply let things go by without questions? (-)	+	-
8.	Do I encourage others towards positive participation and give them due credit? (+) Or am I indifferent to or critical of their efforts? (-)	+	-
9.	Do I prod the group to concentrate on worthy techniques and projects that will improve success? (+) Or am I satisfied to let the group diddle around and the deal with "busy work" projects? (-)	+	-
10.	Am I willing to compromise (when it is ethical and proper) for the good of the group? (+) Or am I inflexible in my point of view? (-)	+	-
11.	Do I help everyone have a fair chance to speak? (+) Or do I tolerate some people "hogging the floor" or perhaps tend to do it myself? (-)	+	-
12.	Do I tend to be a mediator and peacemaker? (+) Or do I tend to allow or cause ill feelings to develop? (-)	+	-
13.	Do I tend to do things which help improve understanding and problem-solving (e.g., listen - ask - suggest - summarize - thank) (+) Or do I tend to show behaviors which disrupt the group (e.g., sarcasm - diversion - asides - pessimism - arguing - excessive joking - pet peeves)? (-)	+	-
14.	Do I tend usually show respect for the leader/facilitator? (+) or do I often show impatience, indifference or hostility? (-)	+	-
15.	For the most part: Do others tend to see me as a positive participant? (+) Or do they tend to view me negatively? (-)	+	-

FIGURE 13.7 **Evaluating your group participation skills**

5. **Use organized campaigns or theme programs.** Give major emphasis to a critical SHE concern for a period of two weeks or two months. For each program, have a theme team, headed by an upper-level manager, with team members from various organizational levels. The team designs and administers the promotional campaign, using several of the following channels:

- Safety talks
- Posters
- Memos from senior management
- Articles in safety bulletins, magazines, and newsletters
- Guest speakers
- Exhibits
- Distribution of pamphlets or flyers
- Banners, buttons, and badges
- Contests or competitions
- Related field observations
- Special inspections or tours

CHECKLIST FOR EVALUATING MEETINGS

		Yes	No	Comments
1	Did the meeting start on time?			
2	Was there an agenda or other evidence of a well planned, organized meeting?			
3	Was the purpose of the meeting made clear to all concerned?			
4	Were questions either answered adequately or noted so that answers could be given after the meeting?			
5	Were necessary facts and information given clearly and succinctly?			
6	Were problems clearly defined?			
7	Did the meeting stay on course rather than veer off into too many tangents?			
8	Were people interrupted too often			
9	Was there evidence of good espirit de corps?			
10	With respect to future action:			
	A. Was the course clearly set?			
	B. Were definite responsibilities assigned?			
	C. Were target dates established?			
11	Was the meeting summarized at the end?			
12	Did the meeting fulfill its purpose?			
13	What one or two things could have done most to improve the meeting?			
	A.			
	B.			
14.	What one or two things were best about the meeting?			

FIGURE 13.8   Meeting evaluation checklist

- Pictures, slides, films, and videos
- Questionnaires.

By having different people on each theme team, it is possible to get all members of management involved in SHE program activities. Thus, they *show* their commitment to all employees.

6. **Accentuate the positive.** In promotional activities, emphasize:
   - What *to do*, more than what *not* to do
   - What is right more than what is wrong
   - The positive more than the negative.

   Group performance can be promoted positively. This involves work sections or departments and is directed at compliance to program standards. These promotions are most effective when they concentrate on performance (learning, remembering, and/or doing) rather than accident-free days. Positive, successful programs have been based on safety suggestions, spot observations, compliance with PPE requirements, attendance at safety meetings, reporting near misses, rule compliance, awareness of specific rules or themes, and other performance indicators.

7. **Add spice with variety.** If you use posters, change them frequently. Stay out of a communication rut; keep things fresh, attention-getting, and interesting. Use a variety of promotion aids such as the A to Z list in Figure 13.9.

PROMOTION AIDS A TO Z

ANECDOTES	GRAPHS	ORDER	STANDARDS
ANNOUNCEMENTS	GUARDS	ORIENTATION	SYMBOLS
AUDIO TAPES	GROUP MEETINGS		SUGGESTION
AUDIT			SYSTEMS
AWARDS		PAINTINGS	SUPERVISION
	HANDBOOKS	PERSONAL CONTACTS	
	HOUSEKEEPING	PERSONAL EXAMPLE	
BADGES		PICTURES	TAGS
BALLOONS		POCKET CARDS	TEAMS
BANNERS	INSPECTION	POLICIES	TELEVISION
BOOKLETS	INSTRUCTION	POSTERS	THEME PROGRAMS
BULLETIN BOARDS	INVESTIGATION	PROCEDURES	TOOLS
		PROJECTORS	TOURS
		PROTECTIVE	TRAINING
	JOB ANALYSIS	EQUIPMENT	TRANSPARENCIES
CAMPAIGNS	JOB INSTRUCTION		
CARTOONS	JOB ORIENTATION		
CHALK BOARDS		QUESTIONNAIRES	UNDERLYING
COACHING		QUIZZES	CAUSES
COMMENDATIONS	KANGAROO CLUB	QUOTATIONS	UNDERSTANDING
COMMITTEES	KEY POINT TIPS		
CONTACTS	KITS		
CONTESTS	KUDOS	RADIO	VARIETY
COUNSELING		RECOGNITION	VIDEOTAPES
		RECORDS	VIGILANCE
		REGULATIONS	VISUAL AIDS
	LEADERSHIP	REINFORCEMENT	VITAL STATISTICS
DEMONSTRATIONS	LEAFLETS	REMINDERS	
DIAGRAMS	LETTERS	REPORTS	
DISCIPLINE		REWARDS	WALLET CARDS
DISPLAYS		RULES	WARNINGS
DRAWINGS			WISE OWL CLUB
	MACHINES		WORKSHOPS
	MAGAZINES	SAFE JOB PRACTICES	
	MOBILES	SAFETY CLUBS	
EQUIPMENT	MOCK-UPS	SAFETY TALKS	X-RAYS
EXAMPLES	MODELS	SAFETY TIPS	
EXHIBITS	MOTIVATION	SCHEMATICS	YARNS
	MOVIES	SIGNS	YOURSELF
		SLIDES	
		SLOGANS	
FEEDBACK			ZEAL
FILMSTRIPS	NEWSLETTERS		ZEST
FIRSTAID COURSES	NEWSPAPERS		ZING
FLANNEL BOARDS	NOTICES		
FLIP CHARTS	NOVELTIES		

FIGURE 13.9   Promotion aids: A to Z

8. **Use proven principles for effective promotion.** Here are five of them:

   ▪ The Goal-Power Principle—motivation to accomplish results tends to increase when people have meaningful goals toward which to work.

   ▪ The Information Principle—effective communication increases motivation.

   ▪ The Principle of Involvement—meaningful involvement increases motivation and support.

   ▪ The Principle of Mutual Interest—programs, projects, and ideas are best sold when they bridge the wants and desires of both parties.

   ▪ The Principle of Behavior Reinforcement—behavior with negative effects tends to decrease or stop; behavior with positive effects tends to continue or increase.

9. **Evaluate promotion results.** Get feedback. Find out what people pay attention to, what they remember, how they apply the information. Use personal contacts, group discussions, structured interviews, questionnaires, spot observations, records analyses, tests, inventories, and random sampling.

10. **Coordinate general promotion activities with other elements of your SHE management system.** Posters, contests, and related promotion programs are not a management system. They are one of many elements in SHE management success; elements such as policies, design, ergonomics, purchasing controls, hiring practices, rules and regulations, orientation, training, investigation, inspection, critical task procedures, safety meetings, emergency preparedness, and leadership example.

As a key closing concept in applying these ten guidelines, always keep in mind these two basics of effective propaganda (or promotion): Simplify and Repeat. Simplify and Repeat. Simplify and Repeat.

REFERENCES

Bird, F.E., Jr., and G.L. Germain. 1996. *Practical Loss Control Leadership*. Loganville, GA: Det Norske Veritas (USA), Inc.

——. 1997. *The Property Damage Accident*. Loganville, GA: FEBCO, Inc.

Covey, S.R. 1989. *The 7 Habits of Highly Effective People*. New York: Simon & Schuster.

Germain, G.L., R.M. Arnold, Jr., R.J. Rowan, and J.R. Roane. 1998. *Safety, Health, and Environmental Management*. Dallas, TX: International Risk Management Institute.

CHAPTER 14

Task Analysis and Observation

Ben W. Sheppard, C.M.S.P.
Ben W. Sheppard and Associates, LLC, Haden Lake, Idaho

INTRODUCTION

Task analysis is one of the most valuable processes available to management, involving not only management, but also every employee working in the process. In fact, task analysis can spell the difference between success and failure for management teams and the companies they represent.

TASK ANALYSIS: NOT TO BE CONFUSED WITH JOB SAFETY ANALYSIS

Although task analysis does bear some resemblance to job safety analysis, the process of task analysis is uniquely more time consuming and far reaching. Generally, job safety analysis (JSA) examines hazards associated with each job. This analysis does not take long for people experienced in performing each job to conduct, and the analysis provides a short list of steps to control apparent job hazards. To put it simply, *JSAs are used to train personnel in recognizing the hazards associated with the job and developing formal guidelines for safe work procedures*.

Task analysis is a relatively complex procedure. It not only identifies items contained within a JSA, it also identifies each intimate detail of each segment of each job. Task analysis may have several hundred steps compared to a dozen steps identified within a JSA.

The Benefits of Task Analysis

The simple description of the benefits of task analysis is accomplishing the job in the safest most efficient way. Having said this, what does it mean? The author of this chapter has used task analysis in varying degrees and/or capacities for nearly 20 years. The benefits have varied according to the effort put into the program. Some mining companies and other heavy industrial companies have advanced to this point in a formal loss control program and are dedicated to the process of task analysis. On average, the author estimates that these companies have been able to achieve an overall 40% to 50% cost reduction. Impossible, you say? Not at all. The author of this chapter has experienced these benefits firsthand.

We all know what productivity means, don't we? Or do we? At least we all think we do. Personal experience has shown that, when stockholders are asked, their definition of production is producing as much as possible to maximize income potential. Many front-line supervisors, after much hesitation, define production as getting the most out of workers. More enlightened CEOs will define production as producing as much as possible for the lowest possible cost, to achieve the maximum return to the stockholder. In this case the CEO's definition is the closest to what we are trying to achieve.

Task analysis performed appropriately will identify areas of waste, in terms of time, resources, production, and dollars. It will also identify areas where efficiency can be improved, thereby increasing productivity. These benefits are achieved while at the same time improving safety and general morale.

Let's review some actual success stories.

Benefit Example #1. At a large gold mine in the western United States, task analysis provided the impetus for management to change their procedures and management style.

Picture if you can a long conveyor belt feeding an ore-leach area. This belt has a take-up pulley on one end. The belt has spilled an excess of material for a period of more than 2 years. Employees have complained about having to shovel every shift to clean up along the belt, and management has consistently placed a small front-end loader with the bucket under the take-up pulley to catch spilling ore. Analysis was responsible for correcting the condition with a $25 scraper, eliminating the need for one piece of heavy equipment and two employees each shift. You ask how this could have happened? Sometimes we have trouble seeing the forest for the trees. In this case management had been told many times, but they continued to put it on a back burner. They had higher priorities, and those priorities allowed a condition to persist for a period of time that cost them hundreds of thousands of dollars. This condition, when eliminated, was one of many that contributed to a 54% reduction in operating costs.

Benefits Example #2. A work process in a refinery area was analyzed. The analysis identified no less than five steps employees were still using that should have been removed years before during a process modification. It also identified that employees were mixing reagents that were no longer necessary and the costs amounted to hundreds of thousands of dollars. A new procedure was written to address the situation. When modified, this procedure, among others, led to a reduction in costs of nearly 50% on the bottom line.

Both of these examples contributed to an overall reduction of the bottom line. In addition to cost reduction, each of these sites achieved amazing safety and health records. Each has gone 3 to 5 years without a lost-time incident.

WHO SHOULD CONDUCT TASK ANALYSIS?

To achieve the benefits we saw in the previous section, we need to conduct an extremely detailed task analysis. To do this, we need to draw on all levels of knowledge and expertise. Task analysis begins with the workers and front-line supervisors.

Every worker has a feel for his or her job. They also know each step of each phase within a particular job. They know what they do better than anyone else, even their immediate front-line supervisor. Once trained on how to conduct a task analysis, the employee has the potential to identify significant items and issues that have been overlooked or unobserved by management.

When employees complete their analysis it should go directly to the front-line supervisor for scrutiny. Next, it should go to each level of management for their examination. All levels of supervision/management will have the authority to send the analysis back to the floor, if they see something that has been left out or not identified.

Generally, the last person to see the analysis is the safety professional. He or she should review the analysis to affirm that all safety issues have been identified and controlled.

GUIDELINES FOR CONDUCTING TASK ANALYSIS

The first step should be to assign or appoint a task analysis coordinator. The outline below has been used by the author to successfully orchestrate task analysis programs at several different locations and companies.

- Establish a standard that indicates which task(s) should be listed as critical. (*Example:* $1,000 potential loss, or any personal injury.)
- Develop a list identifying all tasks (both critical and noncritical).
- Develop a work sheet to identify critical tasks. Evaluate all tasks for loss potential. Prioritize by loss exposure and loss potential. Quantify loss exposures—frequency of exposures and potential cost of loss to people, property, processes, and planet. Sort out those tasks that would be classified as critical.
- Develop a list of critical tasks. This is generally done by middle management, like a superintendent, general foreman, or someone who recognizes the importance of task priorities.

- Develop a task analysis work sheet. This work sheet should identify each critical task. It should then have a means of breaking each task into steps or mini tasks. Once the mini-task is identified and broken into steps, the work sheet should provide a means of quantifying exposures. Identify losses such as:
  - What chemicals are used at each phase of each step?
  - What safety equipment is used during use of the chemicals?
  - What quality measures maximize efficiency of the chemical usage?
- **Train relevant personnel to dissect tasks into steps.** All levels involved should be trained to break each process into multiple tasks, then break each task into mini tasks. For example, operating a haul truck is a task, but checking the oil, accessing the dipstick, and even pulling the dipstick may be considered mini tasks. Checking tires, checking fire extinguishers, and ascending and descending ladders are also mini tasks. Remember, even mini tasks may have several tinier tasks within them.
- **Assign critical tasks to individuals.** Whenever possible the author assigns the same task to two teams. This allows two different points of view to the same job. The front-line supervisor oversees his team's activity and is positioned to assist his team in managing the breakdown of the task. The supervisor is also assigned the responsibility of assuring the analysis is done and pushed up to the next level of management. This level of management is the first to see similarities or dissimilarities of each team's effort. Ultimately each analysis will pass through each level of management to the task analysis coordinator.
- **Management team evaluation.** A team made up of a representative of each management level will meet with the task analysis coordinator to discuss, evaluate, and homogenize the findings of each task.
- **Reassign the homogenized tasks to each team for evaluation.** The homogenized task analysis is returned to the initial teams to reevaluate and comment on. When completed, the task analysis is returned to the task analysis coordinator.
- **Reduce task analysis to a Standard Operating Procedure (SOP).** Develop a thorough written operating procedure for each task. (SOPs should be written as a step-by-step detailed set of operational directions.) An SOP should be so clearly written that an inexperienced person can follow the procedure and do the job. (It should be noted this is a test only and nothing can take the place of actual training and operational practice.)
- **Train employees on the new procedure.** Using the operating procedures developed from the task analysis, thoroughly train the employees in the intricate details of the task.
- **Begin again.** When the task is completely analyzed, an SOP has been developed, and the employees have been trained in the task, have them reanalyze the task. You will be surprised. Task analysis affords the opportunity for continuous improvement in all areas.

TASK OBSERVATION AS A TOOL

Regardless of whether operating equipment, working as a laborer on the floor, or working in management, task observation, when used appropriately, is a valuable tool for improving performance.

History indicates that employees and even management, when left to perform tasks on their own, will develop bad habits and/or develop undesired practices. They may develop undesirable traits from watching or talking to others, or they may gradually develop traits simply through the repetitive rigors of the job.

Formal task observation allows constructive input from trainers or supervisors that observe the employee at work. If possible, the employee should be observed without his or her knowledge. This will allow for a more accurate data collection. Note: As a prerequisite to any observation, assure that all employees are aware a task observation program exists, and that they will be observed at some point. The employees should also be made aware that observation is not for punishment, it is to maintain a higher level of performance and allow for continuous improvement.

MAKING TASK OBSERVATION A FORMAL PROCEDURE

To fully realize the benefits of task analysis and the subsequent improvements (e.g., SOPs, training, and other modifications that have occurred), we must develop a formal procedure to observe the task. This will ensure that old habits and steps don't come back, and it may identify other areas to improve.

Like the majority of tasks, task observation should also have formal procedures written for the observer to follow. The formal procedure should walk the observer through a step-by-step observation procedure.

Management and supervisors are practiced at observing the job site, and perhaps even to an informal level conducting task observations. Generally, however, they do not conduct formal task observation. To conduct a formal task observation program is not too far from what they are already practiced in.

The following steps depict a successful program developed and utilized by the author.

Step 1. Develop a standard observation procedure. Identify who should do formal observations. The author generally makes task observation a two-phase process. Both a qualified trainer (if available) and the front-line supervisor conduct the observation. (Not at the same time. Their notes and/or work sheet are compared later.)

- Identify task(s) to be observed. All critical tasks should be observed. Experience indicates that benefit is gained by observing both tasks that have been fully analyzed and tasks that have not yet been formally analyzed.

- Identify when task(s) are to be observed. **Task observation should be required, and it should be part of the supervisor's and trainer's evaluation.** Tasks should be observed on a regular basis. (A schedule should be followed, and it should be flexible but firm.) In some cases several tasks can be observed at the same time. Those conducting the observation (the frontline supervisor and the trainer) should coordinate their activities to coincide with each other, so the results can be compared at nearly the same time.

Step 2. Develop a task observation work sheet. The work sheet should indicate the date, time, person conducting the observation, observers title, task being observed, checklist of items to be observed, place for comments, and a place for rating proficiency, if appropriate. (The author has developed a successful program where promotion depends on achieving a performance standard for efficiency. The performance is verified through task observation by the trainer and front-line supervisor. With proper training the observers were able to rate operator proficiency on a scale of 1–10. This is done accurately enough and is key to both merit and bonus programs.)

Step 3. Train the observers. Those conducting the observation should be given training in how to conduct task observation. They must learn to utilize the standard observation procedure and the work sheet, as well as generally how to conduct observations.

Step 4. Conduct the task observation. Task observation should be conducted on the employee's regular shift. If possible the employee should not be alerted to the fact that he or she is being observed.

Step 5. Compare observations. Compare the observations of the trainer and the supervisor.

Step 6. Give feedback to the employee or retrain in substandard areas. Finally, as with any successful program, an individual must be responsible and accountable for the coordination and communication aspects (i.e., feedback to all levels of management, employees, and departments) of task management.

CHAPTER 15

Emergency Preparedness and Response

Robert E. Launhardt
Pinehurst, Idaho

INTRODUCTION

Properly and adequately trained mine rescue teams are the heart and soul of emergency preparedness and response. Although mine rescue is usually viewed in the context of an underground mine, surface rescue training may be needed if conditions warrant. In some situations, rescue teams are trained exclusively for surface response.

An emergency response plan provides the framework for maximum utilization of all mine personnel, including mine rescue workers. Frequent testing of the emergency response plan is essential and must involve all key players. Emergency response can then take place at a high level of efficiency.

IDENTIFYING THE POTENTIAL FOR EMERGENCIES

Mine management may want to identify the type of emergency most likely to occur and plan accordingly, focusing on such an emergency. But a word of caution is needed about that concept. Before the Sunshine Mine Fire Disaster, no one believed such a disaster could occur in a hard-rock mine. Unfortunately, that supposition was wrong. The entire mining industry learned many lessons from that disaster.

Emergency preparedness and response require careful advance planning. Before such planning can take place, all potential causes of a mine emergency must be identified. The order in which hazards are listed does not imply an order of importance or the likelihood of a problem involving any particular hazard.

The history of mine disasters in the United States identifies mine fires, especially shaft fires, as the number one cause of mine disasters. By definition, a disaster is an accident or incident resulting in the loss of five or more lives. In coal mine disasters, explosions of methane gas or coal dust often occur in conjunction with or cause a fire.

Although mine fires are the main concern in emergency preparedness, other hazards must also be taken into account. The hazard of methane gas is not limited to coal mines or "gassy" mines. Methane gas has found its way into hard-rock mines in the Coeur d'Alene Mining District as well as into mines in west central Washington State. A methane explosion in the Tarbox Mine near Saltese, Montana, resulted in two fatalities. Occasional mini-explosions of methane gas occurred in the upper workings of the Star Mine north of Wallace, Idaho. Methane gas was detected in the Howe Sound Mine near Holden Village and the Cannon Mine near Wenatchee, both in west central Washington.

An oxygen-deficient atmosphere (apart from mine fires) has occurred in two different inactive development headings in the Sunshine Mine. The oxygen level was inadequate to sustain the flame in a flame safety lamp. No injuries occurred in either instance. But workers in mines near Patterson and

Stanley, Idaho, were not so fortunate. An oxygen-deficient atmosphere caused the loss of one life in each of those mines.

Mines near Cripple Creek, Colorado, and in the East Tintic Mining District in Utah share a unique history of "rock gas." Before the use of mechanical ventilation, rock gas (which consists mostly of nitrogen and carbon dioxide) issued from the mine rock strata during decreasing atmospheric pressure (approach of a low-pressure system) and displaced the mine atmosphere. Early day Cripple Creek miners carried a flame safety lamp that was placed in clear view of the heading in which they were working. They left the mine immediately if the flame started to go out.

Hydrogen sulfide is a very poisonous naturally occurring gas that is frequently found in gypsum ore-bodies. It may migrate from its source into mines, dissolved in ground water. It may occur in sulfide ores. Its rotten egg odor makes it easy to detect. This means of identification, however, is lost when hydrogen sulfide reaches a dangerous concentration. At higher concentrations the gas causes paralysis of the olfactory nerve, leading the person smelling the gas to believe it is no longer present.

Carbon monoxide gas from blasting creates problems more frequently than all other gases identified above. This colorless, odorless, tasteless gas has caused many illnesses and occasional fatalities in underground mines. Perhaps it is the frequent use of explosives and the infrequent problem with dangerous levels of carbon monoxide that leads mine personnel to disregard the hazard; familiarity breeds contempt!

Adequate mechanical ventilation of active mines is of extreme importance in avoiding problems with mine gases. Once one understands the importance of adequate ventilation, that person is much less likely to venture into an unventilated area in a mine.

SECONDARY ESCAPE WAYS AND REFUGE CHAMBERS

Secondary escape ways are required under the Mine Health and Safety Act (the Mine Act). Nevertheless, mine management should look beyond nominal compliance with regulations and verify the reliability of secondary escape ways by occasionally testing the emergency response plan, rather than relying on theory. Such testing is best done in the form of surprise drills in which only the general manager and a mine rescue team captain know in advance that the drill is planned. Either the general manager or the mine rescue team captain plans the surprise drill.

Refuge chambers are required under the Mine Act while a secondary exit is being developed, or when mine personnel cannot reach the surface within 1 hour. Effective emergency preparedness requires regular inspections of refuge chambers and their contents.

VENTILATION RELIABILITY

The ability to control mine ventilation is often the most important element in providing for the safety of personnel in a mine during an evacuation brought about by a mine fire. Emergency preparedness must include having up-to-date mine ventilation maps at headquarters for a mine emergency.

SELECTING EQUIPMENT FOR EMERGENCY USE

Emergency preparedness must include equipment and supplies that will adequately protect personnel in any foreseeable emergency. It must also include research by the purchasing department to determine availability of emergency supplies. Mine rescue equipment should be state of the art and should be well maintained. Telephone service must include one phone system that has an emergency power supply to enable use should electrical power fail.

EMERGENCY RESPONSE PLAN

In an emergency, a mine needs its key personnel or their designees at a central location (headquarters). Each key person must delegate responsibility under the emergency response plan when he or she is unavailable. Personnel not essential to the emergency must be excluded. The same applies to the news media.

In a disaster, the family, relatives, and friends of personnel working in the mine will arrive on the scene, along with members of the public. It is essential, then, that crowd control planning be a part of emergency planning. Some operations may have a well-established security group. If that is not the case, arrangements can be made in advance for personnel from local law enforcement agencies.

Those who are to respond to a mine emergency should be identified by position within the organization, rather than by name. Notification to personnel listed in an emergency response plan starts at the top of the list. The person whose position is at the top of the list is the person in charge of the emergency. If that person is unavailable, the next person in line assumes control.

The emergency response plan should incorporate a brief description of the role played by each person involved in the emergency response. Duties such as contact with the state and federal government agencies and the news media must be preassigned. Crowd control responsibilities should also be assigned to one person.

MINE RESCUE

Well-trained and experienced mine rescue teams are a mine's greatest asset in an emergency. Mine rescue personnel know the mine in which they work and understand the systems that are used in transportation as well as power supplies. They are also trained in advanced first aid and in fire fighting. In all mine emergencies, at least one mine rescue team captain should be called in, even when it has not yet been decided to create a mine rescue team.

Emergency preparedness is best served when candidates for mine rescue teams are carefully selected. Mine management must consider the needs within their mine and select mine rescue personnel capable of meeting anticipated needs in an emergency. Individuals with special skills, such as electricians and mechanics, are needed for mine rescue work. If the mine has hoists underground, hoistmen may be needed. If the mine is heavily timbered, timbermen are needed on the team.

Use of mine rescue teams is almost a certainty in a mine fire involving personnel trapped or missing in the mine. Advance plans must be made for additional mine rescue teams, as well as for acquiring supplies and materials. This need becomes critical in a fire that extends beyond a few days.

It is extremely important that mine management personnel understand the capabilities and limitations of mine rescue personnel. Well-trained mine rescue teams know what they can accomplish. Management personnel who fail to understand the capabilities of mine rescue teams should not attempt to control the activities of the teams.

VENTILATION PLANNING

It is essential that ventilation data is up to date and that current ventilation schematics are on hand at headquarters. The ventilation engineer must have the skills and training to quickly determine how changes in the mine that occur during an emergency will affect air flows throughout the active portions of the mine.

MINE MAPS

Up-to-date maps of all active portions of the mine must be on hand at headquarters. Maps of inactive mine openings must also be provided if there is a possibility of use by mine rescue teams. If there are adjoining mines, maps of such mines must also be at headquarters.

MINE ALARM SYSTEM

A suitable fire alarm system is a Mine Safety and Health Administration (MSHA) requirement. It is mentioned here because of its importance in emergency preparedness and in development of an emergency response plan.

SURPRISE DRILLS

Run drills! Do not give advance notice, but simulate fires in various parts of the mine and challenge personnel to respond. Don't be surprised if the first such drill results in a lot of confusion and "I don't know" responses.

SURFACE FIRE

BASIC PLAN IN ALL CASES

- KNOW THE LOCATION OF ALL EXITS FROM YOUR WORK LOCATION AND FROM EACH BUILDING YOU ENTER DURING WORK.

- The **ONLY ACCEPTABLE RESPONSE** to a fire that is not extinguished by the sprinkler systems or through the use of a hand portable fire extinguisher is **EVACUATION OF PERSONNEL FROM THE AFFECTED BUILDINGS.**

- **NOTIFY SECURITY AS SOON AS POSSIBLE.** Security personnel will ensure that fire alarms are sounded and notify the local fire department.

- ALL SURFACE FIRE FIGHTING WILL BE DONE BY THE LOCAL FIRE DEPARTMENT.

- UNTRAINED PERSONNEL WILL NEVER ATTEMPT TO FIGHT A MAJOR FIRE.

FIGURE 15.1 Example of emergency response plan

Drills offer multiple benefits to the safety of the mine. Deficiencies in the emergency response plan are identified. A drill identifies personnel who have failed to follow through on their responsibilities. A drill also identifies needed changes, if any, in headquarters.

ANALYSIS OF AN EMERGENCY RESPONSE PLAN

Following are key parts of an actual mine emergency response plan. Key personnel are identified by their positions. The original emergency response plan was developed following a mine fire disaster. The plan was most recently updated in July 1999. The plan has been in effect since 1973 and has served reliably in a number of emergencies.

The complete plan includes detailed information about the mine and the surface operations. Portions of the plan are included below as examples of how an emergency response plan is developed.

MINE EMERGENCY

Scope of Plan

This plan is designed as a guideline for all types of emergencies including fires, explosions, entrapment of personnel, loss of electrical power, and natural disasters.

Leadership Qualifications

It is imperative that the person in charge topside understands the layout of the mine, primary and secondary escape way, location of rescue chambers or refuge areas, and the mine ventilation system.

SURFACE FIRE

DETAILED SURFACE PLAN—MILL

911 LOCATION IDENTIFICATION—2227 BIG CREEK ROAD

SPECIAL PRECAUTIONS

Water hoses must NOT be used within the facility until after electrical power has been

shut off.

SHUT-DOWN PROCEDURES

- Kill electrical power at North Substation (5 breakers).

- Push OFF button — green light indicates system is <u>OFF</u>.

- Killing power in the mill also kills power in the machine shop, dry, boiler rooms,

  crushing plant, Jewell top station, old brick office building, and assay office.

- Note: Grinnel system will trip if fire occurs.

RESPONSIBLE PERSON

First Name, Last Name, and Phone Number

SPECIAL CAUTIONS

55-gallon oil drums in area
Acetylene and oxygen bottles in area
Reagents will burn. **Close valves at reagent tanks to keep reagents from flowing**
       through damaged pipes.
Chemicals stored at upper level may cause hazardous fumes when burned.

FIGURE 15.1   Example of emergency response plan (continued)

Chain of Command

The **general manager** or his designee will be in charge of any emergency. If he is not available for a mine emergency, the mine manager will be in charge. If he is not available for a surface emergency, the manager of metallurgy will be in charge. If initially designated personnel are unavailable, the command position will pass down the list of staff personnel to the first available staff person.

Delegation of Responsibility during Absences

Each person whose duties are included in this **Emergency Response Plan** will designate a replacement during any vacation or planned absence. This information shall be provided to the security office. Figure 15.1 is an example of an Emergency Response Plan.

Basic Responsibilities of Key Personnel

- The **general manager** will exercise overall control of operations, making certain that all staff and supervisory personnel are following the **Emergency Response Plan.**

- The **mine manager** will be **in charge of** all emergency response activities involving the **mine facilities**. He will establish headquarters in the mine office and assume control. He will assign supervisory personnel as needed and determine needs for mine rescue personnel or other hourly personnel. In a surface emergency, he will coordinate all operations not involved in the emergency. In his absence, control will pass to the mine superintendent.

- The **chief engineer** will provide and supervise all engineering support requested by the mine manager.

- The **ventilation engineer** will provide ventilation engineering support as the highest priority. The engineer will ensure that current ventilation maps are always maintained in the mine office. (Comment: In a mine emergency, particularly in a mine fire, the ability to control mine ventilation becomes one of the most important functions.)

- The **mine superintendent** will assist the mine manager in identifying problems within the area involved in the emergency. He will also assist the safety director in accounting for personnel affected by the emergency. (Comment: If the mine manager is unavailable, the mine superintendent becomes the key management person during the emergency.)

- The **manager of metallurgy** will evaluate the impact, if any, of the mine emergency on the surface plant and respond accordingly. He will arrange surface transportation of supplies and equipment. (Comment: It is important to take surface operations into account during an underground mine emergency. The opposite is true if the emergency involves surface structures. Possible impacts on the mine must then be considered.)

- The **purchasing agent/services foreman** will arrange for movement of supplies and materials as directed by headquarters control. He will procure additional equipment and supplies as requested by headquarters control. (Comment: Mine emergencies may continue for days or weeks. Acquiring supplies, materials, and replacement equipment becomes a critical function.)

- The **electrical supervisor** will evaluate the emergency relative to control of electrical power. He will advise headquarters control of any potential electrical problems that might occur as a result of the emergency.

- The **mechanical supervisor** will ensure the availability of equipment and maintenance personnel.

CHAPTER 16

Contractor Health and Safety

Timothy M. Biddle and Thomas C. Means
Crowell & Moring LLP, Washington, D.C.

INTRODUCTION

In this chapter, we discuss the use of independent contractors in the mining industry and the mine safety and health law and liability issues to which this gives rise. First, we set the stage by describing the nature of the owner-contractor relationship, the various ways that independent contractors are employed in mining, and the reasons that they are used in mining. Then, we explain the safety and health responsibility and liability issues that bear on the owner-contractor relationship under federal mine safety law and state tort law. After describing the use of mine safety and health partnerships between the Mine Safety and Health Administration (MSHA) and mineral owners as a way to address some of the safety issues created by the use of independent contractors, we then consider how the relationship between the owners and contractors should be structured so as to protect their respective interests in mine safety and health matters. Finally, we offer some suggestions for handling the types of problems that may arise so that the owner-contractor relationship can be maintained for the benefit of both parties.

INDEPENDENT CONTRACTORS: WHEN, WHERE, AND WHY

When a mining company needs a task done that requires specialized skills or equipment, it often hires an "independent contractor." An independent contractor is an entity that performs work with its own equipment and employees for an unrelated person or company (in the remainder of this chapter, we refer to the person or company that employs an independent contractor as the "owner"). Although an owner has the right to specify the results of a contractor's work, the contractor who performs the work is independent—meaning it does not work under the day-to-day supervision and control of the owner. In the mining context, independent contractors often are hired to perform a wide variety of tasks connected with the exploration for minerals, the development of a mine, and the production and processing of resources owned by someone else—usually a mining company or an absentee property owner.

To understand the relationship between an independent contractor and an owner in the context of mine health and safety, it is useful to first focus on the kinds of work commonly done by independent contractors for mining companies. Three principal kinds of independent contractors are employed by owners in the mining industry: construction contractors, service contractors, and production contractors.

Independent contractors performing construction on mine property often are hired to build buildings, sink shafts, construct plants and mills, lay railroad track, build dams, and build roads. Although construction contractors may be on mine property for a lengthy period, once their job is complete, this kind of independent contractor usually leaves the property.

Service contractors may also perform a "one-time" task, such as repairing a hoist or rotary dump, but more often they are at a mine frequently—sometimes constantly—where they may work alongside mining company employees to maintain and repair equipment, survey, monitor miners for medical problems, check for compliance with environmental laws, prepare engineering drawings, and perform similar tasks. Service contractors often will have their own worksites at a mine for their equipment and employees, such as a separate building, a room, or a bay in a maintenance shop.

Independent "production" contractors typically use their own equipment and employees to operate a pit, an entire mine, a preparation plant, or a mill for the owner of a resource, who often is not at the site. These kinds of independent contractors, sometimes called "contract miners," may, in turn, hire other independent contractors to perform construction or services at the mine they are operating for an owner.

Why would an owner hire an independent contractor? The answer is simple: economics and efficiency. Owners hire independent contractors when they conclude that it is more economic or efficient to hire an outsider to do a task instead of accomplishing that task with its own employees or equipment. An owner's employees may not be able to do a task because they do not have the skills, equipment, or time necessary, or the job that needs to be done may be unrelated to the owner's business. Using contractors also enables the owner to get necessary tasks done without having to expand his workforce beyond what is needed generally and then reducing it, thus avoiding additional administrative and labor relations costs, as well as other costs that layoffs would engender. In the mining context, specialized knowledge, skills, and equipment often are important to getting a job done rapidly and safely, without serious interruption of the mining process. Independent contractors can provide that benefit. Sometimes an owner will find it necessary to hire several independent contractors for different projects on the same property.

Independent contractors may *subcontract* work at an owner's property to other independent contractors. This arrangement commonly occurs on construction projects where the owner enters into a contract with an independent contractor to be the "general contractor"—the entity responsible for the entire job. The general (and independent) contractor, in turn, usually will hire other independent contractors to perform various parts of the job, such as site preparation, steel erection, carpentry, electrical work, plumbing installation, and other specialty jobs. Although general contractors will have a written contract with the owner, the subcontractors often have no direct relationship with the owner. Instead, the subcontractors will have a contract with the general contractor, who is responsible to the owner. On large projects, there may be several "layers" or "tiers" of subcontractors, but they all are business entities with employees and equipment not controlled in either a legal or practical manner by the owner or by any other contractor on the property. For the reasons we explain in the next section, however, the owner should keep track of which independent contractors are working on its property, for whom each contractor is working, and what each of them is doing—at least generally.

Occupational accidents and illness are dispiriting, disruptive, and expensive. Both owners and independent contractors who work on an owner's property should share a strong interest in maintaining healthful and safe worksites. Thus, ensuring the safety and health of each entity's employees is a critical element in the independent contractor/owner relationship and in the relationship between general contractors and subcontractors. For this reason, contractor employees must take precautions to protect everyone from hazards in the contractor's workplace; the owner will need to protect employees of contractors from hazards peculiar to its mining activities.

In later sections of this chapter, we will discuss structuring the relationship between independent contractors and owners and maintaining that relationship, with an emphasis on safety and health issues.

LEGAL RESPONSIBILITY AND LIABILITY

At one time, questions of legal responsibility and liability between independent contractors and mine owners had relatively easy answers. In fact, aside from their specialized expertise, and their other advantages as discussed above, independent contractors were employed by mine owners, in part, because the mine owner's liability was limited with respect to the work performed by independent contractors. At bottom (though there were qualifications and exceptions to this general rule), contractors were solely liable for their own conduct or misconduct, as the case may be. Those days are long gone. Under certain circumstances, contractors and owners, and perhaps other entities as well, can be held liable for violations caused by a contractor. The rules of the game have been changing, and remain in flux, as discussed below. We first examine the law under the Federal Mine Safety and Health Act of 1977, and then under state tort law.

Under the Federal Mine Safety and Health Act of 1977

Historically, the federal law applicable to contractor health and safety could be divided into two different categories. One set of principles governed contract mine operators. In contrast, independent contractors performing construction or services for the mine operator (rather than as the mine operator) were governed by a different set of rules as to legal responsibility and liability. Whether those distinctions are still viable today remains to be seen, as discussed below.

Independent Contractors Working for the Mine Operator   As explained in Chapter 7, the Federal Mine Safety and Health Act of 1977 ("Mine Act") makes the "operator" responsible for all safety and health responsibilities and compliance obligations at a mine. Who is a mine operator thus becomes the critical inquiry. Under the Mine Act today, the operator is defined to mean "any owner, lessee, or other person who operates, controls, or supervises a coal or other mine or any independent contractor performing services or construction at such a mine" (30 USC § 802(d)(1994). To fully understand the law in this area, a little history is a must (See Vish et al. 1989; Hardy and McCambley 1997).

The reference to independent contractors in the definition of operator was not added until 1977 when the Mine Act was passed, amending and superceding the 1969 Coal Mine Health and Safety Act ("Coal Act"). Before the passage of the Mine Act, there was an extensive litigation history under the Coal Act over the status of independent contractors working at mine sites. That controversy focused on the fact that most independent contractors by their very nature—not being subject to the control of mine owner as to the method and manner in which they performed their jobs, and generally using their own equipment and their own employees—effectively controlled that part of the mine where their work was being performed. Accordingly, many in the industry took the position that the independent contractor, not the mine owner, was the "operator" with respect to the specific work that the contractor controlled and therefore was the party responsible for workplace safety and health there, as well as for any safety or health violations.

Over time, federal regulatory policy on the issue of independent contractor liability ran from one extreme to the other under the 1969 Coal Act: at one point, the Interior Board of Mine Operations Appeals (*Affinity Mining Co.* 1973) held that the key to liability as "an operator" was determined by the locus of responsibility for the health and safety of the miners in question, and that "while more than one person may fall technically within the definition of 'operator,' only the one responsible for the violations and the safety of employees can be the person served with notices and orders and against whom civil penalties may be assessed." At the other end of the spectrum, after a district court ruling that independent construction contractors were not within the definition of operator and could not be held liable for violations, the Secretary of the Interior (before that district court judgment was reversed in the D.C. Circuit) instructed all federal mine safety inspectors to issue citations for independent contractor violations only to the operator who hired the contractor (*Association of Bituminous Contractors* 1975).

After the coal industry challenged that policy, the U.S. Court of Appeals for the Fourth Circuit held that independent construction contractors could be held liable as operators under the Coal Act, but that a mine owner also could be held responsible for violations of its contractors (*Bituminous Coal Operators' Association* [BCOA] 1977). When the Mine Act was passed in 1977, amending the Coal Act, the current language expressly adding independent contractors to the definition of operator was included and the legislative history stated that this was intended to be consistent with the BCOA holding in the Fourth Circuit.

The issue was also addressed by the U.S. Court of Appeals for the District of Columbia Circuit, which held that, in addition to mine owners or lessees, other persons who operate, control, or supervise a coal mine can be operators as well, and that under the Coal Act an independent contractor doing construction work at a mine can be an operator with respect to the work it performs. The court recognized the importance of placing responsibility on the party in the best position to protect the safety and health of the miners and also stated that the control and supervision that independent contractors have over their work projects is an appropriate basis for holding them liable for their own violations as mine operators. Whereas the Fourth Circuit had stated that it was up to the agency to allocate liability between mine owner operator and independent contractor operator, the D.C. Circuit suggested that only contractors should be liable for their violations ("otherwise, the owner would be constantly interfering in the work of a construction company in order to minimize his own liability for damages. The Act does not require such an inefficient method of ensuring compliance with mandatory safety regulations") (*Association of Bituminous Contractors* 1978).

After the passage of the Mine Act, MSHA continued to cite only mine owners for the violations of independent contractors. Several owners contested such citations before the commission. Although the commission upheld MSHA's citations issued to the mine owners, it cautioned MSHA that the commission has the authority to review MSHA's exercise of prosecutorial discretion to ensure that the secretary's decision to prosecute a mine operator for its independent contractor's violations was made for reasons consistent with the purpose and policies of the 1977 Act, and not merely for administrative convenience (*Old Ben* 1979). This litigation led to the issuance of MSHA's regulations governing procedures for identifying independent contractors as operators and distinguishing them from the "production-operator" that MSHA defined (in 30 *Code of Federal Regulations* [CFR] § 45.2(d)) as the mine operator (owner, lessee, or other person) with overall control of the mine. In addition to issuance of these regulations under 30 CFR Part 45, MSHA also published at the same time enforcement guidelines for the allocation of liability between production operators and independent contractors for contractor violations. Although MSHA indicated that ultimate responsibility for the safety and health of all persons working at a mine remains with the production operator, and that MSHA could take enforcement action against production operators for independent contractor violations, it stated that it would generally hold production operators liable for contractor violations only in certain circumstances (*Federal Register* 1980).

> (1) when the production-operator has contributed by either an act or omission to the occurrence of a violation in the course of an independent contractor's work, or (2) when the production-operator has contributed by either an act or omission to the continued existence of a violation committed by an independent contractor or (3) when the production-operator's miners are exposed to the hazard, or (4) when the production-operator has control over the condition that needs abatement.

That remains MSHA's general policy today, although over time MSHA has increasingly tended to cite the production operator as well when it cites the independent contractor. In its most recent articulation of its policy concerning liability for violations committed by independent contractors, MSHA (1994) reaffirmed that:

> [MSHA's] enforcement policy is to cite independent contractors for violations committed by a contractor or its employees. This policy does not change the production operator's overall responsibility for compliance with the Mine Act, standards, and regulations. Production operators have the responsibility for the health and safety of all persons working at their mine sites. In certain circumstances, enforcement actions may be taken against both a production operator and independent contractor jointly, or against either entity individually.

> Because production operators have the overall knowledge and daily control of a mine operation, they are in the best position to coordinate the contractor's activities and to monitor the contractor's safety performance. When a production operator selects an independent contractor to perform services at a mine, the focus should be not only on the technical ability of the contractor to do the job, but also on whether the contractor has the necessary knowledge, skills, resources, and commitment to ensure the safety and health of the persons they employ.

Additionally, it should be noted that MSHA is not legally obligated to adhere to its enforcement guidelines. The courts have held that, even though those guidelines are published in the *Federal Register*, they are not binding regulations (*Brock* 1986). Accordingly, MSHA has discretion about whether or not to cite the independent contractor, the production operator, or both under the circumstances described in its enforcement guidelines and its enforcement action will not be overturned, even if it is inconsistent with those guidelines, unless it is found to be an abuse of discretion (*Amax* 1994).

Contract Mine Operators (Independent Contractors Working as Mine Operators)   In contrast to the fluid, litigation-driven history of federal regulatory liability for independent contractor violations, the law governing contract mine operators has been constant over time—at least until quite recently. Throughout the history of mining in this country, some mineral owners (including lessees) have chosen not to mine their reserves themselves, but have instead engaged skilled professionals to develop and operate mines on their property. These independent contractors who are hired as mine operators are termed "contract miners." They typically have complete control over the mining operation itself, subject only to any restrictions imposed by the terms of the contract between them and the owner, usually governing what area is to be mined, the specifications for the mineral, delivery schedules, payment schedules, and the like, but reserving to the contract miner exclusive control over the manner and method of mining.

The contract mine operator employs the miners, hiring, firing, disciplining, and directing the workforce. He typically owns mining equipment, files his own legal identity report with MSHA under 30 CFR Part 41, and files his own mining plans (roof control, ventilation, and sediment pond plans, for example). Until recently, contract miners—and contract miners alone (i.e., not the mineral owners)—were always cited by MSHA for all violations occurring in a mine. Indeed, the concept of the "contract miner" was rarely if ever addressed in mine safety law because, for Coal Act and Mine Act purposes, the contract mine operator was *the* operator; that is, the form of legal authority by which a mine operator had the right to run its mine (e.g., whether by contract, lease, or deed) was irrelevant for purposes of determining compliance with MSHA standards or liability for MSHA enforcement actions.

That all began to change in 1994 with the commission's decision in *W-P Coal Company*. In *W-P*, MSHA broke precedent, successfully holding a coal lessee liable for a contract miner's violations. After learning of the bankruptcy of the contract mine operator it had cited for multiple violations, MSHA then issued the same citations to the mineral lessee that had engaged the contract operator. The Federal Mine Safety and Health Review Commission, after protracted litigation, eventually upheld MSHA's citations against the lessee. Although it rejected MSHA's contention that the lessee was a "cooperator," it held that the lessee was substantially involved in the operation of the mine through its involvement in engineering, production, financing, personnel, and health and safety matters there, and that this brought it within the definition of mine operator.

Some industry observers have discounted the ruling in the *W-P* as largely a function of the fact that the mineral lessee had itself previously been the production operator of that mine for many years and had recently brought in a series of small, undercapitalized contractors to operate it, to the extent that the cited contractor was really more of an agent of the lessee than an independent contractor. MSHA, however, subsequently persisted with its aggressive attempt to expand the universe of mine operators who could be held liable for safety and health violations. In *Berwind,* MSHA recently sought to hold liable as operators—in addition to the contract miner—both individually and collectively the mineral lessee that hired the contract miner, the mineral lessor, an affiliated company that performed surveying and spad-setting services, and the parent corporation that owns the latter three, jointly and severally liable as mine operators for more than 200 alleged violations at the mine (*Berwind* 1996 and 1999).

The administrative law judge (ALJ) held that only the lessee (in addition to the contract miner, whose liability was uncontested) could be held liable as a mine operator because none of the other three entities exercised substantial day-to-day control of the mining operation, which he viewed as necessary for "operator" status, nor had MSHA established the necessary legal grounds to hold the related corporate entities liable for each other's violations. With respect to the lessee, the ALJ found that even though the contract mine operator had exercised control over all other aspects of safety and health at the mine, the lessee was nonetheless an operator because the lessee had reserved the right to approve any changes by the contract miner in the direction of mining (in order to ensure that its reserves were efficiently mined, so as to avoid incurring liability to the lessor for waste [*Berwind* 1996]).

On administrative review, the Federal Mine Safety and Health Review Commission upheld the ALJ's decision as to each entity in result, but for somewhat different reasons. Rather than necessarily requiring a showing of day-to-day control, the commission held that whether an entity would be deemed an operator would be based on the totality of the circumstances determined on a case-by-case basis. In a lengthy decision composed of a four-person majority opinion and five additional opinions of the commissioners, concurring in parts of the decision and dissenting in parts, only the lessee (not the lessor, the "spad-setter," or the parent) was held to be an operator under that totality standard. A three-person majority also agreed with MSHA's argument that two or more companies could be treated as a "unitary operator" based on a new test forged by that three-person majority (considering the degree of interrelation of their operations, common management, centralized control over mine safety and health, and common ownership), and that the "spad-setting company" could have been liable as a unitary operator with the lessee. However, no entity was held liable as a unitary operator in this case because a majority believed that MSHA had not given adequate notice that companies could be subject to such liability. Given the badly divided views of the commissioners and the fact that the case was then settled rather than taken to the court of appeals, definitive guidance on the state of the law did not result from this decision (*Berwind* 1999).

As noted above, depending on how MSHA, the ALJ, the commission, and the courts review the facts, violations at the operations of a contract miner may (or many not) result in Mine Act liability for the contractor, the owner, and other entities as well.

Under State Tort Law

If a person breaches a duty of care and a person to whom that duty was owed is injured, the injured person may sue the party who breached the duty and may collect civil damages to compensate him for his injury, and perhaps even punitive damages if the breach of duty was in some way egregious. That is the basic principle of negligence liability in American tort law. It would apply to employees whose employers owe them a duty of care to provide a safe work place, except that virtually every state has adopted a workers compensation system that insulates the employer from such tort liability in exchange for his payment of workers compensation benefits to any of his employees who is injured on the job, regardless of fault. Thus, an employee of an independent contractor generally cannot sue the contractor if he is injured while performing services or construction at a mine. But there is no such clear barrier to the employee's suit against the owner (the mine operator) if the employee can establish the existence of a duty that the operator breached.

Traditionally, mine operators have attempted to avoid conduct that could give rise to such a duty in order to insulate themselves from tort liability for on-the-job injuries to the independent contractor's employee. Because the independent contractor has complete control over the manner and method by which the work is performed, and legal responsibility for the safety of his own employees, mine owners, like other third parties, should generally bear no tort liability when a contractor's employee is injured. However, the law provides that where the owner, for whatever reason, involves himself in the way that the contractor conducts his operations or otherwise interferes with the independence of the contractor with respect to such matters, the owner can be held to have assumed a duty of care and can be held directly liable for the injuries suffered by the contractor's employee through the operator's negligence. For example, where the mine owner has directed the contractor with respect to how to conduct its operations, advised the contractor with respect to the safety of its operations, or otherwise involved itself in the manner and method of the contractors' work, injured employees of the contractor have, with remarkable success, sued the mine owner to recover damages.

It is the fear of such liabilities that substantially deters mine operators from involving themselves in the safety and health aspects of their contractors' operations. This potential liability lies at the heart of the battle between the mining industry and MSHA about the proper role of the mine operator in contractor safety. MSHA, for years, has urged mine owners to take responsibility for the safety and health of their contractors' operations, inspecting for safety, identifying violations, and requiring abatement; at the same time, most mine operators have persistently resisted such responsibilities as open invitations to civil litigation defense costs, if not actual tort liabilities, if contractor employees are killed or injured. The tort liability situation poses a dilemma for mine operators: if they don't involve themselves in contractor safety and health, MSHA is likely to prosecute them for violations that occur on the contractor's worksite; on the other hand, if they do involve themselves in the safety and health of the contractor's operations, they will almost certainly be sued by an injured employee or his estate and survivors in the event of an accident. This tension is unresolved in the law, but, as we discuss below, MSHA has sought to provide a partial answer through the mine safety and health partnership concept.

SAFETY AND HEALTH PARTNERSHIP WITH MSHA

Several major coal companies have entered into "partnership" agreements with MSHA in response to MSHA's concerns about the disproportionately high accident rates of independent contractors on the whole. MSHA points to statistics showing that the use of independent contractors is increasing in the mining industry on the one hand, while accidents attributable to independent contractors continue to substantially exceed industry averages (MSHA 1994).

Because MSHA has long held the view that the larger mine operators who employ independent contractors have the resources, ability, and *responsibility* to improve contractor safety, it has engaged in various tactics to prod those mine operators to proactively take responsibility for contractor safety. In addition to more aggressive enforcement efforts against mine operators for their contractors' violations, MSHA has also promoted the concept of safety and health partnerships between MSHA and mine owners.

Each of the several partnerships with major mining companies into which MSHA has entered thus far is different. All of them, however, are grounded in the mine owners' assumption of responsibility for improving the training of contractors and their employees, as well as for using safety and health criteria in the selection of contractors, and in the subsequent monitoring of their contractual performance.

The two most recent partnership-type agreements illustrate both the existence of these common themes, as well as the fact that each is different. The agreement between MSHA and the A.T. Massey Coal Company, entered into in 1996, is focused on improving the safety of contract mine operators. CONSOL, Inc., by contrast, agreed with MSHA on a program (also entered into in 1996) that focuses instead on independent service and construction contractors, not contract miners. Yet, each commits the mining company to oversight of and assistance in the contractor's safety and health training, the selection of safe and responsible contractors with a good compliance history, and the follow-up auditing of the contractor's accident and violation records with the implicit or explicit understanding that those contractors who perform poorly in these areas will not have their contracts renewed.

In exchange for the mining company's participation in the program, MSHA promises to provide technical assistance and information to them, to allow them to participate in closeout and other health and safety conferences between MSHA and the contractors, and to furnish information about contractors' accident records and violations. In addition, MSHA agrees not to use the fact of the mining company's involvement in its contractor's safety, health, and training as a basis for imposing Mine Act liability on the mining company for its contractor's violations. Importantly, although MSHA makes no binding commitment, it is implied that, in exchange for the mining company's participation in such a program, MSHA will not cite the mining company for the contractor's violations generally absent actual mining company responsibility for such violations.

Unresolved by these partnership agreements, and the likely reason that they have not been more widely adopted, is their effect on the mine owner's tort liability exposure. No assurances from MSHA can protect the owner from tort liability in the event that death or injury occurs to an employee of a contractor that the mine owner has obligated itself to assist in training, for example. The assumption of such responsibilities by the mining company, notwithstanding its disclaimers and protestations to the contrary, will almost certainly be deemed an assumption of a duty by the mining company and result in an increased likelihood of tort liability in the event of an accident (Rajkovich 1998).

Whether the improved safety and health records of contractors and fewer MSHA violations that may be anticipated from these partnerships will justify the increased tort liability exposure remains to be seen. Certainly this is an area where law and policy need to coincide, not conflict.

STRUCTURING THE RELATIONSHIP

From a health and safety perspective, the relationship between an owner and its independent contractor must be carefully structured to protect their respective interests.

The agreement between an owner and an independent contractor should be detailed in a written contract. Before entering into a contract, however, and assuming there is a choice for owners in selecting a contractor, an owner may use a preselection process (sometimes called prequalification) to identify contractors that the owner believes would be able to successfully accomplish the work. In a preselection process, owners may send a request for proposal (RFP) to potential contractors that informs them about the nature of the work, the time in which it is to be accomplished and any special requirements (like proof of financial ability and ability to obtain a performance bond and insurance), makes clear who is to supply the materials required for the work, and asks for a list of prior similar jobs and references from them. To assess a potential contractor's health and safety record, the RFP may also require that the potential contractor provide information about his frequency of lost time accidents and the number and type of violations issued by MSHA during inspections at the contractor's worksites over some specified period, usually a year or two. An owner may also inquire about the contractor's arrangements for MSHA-required safety and health training, because contractor employees who regularly will work on mine property will be considered miners and must be trained in accordance with the kind of job they will be doing and where they will be doing it.

Along with obvious terms such as work specifications, deadline for completion, price, and the way any dispute will be resolved–to name but a few–the written contract between an owner and an independent contractor should cover health and safety obligations, provisions that are particularly important in the mining context. For example, contract terms for work to be done by an independent contractor at a mine worksite often include these following health and safety subjects:

- Whether the independent contractor is obligated to comply with all federal and state health and safety laws and regulations while the contractor works on mine property

- Whether the owner reserves the right to inspect the contractor's worksite and equipment for safety and health hazards

- Whether the owner or the contractor will provide the equipment and material necessary for the job and which of the parties bears the risk if any of that equipment or material causes an accident or results in the issuance of a citation or order by MSHA or state regulatory authority

- Whether the contractor must obtain an MSHA identification number prior to beginning work (contractors may obtain identification numbers from MSHA by following the procedures at 30 CFR Part 45 or by registering online by using MSHA's website at www.msha.gov/FORMS/CONID.htm)

- Whether the contractor is required to report to the owner the issuance of safety or health violations alleged by MSHA (or its state counterpart) at the contractor's work site

- Whether the contractor will be responsible for paying civil penalties assessed for any citations or orders issued by MSHA to the contractor or to the owner for violations alleged by MSHA for conditions at the contractor's worksite or for conditions caused by the contractor's employees or equipment (civil penalties of up to $55,000 per violation are mandatory under the Federal Mine Safety and Health Act. See 30 USC §820(a)(1994)(the maximum penalty was increased to $55,000 by the Omnibus Budget Reconciliation Act of 1997). For civil penalty assessment procedures, see 30 CFR Part 100 (1999)

- Whether the contractor is required to indemnify the owner for any damages for personal injury or death or harm to property caused by the contractor's activities

- Whether the independent contractor, will be responsible for training its own employees before they begin work on the owner's property (see 30 CFR Part 48 (1999) for training requirements), and thereafter as necessary (e.g., new task training or annual refresher training)

- Whether the owner is reserving the right to default the contractor if the contractor's accident and MSHA compliance rate is unacceptable and, if so, an objective standard to apply in determining whether a contractor can be so defaulted

- Whether the owner must review any plans or other MSHA-required written submissions prepared by the contractor relating to work to be done on the owner's property before those plans or other submissions are sent to MSHA for approval.

Although, as discussed above, MSHA may well cite an owner for a contractor's violation, the contractor may be assessed a much higher penalty than the owner if the contractor had actual control over the violation. For these reasons, it is important to make sure that the written contract between the owner and the independent contractor clearly deals with the "control" issue. It also is important that the way the owner and contractor deal with each other while the contractor is working on the owner's property faithfully carries out whatever is provided in the contract on the "control" subject. This is because no matter what a contract may say, the on-site relationship between the owner and the contractor may be critical evidence on the issue of control. In fact, if an owner's control over a contractor's work is so pervasive as to put into question whether the contractor is really independent, the owner may be deemed the operator of the contractor's "mine"; in addition, MSHA may characterize the contractor as an *agent* of the owner. An agent is a person authorized by another (called a "principal") to act for him. The agent is entrusted with the principal's business even though he often works at locations away from the principal's place of business. Wherever he works, the agent has the authority to transact business for his principal. A sales agent for mining company is a good example. Thus, both on paper and in day-to-day actions, a contractor should be treated as an *independent contractor* by an owner, not in a manner that makes the contractor appear to be the owner's agent.

The next section discusses maintaining the relationship between an owner and an independent contractor in a manner to keep separate the independent contractor and the owner in reality, as well as by contract.

MAINTAINING THE RELATIONSHIP

Once an independent contractor is working on mine property, it is important to make the contractor's independence real. At the same time, however, both the owner (if on site) and the contractor must be able to work in a coordinated manner so both can accomplish their work.

Without meddling in the contractor's work, and certainly without exercising the kind of control over the contractor's work that could increase the likelihood of Mine Act liability for the contractor's violations or could lead MSHA to a conclusion that the contractor is really the owner's agent, the owner probably will want to monitor the performance of the contractor as the work is being accomplished, particularly if construction to specifications is involved. Monitoring a contractor's work, however, does not mean that the owner is taking responsibility for protecting the contractor's employees from health and safety hazards. Owners who believe it necessary to closely monitor a contractor's safety and health measures, usually by conducting periodic inspections, are assuming risks that would not otherwise be present if they let the contractor administer his own safety program. Those risks are detailed earlier in this chapter.

It should be emphasized, however, that it should not be considered "control" for an owner to require an independent contractor to submit periodic reports about safety and health compliance (or noncompliance), if the contract between the owner and the independent contractor requires such reports. Similarly, where the owner monitors the performance of the independent contractor, but does not direct the contractor's employees and does not direct when, where or how the work is to be done, the independence of the contractor should not be questioned.

Owners who wish to minimize the risks of being cited by MSHA for contractor-caused safety or health violations or who or who wish to avoid creating a legal duty by becoming involved in a contractor's safety and health activities should carefully plan to keep the contractor's activities separate from the owner's activities. For example, "hands-off" owners will not conduct safety inspections at contractor worksites, will not accompany MSHA inspectors when MSHA inspectors are inspecting at contractor worksites, will require the contractor to do its own training of its own employees, and will, if feasible, keep the work area of the contractor segregated from the areas where the owner's employees are working; in addition, the owner's employees should be instructed to stay away from the contractor's operations. For their part, independent contractors often prefer that the owner take these steps so that there is no confusion about who is in charge of the work, and who is in charge of safety and health measures. A contractor who is working in a clearly definable work area, preferably fenced off with prominent signage prohibiting entry into the contractor's area, should be able to avoid liabilities that might result from the owner's employees being injured or killed at the contractor's worksite.

Of course, owners and independent contractors should both understand that if there are hazards created at the worksite of either entity that may endanger the others' employees, they have a duty to warn about that danger and a duty to take reasonable steps to guard against people accidentally getting in harm's way. The same principle applies to use of equipment and tools by employees of both entities. If an injury or fatality results from use of equipment or tools by an employee of an entity that does not own that equipment or tool, there likely will be claims for damages against the owner of the equipment or tools. For this reason, an owner's employees not only should stay out of the contractor's work area, but they should not be permitted to operate the contractor's equipment or to use his tools. The reverse, of course, is also true.

In summary, the owner wants his job done to specifications, on time, and at the price promised. The contractor wants the same thing. Good relations between the owner and an independent contractor will provide the best opportunity for both to realize their goals.

REFERENCES

Affinity Mining Company. 2 IBMA 57 (1972). *Aff'd as modified,* 2 IBMA 63 (1973).

Amax Coal West Inc. 16 F.M.S.H.R.C. 2489 (1994) (ALJ).

Association of Bituminous Contractors v. Andrus. 581 F.2d 853, 862-63 (D.C. Cir. 1978).

Association of Bituminous Contractors, Inc. v. Morton. No. 74-1058 (D.C.C. May 23, 1975). *Rev'd, Association of Bituminous Contractors, Inc. v. Andrus,* 581 F.2d 853 (D.C. Cir. 1978).

Berwind Natural Resources Corp. 18 F.M.S.H.R.C. 202 (1996), (ALJ), (Berwind 1996). *Aff'd in part and vacated in part,* 21 F.M.S.H.R.C. 1284 (1999), (Berwind 1999).

Bituminous Coal Operators' Association v. Secretary of Interior. 547 F.2d 240 (4th Cir. 1977).

Brock v. Cathedral Bluffs Shale Oil Co. 796 F.2d 533 (D.C. 1986).

Hardy, D., and M. McCambley. "Liability of Owners Under the Federal Mine Safety and Health Act of 1977." Chapter 7 in 16 E. *Min. L. Inst.* (1997).

45 *Federal Register* 44,494, 44,497 (1980).

MSHA Program Information Bulletin. No. P. 94–14 (May 20, 1994).

Old Ben Coal Co. 1 F.M.S.H.R.C. 1480 (1979).

Rajkovich, M. "MSHA Partnership Agreements: A New Approach Toward Enforcement." Chapter 2 in 18 E. *Min. L. Inst.* (1998).

Vish, D., D. McGinley, and T. Biddle, 1 *Coal Law & Regulation* § 3.13[3][b] (Matthew Bender 1989).

W-P Coal Company. 16 F.M.S.H.R.C. 1407 (July 1994).

CHAPTER 17

The Role of Miners in Ensuring Safe and Healthy Working Conditions: A Perspective of Miners and Their Representatives

Joseph A. Main
Administrator, United Mine Workers of America, Department of Occupational Health & Safety
Fairfax, Virginia

Harry Tuggle
Safety & Health Specialist, United Steelworkers of America
Pittsburgh, Pennsylvania

INTRODUCTION

Although mining continues to be one of the most dangerous occupations in America, there has been a significant decrease in the number of accidents and fatalities. Much of the success in decreasing these incidents can be attributed to the enactment of the Federal Coal Mine Health & Safety Act of 1969 and the Federal Mine Safety & Health Act in 1977 (the "Mine Act"). In passing this landmark measure, Congress recognized the miner as the mining industry's "most precious resource." The Mine Act declared that the first priority of the industry is to provide miners with safer and healthier working conditions. To accomplish this goal, the Mine Act established mandatory health and safety standards. It also imposes a penalty system for those mine operators that do not adhere to the required standards.

The Mine Act recognizes the importance of miners' input into building a health and safety culture in the mining industry by providing them with significant rights to participate in these efforts. By exercising these rights, miners have helped to improve safety and health in the mines: indeed, no one is better suited to assist in efforts to ensure safe and healthy working conditions for miners than the miners themselves. Given their firsthand experience in the mines, miners possess an extensive knowledge of the physical mine and the dangers it presents.

This chapter explains the role miners play in the various aspects of a mine's safety and health program, as well as the contributions they can make to the regulatory process. It focuses exclusively on the federal safety and health law. However, it is important to note that the states, pursuant to Section 503 of the Mine Act, may administer many of the powers provided in the Mine Act to ensure safe and healthy standards in mines. However, in doing so, the state must abide by the Mine Act.

ASSISTANCE IN BUILDING A HEALTH AND SAFETY CULTURE THROUGH MINE-SPECIFIC AND INDUSTRY-WIDE INSPECTIONS

First, the Mine Act seeks to ensure safe and healthy work conditions for miners by requiring regular complete inspections of all mines. Through comprehensive inspections, the Mine Safety and Health Administration (MSHA) investigates whether mine operators are complying with the Mine Act. These inspections help to prevent mine accidents by identifying mine hazards. Under the Mine Act, the miners have the right to participate in such inspections and to voice their concerns about the condition of the mine. If miners have concerns about conditions or practices at the mine, they should bring those concerns to the attention of mine management immediately and not wait until an inspector comes to the mine. This is a protected activity under the Mine Act. With the miners' input, the inspectors are able to better understand the conditions of the mine and the dangers it presents to miners.

The Mine Act requires different inspections for different types of mines. For instance, MSHA is required by law to make at least four regular, complete inspections per year at every underground mine in the United States, and at least two regular, complete inspections per year at every surface mine. The purpose of these inspections is to spot imminent dangers, if any; determine regulatory compliance; gather information about the effectiveness of mandatory health and safety standards; and distribute information about health and safety conditions and causes of accidents. MSHA is also required to conduct spot inspections at mines prone to hazardous conditions, such as high methane levels. Spot inspections are required at least once every 5 days at these particular mines.

The miners' right to participate in these MSHA-required inspections is commonly referred to as "walk-around" rights. Those rights are contained in Section 103 (f) of the Mine Act. Miners independently select miner's representatives[1] (without interference from the mine operator) to engage in the walk-around rights, which extend beyond the actual inspection to include conferences with the government officials before and after the inspection. Those are otherwise known as the pre- and postinspection conferences. Throughout the process, the miner's representative has the right to express miners' concerns about health and safety conditions and specific hazards. In addition, the representative can help the inspector look for violations of the law or regulations and help ensure that violations are corrected.

Those miner's representatives who participate in MSHA inspections and are also employees of the particular mine operator being inspected suffer no loss of pay for the time spent assisting in inspections. Moreover, the MSHA inspector can allow additional representatives to participate in the inspection. Though the operator and employees are permitted to have an equal number of representatives participating in the walk-arounds, the law requires that only one representative of miners who is employed by the operator must be paid for accompanying the inspector. However, where two or more inspectors are at a mine at any single time and are conducting separate inspections, one representative of the miners is allowed to travel with each inspector or separate group of inspectors, suffering no loss of pay.

The miner's representatives right to pay for walk-around duties under the Mine Act covers inspections and investigations involving the enforcement of safety and health standards. Miners also can play a large role in technical consultations, equipment demonstrations, and discussions on research under the Mine Act and participate in these activities.

In giving the miners walk-around rights, Congress recognized their extensive knowledge of their individual worksites and the fact that such familiarity can improve the quality of the government's inspections. By allowing miners to participate in the inspection process, miners can give the inspector useful information about the operation of the mine and potential hazards within the mine. Their contribution to MSHA inspections allows the agency to conduct more complete and thorough inspections, creating a safer and healthier work environment. Additionally, participation in the inspection process educates miners about the Mine Act and its important role in ensuring their well-being. At mines where miners do not select walk-around representatives, the MSHA inspector is required to consult with a reasonable number of miners during inspections to find out about the health and safety conditions of the mine.

---

1. The "miner's representative" is any miner, other person, or organization selected by two or more miners at a particular mine to represent them in health and safety matters. In union mines, the safety representative is usually an elected or appointed union representative or officer. In nonunion mines, the safety representative can be designated by two or more miners. Nonunion miners can even select union representatives to serve as their designated representative.

NO ADVANCE NOTICE

Under the Mine Act, "... no advance notice of an inspection shall be provided to any person...." Prohibiting advance notice of these inspections is intended to give a more accurate picture of mine operator compliance with federal regulations. The miner's representatives are to be notified of the inspection when the MSHA inspector arrives at the property. The *Code of Federal Regulations* Title 30 (30 CFR), Part 40, requires that the list of miners representatives be filed with MSHA and the mine operator, so that they know who to contact to prepare for an inspection or other necessary business.

REQUESTING AN INSPECTION UNDER THE MINE ACT

Section 103(g) of the Mine Act guarantees miners the right to obtain an inspection of conditions at the mine. Miners and their representatives can notify MSHA and obtain an immediate inspection when they believe there is a violation of the Act or safety or health standards, or that an imminent danger is present. Upon receiving a miner's complaint, MSHA is required to conduct an inspection. Should MSHA determine that a violation or danger does not exist, MSHA must explain its decision in writing to the miner or representative. That miner or representative has the right to an informal review of this decision. The miner or the miner's safety representative must send a written request for informal review to the MSHA district manager within 10 days of the refusal to issue a citation or order. The district manager may hold an informal conference when the miner or the representative presents the miner's complaint. The district manager determines whether to order an inspection. The district manager must render a decision, to the miner or miner's safety representative in writing stating the reasons for the decision.

CONFIDENTIALITY

It is important to point out that under the Mine Act all miners and their representatives are entitled to confidentiality when requesting a government inspection or an informal review, and throughout the stages involved with each of these requests. This confidentiality is intended to protect miners from retaliation from their employers.

REQUESTING A NIOSH INSPECTION FOR HEALTH PURPOSES

Miners are also given the right to request special studies if they believe a health hazard exists in the workplace. In order to do this, a miner or miner's safety representative can ask for a Health Hazard Evaluation (HHE) from the National Institute for Occupational Safety and Health (NIOSH) (Mine Act, Section 501(a)(11)). A NIOSH representative will then visit the miner's worksite. The miner's safety representative may accompany the NIOSH inspector during this inspection. NIOSH can issue recommendations on correcting hazards. If NIOSH discovers violations of the standards or an imminent danger, they can inform MSHA so they can take appropriate action.

Following an inspection by a NIOSH official, the inspector must submit findings of the inspection to the miner's safety representative and the mine operator. The mine operator is required to either post a copy of the findings at the mine or provide NIOSH with a list of affected miners so that the agency may directly inform these miners of the findings.

ACCIDENT PREVENTION

The Mine Act established safety and health standards for miners and mine operators. Although miners and mine operators both play vital roles in ensuring safe mining conditions, this responsibility falls in large part on the operators. In fact, the Mine Act stipulates that mine operators "with the assistance of the miners, have the primary responsibility to prevent the existence of such conditions and practices" in mines.

Mine conditions are primarily controlled by mine operators. Accordingly, Congress charged operators with ensuring that the miners are protected from dangerous conditions within the mines. The mere operation of a mine operation explains why the operator is primarily responsible for ensuring safe mining conditions. After all, it is the operator that purchases the equipment used in the operation of the mine, trains the miners (including mine management) who use this equipment and work in the mines, and manages the equipment and mine maintenance program.

Given their control over the operation of the mine, it is vital that operators understand their responsibility in providing a safe and healthy work environment and that they take the proper safeguards against the dangerous conditions that are present in mines. These proper safeguards include, but are not limited to, preparing for known hazards, providing adequate training for both management and miners, providing adequate equipment and properly maintaining the equipment, and building in a certain margin of safety.

For their part, miners are aware that any little mistake on their part may lead to an accident, even a fatal one. With this in mind, miners must take extra precautions to ensure their own safety and that of their fellow workers. Additionally, they must be aware of and exercise their rights under the Mine Act and other safety and health regulations to ensure a safe and healthy work environment.

DAILY EXAMINATIONS TO PROTECT MINERS

In addition to regular MSHA inspections, each operator must conduct daily preshift and on-shift examinations each day to prevent unsafe conditions in the mines. These examinations are instrumental in eliminating hazardous conditions in mines.

The Mine Act requires that a competent individual, appointed by the operator, inspect the workplace for possible hazards during preshift and on-shift inspections. Certain restrictions regarding these daily examinations apply to different mines. For instance, examinations must be conducted at underground coal mines before each shift and at least every 8 hours. In underground metal/nonmetal mines, an examination should be made at least once during the shift. Examinations at surface coal mines are required during a shift, but it is recommended that one be conducted before the miners begin to work (30 CFR Parts 75.303 [coal/underground]; 77.1713 [coal/surface]; and 55/56/57.18-2 [metal/nonmetal]).

Should a hazardous or potentially dangerous condition be found in the mine, the examiner must immediately notify the mine operator. Additionally, an operator of a coal mine must post a danger sign in the hazardous area. If an imminent danger exists, the operator must adhere to imminent danger requirements, including the withdrawal of all affected people from the mine.

Records of preshift and on-shift inspections must be kept and made available to miners (as required for coal and metal/nonmetal mines in the 1977 Mine Act section 103(h)). There are other record-keeping requirements for these inspections as well. In underground coal mines, the record must be kept in a book labeled "Preshift, On-shift, and Daily Report," which must be secured in a fireproof repository. In surface coal mines, the daily report must be countersigned by the surface mine foreman, the assistant superintendent of the mine, the superintendent of the mine, or a person designated by the operator as responsible for health and safety at the mine. In metal/nonmetal mines, each working place shall be examined once each shift. Records of preshift and on-shift examinations must be kept for 1 year (coal/underground: 75.1802, 75.1808; coal/surface: 77.1713; metal/nonmetal: 55/56/57.18-2). Record keeping of these examinations allows miners to be aware of them.

Mines may also pose hidden dangers, such as those associated with dust levels or noise. The mine operator and MSHA must keep records of these hidden problems and those records must be made available to miners. Information about previous accidents and investigations in a mine is also available to miners. Information about hidden problems, along with an account of a mine's accident and investigation history and miner access to this information is vital to ensuring a safe and healthy working environment.

CITATIONS, ORDERS, AND PENALTIES

To ensure compliance with the Mine Act and other health and safety regulations, the Mine Act established a system of penalties intended to deter violations of the Mine Act and to penalize mine operators that fail to comply. Given the fact that mine operators are ultimately responsible for the condition of the mines and the training of the miners, mine operators, not the miners (with the exception of Section 110(g) of the Mine Act, which subjects the miner to a civil penalty if that miner violates safety standards related to smoking or smoking materials), are the subject of these citations.

Citations are usually issued following a MSHA inspection, during the postinspection conference. Following the discovery of any violation of the Mine Act, regulation, or any health or safety standard, a MSHA inspector must issue a citation or an order to the mine operator. This citation or order describes the violation and sets a specified amount of time in which the violation must be corrected. In the case of orders, the area affected is closed down until the condition is corrected. The inspector must also determine the penalty to be assessed against the operator. Citations are issued for each individual violation.

There are different types of closure orders. When MSHA inspectors discover a violation so serious that it poses an "imminent danger" to the miners working in the area of the violation, they are required to close the area of the mine and order the withdrawal of miners from the dangerous area of the mine, or even the whole mine should the violation's threat reach that far. The miners are not required to return to work until the mine operator has corrected the violation and obeyed the law.

Miners idled from work because of a withdrawal order are entitled to compensation under Section 111 of the Mine Act. Miners working while the order is executed and idled by it may receive full regular pay for the time lost, for the balance of their shift. If the order is not terminated before the next shift, all miners on the next shift who are idled by the order must be compensated at their regular rate of pay for the time they are idled, up to 4 hours. However, miners idled by a withdrawal order issued because the mine operator failed to comply with any health or safety regulations must be paid for lost time at their regular rate of pay for the time they are idled, up to 1 week. Furthermore, failure of a mine operator to comply with a withdrawal order and remove miners from dangerous conditions at a mine entitles those miners left operating in that particular mine to receive double compensation from the company.

Like other aspects of the daily operation of a mine, miners are legally provided a voice during the citation/order process. In addition to traveling with the MSHA inspector and observing the violations, a miner's representative can be present at postinspection conferences where citations are normally discussed. In addition, MSHA is required to send the safety representative copies of all citations, orders, and penalties issued to their mine operator. The operator is also required to post copies on the mine bulletin board. Providing notice to the miners plays an important role in keeping the miners informed about their working conditions and actions being taken to prevent or correct an unsafe and unhealthy working environment.

Miners or their representatives may appeal the issuance, modification, or termination of any order issued under Section 104 of the Mine Act. They can apply for reinstatement, modification, or vacation of a 107 "imminent danger" order. They can also challenge the abatement time or modification of a citation. Such appeals must be filed with the Federal Mine Safety and Health Review Commission within 30 days of the MSHA decision/action. Mine operators also have the same right to an appeal. During a commission review, miners are afforded the opportunity to be a party to or to testify in any enforcement action contested by the operator of the mine. Miners also have a right to a copy of MSHA's initial review of a citation or order, to submit additional evidence, and to request and attend a conference to review the citation.

The commission assigns the cases to administrative law judges (ALJs). The ALJs schedule hearings and render decisions. Should a miner be dissatisfied with an ALJ's decision, he or she has the right to request a review of the decision by the commission's five commissioners. The commissioners may or may not decide to hear the miner's request for review.

MINERS AND MINER'S REPRESENTATIVES' INVOLVEMENT: PROMULGATION, REVISION, MODIFICATION, AND REVOCATION OF MANDATORY HEALTH AND SAFETY STANDARDS

Under the Mine Act, miners play an integral role in formulating health and safety standards. At each stage of the process, from promulgation to revision to revocation, miners assist MSHA in developing health and safety standards.

Input from miners into the formulation of health and safety standards begins with proposed standards. Pursuant to the Mine Act, MSHA is to provide notice of all proposed health and safety standards by publishing them in the *Federal Register*. Miners have the right to comment on the proposed regulations and may request a hearing to state their views verbally, as well.

Miners also play a part in modifying the application of any safety standard. As operators may, any representative or miner may ask MSHA to modify the application of any safety standard under two conditions. First, the alternative method proposed must guarantee at least the same measure of protection that the safety standard affords. Alternatively, application of the standard can be waived if its enforcement would itself cause a reduction in safety at the mine.

If it is an operator or other entity that seeks to modify a standard, MSHA shall notify the miner's representative when it receives a petition for a modification. The representative will have an opportunity to present his or her views on the proposed modification in writing. In addition, the representative may request a hearing to present his or her views concerning the proposed modification. The Department of Labor ALJs conduct such hearings. ALJ decisions can be appealed to the assistant secretary for Mine Safety and Health. A copy of MSHA's final decision on the modification is sent to the affected miner's representative.

Finally, any person (including a miner or miner's representative) who may be adversely affected by a safety and health standard has the right to file a petition challenging the new standards for the first 60 days after the standard is published in final form in the *Federal Register*. A petition challenging MSHA's standard must be filed in either the U.S. Circuit Court of Appeals for the District of Columbia or the federal judicial circuit where the miner or representative resides. However, the court will not consider, except for "good cause," any objection to the standards that was not previously mentioned to the Secretary of Labor during the proposal period.

PROTECTION AGAINST DISCRIMINATION

Miners and their representatives are protected under the Mine Act from retaliation for exercising their rights under the Mine Act. Section 105(c) prohibits mine operators from taking action against miners or their representatives and applicants for employment for engaging in activities covered by the Mine Act. From filing health or safety complaints to making comments on mining plans or proposed mandatory rules, miners are protected from retaliation. If a miner, miner's representative, or applicant for employment believes he or she has experienced discrimination, a complaint may be filed with MSHA within 60 days. MSHA must begin an investigation of the complaint within 15 days of filing and issue a written finding within 90 days of the filing. If MSHA decides the complaint was valid, the agency will represent the miner in the proceedings that go before the Federal Mine Safety and Health Commission. If MSHA decides the case is frivolous the complainant can file action before the commission on their own within 30 days of the MSHA notice. In cases of discharge, the miner can seek immediate reinstatement pending outcome of the complaint.

TRAINING OF MINERS

Pursuant to Section 115 of the Mine Act, each operator of a coal or other mine must have a health and safety training program that is approved by the secretary. Under 30 CFR Part 48 for coal, metal, and certain nonmetal mines, and under 30 CFR Part 46 for sand, gravel, stone, and certain other related mines, the secretary has promulgated regulations that require each training program there under to meet approval.

At minimum, all new nonexperienced underground miners must receive no less than 40 hours training and all new nonexperienced surface miners must receive no less than 24 hours training. The training includes an array of mine condition subjects, with the most prominent to "include the statutory rights of miners and their representatives" under the Mine Act. Thereafter, each miner is to receive 8 hours of approved "annual refresher training" and upon being reassigned to any new task, the miner must receive new task training, as promulgated and called for in the respective training program.

Accordingly, all safety and health training is to be provided during normal working hours, with miners paid at their normal rate of compensation during training, and with new miners paid at their starting wage rate. Any miner must also be compensated for any additional cost if attending a training session at a location other than their workplace. Upon completion of any portion of a training program, the mine operator must certify on a form provided by the secretary, for each miner trained, that the miner has received the specified training in each subject area of the approved health and safety training plan. With all the foregoing said on the matter of training and in the spirit of "building a health and safety culture" throughout the system, no miner should sign or accept a copy of any certification form that conveys training that has not been provided, since safety and health training is the very essence and foundation of the system to prevent accidents and injuries in mining.

Pursuant to Section 104(g) of the Mine Act, should an inspector find a miner employed at a coal or other mine who has not received the requisite safety training under Section 115 of the act, an order shall be issued for the mine operator to withdraw the miner until the requisite training is provided. Accordingly, any such miner withdrawn, shall not be discharged or otherwise discriminated against, nor shall they suffer any loss of compensation during the period necessary for the miner to receive the requisite training.

CONCLUSION

Mining continues to be one of the most dangerous occupations. To prevent mine accidents and fatalities, it is vital that every member of the mining industry, from the miner to the CEO of a company involved in mining, be concerned and committed to ensuring safe and healthy working conditions for miners. It is no secret that safer and healthier working conditions inevitably mean a more successful and more competitive mining company. The more cooperation from all parties in the mining industry on safety and health matters, the better off the industry as a whole will be.

The Mine Act has had tremendous success in reducing the amount of accidents and fatalities in our nation's mines in part because it guaranteed miners a significant role in ensuring safe and healthy mine conditions. Given the positive impact of miner input, it is imperative that miners be encouraged to exercise their rights to eliminate unsafe working conditions. Without their knowledge of and insight into the conditions and operations of the nation's mines, efforts to build a health and safety culture within the mining industry would be much more difficult.

Safety and Health Hazard Anticipation, Identification, Evaluation, and Control

CHAPTER 18

Hazard Identification, Risk Management, and Hazard Control

R. Larry Grayson
Associate Director, Office for Mine Safety and Health Research
National Institute for Occupational Safety and Health (NIOSH), Washington, D.C.

INTRODUCTION

As outlined in chapter 1, hazards in mining have been recognizable since extraction of coal and ores began in the United States. Of course, the more serious hazards of methane gas and conditions that support combustion, leading to explosions and fires, caused a national conscience to demand health and safety regulations to protect miners. Also described in chapter 1 was the great progress that has been made over this past century in reducing fatalities, serious injuries, and illnesses affecting miners. In spite of this tremendous success, major impediments to future progress persist. Mining continues to be one of the most hazardous occupations in the nation (Grayson 1999). For the preceding decade, mining's average annual incidence rate (per 100,000 workers) of traumatic occupational fatalities was 31.91 versus 25.61 for the construction industry, which was second (Anon. 1993). As we are well aware, serious hazards will always exist in mining. It is the job of mining professionals to anticipate them, plan to eliminate them or reduce their impact, monitor them to ensure they do not adversely affect miners, and make mining system adjustments to address those that do appear.

This scenario sounds easy, but often hazards, even serious ones, are not so obvious. Today, mining operations are complex and highly sophisticated technically. Miners must interface with these complex systems, including with high-tech equipment in confined spaces. There is also an extremely complex cognitive load placed on miners performing their jobs. It is often difficult to maintain awareness of complicated equipment operation sequences as well as exercise vigilance over changing conditions, interactions among miners and mobile machines, and requirements for maintaining or advancing engineered controls to keep workplaces safe and healthy.

In this chapter, we will cover three major topics—hazard identification, risk management, and hazard control in the context of risk management. It will become apparent that well-designed and timely measures must be implemented to mitigate the impacts of mining hazards. This can be achieved comprehensively only if health and safety aspects are considered throughout the planning, organizing, monitoring, and controlling functions of management, including engineering design. Situations and conditions, and the hazards presented by them, are much different for coal and noncoal operations and for underground and surface operations. Thus the potentially hazardous conditions and situations that develop in each setting must be outlined separately. Here we will focus on differences between underground and surface operations, with differences between coal and noncoal brought out within different mine types.

Today it is generally acknowledged, for major operations, that the most efficient mines are also the safest ones. In most major operations, very systematic and comprehensive planning, monitoring, and control processes are implemented, which result in continuous improvements in miners' health and safety, both on and off the job, as well as in productivity and cost. Today a total loss control perspective pervades mine management philosophies, and the general definition of an accident—anything that occurs that was not planned—is adopted.

GENERAL DEFINITION OF ACCIDENT—LOSS CONTROL PERSPECTIVE

Modern managers seek continuous improvement of every aspect of their operations. Extensive planning targets improvements in outcomes such as production, downtime, productivity, health, safety, compliance with environmental and mining regulations, and cost. Any adverse deviation from planned levels of achievement for any of the outcomes is considered a loss. Any event that leads or contributes to any adverse deviation from plan is considered an accident, in the general sense of the word. Thus, in this sense, an accident is an event that is not expected or intended to occur, and it causes a loss of some type. As a note, many safety professionals prefer to use "incident" rather than "accident" when referring to unexpected personal injuries, which avoids misunderstanding of the definition of accident presented above. The types of losses can be classified as follows (Brauer 1990, p. 17):

- Injury, illness, disease, and death to people
- Damage to property, equipment, and materials as well as replacement cost
- Time, production, and sales
- Extended costs.

Extended costs may include increased insurance or workers compensation cost, reporting of accidents, travel, investigation, cleanup at the accident site, legal and medical services, more extensive rehabilitation of the plant, and damage to public image, among others.

Brauer also describes how the costs may be classified as either direct or indirect or as insured or uninsured.

An interesting concept that applies to accidents and losses is the Pareto Principle, or the 80–20 rule (Juran 1974; Humphreys 1991), where 80% of the loss is accounted for by 20% of the incidents. This is an effective tool that can allow safety professionals and operations managers to prioritize targeted areas for interventions, gaining most effect from the major causes of loss. However, this approach to prioritizing interventions does need to be tempered with the need to intervene specifically in high-risk subgroups. Some consideration also needs to be given to the likelihood that success may be achieved in particular interventions.

This general definition of accident encompasses an idea of chance, since accidental events are not supposed to happen but sometimes do. Generally, there is also a consequence associated with the accidental event; in other words, some loss has occurred. Finally, each accidental event has some duration, hopefully short and with little consequence.

Much research has been done to study causes of accidents. Although people believe in "Acts of God," the mine safety professional believes that there are generally controllable causes for accidents. The most common causes of accidents are unsafe acts and unsafe conditions, and most often both come into play. In a study by the Pennsylvania Department of Labor and Industry in 1960, in which 80,000 accidents were analyzed, these two basic causes contributed to greater than 98% of all accidents (Brauer 1990, p. 18). Today engineered technologic controls have been applied widely in mining, and safety professionals have begun to concentrate on the human element. One study of 75,000 industrial accidents indicated that 88% of them were caused by unsafe acts (Heinrich 1959).

At this point, we need to introduce an important concept. Most accidents, considering the general definition, do not involve death, injury, or significant loss. Research on the occurrence of various types of losses from accidents indicates that generally 90% of them have no injury or loss, 9.5% result in minor injury or loss, and the remaining 0.5% result in major loss or injury (Heinrich 1959; Fletcher 1972). Importantly, studies generally indicate that useful information is nonetheless obtained from examination of no-loss accidents, leading to insight on effective prevention measures. Finally, it is also important for the safety professional to emphasize that although no loss occurs in the overwhelming percentage of accidents, just a split second in timing or a slight change in behavior or conditions could have led to significant injury or damage, including death. Thus, to achieve the highest

TABLE 18.1   Number of U.S. mines and their employees in 1995

Mining Sector	U/G Mines	Surface Mines	U/G Miners	Surface Miners
Coal	1,081	1,275	51,777	33,875
Metal	118	176	7,560	17,509
Nonmetal	57	570	3,904	5,832
Stone	102	3,296	1,940	29,028
Sand and Gravel*	—	6,021	—	32,970

*Includes 824 dredge operations employing 4,669 miners.

level of continuous improvement, safety professionals and operations managers should investigate near misses systematically and formulate preventive measures based on the information they yield.

HAZARD IDENTIFICATION OVERVIEW

In beginning a discussion on hazards, a couple of definitions are in order (Anon. 1981a). Safety can be defined as "the state of being relatively free from harm, danger, injury or damage." A hazard poses "the potential for an activity, condition, circumstance, or changing conditions or circumstances to produce harmful effects." A hazard is often considered simply an unsafe condition, but because of the human element, behaviors in situations (unsafe acts in particular) must be considered along with unsafe conditions. In these contexts, hazard identification will be discussed next, specifically as it relates to mining activities.

Identification of hazards in mining requires considerable experience, and the effective assessment of hazards demands good analytical tools and judgment. Many hazards are quite different for underground mining and surface mining, dependent on the complexity of the operational system, with many subsystems, and the interactions of people within the mining complex. Some hazards are nearly the same for different operations, which will be described later. Before identifying hazards for each setting, however, a perspective on the mix of mines and the number of miners will be given.

A Quick Cross-Section of U.S. Mines and Miners in 1995

Table 18.1 gives the number of operations and number of miners employed in the U.S. mining sectors in 1995 (Reich and McAteer 1997a, b, c, d, and e). The number of mines in the aggregates industry dominated (3,398 in stone; 6,021 in sand and gravel), followed by coal (2,356) and nonmetal (627). Employment was dominated by the coal industry (85,652), followed by aggregates (30,968 in stone; 32,970 in sand and gravel). These figures do not include processing facilities, independent shops, and contractors. To place these figures in historical context, refer back to chapter 1.

Identifying Hazards at Mines

(Note: This section is reprinted with permission from Grayson 1999.)

Surface mines employ fewer miners per comparative tonnage handled than underground mines. Injury incidence rates and reported accident rates are generally lower for surface mines than underground mines as well. Some mining methods in underground mines provide greater protection for workers at the extraction area, e.g., longwall mining, which is primarily used in coal mines.

For underground mining, the longwall mining method, used primarily in coal mines, generally has an overall injury incidence rate comparable to surface mining. However, the underground longwall mine still has a much higher incidence rate because of the hazards miners encounter when performing support operations, including room-and-pillar mining to set up longwall panels.

Underground coal mining, in general, has a much higher overall injury incidence rate than underground hardrock mining, as shown in Table 1. There are physical conditions and work situations that account for the differences between the methods, and these differences will be delineated later. As mentioned earlier, the hazardous conditions and situations that impact miners will be presented separately for underground and surface mining. Topics generally covered in mine health and safety conferences include the following:

rock and gas outbursts, or coal mine bumps
strata and roof control;
haulage and transportation;
mine rescue, emergency preparedness and escape;
gas drainage and control;
dust and toxic substance control and ventilation;
mine monitoring;
fires, explosions, and ignitions;
explosives and blasting;
human factors and ergonomics; and
miscellaneous topics.

The hazards, which define unsafe conditions, and situations, which define human interfaces with the hazards, are presented next. Those presented generally encompass the hazards that occur within the aforementioned common content areas, and these hazards are the ones that need to be identified when planning and implementing operations free from loss.

Underground Mining (paraphrased from Grayson 1999)   Hard-rock mining generally employs the unit operations of drilling, blasting, excavating and loading, and hauling, with a few support activities also being required, as needed. The support activities may involve roof/ground support, ventilation, delivery of supplies and materials, maintenance, drainage of water, and advancement of main development workings and support systems. In coal mining, the unit operations of drilling, blasting, excavating, and loading are combined into a single operation by using continuous mining machines or longwall mining systems (shearer- or plough-based, although ploughs have nearly disappeared). However, each type of mining generates similar potentially hazardous conditions and/or work situations. These are outlined separately in the sections that follow.

Dust, Gases, and Fumes   As mining progresses, dusts and possibly other toxic substances are generated from the orebody and the host rock. Particulate matter, gases, and/or fumes may be generated by mining equipment. Distinguishing features between underground hard-rock and coal mining are the omnipresence of methane gas in coal mines, the methods of extraction (and equipment), which generate differential amounts of dust and other toxic substances, and requirements for ground control.

Dusts generated by mining activity include crystalline silica (mostly alpha quartz, but other forms may exist). Crystalline silica was identified as a probable carcinogen to humans by the International Agency for Research on Cancer (IARC), which has recently voted to change the classification to "carcinogenic to humans" (Carroll 1997). As such, it presents a special hazard to miners' health. Silicosis can be a deadly disease, sometimes causing death in very short periods of time (acute or accelerated silicosis). A classical case of uncontrolled exposures to crystalline silica occurred at the Hawks Nest (or Gauley Bridge) tragedy in West Virginia in the early 1930s, where 764 workers died of acute silicosis during excavation of a tunnel (Burtan 1984). The matter of control of free silica dust will be discussed in greater detail later under hazard control.

The uncontrolled exposure of miners to coal mine dust is another hazard, which causes significant disability and mortality from coal workers' pneumoconiosis and progressive massive fibrosis. In the United States, approximately $1.2 billion is currently paid annually to "blacklung" recipients. Blacklung is a U.S. political term that encompasses all coal-related disabling diseases of the lungs, including chronic pulmonary obstructive disease. Extensive worldwide research has been intensively undertaken since World War II by virtually every major mining country to control dust exposures and disease incidence rates. State-of-the-art coal mine dust control methods will be presented later.

Most other dusts are considered nuisance dusts; that is, long and substantial exposure could lead to some health impact, but generally the impact does not result in disability at significant rates under normal working conditions. There are some exceptions, such as dusts containing significant amounts of lead, beryllium, or other toxic metals. The amount of worker exposure to nuisance dusts is generally well controlled.

Of course, methane in coal mines has long been a major cause of mine disasters. Chapter 1 highlighted the extent of the impact of methane explosions. The methods of controlling methane in the mine atmosphere will be discussed in some detail later, including methane drainage.

Other dangerous gases that may be encountered in mining operations include carbon monoxide (poisonous and explosive), carbon dioxide, hydrogen (explosive), hydrogen sulfide (poisonous), oxides of nitrogen (poisonous), sulfur dioxide (poisonous), and other natural gases (explosive). The control of methane and diesel emissions will be the primary focus in the later section concerning hazard control, but dilution by ventilation is the primary method of control for these gases.

With the proliferation of diesel equipment in mining, emissions are a concern. Some of the previously mentioned gases (e.g., carbon monoxide, oxides of nitrogen, and sulfur dioxide) are generated by diesel equipment, but diesel particulate matter (DPM) is also generated, which is classified as a carcinogen primarily because of the polycyclic aromatic hydrocarbons it contains (Anon. 1988; Lowndes and Moloney 1996). The control of diesel emissions will also be discussed later.

Potential exposures of miners to such hazards must be identified, and preferably anticipated, so that effective control and/or administrative measures may be designed into the mining system, considering interactions among complex subsystems, and the proper personal protective equipment may be provided to the miners. This is one of the major roles of the mine safety and health professional. (Note: end of paraphrased section.)

Roof (Back), Floor, and Ribs   As an orebody is extracted, the natural ground condition surrounding it is disturbed, and physical hazards are created. The pressures induced by mining on the ribs (walls), corners, and cores of pillars depends on the following factors:

- The depth of excavation
- The properties of the rock strata
- The configuration of interacting pillars and openings
- The amount of water and gas trapped in pore spaces
- The tectonics and other geologic processes, which can develop high horizontal stresses
- The types of artificial supports used to stabilize the workings.

Methods for analyzing stress conditions, achieving entry closure, and stabilizing the roof, floor, and ribs around excavations will be outlined later. To anticipate and identify hazards, good mine design techniques must be used, comprehensive procedures should be used to select proper equipment, regular inspections must be made, and vigilant work practices must be maintained.

Noise   (Note: This section is reprinted with permission from Grayson 1999.)

Noise is a pervasive hazard in mining that is generated in operations primarily by equipment. Drills, excavators and loaders, haulers, crushers, ventilation fans, and other equipment can generate noise pressure levels well in excess of 90 decibels (dB, on the A scale), which is the level where hazardous exposure to workers begins by the current U.S. mining definition. In a NIOSH study (Anon. 1981b), findings showed that 30% of miners, age 50, who worked approximately 30 years in the coal mining industry lost 40 dB in their hearing, while 50% of them lost 25 dB.

Currently in the United States a new "action" level of 85 dB is proposed that will require training of affected miners placed on noise protection and annual audiometric hearing tests (Mine Safety and Health Administration [MSHA] 1996; Burns 1997). There are many ways to control noise exposures, which will be presented in the section on hazard control.

Heat

The major sources of heat in underground mines are (1) the conversion of potential energy to thermal energy as air descends shafts, (2) machinery, and (3) geothermal heat (Pickering and Tuck 1997). There are numerous other sources of heat, including explosives, oxidation, falling rock, mine lighting, etc. The efficiency of miners in performing work can diminish substantially as ambient effective temperatures exceed 28 °C. Miners can also cramp, faint, and suffer exhaustion when working at elevated temperatures for prolonged periods. Ultimately when a miner works an extended period without body-temperature reduction, a heat stoke may result (body core temperature rises beyond 41 °C). Methods for controlling the ambient work environment temperature and worker exposure to heat will be addressed later.

Workplace Activities

Workers are often exposed to hazardous combinations of conditions and situations in the workplace, e.g., working around equipment, especially when located near deteriorated physical conditions, working on scaffolding, handling materials awkwardly, performing tasks in confined space, etc. Many routine tasks require repetitive motion, which places repeated stress on susceptible parts of the miner's body and leads to chronic motion-related diseases such as carpal tunnel syndrome. Handling materials of various configurations also places stress on key body components, especially the back. Muscle sprains and strains are a particular problem in getting required supplies and materials to and around the workplace. Methods for mitigating the impacts on miners will be discussed later.

Work Shift Design   Many progressive mining companies have designed work shifts to ensure a quality work life for their employees. It is common to see scheduling for four 10-hour shifts in the United States, followed by 3 days off. Many other variations of shift scheduling attempt to arrange favorable combinations of on-duty and off-duty times for workers and meet the companies' demands for production.

Many companies do not manage favorable shift scheduling for their miners. Instead, production demand and cost govern the scheduling of workers, and the numbers of hours worked by employees per week are often quite high. In hazardous situations, it is common to observe miners working 10 or more hours per day, 6 days per week. Many of the miners, usually voluntarily, work the seventh day as well and may travel an hour or more to the mine. In unfavorable scheduling, high cognitive load situations, fatigue, and inattention can become problems, along with a general resentment of forced work hours.

Emergency Preparedness and Response   As described in chapter 1, mine disasters (involving five or more deaths by past definition) persisted, especially in underground coal mines, until approximately 1975 in the United States. Strict enforcement of federal mining regulations began after the Federal Coal Mine Health and Safety Act of 1969, and after the Mine Safety and Health Amendments Act of 1977 for other mining sectors. Although internal vigilance and enforcement are the key components in preventing the hazards that may lead to a mine disaster, emergency preparedness practiced comprehensively in its broadest perspective is also very effective in preventing disasters and in ensuring a swift and effective response when a disaster does occur.

Surface Mining

Hard-rock and coal surface mining methods and unit operations are similar. Generally drilling, blasting, excavating and loading, and hauling, with a few additional support activities, are required. The support activities generally involve maintenance of slope stability, maintenance of haul roads, delivery of supplies and materials (e.g., drill bits, blasting caps, and powder), equipment maintenance, drainage of water, reclamation, and advancement of operations and support systems. Although many of the potentially hazardous conditions are similar to the ones encountered in underground mining, the specific generation of the hazards and the situations in which the miners encounter them are dissimilar. Thus the potentially hazardous conditions are again outlined separately.

Dust, Gases, and Fumes   Silicosis is the major health concern in surface mining, whether hard-rock or coal. In the United States in 1992, a silicosis alert was initiated by NIOSH (Anon. 1992) for drill operators. In 1996 MSHA joined NIOSH for a general alert on silicosis because of an unusually high incidence of silicosis in Pennsylvania among drill operators at surface coal mines (Anon. 1996). The effort involved an intensive information campaign, training program, and call for voluntary chest x-rays.

Coal workers' pneumoconiosis is also a concern at surface coal mines and preparation plants, but not to the extent as in underground mines for high-risk occupations. Dust control measures for surface mines (primarily for dust generated from drilling, hauling, and crushing) are different from the ones implemented in underground mines, and these will be covered in the section on control of hazards.

Slope Stability   The primary ground control concern in surface mines is slope stability, and the handling of unstable slopes when they occur. Generally it is not a problem because of good mine design and operational practices, but when wet conditions occur in a mine, once-stable slopes can become unstable. The methods for designing and maintaining stable slopes will be covered briefly in the section on control of hazards.

Noise   The sources of exposure of miners to noise at surface mines are similar to those at underground mines—equipment. Of course, the equipment used is quite different. The proposed new regulations will apply to both surface and underground mines. The methods of noise control will be discussed later.

Heat   The source of heat stress at surface mines is primarily ambient air temperature and humidity, especially in arid and semi-tropical climates. In addition, areas with little air movement can develop in pits, which intensifies the effect of the heat. Methods for control of the exposure of miners to heat will be discussed later.

Workplace Activities   Surface miners may also be exposed to hazardous combinations of conditions and situations in the workplace (e.g., working around equipment, and especially near high-walls, and performing maintenance tasks in confined spaces). Repetitive motion tasks and materials handling also place stress on important parts of the miner's body, which can lead to chronic motion-related diseases and sprains and strains. Methods for mitigating the impact on miners will be discussed later.

Comments on work shift scheduling for underground workers apply to surface miners as well. No further comments are needed here. Emergency preparedness and effective response to emergencies, although rare for surface mines, are also considerations for surface mines.

RISK MANAGEMENT

Risk, in a mining context, may be defined as a measure of both the likelihood and the consequences of a hazard associated with a mining activity or condition. Risk analysis may involve a subjective evaluation of relative failure potential and the associated loss, or it may involve a more quantitative analysis. The quantitative approach incorporates the probability of injury, damage, or loss occurring as well as the magnitude of the loss. As a quantitative measure, risk is the product of accident frequency and the severity of potential losses.

Every activity in a person's life has some risk associated with it. For occupational safety and health issues, the level of risk society finds acceptable is a moral issue, not just a technical, economic, political, or legal one. In mining, the various members of the mining community participate in setting standards as rule making is pursued by MSHA, and together they determine the acceptable level of risk and the price level associated with achieving it. Standards are not constant, but change over time, and interpretation of them may vary by location (say, by MSHA district office).

A formal loss-control program is closely related to risk management and assessment. Each tries to reduce the likelihood of accidents (unplanned events) and their severities. Risk management, similar to a loss-control program, encompasses the following functions:

- Risk identification
- Risk analysis
- Risk reduction or elimination
- Risk financing
- Process administration.

The objectives of risk management can be broken down by preloss and postloss ones (Brauer 1990, p. 528). Preloss objectives include the minimization of expenditures for loss, reduction of anxiety about loss, meeting externally imposed obligations, and meeting social responsibility. Postloss objectives include economic survival, continuity of operations, earnings stability, continuity of business growth, and meeting social responsibility.

Different strategies can be followed in identifying and reducing risk and in preventing loss. Management may choose to focus on high-frequency events, high-severity losses, or high-cost events. Alternatively, management may use a combination of strategies across a mining complex and the corporation. Regardless of the focus, the Pareto Principle applies well in targeting the areas for emphasis (i.e., 80% of the incidents, losses, or costs can generally be addressed by focusing on 20% of the causes or events).

Regardless of the perspective applied, analysis of events seeks to recognize factors and causes for losses and helps direct preventive efforts. For example, it is well known that a high percentage of accidents happen to miners who are new on a job (within the first 2 years, and especially within the first 3 months). By focusing on new employees in their work environment, a company may effectively address this problem. Of course, in mining, 30 CFR Part 48 requires new-hire training and task training for this reason, but companies must be proactive in designing effective training materials and techniques to make an impact on this problem. In another example, a study by Ross (1981) reported that serious injuries occurred most frequently in construction work, nonproductive activities, in rare and unusual work situations, in nonroutine work, and in work involving high health risks. These are very familiar high-risk scenarios in mining as well.

Risk Identification

The first step in a risk management program is to identify the risks in the operation. Some of the risks are readily apparent, associated with known or anticipated hazards; others are much more difficult to discern, especially when new technologies and associated human interfaces evolve. Risks change as the following factors that affect an operational change:

- Equipment and methods
- Geology
- Mix and availability of employees
- Regulatory climate
- Economy and competitive forces
- Political environment.

Identification of hazards, covered earlier, is an important part of risk identification. Risks accrue to hazards, which are often framed by complicated situations involving conditions and people working in them. Detecting and anticipating both unsafe conditions and unsafe acts requires substantial understanding of the mining complex, its unit operations, the capabilities of its workers, and the changing nature of the plant and equipment, and it requires much experience. Identifying hazards in the planning stage (being proactive) is of utmost importance to drive continuous improvement. In a more reactive mode, hazards can be identified by studying the frequency of unplanned events (accidents), the severity of losses suffered because of these events, and the costs incurred by the operation.

Once hazardous conditions and situations have been identified across an operation, an improved understanding of risks must be developed. Risk analysis will be covered later, but the understanding of risk must be disseminated across groups of people and the situations under which they manage or work. This perspective fosters an awareness of risk throughout the organization, which is a key to culturalizing the approach of risk management. Involving people at all levels of the operation gives much greater power in identifying the factors that most contribute to risk and produce loss. Further, as most employees become involved and come to better understand risk management, the process is more easily generalized and can be extrapolated to other situations and groups of workers.

Risk Analysis

After hazards and their associated risks are identified, a formal analysis of risk allows management to prioritize the losses or events that should be targeted for greatest improvement. Risk analysis may be quantitative or qualitative, and formal techniques may be applied to analyze potential risks that are identified. Through formal risk analysis, uncertainties in measuring and addressing risk are reduced, and a more systematic and objective approach to risk management results. As hinted earlier, all risks cannot be quantified, but risk analysis can still be accomplished in a semiquantitative or a qualitative way and still be systematic and objective. The different approaches will be demonstrated through the examples that follow.

Quantitative Example   In 1993, underground coal mine operators in Mingo County, West Virginia, reported 250 nonfatal days lost accidents to MSHA. Miners working in those mines worked 3,856,409 hours that year, averaging 2,000 hours each for the year. Thus, the probability (a dimensionless number, always < 1) that an underground coal miner in Mingo County would incur a nonfatal days lost accident in 1993, $P(NFDL_{1993})$, is computed as follows:

$$P(NFDL_{1993}) = (250)(2,000)/3,856,409 \qquad \text{(EQ 18.1)}$$
$$P(NFDL_{1993}) = 0.1297$$

This result is the equivalent of a nonfatal days lost incident rate (NFDL IR) of 12.97, which is calculated for 100 miners working 200,000 hours for 1 year. The basic formula for this calculation is given in 30 CFR Part 50.

If the average cost to the Mingo County mine operator for a nonfatal days lost accident in 1993 was $10,000, the overall risk can be calculated thus:

$$\text{Risk}(NFDL_{1993}) = \text{Frequency of Loss} \times \text{Magnitude of Loss} \qquad \text{(EQ 18.2)}$$
$$\text{Risk}(NFDL_{1993}) = 0.1297 \times \$10,000 = \$1,297$$

There are two ways to interpret this result. First, the risk to each underground coal miner in Mingo County in 1993 was $1,297. Second, if a Mingo County underground mine operator employed 100 miners in 1993, the risk to that mine would have been $129,700. For further insight on the bottom-line cost, if the mine produced 500,000 tons, the risk to the mine operator would have been $0.26/ton.

Qualitative Example   Frequently, it is not possible to calculate the probability of a loss event or estimate its severity, especially proactively. A meaningful risk analysis can be done nonetheless, based on the good judgment of the mine operator and/or the safety professional. Insurance companies may also be able to help.

In a qualitative risk analysis, probability categories must be defined. One such definition (Brauer 1990, p. 530) includes the following categories:

- Frequent
- Probable
- Occasional
- Remote
- Improbable.

Severity categories also need to be defined, and one scenario (Brauer 1990, p. 529) follows:

- Catastrophic (death or system loss)
- Critical (severe injury, illness, or damage)
- Marginal (minor loss)
- Negligible (minimal loss).

Using these probability and severity categories, a risk analysis matrix can be developed for any type of event and used to identify unacceptable risks for the operation. It can also be used to prioritize which risks will be addressed—where action is taken to eliminate or reduce them—and in which order. An example risk-analysis matrix is given in Figure 18.1, with high priority cells identified. The highest priority cells are located in the upper left part of the matrix, while the lowest priority cells are in the lower right corner. The approach could be used to compare the impact of many different events, such as roof fall accidents, rock burst events, and mine fires. It can also be used to combine both quantitative and qualitative risks.

Data Sources for Mine Health and Safety Risk Analysis   A number of sources for data can be used in performing a risk analysis of mine safety and health outcomes. The most notable follow:

- MSHA accident and production-employment databases
- State accident and production-employment databases (some states)
- Workers compensation databases (by state)
- Bureau of Labor Statistics databases (which include oil and gas sector data with mining data)

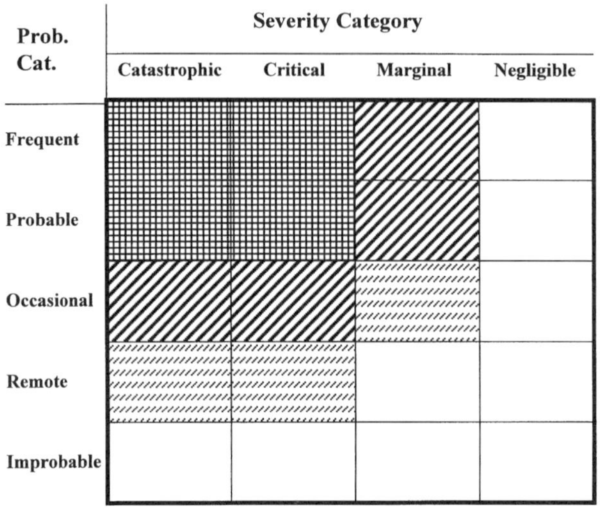

FIGURE 18.1 Qualitative risk-analysis matrix

- Mine or company accident databases
- Mine or company reports on cost and downtime
- MSHA citation/violation databases
- MSHA respirable dust compliance sample database.

Health and Safety Outcome Measures Besides the NFDL IR measure used above in the quantitative risk analysis example, other frequency-based IR measures include:

- Fatal IR
- Serious injury IR (>19 lost or restricted workdays)
- Disabling injury IR
- Total reportable accident IR.

Different severity measures can be developed and applied, too, using the days lost or restricted workdays instead of numbers of accidents in IR calculations. Thus, for example, the Severity Measure, as described in 30 CFR Part 50, gives the incidence of days lost or restricted workdays per 200,000 employee hours for an operation. Another measure mentioned in 30 CFR Part 50 is the Average Severity, which is the number of lost or restricted workdays divided by the number of accidents causing them.

Reducing or Eliminating Risk and Hazard Control

(Note: This section is reprinted with permission from Grayson 1999.)

Once risks have been determined through risk analysis, i.e., either quantitatively or qualitatively, or both, then management must evaluate the estimated risks to determine which occurring or potential losses, and associated events, will be addressed and in which priority. Once priorities are set, then action plans need to be determined to address the targeted risk areas. There are often a number of different ways to address a high-risk area. The three classical ways to address targeted health and safety problems are engineering, enforcement, and education (the three Es). In determining which of various options to employ, a cost-benefit analysis is often done. Each control or intervention strategy has a cost associated with its implementation, but the relative effectiveness of each loss control option must also be considered. For whichever option is ultimately selected, a fourth E, enthusiasm, should be designed to pull management and labor together in addressing the targeted area, and better ensure success.

Commitment by management, which fosters enthusiasm, is important for having much impact, regardless of the type of intervention. Once management manifests its commitment, then continuous improvement of all aspects of mine performance is the goal, reinforced by frequently-changing initiatives aimed at specific objectives concerning successive targeted areas. Specific methods for reducing or eliminating risk, through control of hazards associated with various conditions/situations addressed earlier will be presented next. Elsewhere in this textbook, certain topics will present additional information on some of these topics.

Dusts, Gases, and Fumes   *The primary method of controlling dusts, gases, and fumes in underground mines as well as reducing their adverse impacts in the workplace is dilution through effective ventilation. Mining regulations generally specify permissible exposure limits for specific dusts, gases, and fumes and, often, a minimum quantity of fresh air that is required at various locations in a mine. Usually the ventilation scheme for a mine is carefully planned, often requiring enforcement agency approval, engineered, and implemented. Thorough monitoring of mine ventilation is also required by law, usually on a shift or daily basis, to ensure that the proper quantity and quality of air is moving in the planned directions throughout the mine.*

The second line of defense for maintaining a healthy and safe work environment is enclosures and water sprays for dust-generating equipment, incorporation of surfactants in spray water to enhance capture of dust particles, ventilation control devices, and other dust-allaying methods or work procedures (e.g., sprinkling roadways). Most mining handbooks include various effective methods for controlling and mitigating the effect of dusts. Haney, Ondrey, Stoltz, and Chiz (1988) outline common methods for controlling dust in U.S. underground coal mines, while Mohamed, Mutmansky, and Jankowski (1996) give a general overview of effective methods. These methods are for the most part effective for coal dust or crystalline silica, as well as other entrained dusts. The methods are also generally applicable to surface mines, although they must be adapted to specific situations and equipment in a unique way. For example, adaptation of these general methods to control crystalline silica dust in surface mines was included in the NIOSH Alert of August 1992 (Anon., 1992).

Control of diesel equipment emissions generally requires monitoring of tailpipe gases, the use of effective (preferably regenerative) on-board scrubbers, and specified quantities of air. An excellent review of these techniques is presented by Lowndes and Moloney (1996). Of course, a good maintenance program is required to maintain emissions levels of equipment over time, especially with changing engine duty cycles.

The last line of defense is the use of respirators or other breathing apparatus (e.g., self-contained breathing apparatus, powered-air helmets, etc.). In the U.S., engineering measures must be applied first. When the primary and secondary measures cannot ensure a healthy work environment, then administrative controls may be applied to maintain compliance with dust standards. If, after application of administrative controls, an operation is found in non-compliance with the regulations, the miners must wear personal protective equipment. Even when a working place is in compliance, miners must be provided respiratory protection on request. Many companies require that their workers wear protection regardless of conditions, as good working practice.

Roof, Floor, Ribs, and Slopes   *To ensure the safety of workers in mines, effective design of underground mine entries, pillars, roof, floor and ribs must be incorporated using rock mechanics/ ground control analysis methods. Similarly, stable slopes must be designed for surface mines in consideration of geology, time, and anticipated conditions.*

Mining handbooks and rock mechanics textbooks contain extensive coverage of design principles, techniques, and formulas for a wide variety of conditions. The international literature is replete with technical papers on these topics. Recurring conferences and symposia keep experts on top of the latest developments.

The modern trend in analysis is to examine sites carefully for existing problem phenomena, instrument the site to attain rock properties and magnitudes of deformations, and then perform a detailed engineering analysis using finite element, boundary element, finite difference, or hybrid modeling.

Brady and Brown (1993) provide a comprehensive textbook on general rock mechanics. Peng (1978) provides a textbook dealing more specifically with coal mining.

Often times following analysis, remedial measures of various types are needed to control actively changing conditions. For example in underground coal mines, installation of cribs (of various stiffness and types), trusses, rib or floor bolts, cable bolts, and different types of roof bolts may be used to supplement the initial method of support. In hard-rock mines, supports may be added where none were used initially.

Heat   *Well-designed ventilation and air conditioning are the primary methods for controlling the impact of heat on workers. McPherson (1993) provides an excellent textbook on engineering aspects. Secondly, cool drinking water should be made available for workers in mines where elevated temperatures occur. Light clothing should be worn in such environments, with "ice" jackets being used in onerous climates. As mentioned by Pickering and Tuck (1997), "the workforce which is required to work in hot environments should be trained to recognize the symptoms of heat strain and to adopt sensible work habits...." In practice, workers should also be acclimatized over time, be in good physical condition, and periods of rest and refreshment should be interspersed with work periods.*

Workplace Activities   *Workplace interventions in the area of ergonomics have helped drive continuous improvement in safety performances throughout the mining industry. Companies have been implementing systematic programs to eliminate sprains, strains, and other musculoskeletal injuries (Grayson et al., 1997). Back injuries have been given special attention by the U.S. government (Gallagher, Bobick, and Unger, 1990) as well as companies. Special attention has also been directed at specific problems, such as worker-machine interfaces during roof bolting (Anon., 1994a; Anon., 1994b). Other problem areas such as handling of supplies and materials, operating machinery in confined space, vibration, lack of visibility, using the proper tools for specific tasks, and using proper protective devices for safety in performing work are addressed systematically as well. The NIOSH (Cohen et al., 1997) has published a useful general industry primer for systematically addressing musculoskeletal disorders in the workplace.*

Work Shift Design   *As mentioned earlier, many companies design shift schedules to not be a long-term burden to their workers. One example is evidenced by Mingo Logan Coal Company in West Virginia which studied work scheduling in a number of other industries before deciding on a schedule that would both motivate their workforce and achieve company production demands (Ladd, 1990).*

Emergency Preparedness and Response   *Although the frequency of mining disasters has diminished substantially, as discussed earlier, the conditions and potential for disasters exist nonetheless. Mine fires persist in U.S. mines even though they are generally controlled or extinguished promptly. Thus companies maintain a readiness to respond to emergencies through mine rescue teams, required by regulation, fire brigades, emergency medical technicians, first aid training for all employees, and doctors on-call. Recurring training for first aid (annual) and mine rescue teams (monthly or bimonthly) is required by regulation. Emergency medical technicians must be certified by the state in which a mine is located, and recertification is required for currency (generally every three years).*

In addition, many underground mines have installed a mine-wide monitoring system that can detect incipient fires (generally with CO sensors), including spontaneous combustion in remote or isolated gob (goaf) areas. Further, a reliable fire-fighting system is installed, maintained, and checked periodically for proper functioning and capability.

Financing Risks

In risk management, the method of financing risk is also a consideration since cost is always associated with any intervention. Management may choose to pay directly for the effort to eliminate or reduce risk, in other words, to finance it as a direct cost to operations. Alternatively, a company may elect to use retained earnings or a cash reserve to cover the anticipated loss; the cost could be capitalized.

Finally, certain risks of loss may be covered through insurance, an approach that transfers risk to another business. This covers a fairly low probability event. An example by Brauer (1990 pp. 529, 532) is given next to demonstrate the rationale for insuring losses from automobile accidents.

Assume that the cost of 29.8 million automobile accidents in the United States for a particular year was estimated at $39.3 billion. Also assume that people travel a total of 1.511 billion miles during the year and the average person drives 4,500 miles to and from work. Thus, the average cost per accident is $1,319 ($39,300 million/29.8 million), and the probability of a person having an accident while driving to or from work is 0.089 (29.8 million accidents × 4,500 miles to and from work/1,511 million miles total). Now, given the probability (0.089) of an accident happening to the average person while driving to and from work and the average cost per accident ($1,319), the risk is simply $117.39 per person per year (0.089 × $1,319).

This calculation could form the baseline value upon which the average person would be charged for insurance coverage. As we all know, though, there are many risk factors associated with different drivers, and these risk factors are considered in determining an annual rate for an insurance policy. For example, one automobile insurance company charges a 50-year-old driver of a 5-year-old family car, with no previous accidents and no violations of traffic laws, $250 every six months. On the other hand, it charges a 23-year-old driver of a 3-year-old car, with no previous accidents and one speeding ticket, $650 every 6 months.

In the public arena, other decisions must be made about covering costs associated with automobile accidents, including the cost of fatalities. The basic questions asked include: Is requiring varying levels of insurance enough to control the public cost? Or should roads be repaired more often? Should roads be widened? Should more protective features be required for new cars? Which combination of interventions makes most sense for society, and at what cost?

Administration of Risk

Today, the evaluation of risk and the systematic targeting of high-risk areas for elimination or reduction are ongoing components of managerial responsibility, which is framed by competitive forces that demand continuous improvement in operational performances. Administration of risk embraces all components of an effective risk management program—risk identification, risk analysis, risk reduction or elimination, and risk financing. However, specific steps or functions of each component may vary somewhat from industry to industry. For example, a widely used process of chemical risk assessment, as specified by the National Academy of Sciences (1983), has four steps:

1. Hazard identification
2. Dose-response assessment
3. Exposure assessment
4. Risk characterization.

Many other methodologies exist for risk assessment and management, well beyond the scope of this chapter. See, for example, Fine (1971); Frank and Morgan (1979); and multiple papers in Occupational Injury Risk Assessment (Anon. 1998).

Finally, some general questions may be asked as a part of any public debate on risk assessment:

- What exposures will workers experience?
- What effects will result from the exposures?
- What uncertainties are associated with exposures and effects?
- What assumptions were made in a risk assessment?
- Do animal studies adequately predict impact on humans?

Often there are inadequate scientific data to do definitive risk analysis, and, sometimes, important assumptions are involved. After analysis, either liberal or conservative interpretations can be made of the results, and consensus is reached generally through public processes such as occupational safety and health rule making.

ACKNOWLEDGMENT

The author is grateful to Springer-Verlag for giving permission to reprint major portions of text from *Environmental Science*, chapter 7, Mine health and safety: Industry's march towards continuous improvement—The United States experience, pp. 83–100 (Grayson 1999).

REFERENCES

Anon. 1981a. *Dictionary of Terms Used in the Safety Profession*. Des Plaines, IL: American Society of Safety Engineers.

——. 1981b. *Noise in the Mining Industry—An Overview*. MSHA IR 1129. Washington, DC: U.S. Government Printing Office (GPO).

——. 1988. *Carcinogenic Effects of Exposure to Diesel Exhaust*. NIOSH Current Intelligence Bulletin 50. U.S. Department of Health and Human Services (NIOSH) Publication No. 88-116. Washington, DC: GPO.

——. 1992. *Preventing Silicosis and Deaths in Rock Drillers*. NIOSH Alert. Department of Health and Human Services (NIOSH) Publication No. 92-107. Washington, DC: GPO.

——. 1993. *Fatal Injuries to Workers in the United States, 1980–1989: A Decade of Surveillance*. Department of Health and Human Services (NIOSH) Publication No. 93-108S. Washington, DC: GPO.

——. 1994a. *Report of Findings. MSHA Coal Mine Safety and Health Roof-Bolting-Machine Committee*. Washington, DC: GPO.

——. 1994b. *Human Factors Analysis of the Hazards Associated with Roof Drilling and Bolt Installation Procedures*. Report submitted to West Virginia Board of Coal Mine Health and Safety. Washington, DC: U.S. Bureau of Mines.

——. 1996. *Labor Secretary Calls for an End to Silicosis*. MSHA News Release No. USDL 96-455. URL: www.msha.gov.

——. 1998. Occupational injury risk assessment. *Journal of Human and Ecological Risk Assessment*. 4(6).

Brady, B.H.G., and E.T. Brown. 1993. *Rock Mechanics: For Underground Mining*. London: Chapman and Hall.

Brauer, R.L. 1990. *Safety and Health for Engineers*. New York: Van Nostrand Reinhold.

Burns, K. 1997. MSHA publishes proposed rule on noise exposure. *Stone Review* 13(2): 30–33.

Burtan, R.C. 1984. Silicosis, an ancient malady in a modern setting. *Society of Mining Engineers of AIME Preprint Number 84-81*.

Carroll, D.W. 1997. Crystalline silica update. *Stone Review* 13(2): 14–15.

Cohen, A.L., C.C. Gjessing, L.J. Fine, B.P. Bernard, and J.D. McGlothlin. 1997. *Elements of Ergonomics Programs: A Primer Based on Workplace Evaluations of Musculoskeletal Disorders*. DHHS (NIOSH) Publication No. 97-117. Washington, DC: GPO.

Fine, W.T. 1971. Mathematical evaluation for controlling hazards. *Journal of Safety Research* 40: 157–166.

Fletcher, J.A. 1972. *The Industrial Environment—Total Loss Control*. Willowdale, Ontario, Canada: National Profile Limited.

Frank, K.H., and H.W. Morgan. 1979. A logical process risk analysis. *Professional Safety* June: 23–30.

Gallagher, S., T.G. Bobick, and R.L. Unger. 1990. *Reducing Back Injuries in Low-Coal Mines: Redesign of Materials-Handling Tasks*. Bureau of Mines IC 9235. Washington, DC: GPO.

Grayson, R.L., et al. 1997. Incipient cultural change in safe workplace behaviors. *Transactions of the Society for Mining, Metallurgy, and Exploration, Inc.* 302: 1501–1509.

Grayson, R.L. 1999. Mine health and safety: industry's march towards continuous improvement—the United States experience. Chapter 7 in *Environmental Science*. Edited by J. Azcue. Heidelberg: Springer-Verlag. 83–100.

Haney, R., R. Ondrey, R. Stoltz, and D. Chiz. 1988. Overview of respirable dust control for underground coal mines in the United States. *Proceedings of the VII International Pneumoconiosis Conf.* Vol. I. Washington, DC: U.S. DHHS (NIOSH): 43–45.

Heinrich, H.W. 1959. *Industrial Accident Prevention*. 4th ed. New York: McGraw-Hill.

Humphreys, K.K. 1991. *Jelen's Cost and Optimization Engineering*. 3rd ed. New York: McGraw-Hill.

Juran, J.M., editor. 1974. *Quality Control Handbook*. 3rd ed. New York: McGraw-Hill. 2:16–19.

Ladd, M. 1990. Personal communication.

Lowndes, I.S., and K. Moloney. 1996. A review of diesel exhaust emission monitoring and control technology. *Mining Technology* 78(902): 275–283.

McPherson, M.J. 1993. *Subsurface Ventilation and Environmental Engineering.* London: Chapman and Hall.

Mohamed, M.A.K., J.M. Mutmansky, and R.A. Jankowski. 1996. Overview of proven low cost and high efficiency dust control strategies for mining operations. *Mining Technology* 78(897): 141–148.

MSHA. 1996. Health standards for occupational noise exposure. *Federal Register* 62 (243). Proposed Rules. Washington, DC: GPO. 66, 348–66, 469.

National Academy of Sciences. 1983. *Risk Assessment in the Federal Government. Managing the Process.* Washington, DC: National Academy Press.

Peng, S.S. 1978. *Coal Mine Ground Control.* New York: Wiley.

Pickering, A.J., and M.A. Tuck. 1997. Heat: sources, evaluation, determination of heat stress and heat stress treatment. *Mining Technology* 79(910): 147–156.

Reich, R.B., and J.D. McAteer. 1997a. *Injury Experience in Coal Mining.* 1995. MSHA IR 1242. Washington, DC: GPO.

——. 1997b. *Injury Experience in Metallic Mineral Mining.* 1995. MSHA IR 1243. Washington, DC: GPO.

——. 1997c. *Injury Experience in Nonmetallic Mineral Mining (Except Stone and Coal).* 1995. MSHA IR 1244. Washington, DC: GPO.

——. 1997d. *Injury Experience in Stone Mining.* 1995. MSHA IR 1245. Washington, DC: GPO.

——. 1997e. *Injury Experience in Sand and Gravel Mining.* 1995. MSHA IR 1246. Washington, DC: GPO.

Ross, C.W. 1981. Serious injuries are predictable. *Professional Safety* December: 22–27.

. . . .
CHAPTER 19

Industrial Hygiene in Mining

Kelly F. Bailey, C.I.H.

Corporate SHE Department, Vulcan Materials Company, Birmingham, Alabama

INTRODUCTION

The word "hygiene" is from the Greek word "hygieinios," meaning healthful. When combined with the word "industrial," it becomes apparent what is meant by the words "industrial hygiene"—a healthy workplace. The objective of the industrial hygiene profession is to prevent job-related illness in the workplace.

This objective is reached by successfully accomplishing the four basic principles of industrial hygiene: anticipation, recognition, evaluation, and control of workplace health hazards (American Industrial Hygiene Association [AIHA] 1998). Each of these principles attempts to answer specific questions about the work environment and the potential health hazards that may be present (see Figure 19.1). These principles are intentionally arranged in a particular order because the effectiveness of each step depends on the successful completion of the previous step. If one does not anticipate a potential problem, it may go unrecognized when it exists in the workplace. If a hazard goes unrecognized, it will not be evaluated or controlled until after it has caused harm. In the workplace, where low-level chronic exposures that do not immediately cause adverse symptoms may be present, an unrecognized, unmeasured, and uncontrolled health hazard can permanently affect many people before protective measures are taken. The mining environment is different from most industrial settings, but these principles are just as relevant and necessary as in other workplace environments. This chapter will discuss these principles and other basic concepts of industrial hygiene from the perspective of the mining environment.

As with any profession, industrial hygiene has its own terminology. It is necessary to understand these terms when discussing industrial hygiene concepts. "Exposure" is the dose of a harmful agent that the worker experiences. To have an adverse health effect from a harmful agent, the dose of that agent must be sufficient to overwhelm the body's natural ability to defend and repair itself. Different people have different levels of susceptibility; for this reason, the health effect may not be the same for each individual who experiences the same or similar exposure. Anything can be a poison at some level or degree of exposure. For instance, oxygen, the gas we need to survive, can be lethal at very high concentrations. The degree of exposure is the product of two variables: the concentration of the harmful agent and the duration of exposure to it. Reducing either of these variables will result in decreasing the degree of exposure and the likelihood of becoming injured.

"Toxicity" refers to the potency of an agent or its inherent ability to cause harm. "Hazard" is the product or result of both the agent's toxicity and the degree of exposure to that agent. By reducing the toxicity and/or the exposure, the hazard can be reduced. "Risk" is the probability of a hazard being realized. Risk reduction and, where possible, risk elimination is the ultimate goal of industrial hygiene.

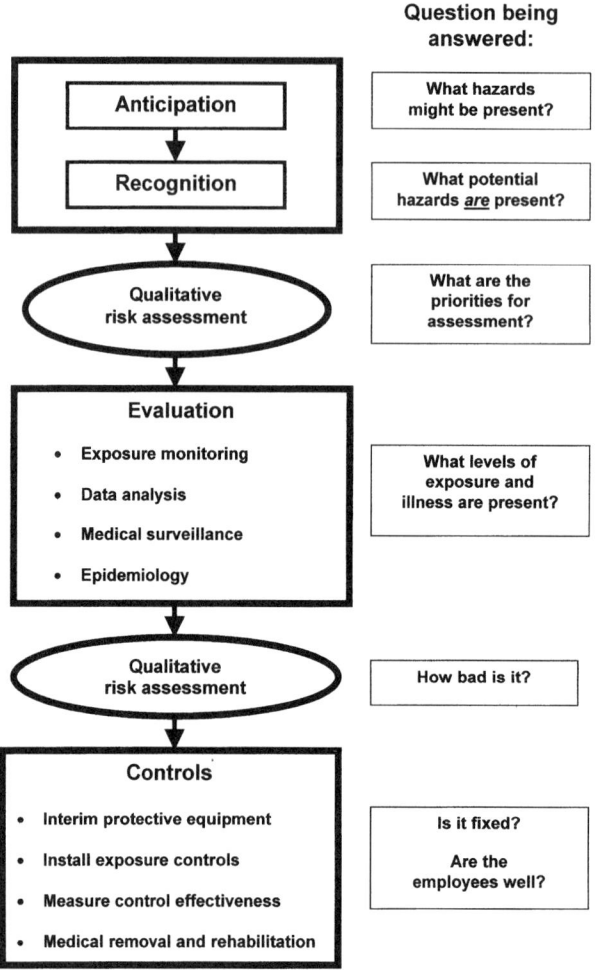

Question being answered:

- Anticipation → What hazards might be present?
- Recognition → What potential hazards *are* present?
- Qualitative risk assessment → What are the priorities for assessment?
- Evaluation
  - Exposure monitoring
  - Data analysis
  - Medical surveillance
  - Epidemiology
  → What levels of exposure and illness are present?
- Qualitative risk assessment → How bad is it?
- Controls
  - Interim protective equipment
  - Install exposure controls
  - Measure control effectiveness
  - Medical removal and rehabilitation
  → Is it fixed? Are the employees well?

FIGURE 19.1 The industrial hygiene process and the questions it seeks to answer about worker exposure and health

FUNDAMENTAL PRINCIPLES OF INDUSTRIAL HYGIENE

Anticipation

The first principle of industrial hygiene is anticipation. The ability to anticipate hazards in a mining environment depends, in large, on one's industrial hygiene experience, understanding of the general production process, and knowledge of important information relevant to the specific mine site. Anticipation is closely related yet different from the second principle, recognition, because anticipation draws on one's knowledge of the potential hazards that ***could be present*** in particular mining environments and, therefore, leads naturally to the ability to recognize those hazards when they are observed. For example, if one did not know that arsenic and lead can coexist with copper in the ore being mined, those potential hazards would not be recognized, evaluated, or controlled. In other words, if one does not know what potential hazards may be present, it is unlikely that important hazards will be recognized and subsequently eliminated. Anticipation essentially draws on one's knowledge and experience to identify the list of possible toxic agents and hazards present. How is this knowledge obtained? By doing your homework, or, to use a more professional phrase, by performing a qualitative risk assessment of the operation.

In all mining, the common denominator is that the process is extracting something from the Earth. Even before the first drill hole is made, several key industrial hygiene questions arise that should be answered:

- What is the geology and mineralogy of the overburden and ore deposit? This material is what most of the miners will have potential exposure to on a daily basis for many years.
- How much crystalline silica is present?
- What do the U.S. Geological Survey or state geological surveys indicate as the primary rock types present?
- If the mine is underground, what is the potential for radon daughter exposure and methane gas generation?
- If the ore is metamorphic or igneous, are the right minerals present for natural asbestos contamination to be present?
- If the mine deposit is in a volcanic zone, are cristobalite and asbestiform zeolites present?

The mineralogy of the deposit will greatly affect potential exposures and which of them need to be controlled. The practice of industrial hygiene in mining requires a basic knowledge of mineralogy so that potential naturally occurring toxic agents and their subsequent hazards will be anticipated.

Most of mining operations have potential exposure to crystalline silica, because silica is one of the most common minerals on earth. Silica can cause the lung disease silicosis. In silicosis prevention, the mineralogy of the ore deposit is a very significant factor in designing an occupational health program. Certain types of rock deposits have naturally higher concentrations of silica than others. For example, quartzite is almost pure silica; sandstone can be 50%–70% or more silica; granite averages around 20%–30%, but can exist as high as 50%–60%; limestone, about 4%, but can be as high as 20% (International Agency for Research on Cancer [IARC] 1997). As the concentration of crystalline silica increases, the risk potential for silicosis increases, because it will take less respirable dust with high silica ore to achieve an unsafe level of exposure. Tighter dust controls will be needed as the crystalline silica concentration in the dust increases.

The geology of the deposit is also important. Most deposits being mined are not geologically uniform or homogeneous. This means that concentrations of potential mineral hazards can differ dramatically in the same mine and even within the active face being mined. In practical terms, a safe exposure today may be unsafe tomorrow and vice versa. An ongoing industrial hygiene program is justified for this reason alone.

In most mining processes, the ore material is steadily reduced in size from solid rock to boulders to smaller rocks, sand, and sediment. Noise and dust are likely to be generated. One important factor in preventing pneumoconioses (lung diseases caused by dusts), is the particle size of the dust present in the air. Pneumoconioses result from inhaling large quantities of particles of respirable size. Respirable particles are those that reach the smallest airways and air sacs (alveoli) in the lungs. Respirable particles are around 0.5 to 2.5 μm in diameter (Morgan and Seaton 1984). Microns are tiny; the period at the end of this sentence is around 500 μm in diameter. When a respirable dust sample is collected, a device (cyclone) is used before the collection filter to separate and to remove particles too large to be taken into the lungs. The size selector on a cyclone is 10 μm of aerodynamic diameter. Obviously, respirable particles are invisible to the unaided human eye.

Understanding the processes that are used to drill and blast, haul the ore, crush and screen the material, leach, wash or treat the material, store and ship the material are all important facets in the anticipation step of industrial hygiene in mining. Each of these production steps will involve processing the ore and thus increases the potential for dust and noise exposure. Some of these processes use chemicals with varying toxicity. It is important to know what chemicals may be used in a particular mining or finishing process so that potential toxic substances can be recognized as one follows the production from ore extraction to final product. A number of maintenance and repair tasks that take place during and after the production shifts also involve chemicals (such as welding, painting, and insulation). Each of these support activities presents a variety of potential hazardous exposures that need to be followed up in the recognition and evaluation steps.

Besides the dust, noise, and chemicals, the mining environment has the potential for a large variety of other hazards as well—exposure to gases, vapors and mists, temperature extremes, ionizing and nonionizing radiation, biological agents, and ergonomic stresses resulting from the miner and machine interface. Knowing that these hazards may be present will enable one to be better able to recognize them in the mining operation.

Finally, as new processes are designed and new regulations are promulgated, one should anticipate the potential impacts and take action to minimize hazards and non-compliance before the new process is installed and operational or the new regulation is enforced.

Recognition

The second principle of industrial hygiene is distinguished from the first in that it involves observing the mining operation and determining if what was anticipated is in fact occurring. The quality of the recognition phase will improve as familiarity with the operation increases. To begin, it is very useful to have a worker roster showing employee names, job titles, and job locations, as well as a simple plot plan that shows the location of major buildings, structures, and equipment, along with a process flow diagram for the specific mine of interest. Recognition activities serve as a continuation of the qualitative risk assessment process initiated during the anticipation step. Recognition activities form a natural bridge to the third principle of industrial hygiene, evaluation, in that it is used to establish priorities for evaluation.

Beginning with mineralogy and geology, one should identify the specific rock types present by examining available literature specific to the mining operation and/or obtaining a site assessment from a geologist. In those rock types where potentially toxic minerals may exist, a mineralogical microscopic assessment on representative samples should be performed.

Next, specific chemicals in the process and how each is generally used should be determined. Material Safety Data Sheets (MSDS) for each chemical used needs to be obtained from the manufacturer of the chemical. Determine which tasks are performed during what jobs, and where and when those tasks are carried out. Employees in the work areas with the highest risk of dust exposure, such as drillers, laborers, baggers, and crusher operators, to name a few, should be especially observed in the initial walk-through survey of the operation. Maintenance and repair jobs that require working in confined spaces should be identified and described, and the frequency of occurrence should be noted.

During recognition, it is also important to get a sense of what exposure controls (i.e., enclosed booths/cabs, air conditioning, and local exhaust ventilation systems) are present. Records of employee complaints about exposures should be given serious attention in subsequent observations and evaluations. Medical surveillance records that indicate occupationally related abnormalities should also be factored into the overall qualitative risk assessment. Mine Safety and Health Administration (MSHA) citations relevant to the industrial hygiene issue of interest and information from previous industrial hygiene studies should be obtained and reviewed. Much of the above information should be gathered before a walk-through of the operation because it will allow one to focus on those parts of the mining operation identified as problem areas.

In the initial walk-through survey, it is important to have a keen eye, a listening ear, and a curious nose. These senses are the qualitative tools that help point the way to areas needing a more quantitative assessment later. The first important observation that can be made at a mining operation during an industrial hygiene survey takes place before one enters the gate. If the vegetation immediately surrounding an operation is covered in dust, it is safe to assume that the dust control for the operation is most likely inadequate or is not commonly used. Visible dust clouds in an operation should immediately draw one's attention to those jobs or tasks performed nearest the dust source. Accumulated dust in work areas or on workers' clothing is further proof of excessively dusty conditions that warrant closer examination. Remember—although evidence of excessive dust is a sure indicator that this hazard is present, its absence is no assurance a dust hazard is *not* present. Respirable dust, the dust that cannot be seen, is the hazardous dust of interest. A dusty operation will have both visible and nonvisible dust. An apparently non-dusty operation will need to be assessed quantitatively in the evaluation step.

During the walk-through survey, the presence of brooms, shovels, and other tools positioned in different work areas such as in a tunnel or on a crusher deck level should be noted. These tools indicate where routine cleanup or other activities take place. Posted areas for required use of protective equipment should be noted on the process flow diagram.

Types of protective equipment (e.g., hearing protection devices, respirator types, protective gloves, and chemical goggles) and where they are used should also be identified at this point. Knowing what protective equipment is available can give insight into what is considered hazardous at the site and may indicate other hazards not anticipated previously. Noting what chemicals and welding materials are present, either by reading labels or by examining purchasing records, will provide very specific information that will be needed in the evaluation phase. During the walk-through, it is advisable to carry a sound level meter to get a quick sense of the noise levels in the operation. These levels can also be recorded directly onto the flow or plot diagrams.

Finally, talking with the employees who do the work is an important part of the initial survey that must not be underestimated or ignored. To do this effectively, one must ask questions of a representative sample of employees in all the different work locations in a mining operation. For example:

- "In your work areas, which jobs, locations, and tasks would you consider to be the dustiest, noisiest, or most irritating to your eyes or throat?"
- "How often is the job or task performed over a year?"
- "Do you ever have to work in a confined space?"
- "Which welding jobs generate the most fumes?"
- "What protective equipment do you wear and what hazards are you being protected against?"
- "What is the heaviest weight that you must lift during your shift?"

Answers to these and other similar questions will assist one's efforts in recognizing the potential hazards present and give some sense of what will be needed to perform an adequate evaluation of the hazards.

In summary, following the anticipation and recognition phases, one should have a fairly solid understanding, at a minimum, of what specific toxic and physically harmful agents are present, how they are used in the process, and what controls and protective equipment are being relied upon to reduce the risks. In addition, a sense of how well the controls are working, and what jobs and tasks have the highest potential for exposure, will have been gained. With this qualitative risk assessment in hand, the priorities for a quantitative risk assessment and the evaluation step can be defined.

Evaluation

The evaluation phase is where judgment, skill, experience, accumulated knowledge, and objective measurements come together to determine whether a health hazard exists or not, and if so, the level of its significance. By the time one has reached this stage of the industrial hygiene process, some preliminary evaluations have already been made (e.g., dusty, not dusty, noisy, not noisy, employees are concerned for their health or not, controls present or not). In the evaluation phase, interest centers on obtaining quantitative assessments of exposures and their impact on the miners. To do this quantitative assessment, the following must be accomplished: certain sampling instruments must be obtained, the samplers must be properly trained in their calibration and use, certified analytical laboratories should be chosen, and a system to manage the incoming exposure information must be established.

A number of industrial hygiene consultants who can perform monitoring functions for the mine operator are available throughout the country. The American Board of Industrial Hygiene maintains a list of practicing consultants (ABIH 1999). In some cases, insurance companies provide industrial hygiene services. For mining operations with more than five mines, it is advisable to establish the industrial hygiene monitoring capability in-house, perhaps with some initial and periodic oversight from a board-certified industrial hygienist.

Extreme care should be taken in the selection of personnel who will conduct the sampling. A detail-oriented person who can perform simple math and write legibly is ideal. Whoever is selected should be thoroughly trained and tested for competence. Because much effort and expense may be spent on the data generated, and because the data will have an impact on worker health and safety, it is critical that the data be accurate and reliable.

Once samplers have been trained, they need to be properly equipped. A set of five constant flow-sampling pumps with battery chargers and the needed respiratory collection devices (cyclones) cost around $5,000 to $6,000. These pumps, equipped with the proper collection filter or device, can be used to collect dusts, welding fumes, mists, mineral fibers, diesel exhausts, and any other particulate of concern. Preweighed sampling filters, which are already loaded in the sampling cassettes specific for the agents of interest, can be obtained from the laboratory performing the analyses.

The choice of laboratory is important. Only AIHA-certified laboratories should be considered (Cohen 1999). Laboratory analytical fees vary greatly. This variation depends in large part on what is to be analyzed, how fast the results are needed, and how many samples need to be analyzed. For respirable silica dust sampling, expect the cost to range from $55 to $85 per filter.

A set of five noise dosimeters will cost approximately $5,000 to $6,000 and a good sound level meter with an octave band analyzer will cost $1,500 to $2,000. The worker typically wears these small pumps and noise dosimeters during the sampling period, and basically, the devices measure the individual's personal exposure. The particulate collection device is attached to the worker's "breathing zone," defined as a spherical area of no more than 18 in. from the nose or mouth. The collection device is connected to the sampling pump with a flexible plastic tube that allows the workplace air to be drawn through the collection media at a known flow rate. For noise sampling, a small microphone attached to the noise dosimeter by a narrow wire is positioned in the "hearing zone" near the worker's ear. Other sampling equipment is available for different exposure concerns (DiNardi 1997), such as Geiger counters, radiation badges, heat stress monitors, detector tube samplers, instantaneous gas detectors for confined space assessment, airflow measuring devices, and others.

The scope of the evaluation step will vary depending on the objective of the investigation. Is sampling being done to address an employee complaint or concern? To measure the effectiveness of installed controls? To determine compliance status with government standards? To collect data for use in medical evaluations or epidemiological studies? A comprehensive industrial hygiene monitoring program, once established, should satisfy all these objectives.

What is a comprehensive industrial hygiene monitoring program? It is a three-stage process that begins by addressing the worst exposures (high risk), evolves into an assessment that ensures that installed controls solve the exposure problems, and ends by implementing an ongoing monitoring program that establishes confidence that exposures are under control over the working lifetime of the miners. How is this done? From the qualitative risk assessment created from the anticipation and recognition steps, a group of mines and jobs or tasks within a mine should be easily identifiable as likely targets for the highest potential risk. This targeted list of mines, jobs, and tasks is where the quantitative assessment of exposures needs to begin.

A targeted sampling strategy is completely biased toward finding the highest exposures, which will represent the highest potential health hazard and the highest risk for an adverse health outcome. Once the highest exposures have been identified, the targeted sampling strategy is continued to ensure that installed controls are effective. When performing targeted sampling, it is important to make sure that the sampling activity takes place either on several days that are representative of the typical workday, or under conditions that may tend to worsen the exposure circumstance.

Before sampling, it is best to predetermine "action levels" (lower exposure levels for the agents being sampled that will trigger appropriate actions or responses). This lower control level, typically set internally by the sampler or the mining company, is below the government exposure limit and represents the level where one begins to take action to more clearly define the exposure source and proceed with reducing exposure levels. For example, a lower control level is typically set where inherent sampling and analytical method errors, if taken into account, may result in an exposure being above the regulated or recommended limit. The lower control level serves as a safety margin to prevent overexposures and noncompliance situations (Leidel and Busch 1994). In setting a lower control level, the current or proposed MSHA exposure limits, the American Conference of Governmental Industrial Hygienists (ACGIH) Threshold Limit Values (TLVs, ACGIH 1998), and the National Institute for Occupational Safety and Health (NIOSH) recommended exposure limits (NIOSH 1997) need to be considered.

If results of sampling show employees' exposures in particular jobs, or doing specific tasks, are less than half the exposure limit, that group of employees may be removed from the high risk list. If exposures fall between 50% of the exposure limit and a preestablished lower control level, collect additional samples to gain a more accurate picture of exposure variability. For employees with exposures that equal or exceed the lower control level, provide personal protective equipment as an interim solution until other exposure reducing controls can be implemented. Of course, gross overexposures must be addressed first, and doing so could mean making an immediate change to the process or task. A system of tracking all exposures and exposure problems from origination to resolution needs to be established to ensure that all identified problems have been addressed.

Once feasible engineering and/or administrative controls have been installed, the job/task will need to be sampled two or three more times to confirm that the exposure is under control. Each group of potentially high risk jobs needs to be systematically sampled in this fashion until exposures of all high risk miners are known and, where necessary, reduced to below the established lower control levels for the agents of concern.

Once overexposure problems have been identified and resolved, the final stage in the three-step industrial hygiene-sampling program is to implement a random sampling strategy where data are collected periodically. Random sampling allows use of sophisticated statistical tools to measure exposure variability and to determine exposure distributions over time. These types of data are very valuable for epidemiological examinations of miners with varying levels of risk. If a job class or mine site in a random sampling program is found to be over the lower control level, targeted sampling will need to be reestablished until controls are shown to be effective once again.

When a sample is taken, a concerted effort must be made to collect and properly record information during the course of the sampling day. Having critical information recorded that clearly describes the exposure circumstance is essential for proper interpretation of the findings and allows for quicker resolution of exposure problems once they occur. If the sample needs to be analyzed in a laboratory, exposure values will likely not be known for 2 weeks or longer. Recall diminishes greatly over this time, particularly if the sample is one in a series of samples or if a series of surveys has been undertaken at different mines. Key information that must be included with each collected sample is listed in Table 19.1. This information not only will give the sampler a head start on identifying what exposure concerns are present to solve an immediate problem, but also will give an epidemiologist, 10 or 20 years later, a clear picture of the exposure circumstances present. In many instances, the toxic agents being monitored present chronic risks to health, meaning the adverse health effect is not seen until many years after the initial exposure. The ability to examine complete and informative exposure records for exposures far back in time is extremely valuable in ascertaining the presence or absence of possible exposure-response relationships.

As essential as industrial hygiene is, it is only half of what is required for an effective, comprehensive occupational health program. Medical surveillance that addresses the potential occupational health risks at the mine is the other half and is also part of the overall evaluation step. Medical surveillance is crucial because it answers the employee's primary question: "Have I been harmed?" In so doing, assuming the answer is "No," the medical component of the occupational health program can bring peace of mind to employees anxious about why industrial hygiene monitoring is being done. The mine operator also benefits because once the program is in place, medical problems, both occupationally related and not, are found at the earliest stages where intervention is most effective and good health outcomes usually result. Another benefit to mine operators and miners is that the medical results for groups of miners can be compiled and used in epidemiological studies to assess long-term health trends. In epidemiological studies, it is important to assess not only the highest potentially exposed, but also those miners with moderate and low exposures. Doing so permits the epidemiologist to determine the presence or absence of possible dose-response relationships in the studied population. This information, along with industrial hygiene data, is very useful in addressing community concerns about a mine's long-term health impact on the surrounding public.

In practically all mining, the potential exists for exposures to noise and dust. Therefore, a medical surveillance program for miners, at a minimum, should include annual hearing or audiometric testing and periodic respiratory screening tests such as a chest x-ray and pulmonary function testing. Comprehensive respiratory, smoking, and hearing histories are also necessary. These medical tests should be performed using standardized procedures established by certifying organizations such as the American Thoracic Society (ATS 1987), the NIOSH program for certifying "B" readers of chest x-rays using International Labour Office (ILO) guidelines (ILO 1980), and the Council for Accreditation of Occupational Hearing Conservation (CAOHC 1993). "B" readers are physicians or radiologists specifically trained to identify dust-related abnormalities, by comparing the miner's x-ray against a set of standardized x-rays.

TABLE 19.1   Key information to be recorded for each sample

- Mine name
- Sample identifier (sample number)
- Sample date
- Substance(s) monitored
- Employee's full name and social security number
- Job employee worked
- Shift time (start and stop)
- Sample time (start and stop)
- Mine location(s) sampled
- Details of employee activities.....................
    - Number of loads hauled
    - Time spent on different tasks
    - Different mine areas worked
    - Unusual events
- Frequency of performing tasks
- Mobile equipment identifiers
    - Make, model, and year
- Presence of exposure controls
    - Working air conditioner
    - Floor mats and noise insulation
    - Integrity of enclosed workstation
    - Doors/windows open or closed
    - Radios (CBs, 2-way, AM/FM)
    - Working muffler
    - Housekeeping in work area
    - SLM levels
    - Ventilation used
- Protective equipment used/how long
- Sampling equipment used
- Laboratory sample identifier
- Average weather conditions
    - Temperature
    - Humidity
    - Wind direction and speed
    - Barometric pressure
    - Weather (sunny, rain, snow, etc.)
- Sampling equipment calibration information
- Diagrams and photographs (especially for welders)
- Analytical method and laboratory used
- Judgment of sample's representativeness
- Sampler's name

For welders:
- Number of rods used
- Type of rods/wire used
- MSDS for rods/wire
- Type of welding performed
- Coating on welding surface
- Polarity and amps used
- Grinding/cutting performed
- Shielding gas used
- Sample filter(s) discoloration

The medical testing program should be expanded to include other tests if additional occupational health hazards are present. For example, in certain types of metal mining, routine blood chemistries and urinalysis may be prudent as well as special tests for blood lead levels and mercury urine levels, among other things. In addition to addressing occupational health hazards, a medical surveillance program can be used to improve the overall health of miners through health fairs and other "wellness" programs. For many mining operations, mobile medical testing vans are the most practical means of conducting a medical surveillance program because they come directly to the mine site (Wolf 1997). Mobile testing services have many advantages: they significantly reduce time off the job, the provide a single contact for all medical testing, they offer a single repository for all records, they ensure a consistent level of testing quality for all mine sites, and they enable the mine operator to accomplish testing needs over a short time period. Finally, mobile medical testing is usually considerably less expensive than sending employees to private clinics or hospitals.

Following the evaluation phase of the industrial hygiene and medical surveillance programs, one should have an excellent picture of where the problems are and a good handle on their significance. After clearly explaining the hazards to the miners, the operator needs to make available appropriate protective equipment to those employees working with exposures at or above the established lower control levels. Personal protective equipment (PPE) must be viewed as a temporary or interim step until a permanent solution to the exposure problem is implemented.

Control

As with evaluation, control efforts must first be targeted on the worst as determined through the three previous phases of the industrial hygiene process. In the profession of industrial hygiene, a hierarchy of controls is recognized. In order of priority, these are: engineering controls, administrative controls (work practices), and as a last resort for routine or daily exposure control, use of PPE. A complete list of all controls for all potential hazards encountered in mining is beyond the scope of this chapter; however, some basic control concepts and examples of different controls follow.

To determine the optimal controls for exposures above the lower control level, a number of important questions must be asked. Recall that the degree of exposure is the product of two variables: concentration and time. A control that reduces either variable reduces exposure. To illustrate how one would go about finding solutions to an exposure problem, an example of a plant clean-up laborer job can be used.

Suppose the plant clean-up laborer is overexposed to dust during his shift. The employee's clothing is obviously dusty, and his answers to various questions posed to him by the industrial hygienist indicate that he believes the dustiest tasks are shoveling up spillage in the conveyor tunnel and around the cone crushers in the secondary plant. These tasks take approximately 7 hours of the 10-hour shift once every week to complete. The first step toward solving this overexposure problem is to find out *why* there is spillage and see if that problem can be eliminated. Many times the solution is simple, such as adding a barrier to direct the product where it was designed to go, decrease the slope or speed of a conveyor belt, or reduce the fall height of product at a transfer point or into a feed hopper of a crusher. These are all examples of different engineering control approaches to solving the problem. The point is that all feasible efforts to eliminate the need for the employee to do the task should be explored first. Is there a smarter way for the process to flow that eliminates the need to manually clean up spillage? This type of engineering solution eliminates the concentration and the duration or time factor of the exposure. The result is no exposure, which means there is no hazard. If the task cannot be eliminated, other options must be explored.

In this example, cleanup is performed while dust- and noise-generating equipment is in operation. If cleanup must continue, can it be done before the plant starts up or after it shuts down? Sometimes this simple change in work practice is all that is necessary. This approach is an example of an administrative exposure control because it involves no engineering. The change in work practice reduces the concentration factor without changing the time factor associated with the exposure. In the tunnel exposure, sometimes the placement of a large fan exhausting to the tunnel vent or escape route will reduce the dust concentration to safe levels. This is an example of an engineering control. When using fans, it is important not to place the worker between the dust source and the exhaust fan. If a fan is improperly positioned, the exposure to the worker can be significantly increased instead of decreased.

Continuing with the plant clean-up laborer example, another solution to the exposure problem may be to apportion the amount of clean-up work over a series of days versus trying to do it all in 1 day. This administrative control will reduce the daily time factor or duration of exposure without affecting the concentration factor. Still, the result is a lower daily exposure and a reduced hazard and risk. Another example of an administrative or work practice control would be to do the job faster with more employees, thereby reducing the time factor of exposure for one person while allowing a lower exposure to more people. In this approach, care should be taken so that increasing the number of employees doing the task does not result in an increase of exposure because of the increased activity in the area. Replacing the shovel with a high-pressure water hose may also resolve the exposure problem.

This may speed up the job (reduce the time factor) and reduce the concentration of dust in the air because the material is less likely to become airborne after it becomes wet. There are many ways to reduce an exposure. Large capital expense is not always necessary. Many times, all that is necessary is close examination of the work environment, an understanding of the tasks involved, and simply doing the job smarter.

In mining, dust suppression is a significant health and environmental issue. The use of water is a very common and effective approach to reducing dust exposure. High-pressure spray nozzles at crushers and key transfer points using recycled and filtered process water is frequently seen. Using water trucks to wet down roadways and for spraying shot rock and stockpiles is also effective in controlling fugitive dust emissions. Many mines pave or apply emulsion coatings to frequently traveled roadways to keep dust emissions down. Stationary spray systems spraying stockpile areas are also used for controlling dust emissions. For drilling rig dust control, water is also commonly used with a backup dry collection system that can be used in low-temperature conditions or when the water system is not operational. Enclosed drill operator cabs are also necessary for both dust and noise control. Where water dust suppression is not an option, duct systems and baghouses are used for dry collection of dust. However, dry control systems are typically more expensive to install and operate and require considerable maintenance. Covered conveyors and screens are also used to reduce dust exposures in processing areas.

Another practice commonly seen in mining is the use of enclosed workstations. These are typically seen in stationary plant process control booths or on mobile equipment in the form of environmentally controlled cabs. This type of control, once the enclosed workstation is air-conditioned and heated, is extremely effective for controlling both dust and noise. Air conditioners should be equipped with high efficiency particulate air (HEPA) filters to filter respirable dust out of the incoming air. HEPA filters need to be routinely checked and replaced as part of a preventive maintenance program. When using an air conditioner in an enclosed booth or cab, the workstation must be cleaned regularly to remove accumulated dust. If dust is allowed to build up, the enclosed workspace becomes a dust chamber and the air conditioner serves to keep the dust suspended in the air the employee breathes. Another engineering control that has been successfully used in enclosed workstations is a simple air purifier or electrostatic precipitator. Of course, keeping the enclosed space sealed to keep out dust and noise is also important. One of the highest dust exposures in enclosed workspaces is the practice of dry sweeping for housekeeping. Using vacuum cleaner systems instead of dry sweeping will eliminate this source of exposure.

With respect to noise control in mining, enclosed production processes and workstations, as mentioned above, are common. When enclosing a production process such as a crusher or a screen tower, noise levels in the surrounding plant areas are reduced; however, levels inside the enclosure can be significantly increased. The design of an enclosed production process needs to consider minimizing the need for employees to enter the enclosure. Use of plastic or rubber screens is an effective method for reducing overall production noise levels.

Barriers and sound-absorbing materials are also commonly used in retrofitting mobile equipment cabs for noise control. When retrofitting cabs, care needs to be taken that noise control materials do not increase other risks such as fire (Bailey and Hartman 1997). A tight-fitting noise barrier floor mat, good window and door seals, and control over radio volume in mobile equipment cabs are necessary for effective noise control. Controlling noise is a difficult job in the mining industry. Many processes are being automated, and remote video cameras are being used more frequently to physically separate the worker from the production process. This trend will increase as noise regulations become tighter and as operations look to reduce labor costs.

Working in a confined space significantly increases the risk of exposure. One of the most common tasks in mining is welding or cutting in confined spaces such as bins, chutes, feed hoppers, and crushers. In these exposure situations, operating a portable exhaust ventilation system is necessary to control fume exposures. Correctly positioning the local exhaust intake so that fumes from the welding rod and any surface coatings are removed from the welder's breathing zone is critically important.

Another type of control approach should always be considered when working with chemical or welding exposures—substituting a less hazardous product for a more hazardous product. MSDS on the various products, as well as employees who have had experience with the alternative products, need to be consulted to ensure that (1) the product is indeed less toxic and (2) the product performs satisfactorily. In this type of control approach, the time and the concentration factor may remain the same, but the toxicity of the exposure is reduced which, in turn, reduces or eliminates the hazard and the risk.

When engineering and administrative controls cannot reduce the exposures to safe levels, PPE will be needed to protect the worker. With particulate exposure, respiratory protection can reduce exposure by physically reducing the amount of particulate inhaled by the employee. When a respirator is used, neither the time factor of exposure nor the concentration factor is reduced, and exposure control is totally reliant on the filtering capacity of the respirator. Proper respirator selection, fitting, and training are needed before relying on this exposure control. When PPE is used as the means to reach a safe exposure, routine exposure monitoring should be conducted to ensure that the protective equipment remains adequate for the exposure conditions. Each job that relies on PPE should be reviewed at least annually to ensure that the equipment is being used properly and to assess whether administrative or engineering controls are feasible.

This chapter was intended to give the reader an understanding of the principles of industrial hygiene and to cover some basic concepts used in the profession. The following chapters on dust, noise, and other important mining health hazard exposures will expand on these fundamental principles as they are applied to specific hazards.

REFERENCES

ABIH. 1999. *Roster of Diplomates of the American Board of Industrial Hygiene and Members of the American Academy of Industrial Hygiene.* Lansing, MI: ABIH.

ACGIH. 1998. *1998 TLVs and BELs, Threshold Limit Values for Chemical Substances and Physical Agents.* Cincinnati, OH: ACGIH.

AIHA. 1998. American Industrial Hygiene Association Mission Statement. *Who's Who in Industrial Hygiene, 1998–1999 Membership Directory of the American Industrial Hygiene Association.* Fairfax, VA: AIHA.

ATS. 1987. Standardization of spirometry–1987 update. Official statement of the American Thoracic Society. *American Review of Respiratory Disease* 136: 1285–1298.

Bailey, K.F., and B.R.G. Hartman. 1997. Noise control–retrofitting mobile equipment to meet MSHA's new noise proposal. *Aggregates Manager* 2: 27–28.

Cohen, H.J. 1999. The American Industrial Hygiene Association IH Accredited Laboratories. *American Industrial Hygiene Association Journal* 60: 692–705.

CAOHC. 1993. *Hearing Conservation Manual.* 3rd ed. Edited by Alice Suter. Milwaukee, WI: Council for Accreditation in Occupational Hearing Conservation Press.

DiNardi, S.R. 1997. *The Occupational Environment–Its Evaluation and Control.* Fairfax, VA: American Industrial Hygiene Association Press. 176–691.

IARC. 1997. *IARC Monographs on the Evaluation of the Carcinogenic Risk to Humans, Volume 68, Silica, Some Silicates, Coal Dust and Para-Aramid Fibrils* 68: 59–80.

ILO. 1980. *Guidelines for the Use of ILO International Classification of Radiographs of Pneumoconioses, Revised Edition.* Geneva, Switzerland.

Leidel, N.A., and K.A. Busch. 1994. Statistical design and data analysis requirements. In *Patty's Industrial Hygiene and Toxicology, Volume III Part A.* Edited by R.L. Harris, L.J. Cralley, and L.V. Cralley. New York: John Wiley and Sons.

Morgan, W.K.C., and A. Seaton. 1984. *Occupational Lung Diseases.* 2nd ed. Philadelphia: W.B. Saunders Company.

NIOSH. 1997. *NIOSH Pocket Guide to Chemical Hazards.*

Wolf, T. 1997. Medics on the move. *Aggregates Manager* 2: 58–59.

CHAPTER 20

Control of Respirable Dust

Fred N. Kissell and Jay F. Colinet

NIOSH Pittsburgh Research Laboratory, Pittsburgh, Pennsylvania

LUNG DISEASES OF MINERS

The two major lung diseases of miners are "blacklung" and silicosis. Blacklung, or pneumoconiosis, was first recognized as a disease of British coal miners in the 1600s. However, investigations into the cause of blacklung disease did not begin until the 1900s. The causative agent of pneumoconiosis in coal miners was thought to be silica until studies in the United Kingdom provided evidence that exposure to coal dust containing minimal silica could also cause pneumoconiosis. In the Federal Coal Mine Health and Safety Act of 1969, coal workers pneumoconiosis (CWP) was defined as "a chronic dust disease of the lung arising out of employment in an underground coal mine."

Diagnosis of CWP is generally based on chest x-ray findings and a patient's history of working in coal mines, usually for 10 or more years. In its early stages, CWP is called "simple CWP." Miners with simple CWP are at increased risk of developing an advanced stage of the disease, called "progressive massive fibrosis" (PMF) or "complicated CWP."

PMF (complicated CWP) is associated with significant decreases in lung function and oxygen-diffusing capacity. PMF is also associated with breathlessness, chronic bronchitis, recurrent chest illness, and episodes of heart failure. Coal miners with silicotic lesions or PMF have an increased risk of tuberculosis and other mycobacterial infections. PMF may progress even in the absence of further dust exposure. This disease is also associated with increased mortality (National Institute of Occupational Safety and Health [NIOSH] 1995).

The most recent study to determine the prevalence of CWP in coal workers was in the mid-1990s. The average prevalence of CWP was 2.8%, but for those with 30 or more years in the industry it was 14%. For the 10-year period from 1987 to 1996, 18,245 deaths were attributed to CWP. The most frequently recorded occupation on the death certificate (70%) was mining machine operator (NIOSH 1999).

Silicosis may develop when inhaled respirable crystalline silica (quartz) is deposited in the lungs. The clinical diagnosis of silicosis is based on (1) recognition by the physician that the level of silica exposure is adequate to cause the disease, (2) the presence of chest radiographic abnormalities consistent with silicosis, and (3) the absence of other illnesses (e.g., tuberculosis or pulmonary fungal infection) that may mimic silicosis. The radiographic patterns are often the same for CWP and silicosis; thus, these diseases are sometimes distinguishable only by work history or pathological examination.

Chronic silicosis commonly involves 15 or more years of exposure to silica. The characteristic microscopic feature is the silicotic nodule. Chronic silicosis is often asymptomatic and may manifest itself as a radiographic abnormality with small, rounded opacities of less than 10 mm in diameter, predominantly in the upper lobes. Lung function may be normal or show mild restriction. Chronic silicosis is also associated with a predisposition to tuberculosis and other mycobacterial infections and with progression to complicated silicosis.

Complicated silicosis, also called PMF, occurs when the nodules coalesce and form large conglomerate lesions. Complicated silicosis is characterized radiographically by the presence of nodular opacities greater than 10 mm in diameter on the chest x-ray. Complicated silicosis typically causes respiratory impairment. Recurrent bacterial infection may occur, and tuberculosis is a concern (NIOSH 1995).

For the 10-year period between 1987 and 1996, 1,054 deaths occurred in the United States from silicosis. About 40% of these were in mining and construction. The most frequently recorded occupation on the death certificate (14.7%) was mining machine operator (NIOSH 1999).

PERMISSIBLE EXPOSURE LIMITS

In coal mines, dust samples are collected by both coal mine operators and the Mine Safety and Health Administration (MSHA) using a size-selective sampling device (cyclone) that separates out dust in a way that reflects the efficiency of deposition in the gas-exchange region of the lungs. This so-called "respirable size fraction" has a lung deposition efficiency of 100% at 1 μm or below, 50% at 5 μm, and zero efficiency for particles of 7 μm and upward (NIOSH 1995).

The permissible exposure limit (PEL) is 2 mg/m^3 for respirable coal mine dust, which is measured gravimetrically as an 8-hour time-weighted average (TWA) concentration. This limit is reduced when the respirable silica (quartz) content exceeds 5%. A formula of 10 divided by the percentage of respirable silica is used to determine the reduced PEL for respirable coal mine dust. For example, a sample with 10 pct silica would have a dust PEL of 1 mg/m3 (*Code of Federal Regulations*, 30 CFR 70.101 and 71.101). For the 10-year period from 1987 to 1996, 7.4% of coal mine inspector samples exceeded the PEL.

A respirable dust PEL has not been established for noncoal mines, but a nuisance dust standard of 10 mg/m^3 is regulated. The nuisance dust sample is comprised of "total dust," which represents airborne particles that are not selectively collected with regard to their size. However, respirable dust sampling is conducted in non-coal mines if potential exposure to silica dust is suspected. If the silica content of the respirable dust sample exceeds 1%, the formula used to establish the dust PEL is 10 divided by (the percentage of silica + 2). Thus, a sample with 8 pct silica would have a dust PEL of 1 mg/m^3.

For the 10-year period between 1987 and 1996, 15.6% of the dust samples in the metal mining industry taken by MSHA inspectors exceeded the PEL because of silica. For coal mining, it was 23.4%, and for stone products, it was 22.5% (NIOSH 1999).

DUST CONTROL TECHNOLOGY AND PRACTICES

In underground coal mining operations, ventilating air and water sprays are the primary controls used to limit respirable dust generation and worker exposure. The quantity of ventilating air supplied has a direct impact on the dilution of the dust cloud as it is generated, while the velocity of the ventilating air determines the rate at which dust can be moved away from the mine workers. Water is applied to coal as it is being mined or crushed to wet the coal particles and minimize the quantity of dust that becomes airborne. After dust is entrained in the ventilating air, water sprays are also used to direct dust-laden air away from workers and/or remove dust particles from the airstream. In addition to these basic controls, mine operators use more advanced control technologies (such as dust collectors, scrubbers, and enclosed cabs) and improved operating practices/administrative controls to further reduce the dust exposure of mine workers.

Dust Control Practices in Room and Pillar Coal Mining

Face Ventilation   To ventilate the working face, line brattice (plastic curtain) is installed along the coal rib, or tubing (fiberglass ductwork) is hung from the mine roof and used to supply fresh air. Federal regulations require a minimum of 1.4 m^3/s (3,000 cfm) of air to be directed to each working face to provide protection from dust and methane gas. In today's high-production mining operations, significantly larger quantities of air are often supplied to the working face. Exhaust and blowing ventilation systems are the two types of face ventilation techniques commonly used in room and pillar operations.

With exhaust ventilation, fresh air is forced up the mine entry to the face to dilute and entrain dust. Dust-laden air is then pulled from the face area and carried behind the curtain or into the tubing and out of the face area. The quantity of air and the distance from the end of the line brattice or tubing to the face are critical, particularly with exhaust ventilation. Studies have shown that dust levels are lower when the brattice or tubing is located close to the face. For this reason, the end of the exhaust brattice or tubing should be maintained within 3 m (10 ft) of the face. Also, when using exhaust ventilation, mean entry air velocities above 0.3 m/s (60 fpm) have been shown to minimize dust. Both of these criteria—3-m setback and 0.3 m/s velocity—are required by MSHA coal mine regulations (30 CFR 75.326 and 75.330).

Historically, continuous miner operators were positioned on the back corner of the mining machine. In this situation, dust exposure could be reasonably controlled with exhaust ventilation. However, if the dust cloud rolls back toward the operator, remote control can be used to lower the operator dust exposure. Operator positioning when using remote control can have a significant impact on dust exposure. For exhaust ventilation, an operator using remote control should be positioned on the off-curtain side of the entry and stand as far outby as practical (Colinet and Jankowski 1997).

Recently, room and pillar coal mining has adopted blowing ventilation in conjunction with dust scrubbers and remote control. This technological development does a better job of clearing out methane gas, and so it has allowed for the extraction of extended cuts up to 12 m (40 feet) in depth. When using blowing ventilation, fresh air is directed behind line brattice or in tubing and then discharged from the end of the curtain/tubing toward the face. This fresh air dilutes and entrains dust at the mining face and the dust-laden air then passes out of the immediate face area and into the dust scrubber. For operations with blowing ventilation, the operator should be positioned at the discharge of the line curtain or tubing in the fresh air stream to minimize dust exposure.

As a general rule, especially in older mines, reducing stopping leakage is the most cost-effective technique to get more air to the face. Varying degrees of airtightness can be realized with different stoppings and the quality of construction used to erect the stoppings. Step-by-step instructions for building three types of stoppings are available in a U.S. Bureau of Mines (USBM) handbook (Timko 1983).

Water Spray Systems for Continuous Miners   Continuous miners are equipped with water supply systems designed to suppress dust, cool motors and bits, and serve as emergency fire-suppression systems. Spray nozzles mounted on the machine body deliver water to strategic areas for dust control. The purpose of these sprays is to wet the coal as it is cut. Once the liberated dust has been entrained in the ventilating air, the dust capture or "knockdown" afforded by the sprays is moderate. Ideally, all spray systems are turned on before cutting and left on for a short period after cutting. Tests have shown that the best spray systems can reduce respirable dust by 60%; typical reductions average 30% (Courtney and Cheng 1977).

Continuous miners utilize three general types of spray systems: conventional, anti-rollback, and spray fan. The conventional spray system is recommended for all blowing ventilation sections and for exhaust ventilation sections with high airflow. The quantity of water needed depends upon the operating conditions of the individual section. Flow rates usually range from 1.3 to 1.9 L/s (20 to 30 gpm). Nozzles are typically located on top of the boom (directed at the top of the drum), beneath the boom (directed at the bottom of the drum and at the gathering arms), and in the conveyor throat. Sprays can also be located on both sides of the boom. Either full- or hollow-cone nozzles are typically used on the top to provide adequate coverage across the total width of the drum. These types of nozzles should also be used below the boom and should be uniformly spaced to maximize coverage of the area between the sprays and the bottom of the drum. Sprays are suggested for the conveyor throat to prevent dust dispersion from the conveyor to the operator.

When exhaust ventilation is used and air velocities are low, turbulence created by the sprays can roll the dust cloud back toward the operator. This is called rollback. High spray pressure (over 692 kPa or 100 psi) and the use of wide-angle top and side sprays that overspray the drum or are set too far from the drum promote this condition. Whether rollback exists can usually be determined by temporarily shutting off the sprays. If the rollback is reduced when the sprays are shut off, one or more of the following measures is taken: (1) face airflow is increased; (2) extension and tightening of brattice or tubing; (3) a reduction in spray pressure; (4) removal of any nozzles pointed outby; or (5) installation of an anti-rollback spray system if the mine is not gassy.

The anti-rollback water spray system (USBM 1985a) is particularly suited for exhaust ventilation faces without a methane problem, with low face airflow, and where dust standards are more stringent because of silica. With this system, a moderate spray pressure of 692 kPa (100 psi), measured at the nozzle, is a practical maximum. Although higher pressure sprays have the potential to knock down more dust, they can also increase the dust blown back to the operator. However, water-flow rates should be as high as possible, within a 1.6- to 2.2-L/s (25- to 35-gpm) range.

As shown in Figure 20.1, the top and side nozzles of the anti-rollback system are arranged for "low" reach (about 300 mm or 12 in.) from the cutting head. This location prevents overspray that would increase rollback. Flat spray patterns, as opposed to cone spray patterns, are better because the entire flow from the nozzle can be directed to the cutting head. On the boom top, horizontal flat spray patterns near the cutting head cause the least air disturbance; on the sides, vertical flat spray patterns are best.

The dust collection efficiency of the anti-rollback system can be greatly improved by using under-boom sprays. These are located on the rear corners of the shovel at the sides of the machine and they are aimed towards the front of the gathering arms (Figure 20.2). Pressures can be as high as 1380 kPa (200 psi) with flow rates of 0.25 to 0.31 L/s (4 to 5 gpm) (USBM 1989).

Another water spray system, designed for use with exhaust ventilation, is the spray fan system (Ruggieri et al. 1984; Ruggieri et al. 1985). The spray fan system is designed to reduce face methane concentrations by using the air-moving properties of ordinary water sprays. A series of water sprays working in concert directs the main ventilation flow to the face and sweeps contaminated air and gas across the face toward the return. The spray fan system should only be used with good face ventilation (mean entry air velocities above 0.3 m/s (60 fpm). It is also effective with curtain setback beyond 3 m (10 ft). Proper operation of the spray fan system requires a minimum pressure of 1034 kPa (150 psi) measured at the spray nozzles. This usually requires that the pressure loss in the supply hose be minimized by the selection of a supply hose with an inside diameter of at least 38 mm (1.5 in.).

The spray fan system was designed for use with exhaust ventilation only. A different system, designed for use with blowing ventilation, was designed by Volkwein and Wellman (1989). It also uses directional sprays to induce air movement around the cutter head. The authors report an improvement in ventilation by a factor of 2 to 3.

A major problem associated with water spray systems is the frequent clogging of spray nozzles caused by particulate matter in the water line. Nozzle blockage can be minimized by using fewer nozzles, but with larger orifice diameters of at least 1.6 mm (1/16 in.). The USBM developed a simple, nonclogging, water filtration system to replace conventional spray filters (USBM 1981a). The system consists of an in-line Y-strainer to remove the plus 3.2-mm (1/8-in.) material, a hydrocyclone to remove virtually all of the remaining particulates, and a polishing filter to remove traces of particulates that are carried over the hydrocyclone overflow during the startup and shutdown of the spray system.

Flooded-Bed Scrubbers   Flooded-bed scrubbers are fan-powered dust collectors installed on continuous miners to collect dust-laden air through an inlet(s) near the front of the miner and discharge cleaned air at the back of the miner. The dust-laden air passes through a filter panel that is being wetted with water sprays, which allows the dust particles to be captured by the water. After passing through the filter panel, the airstream then enters a demister, which removes the dust-laden water droplets from the airstream. The cleaned air is then discharged at the back of the scrubber unit and typically can be directed toward either side of the entry with a louvered discharge on the miner. Approximately 90% of miners now being fabricated are equipped with flooded-bed scrubbers (Armour 1999).

The overall effectiveness of a flooded-bed scrubber is determined by the proportion of face air that is drawn into the scrubber (capture efficiency) and the proportion of respirable dust removed from the captured air (collection efficiency). Scrubbers are primarily used on continuous miner sections employing extended cuts with blowing face ventilation. The scrubber assists in pulling the ventilating air into the face as the miner moves deeper into the cut and away from the line brattice/tubing. In these operations, the face airflow is typically matched to the capacity of the flooded-bed scrubber in an effort to allow 100% capture of the air ventilating the face. Today, scrubbers are also being used

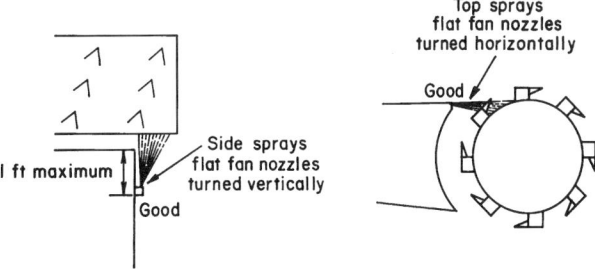

FIGURE 20.1   Top and side nozzles arranged for low reach. Overspray causes rollback

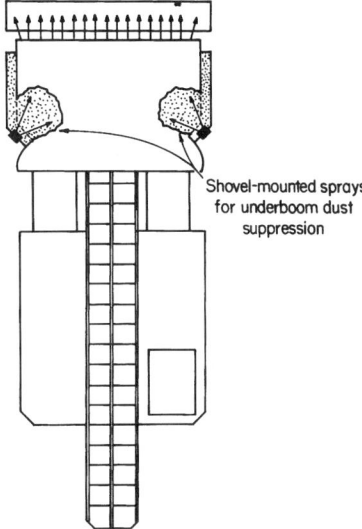

FIGURE 20.2   Underboom sprays

in conjunction with exhaust face ventilation in an effort to further reduce the dust exposure of face workers.

Research has shown that flooded-bed scrubbers can remove more than 90% of respirable-sized coal and silica dust (Colinet et al. 1990). However, the collection efficiency is affected by the density of the filter panel. The original filter panel was fabricated with 40 layers of fine stainless steel mesh. Filter panels containing 30, 20, and 10 layers of stainless steel mesh are now available. The reduced filter density allows larger quantities of air to be moved by the scrubber, potentially improving capture efficiency, but can reduce the collection efficiency. In one study, the 30-layer panel was shown to maintain respirable dust collection efficiency above 90% but the collection efficiency dropped when less dense panels were used (Colinet and Jankowski 2000). When using flooded-bed scrubbers, the balance between the capture efficiency and collection efficiency must be optimized to minimize dust levels.

Bit Replacement   The condition of the cutting bits, design of the cutting drum, and sump rate have a major impact on the quantity of dust of respirable size that will be generated. Routine inspection of the cutting drum and replacement of dull, broken, or missing bits improves cutting efficiency and helps to minimize dust. Also, research results indicate that bits that are designed with large carbide inserts and smooth transitions between the carbide and steel shank typically produce less dust over the life of the bit (Organiscak et al. 1995).

Modified Cutting Cycle   Studies have shown that cutting rock can contribute five times the respirable dust compared with cutting coal. When roof rock has to be cut, an alternative to the usual cutting pattern is to sump into the face 0.3 to 0.6 m (1 to 2 ft) below the roof and to shear down to the floor. This should be continued for at least two sump-shear sequences (more if roof conditions and seam and/or miner height requirements allow). Then the machine is pulled back to cut the remaining top coal and roof rock. This procedure reduces respirable dust levels by allowing the roof rock to be cut to a free face, which generates less respirable dust (USBM 1985).

Roof Bolting   Systems to control dust from roof bolting machines use either a dry collector or water injection to achieve lower dust levels. In either case, a problem with the system can be easily detected and remedied with a few simple maintenance procedures.

If a dry collector is used, dust in the blower exhaust is the most common problem encountered, a sign that dust is bypassing the filters. Common causes of this are damaged or improperly seated filters. Cloth-bag-type filters are less efficient dust collectors than the pleated-paper cartridge-type and allow dust to bleed through the system and escape through the exhaust. Accumulations of dust between the filters and the blower (clean side) are a result of filter leaks. Finally, a visible dust plume from the collar of the drill hole is a sign of inadequate airflow to the chuck or bit and is often a result of air leaks within the system. These occur primarily through loose connections (especially at the chuck hose), air-pressure relief valves, poorly fitting dust-collector access doors, and worn and damaged hoses. Replacement of overloaded and clogged filters will generally increase airflow at the bit by more than 30% (Divers et al. 1987).

Studies have shown that a roof bolter's dust exposure can be substantially reduced by changing from a shank-type bit to a "dust hog" bit (air inlet port located on the bit instead of on the drill steel) (USBM 1985b). Generally, this difference can be attributed to the initial few centimeters of bit penetration when the shank-type bit allows far more dust to become airborne. Underground evaluations of the two bit types showed that the dust hog bit reduced bolter dust exposure by more than 80%, and it also drilled faster and cooler.

In wet systems, hollow drill steels are used to deliver low-pressure water (0.13 L/s or 2 gpm per chuck) to the bits. These systems offer improved bit life, faster drilling, and excellent dust control. However, wet drilling can create problems in sections that cannot tolerate additional water accumulation on the mine floor. Also, use of wet drilling may aggravate the working conditions for the roof bolter operators. As a result, good maintenance of all seals is important to minimize leakage.

Double-Split Ventilation   The roof-bolter operator's dust exposure frequently derives from upwind dust sources, particularly the continuous miner. The use of a double-split ventilation system to provide the bolter operator with a clean split of air is the most effective way to combat this problem. In single-split sections, the mining-bolting cycle must be carefully designed to keep the roof bolter upwind of the continuous miner whenever possible.

Conveyor Belts   The first step in minimizing the amount of dust generated during coal conveyance is to ensure that the coal is wetted adequately at the face. Rewetting the coal at intervals along the belt may also be necessary. This is best accomplished by uniformly wetting the coal stream with flat-fan sprays operating at 280 to 350 kPa (40 to 50 psi). The accumulation of coal and dust particles on the top and bottom sides of the returning belt can be controlled by mounting belt scrapers or wipers near the drive, or by spraying the belt with a low-quantity water nozzle. Maintaining the conveyor system (alignment, rollers, and splices) in good working condition will also reduce dust.

Transfer Points   Transfer points can be the greatest source of dust in outby areas; transfer points include shuttle-car-to-belt, belt-to-belt, and belt-to-mine-car. A major cause of dust at transfer points can be the dislodgment of dust adhering to the underside of the belt. Nozzles projecting a flat, fan-type spray directly at the underside of the belt have been shown to reduce dust levels in this area by as much as 60% (Kost et al. 1981); water quantities of 0.019 to 0.032 L/s (0.3 to 0.5 gpm) are typical for this application. It is also important that the coal be wet prior to its reaching the transfer point. Hoods and chutes may also be used to prevent the ventilating air from agitating dust and to reduce the amount of coal fragmentation and breakage associated with excessive free-fall distances.

Haul Road Dust Control   Good housekeeping practices—such as scooping up excess coal when a cut is finished, shoveling coal along the ribs to the middle of the entry where the machine can readily reach it, and minimizing shuttle car spillage—form a basic and effective approach to the problem of haul road dust control. Another method is to wet the roadway with water. However, this is usually a temporary measure because the water can rapidly evaporate. To keep the moisture content of the roadway dust at a desired 10% level, the use of a hygroscopic salt, such as calcium chloride, is frequently required. It should be spread in two applications: three-quarters applied 1 hour after wetting the dust with water, and the remaining one-quarter applied about 1 week later. Depending upon mining conditions, retreatment of the roadway should not be necessary for about 6 months, but spraying the roadway with water after 3 months is recommended.

Dust Control in Longwall Coal Mining

The number of operating longwall faces in the United States has decreased from more than 90 ten years ago to 59 in the year 2000, yet production from longwall mines now accounts for more than 50% of the coal produced in underground U.S. mines. Advancements in equipment design, equipment reliability, operating practices, and longwall layout have allowed U.S. longwall mining operations to steadily increase production. In 1980, average shift production as reported to MSHA was equal to 890 metric tons, and production has increased to an average of 4,600 metric tons per shift in 1999 (Niewiadomski 2000). High production longwalls are capable of producing more than 15,000 tons per shift on a recurring basis.

Two factors that have contributed to increased production are the increase in longwall face lengths and the widespread adoption of bidirectional cutting sequences. These combine to increase the cutting time during a shift. Currently, about 90% of operating sections use a bidirectional cutting sequence where the shearer extracts full-face cuts in both directions. Typically, the lead drum takes a full cut in the raised position, while the trailing drum cuts the remainder of the coal along the floor. For unidirectional cutting, a full-face cut is only taken in one direction across the face (cutting pass). For the clean-up pass, both shearer drums are lowered to "clean" the coal remaining along the floor, with minimal additional cutting. However, the increase in face length that has occurred in the last 15 years has made the use of unidirectional cutting less popular because of the low production that results during the clean-up pass. The substantial improvement in longwall production provides the potential to increase the quantity of respirable dust generated and thus the dust exposure of mine workers.

However, despite the substantial increase in production, compliance with the 2 mg/m^3 dust standard for longwall mines has actually improved. In the early 1980s, 31% of MSHA dust samples collected for the designated occupations (DO) from longwalls were out of compliance; in 1999, 18% of the DO samples were out of compliance (Niewiadomski 2000). This improvement can be attributed to dust control research that has identified a number of successful control technologies and to longwall operators that have adopted multi-faceted approaches to dust control. Successful dust control in the U.S. longwall industry has been achieved by the following practices: minimizing the quantity of dust liberated into the airstream, preventing airborne dust from reaching the breathing zone of mine workers, removing airborne dust from the ventilating air, and providing workers with the knowledge to protect themselves from excessive dust exposure.

Shearer-Clearer   A poorly designed external water spray system on the shearer body can actually raise operator dust levels. Poorly designed systems have nozzles directed upwind at the cutting and loading zone of the intake-side drum. Airflow generated by these sprays pushes dust away from the face and upstream of the drum. Here, dust mixes with the clean intake air and is carried out into the walkway over the shearer operators.

To prevent this, the USBM has developed a novel shearer spray system, called the shearer–clearer. It takes advantage of the air-moving capabilities of water sprays. The system consists of several shearer-mounted water sprays, oriented downwind, and one or more passive barriers, that split the airflow around the shearer into clean and contaminated air (Figure 20.3).

The air split in the shearer–clearer system is initiated by a splitter arm, with conveyor belting hanging from the splitter arm down to the panline. This belting extends from the top gob side corner of the shearer body to 460 mm (18 in.) beyond the cutting edge of the upwind drum. A spray manifold mounted on the splitter arm confines the dust cloud generated by the cutting drum, further enhancing the air split. The dust-laden air is drawn over the shearer body and held against the face by two spray manifolds positioned between the drums, on the face side of the machine. The air is then redirected around the downwind drum by a set of sprays located on the downwind splitter arm. Operating pressure must be about 1034 kPa (150 psi), measured at the nozzle, to ensure effective air movement. Total water flow rate with all sprays operating is about 0.76 L/s (12 gpm). In underground tests, the shearer–clearer reduced operator exposure from shearer-generated dust by at least

Conventional water spray system pushes dust upstream

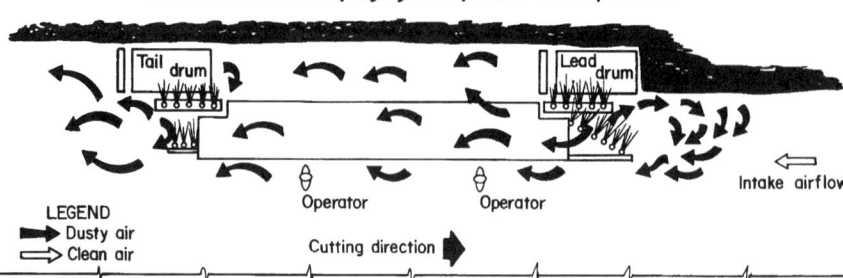

Water sprays can force dusty air toward face

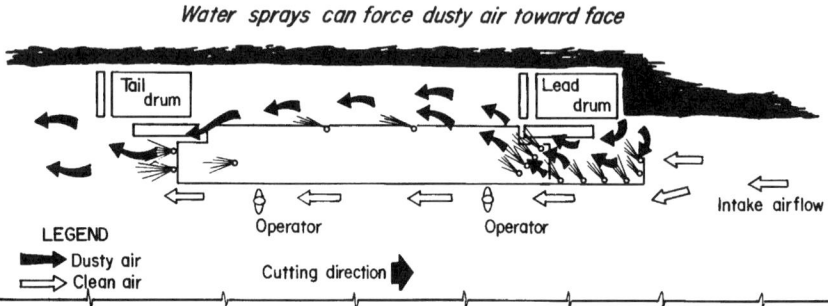

FIGURE 20.3   Air currents with conventional sprays (top) and shearer-cleaner system (bottom)

50% when cutting against the ventilation, and 30% when cutting with the ventilation (Shirey et al. 1985; Ruggieri and Babbitt 1983).

Spraying Water on Shearer Drums   Dust generated by the shearer is reduced by increasing the quantity of water supplied to the shearer drums, so it is important to supply as much water as possible. In two separate studies, water flow to the shearer was increased about 50% and dust levels at the shearer were reduced about 40% (Shirey et al. 1985).

Dust exposure of the shearer operators may be affected by the operating pressure of the water supplied to drum sprays. In two separate studies (Piemental et al. 1984; Kok and Adam 1986), water pressure of the drum sprays was increased from 517 to 793 kPa and 552 to 1,034 kPa (75 to 115 psi and 80 to 150 psi), respectively. In both instances, dust exposure of the shearer operators increased by 25%. Thus, the maximum drum spray pressure to optimize dust control appears to be in the range of 483 to 690 kPa (70 to 100 psi). Also, the water flow rate should be increased by increasing the nozzle orifice size rather than the operating spray pressure.

The type of spray nozzle chosen is important for optimum performance (Kost et al. 1985). The pick-point flushing system with solid-stream (jet) nozzles is the most effective at suppressing respirable dust near the shearer operator's position. The pick-point system with cone-type sprays has been shown to be only 70% as effective. In the Kost study, downwind concentrations were essentially the same for all systems.

Remote Control   Use of remote control on shearers can significantly reduce dust exposure of the machine operators. With remote control, operators control the machine from positions along the face less contaminated than their normal work positions. A survey shows that exposure was reduced 68% by moving the operator just 6 m (20 ft) upwind of the shearer body (USBM 1984).

Controls at the Headgate State Loader and Crusher   Dust generated at the headgate can have a significant impact on the full-shift dust exposure of all face personnel. The major source of dust in the headgate entry is the stage loader/crusher. A basic approach to dust mitigation is to mount water sprays in the stage loader/crusher. Several sprays are mounted in spray bars, which usually span the width of the conveyor to ensure uniform spray coverage of the coal stream.

Recommended spray bar locations include the mouth of the crusher, the discharge of the crusher, and at the stage loader-to-belt transfer point (USBM 1985c). The dust capture efficiency of these sprays may be enhanced by enclosing the stage loader, either with steel plates or strips of conveyor belting. The enclosure also isolates the conveyed material from the airstream, thus reducing dust entrainment. The goal of the water sprays and the enclosing of the stage loader is to wet the coal and confine generated dust. Consequently, water quantity is more critical than water pressure. High-pressure water sprays may actually force dust out of the stage loader/crusher and into the intake air. Water pressure should be maintained below 60 psi. During underground trials with a fully covered stage loader and additional water-spray manifolds, improvements at the headgate operator and at support 20 locations were 80% and 45%, respectively (Jayaraman et al. 1992).

Ventilation   Ventilation is one of the principal methods used to control dust on longwalls. Face air velocities of 2.0 to 2.3 m/s (400 to 450 fpm) are minimum levels appropriate for effective longwall dust control. Adequate longwall panel ventilation involves more than supplying the required volume of air to the headgate entry. Maintaining that airflow along the entire face is just as critical. Air leakage is greatest in the headgate area because there is often a large gap between the first shield and the adjacent rib. Also, the gob behind the first few shields remains open because the headgate entry is supported with roof bolts. This air loss prevents maximum use of the air available to ventilate the face. In addition, dust generated during gob falls may be entrained by this airflow and carried back into the face area. A gob curtain, installed from the roof to the floor between the first support and adjacent rib in the headgate entry, forces the ventilation airflow to make a 90° turn and stay on the face side of the supports (Figure 20.4). During underground trials, the average face air velocity with the curtain installed was 35% greater than that without the curtain (USBM 1981b). The most significant improvement was seen for the first 25 to 30 supports.

Despite the above success, misapplication of the primary ventilation airflow can increase dust exposure. Shearer operators are often exposed to very high concentrations as the headgate drum cuts into the headgate entry. The high-velocity primary airstream passing over and through the drum entrains and carries large quantities of dust out into the walkway and over both operators. An effective solution is to install a wing curtain between the panel-side rib and the stage loader (Figure 20.5). This curtain shields the headgate drum from the airstream as it cuts out into the headgate entry. It is typically located 1.2 to 1.8 m (4 to 6 ft) back from the corner of the face to provide maximum shielding without interfering with the drum. The curtain is only in place during the cutout operation and is generally advanced every other pass. The curtain can reduce operator dust exposure by 50 to 60% during the headgate cutout (USBM 1982a). Shearer operators can further reduce their dust exposure by moving as far upwind at the headgate as possible as the shearer cuts out at the headgate.

Site-Specific Longwall Controls

There are several control techniques that are site-specific, and therefore, cannot be successfully applied at every longwall installation.

Deep Cutting   Reducing drum speed is one of only a few changes a longwall operator can make to increase output, reduce respirable dust, and decrease machine power consumption (Ludlow and Jankowski 1984). Deep cutting is a function of drum speed and machine advance rate. Pick spacing must be increased and gauge length must be adjusted to take full advantage of deep cutting. The rotational speed of the drum is reduced (typically to 30 to 40 rpm). The depth of cut is increased by using large bits with wider spacing of the bit lines while maintaining the same advance rate used at higher rpm.

Field tests have confirmed the benefits of slow-speed deep cutting (Ludlow and Wilson 1982). A 60% reduction in dust generation was achieved by reducing the drum speed from 70 to 35 rpm. This effectively increased bit penetration from 43 to 86 mm (1.7 to 3.4 in.).

Drum Water Proportioning   Increasing the water flow to the drums usually reduces airborne dust levels produced by the shearer. Some operations, though, cannot tolerate an increase in water flow because of clay floors. Excess water in the coal reduces the run-of-mine Btu value. It can also cause problems in the coal transport system and in the coal preparation plant. For operations with these conditions, supplying larger quantities of water only to the upwind cutting drum can have a significant impact on the amount of water used while still reducing the operator dust exposure (USBM 1982b).

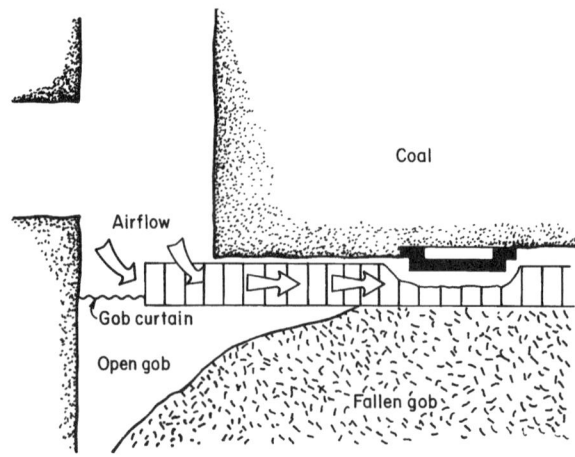

FIGURE 20.4   Gob curtain forces air to stay on longwall face

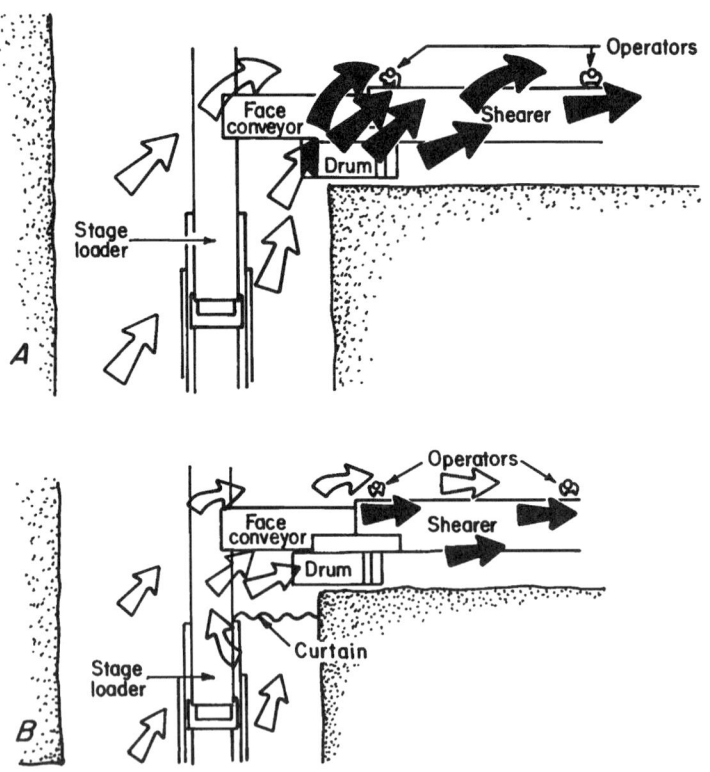

FIGURE 20.5   Airflow at longwall headgate without (a) and with (b) a wing curtain

Support Movement Practices   During bidirectional cutting, shield advance will occur in both cutting directions. In these cases, supports are moved on the intake-air side of the shearer as it cuts head-to-tail (downwind). Shearer operators are then exposed to any dust generated by support movement. Under these circumstances, some mine operators find that support-generated dust can be effectively diluted before it reaches the shearer operators by increasing the distance between support advance and the shearer from 6 to 15 m (20 to 50 ft).

Water application on the immediate roof may also help to suppress some of the support dust generated during lowering, advancing, and resetting the roof supports. The immediate roof can be wetted by: (1) spraying the roof with one or more water sprays mounted on top of the shearer body, directing water downwind, at an upward 45-degree angle; (2) supplying enough water at the shearer drum sprays to wet the roof while the face is being cut.

In addition, shield supports can now be equipped with water sprays in the shield canopy that are used to wet the roof material on top of the shields. Typically, these sprays are automatically activated during the shield advance cycle. The shield spray systems have the potential to reduce dust liberation during shield advance, but require diligent maintenance and upkeep to ensure proper operation.

Finally, roof support automation can contribute to reduced dust exposure. Automation allows jacksetters to minimize their time downwind of dust sources.

Personal Protection Devices

The Federal Coal Mine Health and Safety Act of 1969 mandated that approved respiratory equipment be made available to personnel when exposed to respirable dust concentrations greater than 2.0 mg/m^3. However, this equipment cannot be used in lieu of achieving the 2.0 mg/m^3 standard.

Air Helmet   The air helmet is a redesigned hard hat equipped with a battery-powered fan, filtering system, and face visor, thus providing protection for the head, lungs, and eyes within one unit. Although the air helmet is slightly larger and heavier than conventional hard hats, weighing approximately 1.4 kg (3 lb), wearer acceptance has been favorable in high coal seams.

A small fan is mounted in the rear of the helmet to draw dust-laden air through a filtering system; the resulting cleaned air is directed behind a full-face visor and over the wearer's face. Seals are provided along both sides of the visor so that exhaled air and excess clean air are allowed to exit the helmet at the bottom of the visor. Also, these face seals and additional seals inside the helmet limit contamination from unfiltered air. The fan is externally powered by a rechargeable battery smaller than a conventional cap-lamp battery to be worn on the miner's belt.

The air velocity outside of the helmet and the direction of air impact on the helmet can have a major impact on the effectiveness of the helmet (Cecala et al. 1981). For example, at a longwall face with an air velocity less than 2.0 m/s (400 fpm), the air helmets reduced respirable dust by an average of 84%. However, at another longwall with an air velocity of 6.0 m/s (1200 fpm), the air helmet was not as effective, with an average reduction of 49%. The sampling included periods when the face visor was lowered and periods when it was raised, according to normal underground use; this would tend to minimize differences between inside and outside samples, thus reducing the apparent effectiveness of the helmet.

Replacement Filter Respirators   The replacement filter respirator consists of a filter-holding unit, typically fabricated from plastic, metal, or hard rubber, which also contains intake and exhaust valves. Soft rubber or cloth is used to form a face piece around the filter-holding unit, forming a seal against the wearer's face in an attempt to prevent dust-laden air from bypassing the filter. With a reasonably leak-tight face piece fit, the respirator should remove up to 95% of the respirable dust. During one respirator evaluation program (Cole 1984), two models of face-mask respirators were tested on four longwall sections. The dust exposure of workers was reduced by 80% to 92%.

Although the replacement filter respirator does an excellent job of dust removal when properly fitted, some personal discomforts may arise, including increased breathing resistance, aggravated by dust loading on the filter, facial irritation caused by the face seal, inference with normal voice communication, and interference with eye glasses or goggles.

Single-Use Respirators   The single-use respirator employs a much lighter and simpler design than the replacement filter respirator. The entire mask is fabricated from filter material and covers the mouth and nose, similar to a surgical mask. Single-use respirators offer some advantages when compared to the replaceable-filter respirators. They are more comfortable and require no maintenance. However, single-use respirators usually do not form as tight a seal against the wearer's face as replaceable-filter types, thus allowing more leakage. As a result, they are much less effective than replacement-filter types.

Underground Metal Mine Dust Control

The exposure of workers to respirable dust in hard-rock mines, including both metal and nonmetal mines, may be reduced by a systematic approach that includes all or some of the practices discussed in this section.

Proper Use of Water in Drilling and Blasting   Adequate water suppresses drilling dust. Enough must be provided to keep the rock surface wet all the time, so that the rock is actually broken under a film of water. This does not, however, prevent dust from entering the air during the initial collaring period. Various means have been tried to prevent the escape of dust during collaring, ranging from simple hand-held sprays to elaborate types of suction traps around the end of the drill steel, but no single method has been found to be very efficient.

If some of the compressed air operating the drill leaks into the front head of the drill and escapes down the drill steel, it will cause dry drilling and carry dust out of the hole. Also, compressed air escaping through the front head release ports will atomize some of the water in the front head. This atomized water, which forms a fog at the front head release ports of many rock drills, evaporates rapidly; if the water gets dirty, as it often is, many dust particles will remain in the air.

Water is also important in controlling dust generated by blasting. The first step in controlling blasting dust is to ensure that the area surrounding the blast (walls, floor, and back) is thoroughly wetted beforehand. This precaution will prevent dust settled out during previous operations from becoming airborne. Furthermore, some of the dust created by the blast will adhere to the wet surfaces in the area, thereby reducing the concentration in the airstream. To improve the effectiveness of water when wetting down the area, a spray nozzle ensures an adequate spread of water over a greater area and prevents the settled dust from being stirred up. An alternative is to use a two-phase fog spray nozzle that employs both water and compressed air. These nozzles are effective at reducing dust and the amount of nitrous fumes (because of their solubility in water).

A moisture content of the rock of only 1% produces a very significant reduction in dust production when compared with dry rock. As it is difficult to maintain a uniform moisture content of 1% under conditions encountered underground, the optimum moisture content should be maintained at about 5%. The water used for dust suppression, particularly in drilling and in blasting, should be as clean as possible, in that the evaporation of dirty water can release considerable quantities of dust.

Preventing Dispersal of Dust   The dispersal of respirable dust from crushers, conveyors, and similar equipment can be eliminated in most instances by confining the dust-producing operation within an enclosure and controlling the air contained therein. The air from within the enclosure can be exhausted directly to the upcast airway or, if this is not feasible, it can be filtered. The section of this chapter entitled "Minerals Processing Dust Control Devices and Systems" gives guidelines for dust collection systems.

Ore and waste passes produce large quantities of airborne dust. The broken rock delivered to the passes contains a considerable amount of inherent dust as a result of the preceding operations, which include blasting and loading. Furthermore, the autogenous grinding action of the rock as it is dumped and falls down the pass produces more dust. The first line of defense is to ensure that the rock is thoroughly wetted before delivery to the dump. More wetting can be obtained at the dump site by installing a mist-type atomizer to spray the rock as it falls into the pass. However, excessive use of water at the orepass can be objectionable for many reasons: (1) adverse impact on crushing and milling, (2) a large quantity of water may accumulate on top of the material in the chute, creating a hazard for workers on the lower levels, and (3) plugging of clay minerals.

The second step in lessening dust at ore and waste passes is to prevent its escape and dispersal into working areas by confining it within the passes. This can be accomplished by a system of stoppings and airtight doors over the dumps or "tipping" points. The maintenance of these doors is of prime importance.

A third step in lessening dust, difficult to accomplish in practice, is providing means to keep the confined ore or waste pass under negative pressure to ensure that all leakage paths are in draft, and to capture the air displaced when rock enters the raise. A suitable fan is used to exhaust air from a convenient point in the raise. The contaminated air is filtered or sent via a direct untraveled route to the return air raise.

Dilution Ventilation   Ventilation is the best method for controlling contaminants at underground operations. Ventilation is undertaken in producing areas, such as stopes or scraper drifts, by directing an air split from the main ventilating stream through the workings. The design criterion is 0.15 to 0.25 m/s (30 to 50 fpm), depending upon the type of operation and other local conditions. Volume may have to be increased greatly in some instances—for example, high-speed drives or scraper drifts, where the severe dust-producing operations may require as much as 0.75 m/s (150 fpm).

In headings and raises, the design volume also is based on providing an air velocity of 0.15 to 0.25 m/s (30 to 50 fpm). In most cases, an overlap system will provide a satisfactory environment in most headings. An overlap system consists of a main ventilating duct that exhausts dusty air and a small fan and blowing line kept to within 6 to 9 m (20 to 30 ft) of the face. The length of the overlap of the exhaust and blowing lines depends upon the size of the drift and, in any case, should be at least 9 m (30 ft). The blowing volume should not exceed approximately 60% of the exhaust volume to avoid recirculation. The exclusive use of exhaust systems for auxiliary ventilation should be discouraged, since it is impractical to keep the end of the duct near the dust-producing operation, particularly when blasting.

Proper ventilation is critical since water alone is inadequate. Blasting dust and fumes should be diluted and exhausted to surface via an untraveled route, preferably an upcast raise designed for that purpose. If this is not feasible, the blasting schedule should be arranged so that the contaminated air will pass through working places when the miners are absent.

Avoiding Dust   Dust avoidance is often the best way to prevent exposure to respirable dust. It is applied mainly after blasting by requiring a minimum reentry period, by arranging a fixed blasting time for each working place so that other workers are not exposed to the blasting dust and fumes, and by ensuring that blasting takes place only at the end of the shift when most other workers have already been withdrawn.

Other ways in which workers are kept out of dusty air are by arranging that they travel downcast shafts and by locating all underground waiting places in fresh air. Also, work may be scheduled in such a way as to reduce dusty operations upstream of a designated location.

Dust Control in Water Soluble Ores

This section reviews strategies to suppress and collect dust on cutter machines and face drills, where water usage must be restricted to very low flow rates because the ore is water-soluble. Typical flow rates are 0.063 L/s (1 gpm).

Cutting Machine Dust Control   Achieving effective dust control on cutter machines can be difficult because there are five major dust sources. These are (1) the cutter chain during cutting, (2) the star wheel, (3) the cutter chain reentering the kerf, (4) the bug duster, and (5) a recirculation loop that develops within the kerf. The cutter chain during cutting and the recirculation loop are probably the most severe dust sources.

Wet-bar type cutting techniques are used to help control mine dust by keeping the cutting chain wet. As the chain cuts the kerf, it dampens the dust produced by the cutting action at the point of generation.

Three basic wet-bar techniques are used (Figure 20.6). Water-trickle system A uses a gravity-feed or low-pressure (less than 345 kPa or 50 psi) pump to send water through the bar and to discharge it at the bar tip. Water-spray system B uses a low-pressure spray nozzle located at the front of the cutter head. For protection, the nozzle can be located within the cutter head. Water-trickle system C used a gravity-feed or low-pressure pump to discharge water onto the cutter chain on either or both sides of the cutter head.

Tests on all three wet-bar designs conducted in two salt mines revealed no significant difference in their dust control performance. While there are many variations of the three designs, it is not expected that any one type will be more effective at controlling dust. Also, the performance of the three systems is independent of water flow rate when operated between 0.016 and 0.063 L/s (0.25 and 1.0 gpm). At these water flow rates, the average total dust reduction of the three systems is 60% to 70%.

Dust control efficiency deteriorates significantly when water flow is less than 0.016 L/s (0.25 gpm). Higher water flow rates (more than 0.032 to 0.063 L/s or 0.5 to 1.0 gpm) are not likely to improve the performance of the wet-bar system. Also, excess water causes the dust to cake and solidify on the bit

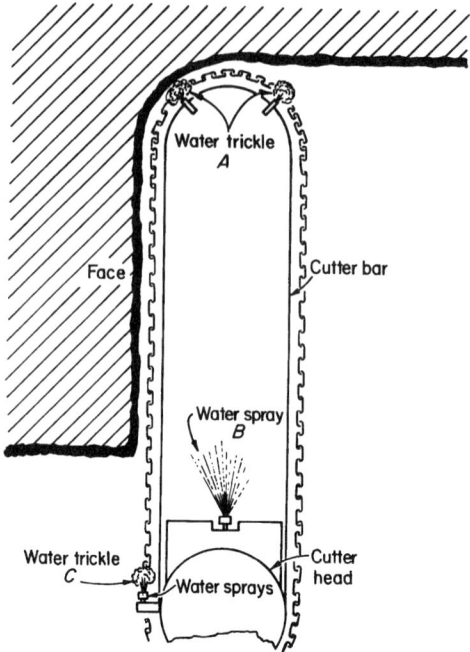

FIGURE 20.6   Wet-bar water spray systems

blocks, increasing bit-changing times. However, cutting the last few feet (meters) of the kerf dry helps to clean the bit blocks without producing a significant amount of dust.

Several dry collection systems on cutter machines have been tried but have been generally unsuccessful. The reasons are (1) they involve a large number of nonlocalized dust sources, (2) the tremendous amounts of dust produced are more than a machine-mounted collector can handle, and (3) the size of a suitable collector is not practical for machine mounting. More information on cutter machine dry collection systems is available in the literature (Page 1983).

Face-Drill Dust Control   Dust control on face drills used in water-soluble ores is generally easier to accomplish than on cutter machines because there are fewer sources. Techniques include both wet and dry systems.

Wet dust suppression systems include external water sprays, water injection through the drill, and foam injection though the drill. External boom-mounted systems are typically homemade and reduce dust by about 50%. Water-mist injection through the drill is available from several manufacturers. The resulting dust reduction is much better, typically 90% or more. A homemade foam system has also been used successfully (USBM 1982c). It achieved 95% dust reduction at lower water flow rates.

Dry collection systems are generally inferior to wet suppression systems. This is due primarily to the inability of dry collection systems to maintain effective intake dust capture because of face irregularities. The overall dust reduction is a product of the inlet capture efficiency and the filtration efficiency of the collector. Therefore, high filtration efficiency is pointless unless the inlet dust capture efficiency is also very high.

An additional reason why dry systems are generally inferior to wet systems is maintenance. Dry systems require that the dust collected be disposed of in some convenient manner. Wet systems require no material handling; the wetted material merely dribbles down the face. One dry collector tested has shown 76% respirable dust efficiency (Page 1983).

Surface Mine Dust Control

Personal exposure to respirable dust at surface mines primarily results from overburden drilling. Both wet and dry methods are available to suppress dust from this source. Haul road dust control is also important.

Overburden Drilling/Wet Suppression   Wet drilling systems consist of a water tank mounted on the drill from which water is pumped into the downhole airline. The water droplets in the bail air conglomerate dust particles as they travel up the annular space of the drilled hole, thus controlling dust as the air bails the cuttings from the hole.

In wet drilling systems, typical water flow rates are 0.0063 to 0.126 L/s (0.1 to 2.0 gpm) depending upon the size and type of drill, as well as the condition of the material being drilled. Flow rate is controlled manually by the drill operator by means of a control valve located in the cab. Some drills may also be equipped with a flow meter to give the operator a visual indication of the flow rate. The operator simply watches the cuttings as they are bailed from the hole and adjusts the flow rate according to how moist the cuttings appear to be. This technique can be effective; however, the delay between the time the valve is opened and the time the cuttings are expelled from the hole can be several seconds. This makes it difficult for the operator to find the proper flow setting. This is especially true when drilling through alternating dry and wet strata.

Too much water pumped into the bail air wets the drill cuttings to a point where they are too heavy to be bailed up the hole. This can result in undesirable regrinding of the cuttings as well as the drill string becoming seized in the hole. Excessive water in the hole may also result in plugging the air orifices of the bit and hastening bit degradation. The most obvious drawback to wet system drilling occurs when the outside temperatures drop below freezing. The entire system must then be heated while the drill is in operation, and during downtime the system must be drained.

Tests show that wet suppression systems can effectively control respirable dust (USBM 1987). Control efficiencies for 200-mm (8-in.) holes varied from a low of 9.1% at a flow of 0.013 L/s (0.2 gpm) to a high of 96.3% at a flow of 0.076 L/s (1.2 gpm). The most significant increase in efficiency is generally between 0.013 and 0.038 L/s (0.2 and 0.6 gpm). The rate of increase of efficiency then decreases until the drill's upper flow limit is reached. In the case of the drills tested, a flow rate approaching 0.063 L/s (1.0 gpm) began to cause operational problems.

To operate at close to the optimum water flow rate, the operator slowly increases the amount of water just to the point where visible dust emissions abate. Due to the initial sharp increase of dust control effectiveness, the visible dust abatement point is easy to identify. Increasing water flow beyond this point does not yield any significant improvements in dust control, but will most likely cause increased bit degradation and possible seizing of the drill stem.

Overburden Drilling/Dry Collection   The use of a dry system involves enclosing the area where the drill stem enters the ground. This enclosure is usually accomplished by hanging a rubber or cloth "shroud" from the underside of the drill deck. This enclosure is ducted to a dust collector, the clean side of which is equipped with a fan. The fan creates a negative pressure inside the entire system, thus capturing dust as it exits the hole during drilling. The dust is removed in the collector device and clean air is exhausted through the fan.

The integrity of the drill stem shroud, including how well it seals to the ground, is probably the single most important factor contributing to the effectiveness of a dry collection system. The shrouded volume under the drill deck should be at least 1.8 times the volume of the hole and should be at a negative pressure of at least 50 Pa (0.2 in. of water). The air is ducted out of the drill stem shroud either from the top of the shroud near the outside edge or from the side of the shroud near the top. Varying the open area of the shroud changes the shroud's dust capture efficiency. As the open area is reduced, the velocity in the open area increases. The most common open area is the gap between the bottom of the shroud and the ground, which is called the shroud height. With a shroud height of 150 to 225 mm (6 to 9 in.) or lower, it is apparent that the control system works well. However, as the height increases, the control efficiencies decrease.

During drilling, it is sometimes necessary to raise the drill shroud. This is done for two reasons: (1) the driller/helper needs to shovel the cuttings to prevent them from falling back into the hole, and (2) the operator must be able to observe when the coal seam has been reached and stop drilling. As a result, there are times when a broken seal between the shroud and the ground or cutting cannot be avoided. Therefore, it is important for the driller to keep the open area to a minimum. This involves raising the drill shroud frequently.

Dust collection efficiency also decreases if significant leaks are present from gaps or holes in the shroud. Most deck shrouds are rectangular and constructed from four separate pieces of rubber belting attached to the deck. Consequently, leakage can often occur at the corner seams as the individual pieces of belting separate from one another.

Testing was completed by NIOSH (Page et al. 1998) to evaluate a circular drill shroud design that was capable of being hydraulically raised and lowered. The circular shroud is attached to the drill deck with steel banding, which is also used to seal the one seam in the sheet rubber material used to fabricate the shroud. A steel band is also attached to the bottom of the shroud to maintain shape and provide weight for lowering the shroud to the ground. The shroud can be raised and lowered through activation of a hydraulic cylinder and guide wires attached to the bottom steel band. The cylinder is controlled by a hand valve located near the drill controls. The shroud is also equipped with a small trap door that can be manually opened to allow cuttings to be shoveled from inside the shroud without having to raise the shroud above the ground. Sampling results indicated that, when drilling with the shroud lowered to the ground, this type of shroud design maintained dust levels below 0.5 mg/m^3.

Enclosed Cabs   Enclosed cabs on mining equipment can also offer substantial protection for the drill operator from outside dust sources. The most effective protection is achieved when filtered air is blown into the cab and all cab seals are well maintained. Filtered air conditioning/heating units are available to control the working environment in the cab. The filtered air units provide a clean air source and, if adequate seals are in place, the positive air pressure will prevent dust leakage into the cab. To ensure the effectiveness of filtered air units, the operator must minimize the time that cab doors and windows are opened.

Haul Road Dust Control   Many methods are available for haul road dust control. Water is the most obvious, but there are many others, including:

- **Salts**—hygroscopic compounds, such calcium chloride, magnesium chloride, hydrated lime, and sodium silicates
- **Surfactant**—substances capable of reducing the surface tension of the transport liquid, such as soaps, detergents, and dust-set monawet
- **Soil cements**—compounds that are mixed with the native soils to form a new surface; for example, calcium lignon sulphonate, sodium lignon sulfonate, ammonium lignon sulphonate, and portland cement
- **Bitumens**—compounds derived from coal or petroleum, such as coherex peneprime, asphalt, and oils
- **Films**—polymers that form discrete tissues, layers or membranes, such as latexes, acrylics, vinyls, and fabric

Salts increase roadway surface moisture by hygroscopically extracting moisture from the atmosphere. Surfactants decrease the surface tension of water, which allows the available moisture to wet more particles per unit volume. Soil cements, bitumens, and films generally form coherent surface layers that seal the road surface and thereby reduce the quantity of dust generated.

A study by Rosbury and Zimmer (1983) showed that the highest control efficiency measured for a chemical dust suppressant, 82%, was for calcium chloride two weeks after application. Generally, however, the control efficiencies hovered in the 40% to 60% range over the first 2 weeks after application, then decreased with time. After the fifth week beyond application, the limited number of data points suggests a control efficiency of less than 20%. Composite watering data were fairly uniform. Watering once per hour resulted in a control efficiency of approximately 40%. Doubling the application rate increased the control effectiveness by about 15% to 55%. The study also showed that chemical dust suppressants (primarily salts and lignons) can be more cost-effective than watering under some conditions.

The cost of using a dust suppressant is very site-specific. Certain types of dust suppressants work better in certain types of road aggregate. Recommendations are:

- **Gravel.** In road surfaces with too much gravel, only watering will be effective. Chemical dust suppressants can neither compact the surface because of the poor size gradation, nor form a new surface, and water-soluble suppressants will leach.

- **Sand.** In compact sandy soils, bitumens, which are not water-soluble, are the most effective dust suppressant. Water-soluble suppressants such as salts, lignons, and acrylics will leach from the upper road surface. However, in loose, medium, and fine sands, bearing capacity will not be adequate for the bitumen to maintain a new surface.

- **Good gradation.** In road surfaces with a good surface graduation, all chemical suppressant types offer potential for equally effective control.

- **Silt.** In road surfaces with too much silt (greater than about 20% to 25% as determined from a scoop sample, not a vacuum or swept sample), no dust suppression program is effective, and the road should be rebuilt. In high silt locations, the chemical suppressants tend to make the road slippery and are not able to compact the surface nor maintain a new road surface because of poor bearing capacity. Further, rutting under high moisture conditions requires that the road be regraded, which almost completely destroys chemical dust suppressant effectiveness. If the road cannot be rebuilt, watering is the best program.

All chemical dust suppressants (with infrequent watering) share one common failing as compared with frequent watering. Material spillage on roadways is very common, and the material spilled is subject to reentrainment. With frequent watering, newly spilled material is moistened at close intervals. With chemicals and infrequent watering, newly spilled material could go for long periods before being moistened. Therefore, in mines where spillage cannot be controlled, watering is more effective for dust control.

In locations where trackout from an unpaved road to a paved road is a problem, chemical suppressants are generally a good choice. Watering aggravates the trackout problem with moisture and mud, whereas chemical suppressants, particularly bitumens and adhesives, leave the road dry. Finally, some mines have a dust problem in winter when temperatures are subfreezing but little moisture is present. The case for chemical suppressants over water in this case is clear.

Minerals Processing Dust Control Devices and Systems

Belt Conveyors   Belt conveyors can be a major source of dust. To minimize dust emissions, the material being carried should be loaded onto the center of the belt. Ideally, the belt conveyor should be designed to operate at 75% of its full rated capacity. Closely spaced impact idlers (0.3-m or 1-ft centers) should be located at transfer points. These absorb the force of impact and prevent deflection of the belt between the idlers, thus preventing dust leakage under the skirting rubber seal. Skirtboards are used to keep the material on the belt after it leaves the loading chute. They are equipped with flat rubber strips that provide a dust seal between the skirtboards and the moving belt. Improved skirtboard designs are also available (Mody and Jakhete 1987).

Muckshelves can be installed in the belt conveyor's material impact zone to load the material centrally on the belt. A belt scraper should be installed at the head pulley to dislodge fine dust particles that may adhere to the belt surface. A scrapings chute should also be provided to redirect the material removed by the belt scraper into the process stream or a container. A V-plow installed on the noncarrying side of the belt will clean the belt and prevent buildup of material and dust on the tail pulley, thus keeping the belt properly aligned.

Water applied to the belt can go a long way in reducing dust. A small quantity sprayed onto the noncarrying side of the return belt will reduce dust (Ford 1973). Water washing belt scrapers are used to clean the carrying side of the return belt (Planner 1990).

A good general reference on conveyor belt dust control is *Foundations 2–The Pyramid Approach to Control Dust and Spillage from Belt Conveyors* (Swinderman et al. 1998).

Transfer Chutes   Transfer chutes transport ore from one piece of equipment to another. The following specifications should be used when designing a transfer chute: (1) the chute depth should be at least three times the maximum lump size to avoid jamming; (2) the chute should be designed so that the material falls on the sloping bottom of the chute and not on the succeeding equipment; (3) wherever possible, the material should fall on a local rockbox or stonebox rather than on the metal surfaces; (4) abrupt changes of direction must be avoided to reduce the possibility of material buildup, material jamming, and dust generation; (5) curved, perforated, or grizzly chute bottoms should be used when the product stream consists of fines and lumps—placing a layer of fines ahead of the lumps on the belt helps prevent heavy impact of material on the belt, which reduces belt wear and dust generation; (6) spiral chutes should be used to prevent breakage of fragile or soft material; and (7) bin-lowering chutes should be used to feed bins and hoppers without generating large amounts of dust.

Enclosures   Enclosures are used to contain dust emissions around a dust source. When designing an enclosure for a dust source, the following parameters should be employed: (1) enclosures should be spacious enough to permit internal circulation of the dust-laden air; (2) enclosures should be arranged in removable sections for easy maintenance; (3) a hinged access door should be provided to aid routine inspection and maintenance; and (4) dust curtains should be installed at the open ends of the enclosures to contain dust and reduce airflow.

Crushers   Crushers emit dust primarily from two points, the discharge and the feed. Dust control measures are not usually considered in the design of a crusher. However, the use of shrouds or enclosures for crushers can contain the dust so that a dust control system can operate more efficiently. In installing crushers, the following measures are recommended: (1) a crusher feedbox with a minimum number of openings should be installed, and rubber curtains should be used to minimize dust escape and airflow; and (2) the crusher should be choke-fed to reduce air entrainment and dust emission. Dust escape at the crusher discharge end can be minimized by properly designed and installed transfer chutes.

Screens   The rate of dust generated by screens cannot be altered. However, properly enclosing the screen can reduce dust emissions. A complete enclosure that can be easily removed for maintenance and inspection should be used. Some screen manufacturers provide sheet-metal covers to enclose the top of the screen. These covers are effective when properly maintained. However, they do not provide a dust seal between the moving screen surfaces and the stationary chutes.

Storage Bins and Hoppers   Dust emissions during feeding operations can be minimized by installing a bin-lowering chute and by completely enclosing the bin or hopper. Also, dust emissions can be minimized by installing a telescopic chute or by installing a loading spout. Loading spouts are sophisticated versions of the telescopic chute and are used to load and stack ore into barges, trucks, and railroad cars. The falling material is enclosed by a flexible duct, acting as a chute, which retracts as the height of the material pile increases. The duct also prevents airflow during free fall of material between the chute and stockpile. The generated dust is captured by the same flexible duct and is conveyed, countercurrent to the material flow, to a dust collector.

Bucket Elevators   Bucket elevators emit dust from two points, the boot where material is fed and the head wheel where material is discharged. The steel casing that encloses the buckets and chain assembly contains dust effectively unless there are holes or openings in the casing. Emissions at the boot of the bucket elevator can be reduced by proper design of a transfer chute between the feeding equipment and the elevator. Dust production can be reduced significantly by keeping the height of material fall to a minimum and by gently loading material into the boot of the elevator. Proper venting to a dust collector will control dust emission at the discharge end of the bucket elevator.

Screw Conveyors   Normally, screw conveyors are totally enclosed except at the ends, where emissions can be controlled by proper transfer chute design. To maintain a proper dust seal, a neoprene rubber gasket should be installed on the trough cover. Many manufacturers provide two-bar flanges and formed-channel cross members that make a continuous pocket around the trough. The flange-cover sections are set in this channel. Once the channel section is filled with dust, an effective dust seal is created.

Stockpiles   All types of stockpiles can be a significant dust source. Generation of dust emissions from stockpiles is due to the formation of new stockpiles and wind erosion of previously formed piles. During formation of stockpiles by conveyors, dust is generated by wind blowing across the stream of falling material and separating fine from coarse particles. Additional dust is generated when the material hits the stockpile.

Dust from stockpiles can be reduced by:

- Minimizing height of free fall of material and providing wind protection using:
  - Stone ladders, which consist of a section of vertical pipe into which stone is discharged from the conveyor. At different levels, the pipe has square or rectangular openings through which the material flows to form the stockpile. In addition to reducing the height of free fall of material, stone ladders also provide protection against wind.

- Telescopic chutes, in which the material is discharged to a retractable chute. As the height of the stockpile increases or decreases, the chute is raised or lowered accordingly. Proper design of the chute can keep the drop to a minimum.
- Stacker conveyors, which operate on the same principle as telescopic chutes.

- Minimizing wind erosion of the stockpile by locating stockpiles behind natural or manufactured windbreaks, locating the working area on the leeward side of the active piles, and covering inactive piles with tarps or other inexpensive materials.
- Minimizing vehicle traffic on or around the stockpile.
- Using specialized equipment such as a reclaimer to minimize the disturbance of the stockpile or providing a tunnel underneath to reclaim the material.

Dust Collection Systems   A dust collection system is one of the most effective ways to reduce dust emissions. The rate of airflow through the exhaust hood is the most important factor for all types of hoods. For local, side, downdraft, and canopy hoods, the location is also important because the rate of airflow is based on the relative distance between the hood and the source. The shape of the exhaust hood is another design consideration.

Ductwork design includes the selection of duct sizes based on the velocity necessary to carry the dust to the collector without settling in the duct. To prevent dust from settling and blocking the ductwork, transport velocities should range from 17.5 to 20 m/s (3,500 to 4,000 fpm) for most industrial dust (such as granite, silica flour, limestone, coal asbestos, and clay) and from 20 to 25 m/s (4,000 to 5,000 fpm) for heavy or moist dust, such as lead, cement, and quick lime.

Recommended minimum transport velocities for different types of dust are shown in Table 20.1.

Wet Dust Suppression Systems   These systems fall into three categories:

1. **Plain water sprays.** This method uses plain water to wet the material. Advantages are low cost and simplicity of operation. However, large quantities of water may not be tolerable.

2. **Water sprays with surfactant.** This method uses surfactants to lower the surface tension of water. The droplets spread further and penetrate deeper into the material pile.

3. **Foam.** Water and a special blend of surfactant make the foam. Less water is necessary to achieve a given level of dust control. However, operating costs can be high.

Background Dust Sources   Background dust sources can expose workers at mineral processing facilities to more significant dust concentrations than from their normal job functions. These background dust sources include such things as soiled work clothes, blowing clothes off with compressed air, broken bags of product material both at the fill station and during the conveying process, bag hoppers overflowing with product, improper housekeeping techniques such as dry sweeping of floors, and dusty makeup air that may flow into mill buildings from outside sources.

The best way to detect background dust sources is to use an instantaneous dust monitor with data logging capability. By monitoring the worker's exposure throughout the entire workday, significant dust-producing events can be identified and controlled.

Research has shown that total mill ventilation systems (Cecala et al. 1993) can be a cost-effective means of reducing background dust levels found in mineral processing operations. Fans are placed near the top of the mill and air intakes are strategically placed on lower levels to provide desired airflow movement through the structure. Test results indicated that dust reductions of 40% to 60% were achieved.

A good general reference for minerals processing dust control is the *Dust Control Handbook for Minerals Processing* (Mody and Jakhete 1987).

TABLE 20.1   Recommended minimum transport velocities

Material	Minimum Design Velocity, m/s	fpm
Very fine, light dusts	10	2,000
Fine, dry dusts and powders	15	3,000
Average industrial dusts	17.5	3,500
Coarse dusts	20 to 22.5	4,000 to 4,500
Heavy or moist dust loading	>22.5	>4,500

REFERENCES

Armour, D. 1999. Joy Mining Machinery, private communication.

Cecala A.B., J.C. Volkwein, E.D. Thimons, and C.W. Urban. 1981. Protection factors of the airstream helmet. RI 8591. USBM. 17 pp.

Cecala, A.C., G.W. Klinowski, and E.D. Thimons. 1993. Reducing respirable dust concentrations at mineral processing facilities using total mill ventilation systems. RI 9469. USBM. 11 pp.

Code of Federal Regulations, 30 CFR 70.101 and 71.101, 30 CFR 75.326 and 75.330.

Cole, D.E. 1984. Longwall dust control-respirators. *Proceedings of the Coal Mine Dust Conference.* Morgantown, WV.

Colinet, J.F., J.J. McClelland, L.A. Erhard, and R.A. Jankowski. 1990. Laboratory evaluation of quartz dust capture of irrigated-filter collection systems for continuous miners. RI 9313. USBM. 14 pp.

Colinet, J.F., and R.A. Jankowski. 1997. Dust control considerations for deep-cut faces when using exhaust ventilation and a flooded-bed scrubber. *SME Transactions* 302: 104–111.

———. 2000. Silica collection concerns when using flooded-bed scrubbers. *Mining Engineering* 52(4): 49–54.

Courtney, W.G., and L. Cheng. 1977. *Control of Respirable Dust by Improved Water Sprays.* IC 8753. USBM. 92–108.

Divers, E.F., N.I. Jayaraman, S. Page, and R.A. Jankowski. 1987. Guidelines for dust control in small underground coal mines. In *U.S. Bureau of Mines Handbook.*

Ford, V.H.W. 1973. Bottom belt sprays as a method of dust control on conveyors. *Mining Technology (UK)* 55(635): 387–391.

Jayaraman, N.I., R.A. Jankowski, and J.A. Organiscak. 1992. Update on stage loader dust control in longwall operations. *Proceedings of Longwall USA.* Pittsburgh, PA.

Kok, E.G., and R.F.J. Adam. 1986. Research on Water Proportioning for Dust Control on Longwalls. OFR 56-86. USBM. 138 pp.

Kost, J.A., J.C. Yingling, and B.J. Mondics. 1981. *Guidebook for Dust Control in Underground Mining.* NTIS PB 83-109207. USBM.

Kost, J.A., J.F. Colinet, and G.A. Shirey. 1985. *Refinement and Evaluation of Basic Longwall Dust Control Techniques.* OFR 129-85. USBM. 263 pp.

Ludlow, J., and R.J. Wilson. 1982. Deep cutting—key to dust-free longwalling. *Coal Mining and Processing* 19(8): 40–43.

Ludlow, J., and R.A. Jankowski. 1984. Use lower shearer drum speeds to achieve deeper coal cutting. *Mining Engineering* 36(3): 251–255.

Mody, V., and R. Jakhete. 1987. *Dust Control Handbook for Mineral Processing.* NTIS PB 88-159108. Denver: Martin Marietta Laboratories.

Niewiadomski, G.E. 2000. MSHA, private communication.

NIOSH. 1995. Criteria for a Recommended Standard—Occupational Exposure to Respirable Coal Mine Dust.

———. 1999. Work Related Lung Disease Surveillance Report 1999.

Organiscak, J.A., A.W. Khair, and M. Ahmad. 1996. Studies of bit wear and respirable dust generation. *Trans Soc Min Eng* 298: 1874–1879.

Page, S.J. 1983. Machine-mounted drill and cutter dust control in mines extracting soluble ores. *Transactions, AIME* 276.

Page, S.J. 1998. New Shroud Design Controls Silica Dust from Surface Mine and Construction Blast Hole Drills. DHHS (NIOSH) Publication No. 98-150. Hazard Control 27. 4 pp.

Piemental, R.A., R.F.J. Adam, and R.A. Jankowski. 1984. Improving dust control on longwall shearers. *Proceedings of 1984 SME-AIME Annual Meeting.* Los Angeles, CA.

Planner, J.H. 1990. Water as a means of spillage control in coal handling. In *Proceedings Coal Handling and Utilization Conference.* Sydney, Australia. 264–270.

Rosbury, K.D., and R.A. Zimmer. 1983. *Cost Effectiveness of Dust Control Used on Unpaved Haul Roads.* NTIS PB 86-115201 and NTIS PB 86-115219 (2 volumes).

Ruggieri, S.K., and S. Babbitt. 1983. *Optimizing Water Sprays for Dust Control on Longwall Shearer Faces.* NTIS PB 86-205416. Waltham, MA: Foster-Miller.

Ruggieri, S.K., D.M. Doyle, and J.C. Volkwein. 1984. Improved sprayfans provide ventilation solutions. *Coal Mining* April: 94–98.

Ruggieri, S.K., C. Babbitt, and J. Burnett. 1985. *Improved Sprayfan System Installation Guide*. NTIS PB86-165065. Waltham, MA: Foster-Miller.

Shirey, C.A., J.F. Colinet, and J.A. Kost. 1985. *Dust Control Handbook for Longwall Mining Operations*. NTIS PB-86-178159/AS. USBM.

Swinderman, R. Todd, L.J. Goldbeck, R.P. Stahura, and A.D. Marti. 1998. *Foundations 2–The Pyramid Approach to Control Dust and Spillage From Belt Conveyors.* Neponset, IL: Martin Engineering.

Timko, R.J. 1983. Techniques for constructing concrete block stoppings. In *U.S. Bureau of Mines Handbook*.

USBM. 1981a. Improved filtering system for water sprays resists clogging. *Technology News No. 20.*

——. 1981b. Reduce dust on longwall faces with a gob curtain. *Technology News No. 119.*

——. 1982a. Ventilation curtain reduces dust from cutting into longwall entry. *Technology News No. 137.*

——. 1982b. More water on upwind drum reduces exposure of shearer operator to dust. *Technology News No. 155.*

——. 1982c. Effective wet dust controls for face drills in non-coal mines. *Technology News No. 148.*

——. 1984. How to reduce shearer operators' dust exposure by using remote control. *Technology News No. 203.*

——. 1985. How twelve continuous miner sections keep dust levels at 0.5 mg/m^3 or less. *Technology News No. 220.*

——. 1985a. Anti-rollback water spray system. *Technology News No. 221.*

——. 1985b. Reducing dust exposure of roof bolter operators. *Technology News No. 219.*

——. 1985c. Improved stageloader dust control in longwall mining operations. *Technology News No. 224.*

——. 1987. Optimizing dust control on surface coal mines drill. *Technology News No. 286.*

——. 1989. Underboom sprays reduce dust on continuous mining machines. *Technology News No. 323.*

Volkwein, J.C., and T. Wellman, 1989. *Impact of Water Sprays on Scrubber Ventilation Effectiveness*. RI 9259. USBM. 12 pp.

CHAPTER 21

Noise

Christopher J. Bise
Centennial Professor and Program Chair of Mining Engineering
Pennsylvania State University, University Park, Pennsylvania

INTRODUCTION

Noise-induced hearing loss (NIHL) is an insidious condition because it usually begins as a gradual, progressive reduction in the quality of communication with other people and responsiveness to the environment. Ultimately, NIHL can result in permanent loss of hearing (deafness). Usually, there is no outwardly visible effect and, in most cases, little or no pain, which may be the reason it is such an underrated debility.

In occupational settings, such as mining, the inability to properly hear various environmental noises results in diminished sensitivity to potentially hazardous sounds. The inability to discriminate between "sounds," which are meaningful and wanted, and "noises," which are annoying and unwanted, further diminishes occupational safety. Much like the other human senses, we often take good hearing for granted until it is lost.

The human ear is divided into three main sections: (1) the external ear, (2) the middle ear, and (3) the inner ear (Figure 21.1). The external ear starts at the pinna, the visible portion, which focuses sound toward the external auditory canal; in the process, the arriving sound can be amplified by as much as 23 decibels (dB) (Brauer 1994). The tympanic membrane (eardrum) separates the external ear from the middle ear; this membrane transfers sound energy to motion. The middle ear is a cavity between the tympanic membrane and the bony wall of the inner ear and contains three ossicles (bones) called the malleus (hammer), the incus (anvil), and the stapes (stirrup). These ossicles form the middle ear's sound-conducting mechanism. The middle ear also contains the eustachian tube, which vents to the throat and enables the pressure in the middle ear to equalize with the external ambient pressure. Finally, the inner ear holds the bony and membranous labyrinths where the hearing receptors are located (Wentz 1998). The major components of the inner ear are the cochlea and the vestibular receptive system (Benjamin and Benjamin 1996). The cochlea, which houses the organ of Corti—the actual hearing organ—is a fluid-filled coil with thousands of hair cells that convert the incoming mechanical sound vibrations into nerve impulses. These nerve impulses are then transmitted to the brain; when these hair cells become damaged by aging, disease, medication, blows to the head, or exposure to high noise levels, hearing loss results (Lichtenwalner and Michael 1999). The vestibular receptive system contains sensors for orientation and balance. The system contains three fluid-filled semicircular canals, which are near the cochlea and perpendicular to each other. These canals respond to movement and provide information to the brain about body position.

There are three principal categories of NIHL: (1) temporary threshold shift (TTS), (2) permanent threshold shift (PTS), and (3) acoustic trauma. TTS occurs when exposure to sound damages the organ of Corti and its receptor cells. However, if the exposure is of relatively short duration, hearing sensitivity returns to preexposure levels after a recovery period (Brauer 1994). PTS, on the other

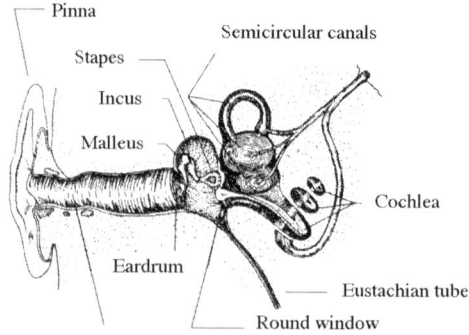

FIGURE 21.1   Major anatomical features of the human ear (Ward 1986)

hand, results from continued exposure to noise; hearing sensitivity does not return to preexposure levels after a recovery period. Finally, acoustic trauma is caused by a single event, such as an explosion or another form of high-pressure wave. It can result in eardrum rupture or structural damage to the middle ear. Postexposure hearing sensitivity can range from temporarily lost to permanently lost.

According to Wentz (1998), many factors influence occupational hearing loss, including:

- Age of the employee
- Preemployment hearing impairment
- Diseases of the ear
- Sound pressure level of the noise
- Length of daily exposure
- Duration of employment
- Ambient conditions of the workplace
- Distance from the noise source
- Employee lifestyle outside the workplace.

The link between noise and hearing loss has been established for several centuries, but efforts to control or eliminate the basic causes for occupational hearing loss have only existed for the last few decades. Possibly, this could be attributed to the fact that occupational settings represent only some of the risk factors associated with hearing loss. Employee lifestyle outside the workplace, such as hobbies, can also contribute to NIHL:

- Listening to loud music, particularly with earphones
- Exposure to gunfire
- Use of equipment such as chain saws.

One of the first documented descriptions of NIHL was written by Bernardo Ramazzini, an 18th century Italian physician who is often called the "Father of Industrial Hygiene." In a book he wrote in 1700—*De Morbis Artificium Diatriba (The Diseases of Workers)*—Ramazzini described workers who hammered copper as having "their ears so injured by the perpetual din ... that workers of this class become hard of hearing, and if they grow old at this work, completely deaf" (Standard 1996). In 1825, C.H. Parry described how artillery fire contributes to NIHL. In one instance in 1782, a British admiral became almost entirely deaf for 2 weeks after 80 broadsides were fired from his ship, the H.M.S. Formidable (Suter 1986). However, NIHL did not become widespread until the Industrial Revolution. The new dependence on machinery and the inherent noise associated with manufacturing operations were the underlying factors. For example, even the construction of the coal-fired steam engines used to drive the machinery required riveted boilers. As a result, the term "boilermaker's ear," which still exists today, was introduced into the occupational health and safety lexicon. We can see from these examples, then, that the vast majority of noises that can cause NIHL are manmade.

Current concerns about NIHL among mineworkers are based on the fact that, even with decades of efforts to deal with the issue, the problem persists. In 1999, it was estimated that the average age of U.S. mineworkers was 48. As the workforce continues to age, mine health and safety specialists will

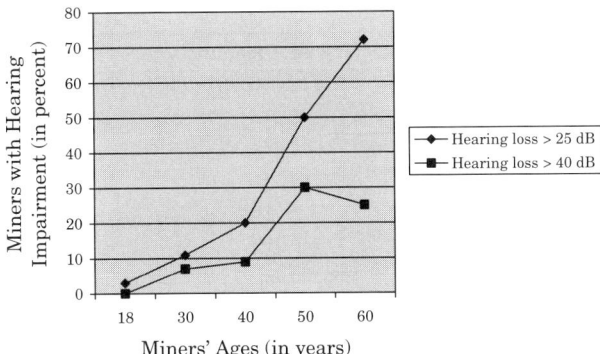

FIGURE 21.2   Results of NIOSH's 1976 study of hearing loss among underground coal miners (after Bobick and Giardino 1976)

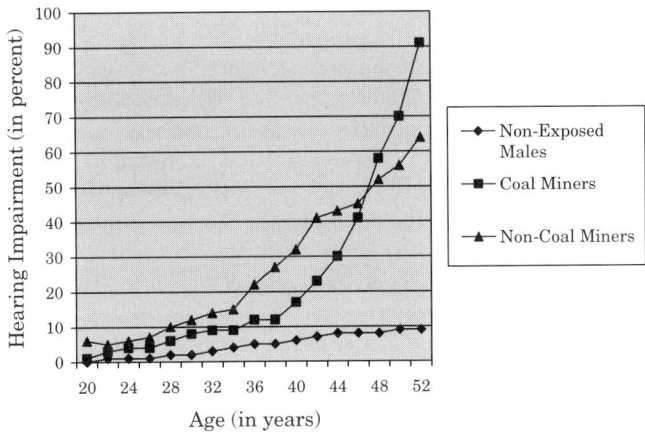

FIGURE 21.3   Hearing impairment greater than 25 dB (after Franks 1996)

be confronted with an ever-increasing problem. Underscoring the situation, the National Institute of Occupational Safety and Health (NIOSH) conducted a hearing survey of 1,500 underground coal miners during the 1970s (Bobick and Giardino 1976). The subjects had no history of significant nonoccupational noise exposure, severe head trauma, or chronic ear infections. When they were tested, they had been out of the working environment a minimum of 14 hours. Figure 21.2 presents the results. At the important frequencies for speech perception—1,000, 2,000, and 3,000 Hz—the percentages of miners who suffered hearing losses of more than 25 and 40 dB at age 48 were approximately 48% and 8%, respectively.

Twenty years later, NIOSH analyzed NIHL in coal and noncoal miners and compared the percentages of hearing impairment (> 25 dB) with those of nonexposed males, by age; the results are shown in Figure 21.3 (Franks 1996). Significantly, the percentage of miners with a hearing impairment greater than 25 dB was found to be approximately 8 to 10 times greater at the age of the average mineworker (48 years) than that percentage for nonexposed males at the same age. Clearly, after more than 2 decades, much work still needs to be done in this area.

THE PHYSICS OF SOUND

To fully understand the concepts of sound, noise, and NIHL, we must become familiar with the terminology and the relationships. **Sound**, with an approximate speed in air of 1,130 ft/s at 70°F, is the auditory sensation caused by the oscillations in pressure in a medium with elasticity and viscosity (Ostergaard 1986). As previously noted, **noise** applies to undesired auditory sensations. In an industrial

TABLE 21.1   Full octave bands

Center Frequency	Lower Band Edge Frequency	Upper Band Edge Frequency
31.5 Hz	22.4 Hz	45.0 Hz
63.0 Hz	45.0 Hz	90.0 Hz
125.0 Hz	90.0 Hz	180.0 Hz
250.0 Hz	180.0 Hz	355.0 Hz
500.0 Hz	355.0 Hz	710.0 Hz
1,000.0 Hz	710.0 Hz	1,400.0 Hz
2,000.0 Hz	1,400.0 Hz	2,800.0 Hz
4,000.0 Hz	2,800.0 Hz	5,600.0 Hz
8,000.0 Hz	5,600.0 Hz	11,200.0 Hz
16,000.0 Hz	11,200.0 Hz	22,400.0 Hz

environment, noise can be either **continuous** (i.e., a steady sound, such as a running fan) or **intermittent** (i.e., a broken sound or a sound burst, such as that generated by a drill). **Frequency** is the time rate at which complete cycles of high and low pressure regions are produced by the source; the most common unit is the **Hertz (Hz)**, which is the number of complete cycles that occur in 1 second (Finucane 1998). The usual range of frequencies of interest to hearing specialists extends from approximately 20 to 20,000 Hz; the range of human conversation is from about 300 to 3,000 Hz (Davis and Hamernik 1995). A sound can consist of only one frequency (i.e., a tuning fork), or, more commonly, a combination of two or more. This combination is referred to as a **frequency band**. Normally, a frequency band is identified by the lowest and highest frequency in the combination. The most commonly used frequency band is the **octave band**; Table 21.1 lists the individual **bandwidths** for the full octave bands, identified by the lower band-edge frequency, the center (i.e., geometric mean) frequency, and the upper band-edge frequency, which is always twice the value of the lower band-edge frequency.

Several characteristic parameters and measurements apply to sound and noise. A source's **sound intensity**, measured in joules per square meter per second or watts per square meter, is the average rate at which sound energy is transmitted through a unit area that is normal to the direction the sound is traveling. Sound intensity is commonly expressed by its level, usually in terms of 10^{-12} watts/m^2. **Sound pressure** refers to the root-mean-square values of the pressure changes above and below atmospheric pressure, which are used to measure continuous noise. Sound pressure is measured in Newtons per square meter (N/m^2) or pascals (Pa), where 1 N/m^2 = 1 Pa.

A healthy human ear can hear a wide range of sound pressures—from 20 µPa to 200 Pa—without incurring damage (Finucane 1998). Because of this wide range, the **sound pressure level** was established as the ratio of the measured sound pressure to a reference base (20 µPa). In this manner, the results can be expressed in **dB**, where 0 dB corresponds to 20 mPa. The decibel (10% of a **Bel**) approximately equals the smallest difference in acoustic power the human ear can detect (Koren 1996). Because the Bel scale is logarithmic, it is more advantageous for dealing with the wide range of human hearing.

The human ear, however, is not equally sensitive to all sound frequencies. To account for this, sound level meters have frequency-response weighting networks to attenuate sounds of certain frequencies, resulting in a weighted total sound pressure level. Three scales are commonly used for these networks: A, B, and C (Figure 21.4). Of the three scales, the A scale comes closest to approximating the ear's response characteristics or, in other words, the A-weighting curve is an approximation of equal loudness perception characteristics of human hearing for pure tones relative to a reference of 40 dB sound pressure level at 1,000 Hz (Earshen 1986). The A scale also approximates the damage potential for high-level sounds. Because of this, regulatory agencies such as the Mine Safety and Health Administration (MSHA) and the Occupational Safety and Health Administration (OSHA) use this scale, and subsequent references to A-weighted sound levels will be in **dBA**. Table 21.2 lists the correction values to convert physical sound pressure levels (in dB) to dBA.

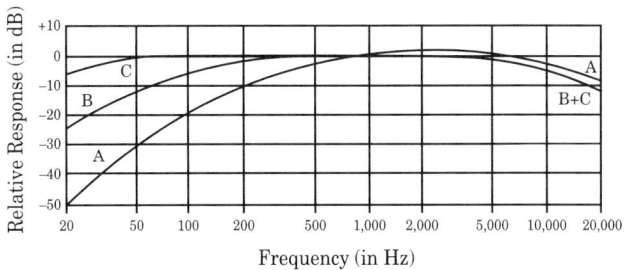

FIGURE 21.4   Sound-level meter weighting curves (after Earshen 1976)

TABLE 21.2   Conversion of dB to dBA

Octave Band Center Frequency	Correction (dB to dBA)
31.5 Hz	−39.4
63.0 Hz	−26.2
125.0 Hz	−16.1
250.0 Hz	−8.6
500.0 Hz	−3.2
1,000.0 Hz	0.0
2,000.0 Hz	+1.2
4,000.0 Hz	+1.0
8,000.0 Hz	−1.1
16,000.0 Hz	−6.6

Sound Power Level (dB re 10^{-12} Watts)		Sound Power (Watts)
TURBOJET ENGINE	160	10,000
	150	1,000
	140	100
	130	10
COMPRESSOR	120	1
LOUD RADIO	110	10^{-1}
	100	10^{-2}
VOICE SHOUTING	90	10^{-3}
	80	10^{-4}
CONVERSATION	70	10^{-5}
	60	10^{-6}
	50	10^{-7}
	40	10^{-8}
VOICE WHISPER	30	10^{-9}
	20	10^{-10}
	10	10^{-11}
	0	10^{-12}

FIGURE 21.5   Relationship between sound power level and sound power (Lichtenwalner and Michael 1999)

Now that the relationships between the various levels have been established, we can relate them to everyday life. The **threshold of hearing** for a healthy human ear is considered to be 0 dB at 1,000 Hz. The **threshold of pain** is considered to be 140 dB at nearly all frequencies.

The relationship between sound power level and sound power is shown in Figure 21.5, and Figure 21.6 shows the relationship between the A-weighted sound pressure level and sound pressure.

When two or more sources of noise are in close proximity, their individual levels cannot be added directly, because of the logarithmic scaling of decibels. To determine the net effect of two noise sources, we can use Table 21.3. To use the table, take the dB readings of the two sources, find the difference between the two (Column 1), and add the corresponding value in Column 2 to the higher of

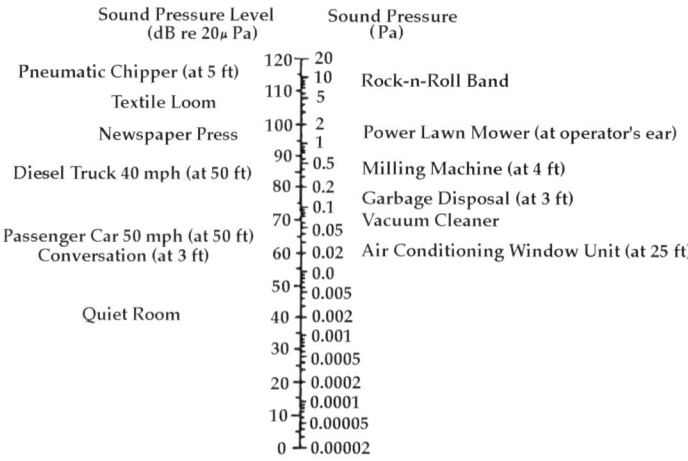

FIGURE 21.6   Relationship between A-weighted sound pressure level and sound pressure (Lichtenwalner and Michael 1999)

the two readings. The result is the net effect of the two sources. When there are three or more sources, start with the two highest readings, find the net effect of that pair, and then use that calculated value of the pair with the next highest reading. Continue in this manner until all levels have been added, or until the difference between the calculated sum and any remaining levels is greater than 20 dB.

DIAGNOSING NOISE-INDUCED HEARING LOSS

To determine if an individual has suffered an NIHL, an audiologist must conduct identification and measurement tests. The audiologist measures auditory thresholds in decibels (relative to normal hearing), for pure tones at various frequencies with an audiometer, and records the results on an audiogram (a frequency-intensity graph). The subject should be seated in a test room where background noise is limited and wear headphones that are connected to the audiometer. Figure 21.7 shows a typical normal audiogram (upper tracings), along with an audiogram from an individual with an NIHL (lower tracings). For an individual with normal hearing (upper two plots of Figure 21.7), all thresholds are less than 25 dB. However, with an NIHL (lower two plots of Figure 21.7), loss is quantifiable across the range of testing.

The maximum loss usually occurs at 4,000 Hz. People usually do not indicate hearing difficulty until a hearing loss greater than 25 dB at a frequency ≤4,000 Hz has occurred (Davis and Hamernik 1995).

NOISE STANDARDS

The origin of the regulatory standards that MSHA enforces in U.S. underground and surface mines was the Walsh-Healy Public Contracts Act. In 1936, the federal government took its first steps toward protecting workers from unhealthy working environments through the act's criteria. However, the act focused on hazardous work conditions for companies that received federal work contracts. Although the act was updated in 1960, several flaws relating to enforcing the provisions remained.

In 1968, the Department of Labor's Bureau of Labor Standards proposed a regulation limiting exposures to steady noise at an 85 dBA level (Lipscomb 1988). It was based upon a threshold limit value (TLV) proposed by the American Conference of Governmental Industrial Hygienists (ACGIH). Eventually, this regulation became known as the Walsh-Healy Noise Standard of 1969 and became known as the "backbone" for many modern noise standards.

MSHA regulates noise in metal and nonmetal mines (30 *Code of Federal Regulations* [CFR] 56.5050; 30 CFR 57.5050) and coal mines (30 CFR 70.500 to 30 CFR 70.511; 30 CFR 71.800 to 30 CFR 71.805). Regardless of the method of mining, MSHA establishes the permissible noise exposures, which are shown in Table 21.4. In addition, no exposure shall exceed 115 dBA, while impact or impulsive

TABLE 21.3 Values for combining two noise sources

Difference Between Two Sound Sources (dB)	Amount to be Added to Greater Sound Source (dB)
0.0–0.1	3.0
0.2–0.3	2.9
0.4–0.5	2.8
0.6–0.7	2.7
0.8–0.9	2.6
1.0–1.2	2.5
1.3–1.4	2.4
1.5–1.6	2.3
1.7–1.9	2.2
2.0–2.1	2.1
2.2–2.4	2.0
2.5–2.7	1.9
2.8–3.0	1.8
3.1–3.3	1.7
3.4–3.6	1.6
3.7–4.0	1.5
4.1–4.3	1.4
4.4–4.7	1.3
4.8–5.1	1.2
5.2–5.6	1.1
5.7–6.1	1.0
6.2–6.6	0.8
6.7–7.2	0.7
7.3–7.9	0.6
8.0–8.6	0.5
8.7–9.6	0.4
9.7–10.7	0.3
10.8–12.2	0.3
12.3–14.5	0.2
14.6–19.3	0.1
≥ 19.4	0.0

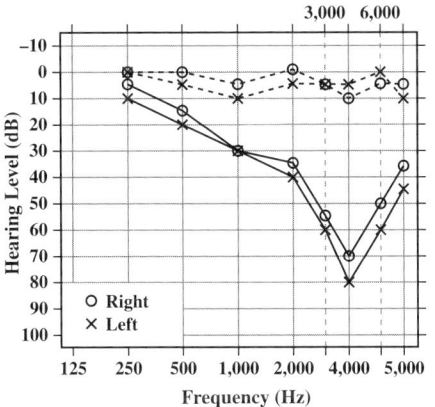

FIGURE 21.7   A typical audiogram from a normal individual and an individual suffering a hearing loss from excessive noise exposure (Davis and Hamernik 1995)

noises shall not exceed 140 dB (the peak sound pressure level). In those instances where the daily exposure comprises two or more periods of noise exposure at different levels, their combined effect shall be considered rather than the individual effect of each using the following equation:

$$(C_1 / T_1) + (C_2 / T_2) + ... (C_n / T_n) \qquad \text{(EQ 21.1)}$$

where C_n indicates the total time of exposure at a specific noise level, and T_n indicates the total time of exposure permitted at that level, as indicated in Table 21.4. If the value calculated in Equation 21.1 exceeds 1.0, then the mixed exposure shall be considered to exceed the permissible exposure. Interpolation between the values shown in Table 21.4 may be determined by the following equation:

$$\log T = 6.322 - 0.0602 \; SL \qquad \text{(EQ 21.2)}$$

where T is the time in hours and SL is the sound level in dBA.

For some time, scientists have attempted to identify the relationship between noise level and duration that will best predict hearing impairment. A closer inspection of the values in Table 21.4 indicates that, as the sound level decreases by 5 dB, the permissible hours of exposure doubles. This relationship, known as the exchange (or doubling) rate, attempts to quantify this potential. Not all organizations use a 5-dB exchange rate. The U.S. Environmental Protection Agency, the United Kingdom, and many European countries use a 3-dB rate because it corresponds to the equal-energy rule, which states that equal amounts of sound energy will produce equal amounts of hearing impairment, regardless of time distribution. On an energy basis, the 3-dB exchange rate enables a true time-weighted average noise exposure to be calculated. The 5-dB exchange rate that MSHA and OSHA use is less conservative than the equal-energy rule because it attempts to account for intermittence in noise exposures that occur in a typical workday. Although NIOSH recommended a 5-dB exchange rate in 1972, it has since recognized the equal-energy rule as being sound scientific practice and now recommends the use of a 3-dB exchange rate (NIOSH 1972; NIOSH 1998).

HEARING CONSERVATION PROGRAMS

With the increased emphasis on combating mining-related noise and NIHL among mineworkers, industry heath and safety specialists will need to incorporate the best practices of well-run hearing conservation programs in other industries into their own programs.

For example, in 1983, OSHA amended the Occupational Noise Exposure Standard by adding a Hearing Conservation Amendment. The standard for exposure was not changed; instead, a time-weighted average "action level" of 85 dBA was instituted. Exposure above this level triggers employer action—the establishment of a hearing conservation program (HCP)—which must incorporate the following components:

- The employer must design and implement workplace noise monitoring.
- The employer must identify specific employees, whose exposure exceeds the action level, to be included in the HCP.
- Employees in the HCP must be provided, at no cost, appropriate hearing protection.
- Employees in the HCP must be provided training and be included in an audiometric testing program.

According to Lichtenwalner and Michael (1999), the characteristics of a well-designed and implemented HCP are:

- Identifying noise hazard areas by taking noise-exposure measurements
- Reducing the noise exposure to safe levels through engineering controls (preferred), administrative controls, or hearing protection devices
- Measuring exposed workers' hearing thresholds to monitor the program's effectiveness
- Educating and motivating employees and management about the need to protect hearing, along with the proper care of personal hearing protectors
- Keeping accurate and reliable records of hearing and noise exposure measurements
- Referring employees with abnormal hearing thresholds for examination and diagnosis.

TABLE 21.4   Permissible noise exposures

Hours of Exposure	Sound Level in dBA (Slow Response)
8.0	90
6.0	92
4.0	95
3.0	97
2.0	100
1.5	102
1.0	105
0.5	110
0.25 or less	115

The most commonly used measurement device for an effective hearing conservation program is a simple sound level meter. Sound level meters capture sound through a microphone, amplify and filter the signal, and present the results, using a digital display or a moving indicator needle. The user has a choice of filters or weighting values and response characteristics (A, B, or C; fast or slow). Impulse meters are used to capture peak levels of impulse sound. Workers wear pocket-sized dosimeters to continuously record and integrate sound levels over time, which facilitates the measurement of cumulative noise dose (Brauer 1990). Obviously, sound level meters are used for area surveys to pinpoint locations of noise hazards; dosimeters are intended to identify individuals having an excessive cumulative exposure.

If a noise hazard cannot be controlled through engineering design or administrative actions, wearing proper hearing protection is the last line of defense. Unfortunately, more emphasis (and therefore money) is often placed on noise measurement than on properly selecting, fitting, and wearing hearing protection (Lichtenwalner and Michael 1999). Hearing protectors usually come in two varieties: (1) insert types, which seal against the walls of the ear canal; and (2) muff types, which seal against the head around the ear. Although there is no "best" protector for all situations, NIOSH has published a document that describes all hearing protectors currently marketed in the United States (Franks et al. 1994).

SUMMARY

As an indication of the importance of noise control and hearing conservation in the mining industry, MSHA recently issued new health standards to protect coal, metal, and nonmetal mineworkers from hearing loss resulting from prolonged exposure to damaging noise levels. The standards appeared in the *Federal Register* on September 13, 1999. For the first time, the new rules require mine operators to enroll mineworkers in an HCP if they are exposed to an average sound level ≥85 dBA over an 8-hour period. Each program must include training, voluntary hearing tests, and voluntary use of operator-provided hearing protection in most cases, although hearing protection is mandatory in particular instances. The 90 dBA per 8 hours exposure limit remains unchanged. Where feasible engineering and administrative controls at the workplace cannot reduce the noise to the exposure limit, the new standard requires hearing protection.

A significant amount of research has explored the damage risk for human exposure to noise. However, as with many other public health issues, not only are there scientific questions to be answered, but there are also many social, economic, and legal considerations. Various controversies, such as the efficacy of an 85-dBA versus a 90-dBA upper limit for an 8-hour workday, or a 3-dB versus a 5-dB exchange rate, will only be resolved as more attention and research is given to the issues. However, the current steps being taken by the mining industry should enable future generations of mineworkers to lead productive and safe lives without the fear of suffering from occupationally based NIHL.

ACKNOWLEDGMENT

The author wishes to express his sincere appreciation to David C. Byrne, research audiologist for NIOSH, and Dr. Kevin Michael, president of Michael & Associates, for their careful review of this chapter.

REFERENCES

Alexander, R.D., J.B. Vaughn, and C. Jones. 1974. The evolution of social behavior. *Annual Review of Ecology and Systematics* 5: 324–83.

Benjamin, G.S., and B.J. Benjamin. 1996. The ears. In *Fundamentals of Industrial Hygiene*. Edited by B.A. Plog, J. Niland, and P.J. Quinlan. Itasca, IL: National Safety Council.

Bobick, T., and D. Giardino. 1976. *Noise Environment of the Underground Coal Mine.* MSHA IR 1034.

Brauer, R.L. 1990. *Safety and Health for Engineers*. New York: Van Nostrand Reinhold.

Davis, R.I., and R.P. Hamernik. 1995. Noise and hearing impairment. In *Occupational Health*. New York: Little, Brown and Company.

Earshen, J.J. 1986. Sound measurement: instrumentation and noise descriptors. In *Noise and Hearing Conservation Manual.* Edited by E.H. Berger, W.D. Ward, J.C. Morrill, and L.H. Royster. Fairfax, VA: American Industrial Hygiene Association.

Finucane, E.W. 1998. *Definitions, Conversions, and Calculations for Occupational Safety and Health Professionals.* Boca Raton, FL: CRC Press.

Franks, J., C. Themann, and C. Sherris. 1994. *The NIOSH Compendium of Hearing Protection Devices.* NIOSH Publication 95-105. Cincinnati: NIOSH.

Franks, J.R. 1996. *Analysis of Audiograms for a Large Cohort of Noise-Exposed Miners.* Internal Report. Cincinnati: NIOSH.

Kohn, J.P., M.A. Friend, and C.A. Winterberger. 1996. *Fundamentals of Occupational Safety and Health*. Rockville, MD: Government Institutes, Inc.

Koren, H. 1996. *Illustrated Dictionary of Environmental Health and Occupational Safety.* Boca Raton, FL: CRC Press.

Lichtenwalner, C.P., and K. Michael. 1999. Occupational noise exposure and hearing conservation. In *Handbook of Occupational Safety and Health.* Edited by L.J. DiBerardinis. New York: John Wiley & Sons.

Lipscomb, D.M. 1988. *Hearing Conservation in Industry, Schools, and the Military.* Boston: College-Hill Press.

NIOSH. 1972. *Criteria for a Recommended Standard: Occupational Exposure to Noise.* Publication No. HSM 73-11001. Cincinnati: NIOSH.

———. 1998. *Criteria for a Recommended Standard: Occupational Noise Exposure, Revised Criteria 1998.* Publication No. 98-126. Cincinnati: NIOSH.

Ostergaard, P.B. 1986. Physics of sound. In *Noise and Hearing Conservation Manual.* Edited by E.H. Berger, W.D. Ward, J.C. Morrill, and L.H. Royster. Fairfax, VA: American Industrial Hygiene Association.

Plog, B.A. 1996. Overview of industrial hygiene. In *Fundamentals of Industrial Hygiene.* Edited by B.A. Plog, J. Niland, and P.J. Quinlan. Itasca, IL: National Safety Council.

Sanders, M.S., and J.M. Peay. 1988. *Human Factors in Mining.* IC 9182. Washington, DC: U.S. Department of the Interior, Bureau of Mines.

Scott, R. 1997. *Basic Concepts of Industrial Hygiene.* Boca Raton, FL: CRC Press.

Standard, J.J. 1996. Industrial noise. In *Fundamentals of Industrial Hygiene*. Edited by B.A. Plog, J. Niland, and P.J. Quinlan. Itasca, IL: National Safety Council.

Stern, M.B., and S.Z. Mansdorf. 1999. *Applications and Computational Elements of Industrial Hygiene.* Boca Raton, FL: CRC Press.

Suter, A.H. 1986. Hearing conservation. In *Noise and Hearing Conservation Manual.* Edited by E.H. Berger, W.D. Ward, J.C. Morrill, and L.H. Royster. Fairfax, VA: American Industrial Hygiene Association.

Ward, W.D. 1986. Anatomy and physiology of the ear: normal and damaged hearing. In *Noise and Hearing Conservation Manual.* Edited by E.H. Berger, W.D. Ward, J.C. Morrill, and L.H. Royster. Fairfax, VA: American Industrial Hygiene Association.

Wentz, C.A. 1998. *Safety, Health and Environmental Protection*. New York: WCB McGraw-Hill.

CHAPTER 22

Other Industrial Hygiene Concerns

Melinda Pon
Manager, Occupational and Environmental Health, BHP Minerals

Illa Gilbert-Jones, C.I.H., C.S.P.
Phelps Dodge Corporation, Phoenix, Arizona

In earlier sections of this book, whole chapters were devoted to industrial hygiene concerns common throughout the mining industry—noise and dust. This chapter covers many other concerns, although they are not necessarily found throughout the industry. Among those we discuss in this chapter are metals, welding, diesel exhaust emissions, solvents, sulfuric acid, cyanides, thermal stressors, work at high altitudes, and biohazards. Although there may be many more associated with mining, it is beyond the scope of this chapter to address all other industrial hygiene concerns. Each section provides an overview of the associated mining application, the health effects, and the risk management practices.

METALS

During mechanical extraction of ores or minerals, there is potential exposure to the metals present. The extent of exposure depends on the metal concentration in the ore matrix, the concentration of airborne dust, and the time of exposure. In metal mining, the base metals are usually considered to be copper, lead, zinc, tin, mercury, and antimony. The ores containing these metals are often complexed with minor metals such as arsenic, cadmium, bismuth, indium, selenium, and tellurium, and with precious metals such as gold, silver, and platinum. Once the mineral is extracted, it moves through a series of processing steps: cleaning or washing for coal, and crushing and milling to concentrate metal ore. Throughout the concentration process, the metallic percentage in the mixture may increase, thereby raising the potential for metal exposure. In the extraction and processing stages of mining, potential exposure to metals can occur when airborne dust is created, or in the generation of fumes when heat is applied to the concentrate or to equipment contaminated with metal dust. Other potential sources of metal fume exposure include assay furnaces and welding, discussed in more detail later in this chapter.

Industrial hygienists face the task of determining the health risks associated with hazardous materials in the work environment and providing management with information to manage these risks. Understanding toxicity and exposure are critical in determining health risks and because all metals cannot be covered in this chapter, we used toxicity and relevant regulations as factors in the selection process. Of the four metals selected, arsenic, cadmium, and lead all have specific Occupational Health and Safety Administration (OSHA) standards and established occupational exposure values. Mercury is included because of its toxicity and its inclusion by the Mine Safety and Health Administration (MSHA) in its recent draft guideline on biological monitoring (MSHA 1999). The exposure values for metals discussed in this chapter are presented in Table 22.1 and include those established by MSHA, the National Institute for Occupational Safety and Health (NIOSH), and the

TABLE 22.1   Occupational exposure values for various metals (ACGIH 1998)

Metal	MSHA (mg/m^3)	OSHA (mg/m^3)	NIOSH (mg/m^3)	ACGIH* (mg/m^3)
Inorganic arsenic	0.50	0.01	0.002†	0.01
Cadmium (inhalable)	0.20	0.005	Lowest‡	0.01
Cadmium (respirable)	—	—	—	0.002
Copper (dust and mists)	1	1	1.0	1.0
Copper (fume)	1	0.1	0.1	0.2
Lead	0.15	0.050	< 0.1	0.05
Mercury	0.05	0.1§	0.1§	0.025
Nickel (elemental/metal)	1.00	1	0.015	1.5
Silver	0.01	0.01	0.01	0.1

*From American Conference of Governmental Industrial Hygienists, Inc., 1998 *Threshold Limit Values (TLVs®) for Chemical Substances and Physical Agents and Biological Exposure Indices (BEIs®).* Reprinted with permission.

†15-minute exposure

‡Lowest feasible concentration

§Ceiling

American Conference of Governmental Industrial Hygienists (ACGIH). MSHA standards incorporate by reference the 1972 (coal) and 1973 (metal/nonmetal) editions of the ACGIH publication "TLVs (Threshold Limit Values) for Chemical Substances in Workroom Air Adopted by ACGIH."

Measurement

The values in Table 22.1 are airborne concentrations, and unless indicated they are 8-hour time-weighted averages (TWA). In the typical work environment, airborne concentrations are measured to assess the worker's inhalation exposures. The most popular air sampling method for determining airborne concentrations of metals involves the use of a solid sorbent, cellulose ester membrane filter, with a pore size of 0.8 micrometer (μm). The filter, held in a plastic cassette, is connected by plastic tubing to a battery-operated pump. The pump is worn on a belt and the filter cassette is placed in the breathing zone (e.g., clipped to the lapel of the worker). The pump is set at a known flow rate between 1 and 4 L per minute (NIOSH 1994) with a run time of up to 8 hours. In determining the 8-hour TWA, all operations likely to generate metal dust or fume must be included in the sampling period. The metals collected on the filter are determined by a variety of techniques; however, the sample filter must first be dissolved in an aqueous medium. The solution is then analyzed. To date the most common techniques for metal analysis used are flame atomic absorption (AA) spectroscopy and inductively coupled plasma, atomic emission spectroscopy (ICP).

As mentioned earlier, air sampling provides data on potential inhalation exposure. However, there are other routes of exposure to metals such as ingestion and to a lesser degree skin absorption. Biological monitoring, which includes exposure on and off work, can indicate overall exposure or the body burden. Thus, it should be conducted in conjunction with, and to substantiate, air monitoring. Biological monitoring procedures require the collection of a biological specimen (urine, blood, or exhaled air) at specified times. These sampling times are based on the uptake and elimination of the chemical and their metabolites. Table 22.2 presents the ACGIH Biological Exposure Indices (BEI) and the OSHA levels that require employee action for the metals discussed in this section. The BEI values for contaminant or metabolites are expressed as micrograms per deciliter (μg/dL), per liter (μg/L), or per gram (μg/g) of whole blood and as micrograms per gram (μg/g) of creatinine in urine.

Health Effects

Arsenic   Arsenic is ubiquitous and is found in trace quantities in plants, animals, the atmosphere, and weather and geologic formations. Human exposure can be through food such as vegetables, grains, fruits, seafood, meats, and tobacco products, as well as arsenic-contaminated drinking water. It is rarely found in nature as a pure element. Instead, it is usually associated with lead, zinc, copper, and gold-bearing minerals and occurs as a trisulfide or in arsenopyrites (Nelson 1983). Inorganic and

TABLE 22.2 ACGIH BEIs and OSHA levels that trigger employer action

	Urine		Blood	
	ACGIH*	OSHA	ACGIH	OSHA
Inorganic arsenic	50 µg/g	None	None	None
Cadmium	5 µg/g	3 µg/g	5 µg/L	5 µg/L
Lead	None	None	30 µg/100 mL	40 µg/100 g
Inorganic mercury	35 µg/g	None	15 µg/L	None

*From American Conference of Governmental Industrial Hygienists, Inc., 1998 *Threshold Limit Values (TLVs®) for Chemical Substances and Physical Agents and Biological Exposure Indices (BEIs®)*. Reprinted with permission.

organic forms of arsenic are present in coal and oil shale and it is a minor constituent of crude petroleum. Occupational exposure to arsenic is primarily through the burning of coal or smelting of metal ores containing arsenic.

It is important to note that arsine (AsH_3, arsenic hydride) gas is the most acutely toxic form of arsenic and that inhalation of 250 ppm (parts per million) is instantly lethal (NIOSH 1979). Arsine gas can evolve when metallic arsenide reacts with water or when nascent hydrogen is generated in the presence of arsenic. The sampling method for arsine gas is different from the method previously described for metals. Rather than a filter, the media is a solid sorbent tube with a sampling rate of 0.01 to 0.2 L/min, NIOSH Method 6001 (NIOSH 1994). Another form of arsenic is arsenic trioxide (As_2O_3), which can be produced as a byproduct of smelting ores containing arsenic. In such an environment it can be present as a vapor. Air sampling for total arsenic in the presence of arsenic trioxide requires a treated filter to assure that the vapor is captured on the sampling media, NIOSH Method 7901 (NIOSH 1994).

Routes of exposure to arsenic compounds can be by way of absorption through the gastrointestinal tract, lungs, and skin. Once absorbed it is distributed to various organs and excreted mainly through urine (Wang 1996). Symptoms of acute arsenic poisoning are burning and dryness of the oral and nasal cavities, gastrointestinal disturbances, and muscle spasms. In extreme overexposures, vertigo, delirium, and coma may occur. Chronic exposure can result in malaise and fatigue and may also result in gastrointestinal disturbances, hyperpigmentation, and peripheral neuropathy (Goyer 1991). Evidence of carcinogenic effects from chronic exposure to arsenic came from studies on lung cancer in smelter workers and skin cancer in people exposed to arsenic-containing drinking water (Wang 1996).

Arsine combines with hemoglobin and destroys the red blood cells. The initial symptoms of acute arsine poisoning are headache, malaise, weakness, dizziness, difficulty breathing, abdominal pain, nausea, and vomiting. Chronic exposure to arsine has been reported to cause shortness of breath and a feeling of weakness.

Cadmium   Cadmium can enter the food chain and reside in the organs of animals such as the liver and kidney. Compared to other metals, it is more readily taken up by plants such as tobacco. As a result, cadmium in cigarettes can be a major nonoccupational source of exposure. One cigarette can contain 1 to 2 µg and approximately 10% of the cadmium can be inhaled during smoking (Elinder et al. 1983). In ambient air in rural areas typical cadmium concentrations are 0.001 to 0.005 $µg/m^3$ and up to 0.06 $µg/m^3$ in urban areas (Kneip et al. 1970). Cadmium from diet and ambient air in North America and Europe has been estimated to be about 10 to 40 µg/day (Goyer 1991).

Little is known about the mechanism of cadmium toxicity. Early symptoms of acute inhalation exposure include upper respiratory irritation and cough. After 1 to 10 hours, shortness of breath, chest pain, and flu-like symptoms (fever, headache, and chills) may occur. Acute pulmonary edema may develop. Nausea, vomiting, and abdominal pain were observed after ingestion of relatively high concentrations of cadmium-contaminated beverages (Nordberg 1972). The kidney contains a major part of the body burden and is the critically affected organ when long-term chronic exposure occurs. Epidemiologic studies on the relationship between long-term inhalation exposure to cadmium and lung and prostate cancer led the International Agency on Research on Cancer (IARC) to conclude in 1987 that long-term occupational exposure to cadmium may contribute to lung cancer. Confounding exposures to arsenic, nickel, and possibly other respiratory carcinogens, including cigarettes, prevented a definitive conclusion (IARC 1987).

Lead   Lead is the most ubiquitous toxic metal and at high doses is toxic to most living things. In humans, its toxicity depends on its solubility in body fluids and the size of the particles. For example, lead sulfide is slightly soluble in gastric juice and poorly absorbed when inhaled (Carlson 1913), whereas, lead carbonate or sulfate is more soluble and pose a greater hazard during mining extraction and processing. Galena contains lead sulfide and lead poisoning is rare among miners of galena (Finkel 1983), although it has been significant when mining oxidized ores, sulfates, or carbonates, that are near the surface.

Occupational exposures to lead are rarely acute. They are chronic in nature and affect the central nervous, the heme, and the gastrointestinal systems. Symptoms include dulled senses, depression, irritability, insomnia, memory loss, muscle and joint pain, tremor, abdominal pain, anemia, and peripheral neuropathy. The kidney may also be affected resulting in elevated blood pressure (Goyer 1991). "Lead line," a bluish-black stippling that appears along the margin of the gums, usually evident along the lower incisors, but in some cases on the lining of the cheeks, may develop. The reproductive system of both men and women can be affected by lead exposure. Sperm abnormalities (Lancrajan 1975), depressed libido, and impotence may result from overexposure. Reports on miscarriage, stillbirth, and menstrual abnormalities have been documented for women who were exposed directly and as a result of exposure to contaminated clothing. Thus, it is extremely important that controls are in place to prevent transporting lead via contaminated clothing from the workplace to the home. An additional concern for preventing home contamination is that children are most susceptible to the effects of lead, in part because they can more readily absorb lead than can adults.

Along with blood lead and urine, effects on the heme system can be used as indicators of exposure to lead. Elevations of zinc protoporphyrin (ZPP) or free erythrocyte protoporphyrin (FEP) can indicate past lead exposures while blood lead will indicate a recent exposure. As shown in Table 22.2, OSHA requires action when blood lead is 40 µg/100 g of whole blood and removal from lead exposure when the blood lead reaches or exceeds 60 µg/100 g of whole blood or if the average of three consecutive blood lead levels are over 50 µg/100 g of whole blood.

Mercury   In nature, mercury exists in three chemical states—elemental metallic, divalent, and trivalent. Divalent inorganic mercury may be reduced to metallic mercury or may be converted to dimethyl mercury by anaerobic bacteria and enter the food chain by fish uptake. Nonoccupational exposure to mercury can result from the burning of fossil fuels that contain mercury and consumption of food that contains organic mercury.

Metallic mercury volatilizes to mercury vapor at ambient air temperatures and as a result is the most likely means by which a worker can be exposed. Mercury can be found in the ore that contains gold and silver. The process of recovering the precious metals from the ore concentrates mercury, and as a result, the potential for miner exposure to mercury can occur throughout the concentration and refinery process. Concentrating the precious metals will also concentrate mercury by a factor of 3,000 to 4,000 (Marsden et al. 1992).

Acute exposure affects the pulmonary and the central nervous systems. Effects on the respiratory system can manifest themselves as pneumonitis, bronchitis, chest pain, cough, and shortness of breath. Mouth sores and skin rashes have also been reported (Lillis et al. 1985; Levin and Polos 1988). Symptoms associated with acute central nervous system effects are tremors and increased excitability (Goyer 1991). Miners are more likely to be chronically exposed to elemental mercury and the critical organ associated with chronic exposure is the central nervous system. Symptoms of chronic exposure that have been observed are tremors, depression, personality or memory changes, fatigue, and irritability. Similar to lead, a dark discoloration at the gum and tooth interface may appear. The kidney will contain the greatest concentration following exposure to mercury vapor and damage to the kidney can be detected in urine (Bouchet 1980). Unlike the other metals, skin absorption of mercury because of poor hygiene can contribute to overall exposure.

Risk Management

Exposure to metals in the mechanical extraction and processing stages of mining would primarily be as a result of exposure to dust. Other constituents of the dust may pose a greater hazard because of its concentration in the ore. For example, the presence of silica in the ore matrix may be the greater inhalation hazard when physical forces create dust. Accordingly, controlling exposure to the major constituents of the dust will likely result in reducing the potential for metal dust exposure. Dust control can be accomplished with the use of one or a combination of techniques: dust collection systems, wet dust suppression systems, airborne dust capture through water sprays, and isolation. Dust collection systems capture airborne dust from the source and then transport the dust to a collector that cleans the air. Liquids, usually water, are used in a wet dust suppression system to wet the material and immobilize the dust, which prevents the particles from becoming airborne. Isolation separates the worker from the dust. For example, the worker can be placed in an enclosed cab or control room and supplied with fresh, clean, filtered air (Mody et al. 1988). For additional information on dust control, refer to chapter 20.

If heat is applied such as in welding, soldering, or cutting, airborne metal fumes can become a significant inhalation concern. Controlling toxic metal fumes at the source is the most prudent measure for protecting the worker. It employs the first level of the control hierarchy, engineering controls. The overall toxic metal exposure prevention program must incorporate local ventilation. If feasible engineering controls cannot control airborne levels below established limits, respirator use for additional protection can be considered.

Medical surveillance as an administrative control enhances the prevention program by enabling the employer to detect and eliminate underlying causes (i.e., inadequate controls or improper use of personal protective equipment [PPE]). It is aimed at detecting an illness or organ dysfunction at an early treatable phase. The OSHA substance-specific standards for lead, cadmium, and arsenic require a medical surveillance program. MSHA recently issued a draft guideline for medical surveillance and biological monitoring for these three metals and mercury (MSHA 1999).

Exposure can continue beyond the work environment as a consequence of contaminated clothing or poor personal hygiene. Contaminated clothing worn outside of the work area can transport the contaminants to personal vehicles and belongings, lunchrooms, and home, potentially exposing others. Clothing contaminated with lead, arsenic, cadmium, and mercury should be stored in a controlled area and laundered by a person or service trained in the hazards and proper handling of contaminated clothing. Showers and a clean room should be provided to separate uncontaminated street clothes from contaminated work clothes. Poor personal hygiene can result in ingesting contaminants by handling of beverages, food, and cigarettes with soiled hands. A separate lunchroom with hand washing facilities available should be provided to prevent these exposures.

WELDING

Welding describes the union of metal pieces at joint faces that are rendered plastic or liquid by heat or pressure or both. The three common direct sources of heat are flame produced by the combustion of fuel gas with air or oxygen, electrical arc, and electrical resistance (Platcow and Lyndon 1998).

There are more than 80 different types of welding and allied processes in commercial use (NIOSH 1988). These include the major categories of arc welding, oxyfuel gas welding, resistance welding, brazing, and thermal cutting. Welding, brazing, and thermal cutting processes generate exposures to gaseous and particulate contaminants as well as physical agents. Table 22.3 summarizes the description and hazards associated with various welding processes.

Table 22.4 (American Welding Society [AWS] 1973) is an adaptation of an AWS schematic representation of the "possible constituents of welding fumes" (i.e., toxic air contaminants that are characterized into toxicological subgroups). The "family" of welding fumes and gases is categorized into particulates with potential for pneumoconioses, and pulmonary irritation or toxic inhalation; and gases with potential for primary pulmonary or nonpulmonary health effects.

TABLE 22.3   Description and hazards of welding processes

Welding Process	Description	Hazards
Gas Welding and Cutting		
Welding	Torch melts metal surface and filler rod, causing a joint to be formed.	Metal fumes, nitrogen dioxide, carbon monoxide, noise, burns, infrared radiation, fire, explosions
Brazing	Two metal surfaces are bonded without melting the metal. Melting the filler metal is above 450°C. Heating is done by flame heating, resistance heating, and induction heating.	Metal fumes (especially cadmium), fluorides, fire, explosions, burns
Soldering	Similar to brazing, except the melting temperatures of the filler metal are lower. Heating is done using a soldering iron.	Fluxes, lead fumes, burns
Metal cutting and flame gouging	The metal is heated by a flame, and a jet of pure oxygen is directed onto the point of cutting and moved along the line to be cut. In flame gouging, a strip of surface metal is removed but the metal is not cut through.	Metal fumes, nitrogen dioxide, carbon monoxide, noise, burns, infrared radiation, fire, explosion
Gas pressure welding	Parts are heated by gas jets while under pressure, and become forged together.	Metal fumes, nitrogen dioxide, carbon monoxide, noise, burns, infrared radiation, fire, explosions
Flux-Shielded Arc Welding		
Shielded metal arc welding (SMAC); "stick" arc welding, manual metal arc welding (MMA), open arc welding	Uses a consumable electrode consisting of a metal core surrounded by a coating.	Metal fumes, fluorides (especially with low-hydrogen electrodes), infrared and ultraviolet radiation, burns, electrical fire, noise, ozone, nitrogen dioxide
Submerged arc welding (SAW)	A blanket of granulated flux is deposited on the workplace, followed by a consumable bare metal wire electrode. The arc melts the flux to produce a protective molten shield in the welding zone.	Fluorides, fires, burns, infrared radiation, electrical, metal fumes, noise, ultraviolet radiation, ozone, nitrogen dioxide
Gas-Shielded Arc Welding		
Metal inert gas (MIG), gas metal arc welding (GMAC)	The electrode is normally a bare consumable wire of similar composition to the weld metal and is fed continuously to the arc.	Ultraviolet radiation, metal fumes, ozone, carbon monoxide (with carbon dioxide gas), nitrogen dioxide, fire, burns, infrared radiation, electrical, fluorides, noise
Tungsten inert gas (TIG), gas tungsten arc welding (GTAW), heliarc	The tungsten electrode is nonconsumable and the filler metal is introduced as a consumable into the arc manually.	Ultraviolet radiation, metal fumes, ozone, nitrogen dioxide, fires, burns, infrared radiation, electrical, noise, fluorides, carbon monoxide
Plasma arc welding (PAW) and plasma arc spraying, tungsten arc cutting	Similar to TIG welding, except that the arc and stream of inert gases pass through a small orifice before reaching the workplace, creating a "plasma" of highly ionized gas which can achieve temperatures of more than 33,000°C. This is also used for metallizing.	Metal fumes, ozone, nitrogen dioxide, ultraviolet and infrared radiation, noise, fire, burns, electrical, fluorides, carbon monoxide, possible x-rays

Continues next page

TABLE 22.3   Description and hazards of welding processes (continued)

Welding Process	Description	Hazards
Gas-Shielded Arc Welding (continued)		
Flux core arc welding (FCAW), metal active gas welding (MAG)	Uses a flux-cored consumable electrode; may have carbon dioxide shield (MAG)	Ultraviolet radiation, metal fumes, ozone, carbon monoxide (with carbon dioxide gas), nitrogen dioxide, fire, burns, infrared radiation, electrical, fluorides, noise
Electric Resistance Welding		
Resistance welding (spot, seam, projection, or butt welding)	A high current at low voltage flows through the two components from electrodes. The heat generated at the interface between the components brings them to welding temperatures. During the passage of the current, pressure by the electrodes produces a forged weld. No flux or filler metal is used.	Ozone, noise (sometimes), machinery hazards, fire, burns, electrical, metal fumes
Electro-slag welding	Used for vertical butt welding. The work pieces are set vertically, with a gap between them, and copper plates or shoes are placed on one or both sides of the joints to form a bath. An arc is established under a flux layer between one or more continuously fed electrode wires and metal plate. A pool of molten metal is formed, protected by a molten flux or slag, which is kept molten by resistance to the current passing between the electrode and the work pieces. This resistance-generated heat melts the sides of the joint and the electrode wire, filling the joint and making a weld. As welding progresses, the molten metal and slag are retained in position by shifting the copper plates.	Burns, fire, infrared radiation, electrical, metal fumes
Flash welding	The two metal parts to be welded are connected to a low-voltage, high-current source. When the ends of the components are brought into contact, the large current flows, causing "flashing" and bringing the ends of the components to welding temperatures. A forged weld is obtained by pressure.	Electrical, burns, fire, metal fumes
Other Welding Processes		
Electron beam welding	A work piece in a vacuum chamber is bombarded by a beam of electrons from an electron gun at high voltages. The energy of the electrons is transformed into heat upon striking the work piece, thus melting the metal and fusing the work piece.	X-rays at high voltages, electrical, burns, metal dust, confined spaces
Arcair cutting	An arc is struck between the end of a carbon electrode (in a manual electrode holder with its own supply of compressed air) and the work piece. The molten metal produced is blown away by jets of compressed air.	Metal fumes, carbon monoxide, nitrogen dioxide, ozone, fire, burns, infrared radiation, electrical
Friction welding	A purely mechanical welding technique in which one component remains stationary while the other is rotated against it under pressure. Heat is generated by friction and at forging temperature, the rotation ceases. A forging pressure then affects the weld.	Heat, burns, machinery hazards

Continues next page

TABLE 22.3   Description and hazards of welding processes (continued)

Welding Process	Description	Hazards
Other Welding Processes (continued)		
Laser welding and drilling	Laser beams can be used in industrial applications requiring exceptionally high precision, such as miniature assemblies and micro techniques in the electronic industry or spinnerets for the artificial fiber industry. The laser beam melts and joins the work pieces.	Electrical, laser radiation, ultraviolet radiation, fire, burns, metal fumes, decomposition products of work piece coatings
Stud welding	An arc is struck between a metal stud (acting as the electrode) held in a stud welding gun and the metal plate to be joined, and raises the temperature of the ends of the component to melting point. The gun forces the stud against the plate and welds it. Shielding is provided by a ceramic ferrule surrounding the stud.	Metal fumes, infrared and ultraviolet radiation, burns, electrical, fire, noise, ozone, nitrogen dioxide
Thermite welding	A mixture of aluminum powder and a metal oxide powder (iron, copper, etc.) is ignited in a crucible, producing molten metal with the evolution of intense heat. The crucible is tapped and the molten metal flows into the cavity to be welded (which is surrounded by a sand mold). This is often used to repair castings or forgings.	Fire, explosions, infrared radiation, burns

Source: Platkow and Lyndon 1998

TABLE 22.4   Possible constituents of welding fumes

Particulates				Gases		
					Primary	
			Pulmonary Irritants or Toxic Inhalants		Pulmonary	Nonpulmonary
	Pneumoconiosis					
Fibrotic	Nonfibrotic	Relatively harmless				
Silica	Beryllium	Carbon	Cadmium		Ozone	Carbon monoxide
Asbestos		Tin	Chromium		Phosgene	Carbon dioxide
Copper		Iron	Fluorides		Phosphine	
		Aluminum	Lead		Oxides of nitrogen	
			Manganese			
			Mercury			
			Molybdenum			
			Nickel			
			Titanium			
			Vanadium			
			Zinc			

Source: AWS 1973

Health Effects

In addition to safety hazards posed by fire, explosion, projectiles, heat and burns, and electrical and energy sources, welding produces a number of health hazards. Among these are physical and chemical hazards.

Physical Hazards   Physical hazards that may arise from welding include:

Ultraviolet radiation—The bright light generated by the electric arc contains ultraviolet radiation. Without a shield or helmet outfitted with the correct filter grade, exposure can produce painful conjunctivitis or photoophthalmia, known as "eye flash" or "arc eye." Immediate medical attention must be provided because overexposure may also cause overheating and skin burn. Because of this sunburn effect, exposed areas such as the face and other parts of the body should be properly protected. Workers near arc welding operations should be separated by screens to protect them from ultraviolet radiation hazards.

Ionizing radiation—X-ray or gamma-ray equipment, used to inspect welds, can generate exposures to ionizing radiation from equipment with insufficient shielding and locking mechanisms. Strict adherence to safe radioactive source procedures must be implemented to protect workers from ionizing radiation hazards.

Noise—Several welding processes, such as plasma welding, resistance welding machines, gas welding, and the use of compressed air can generate noise levels above 90 dBA. Individuals potentially exposed to these noise levels should be included in a hearing conservation program as described in a previous chapter on noise.

Chemical Hazards   A variety of welding sources generate airborne contaminants including the base metal, the metal in the filler rod or steel constituents, constituents of the coating or paint and grease on the base metal, flux coating on the filler rod, the reaction of heat or ultraviolet light on the air or chlorinated hydrocarbons, and inert gas used as a shield. Local exhaust ventilation should be used to capture welding fumes and gases such as ozone, carbon monoxide, and nitrogen dioxide. When ventilation is inadequate, additional measures such as appropriate respiratory protection may be necessary to protect the welder from increased exposure to toxic fumes.

Metal Fume Fever   Metal fume fever is an acute condition that occurs several hours after inhalation of metal particulates or its oxides. Marked by a bad taste in the mouth, dryness and respiratory irritation, cough, shortness of breath (dyspnea), and chest tightness may result. Severe cases may be accompanied by nausea, headache, severe flu-like symptoms such as chills and fever that can present 10 to 12 hours after exposure. The common welding oxides associated with metal fume fever are:

Iron oxide—Siderosis, fibrosis caused by iron oxide particles, is a form of pneumoconiosis. The ACGIH TLV-TWA for iron oxide dust and fume is 5 mg/m^3 (ACGIH 1998).

Zinc oxide—Overexposure to zinc oxide fumes can result in flu-like symptoms associated with metal fume fever. The ACGIH TLV-TWA for zinc oxide fume is 5 mg/m^3 and short-term exposure limit (STEL) of 10 mg/m^3. For zinc oxide dust, the TLV-TWA is 10 mg/m^3 (ACGIH 1998).

Other Toxic Air Contaminants   Other toxic air contaminants that may arise from welding processes include:

Manganese—affects the central nervous system and lungs. The TLV-TWA is 0.2 mg/m^3 (ACGIH 1998).

Copper—produces irritation of the gastrointestinal tract. The TLV-TWA is 0.2 mg/m^3 for fumes and 1 mg/m^3 for dusts (ACGIH 1998).

Fluorides—cause irritation and affect the bones; fluorosis can develop. The TLV-TWA is 2.5 mg/m^3 (ACGIH 1998).

Other metallic air contaminants may include aluminum, beryllium, cadmium, lead, and nickel. The health effects of some of these metals have been discussed previously.

Carbon monoxide—produces anoxia and affects the cardiovascular and central nervous systems. The TLV-TWA is 25 ppm (ACGIH 1998).

Ozone—affects pulmonary function; produces respiratory irritation, wheezing and pulmonary edema, headaches, and other effects. The TLV-TWA is work dependent: 0.05 ppm for heavy work, 0.08 ppm for moderate work, and 0.1 ppm for light work (ACGIH 1998).

Oxides of nitrogen—nitric oxide and nitrogen dioxide, causing irritation, chronic bronchitis, emphysema, and pulmonary edema. The TLV-TWA concentration of nitric oxide is 25 ppm. Nitrogen dioxide's TLV-TWA is 3 ppm with a STEL of 5 ppm (ACGIH 1998). The MSHA permissible exposure limit concentration is 5 ppm; however, it is a ceiling limit rather than a STEL and cannot be exceeded during any part of working exposure.

Confined Spaces   If welding is required in a confined space, it is critical that a confined space entry program be implemented to ensure that the space is safe for entry and work. Atmospheres in confined spaces can be toxic, explosive, and/or oxygen deficient. Because welding processes can produce toxic air contaminants or decrease oxygen content, or both, monitoring the atmosphere and providing adequate ventilation are crucial to prevent buildup of hazardous fumes and gases and to ensure sufficient oxygen levels.

Measurement

Routine monitoring should be conducted in the workplace for exposure determinations. Because of the myriad airborne gaseous and particulate constituents in welding processes and the physical agents such as noise, ultraviolet, and x-ray radiation, a sound workplace sampling strategy should be developed and implemented. Specific air sampling and analytical methodologies, and physical agent monitoring techniques are available and have been described in other sections of this book. A trained industrial hygienist should conduct the sampling and interpret the results.

Because of the health risks associated with welding, biomonitoring may be useful for assessing overall exposures to cadmium, chromium, aluminum, fluoride ions, and lead. In a medical monitoring program, particular attention should be paid to the respiratory system, eyes, and skin during pre-placement, periodic monitoring, emergencies, and termination.

Risk Management

Local exhaust ventilation should be the primary engineering control to capture gases and fumes at the source. If feasible ventilation cannot control exposure to below established limits, respirators should be worn to provide added protection against toxic air contaminants. Welders should be provided with the appropriate PPE including welding helmets with appropriate filters and shields; eye, face, and respiratory protection; and protective work clothing. Workers near welding processes may also need protection from ultraviolet radiation, noise, and air contaminants with proper screens, engineering controls, and PPE.

DIESEL EXHAUST EMISSIONS

Diesel-powered equipment has been commonplace in the mining industry for decades. The preference for diesel units over electrical trailing cable, trolley wire, or battery-powered equipment has resulted from improved safety, enhanced mobility, increased productivity and efficiency, and increased power. In spite of these benefits, diesel engines generate exhaust emissions that if not controlled may pose a health risk to miners.

Diesel exhaust is a complex mixture of thousands of chemicals in solid and gaseous forms. This mixture contains gases such as carbon monoxide, carbon dioxide, the oxides of nitrogen (i.e., nitric oxide and nitrogen dioxide), and sulfur dioxide; hundreds of different hydrocarbons; and diesel particulate matter (DPM). DPM is a mixture of chemical compounds composed of nonvolatile elemental carbon; hundreds of different adsorbed or condensed hydrocarbons such as polycyclic aromatic hydrocarbons (PAHs) and nitro PAHs; sulfates; and trace quantities of metallic compounds.

Health Effects

Miners working in an underground environment where diesel equipment is used are exposed to a myriad of pollutants (Watts 1987, 1992; MSHA 1997; New South Wales [NSW] Minerals Council 1996, 1999). Because of the chemical complexity of the exhaust, evaluating the health risk to miners from exposure to diesel exhaust is particularly difficult. This has been the subject of evolving knowledge, research, and controversy. The controversy arises from the different assumptions and models that have been used to interpret the data—data that have been either inadequate or unavailable. On the other hand, what is not controversial is that diesel exhaust produces complaints about headaches, eye and throat irritation, and unpleasant odors.

Diesel Particulate Matter   Ninety percent of the diesel particulates, by mass, have an equivalent aerodynamic diameter of less than 1.0 μm. DPM contains solid carbon particles that are respirable and small enough to penetrate the deepest regions of the lung. Additionally, the carbon cores of DPM are coated with thousands of complex chemicals, some of which are known to cause cancer in experimental animals and are mutagenic in toxicological assays. These characteristics of DPM give rise to concern about its potential to cause or contribute to the development of lung disease. Exposures to high diesel particulate levels may also result in eye and throat irritation.

The potential carcinogenicity of DPM has been the subject of many reviews (NIOSH 1988; IARC 1989; HEI 1999; ACGIH 1998; WHO 1996; NTP 1998; OEHHA 1998; U.S. EPA 1998) and these reports have identified diesel exhaust as a probable human carcinogen or comparable classification.

NIOSH's *Current Intelligence Bulletin* (1988) recommended that "whole diesel exhaust be regarded as a potential occupational carcinogen." The IARC (1989) classified "diesel engine exhaust as probably carcinogenic to humans." However, these findings continue to be a subject of debate in the scientific community. In the absence of clear and confirmed evidence of DPM as a known, human lung carcinogen, it is prudent that DPM exposures be reduced as low as reasonably practical.

The ACGIH TLV-TWA for diesel particulate matter <1 μm is 0.15 mg/m^3. ACGIH has added DPM to the Notice of Intended Changes for 1999–2000 with a TLV recommendation of 0.05 mg/m^3.

Diesel Exhaust Gases   The gaseous components of diesel exhaust include carbon monoxide, carbon dioxide, oxides of nitrogen, and sulfur oxides. These gases have the potential to cause sensory irritation, asphyxiation, and suffocation (Proctor and Hughes 1996; NSW Minerals Council 1996, 1997).

Carbon monoxide (CO) reduces the blood's capacity to carry oxygen and affects the cardiovascular and central nervous systems. With increased carbon monoxide levels in the body, there is the potential loss of consciousness, asphyxiation, and death.

Carbon dioxide (CO$_2$) displaces oxygen in the lungs. Asphyxiation resulting in death can occur when miners are exposed to high concentrations of CO$_2$ in confined spaces and coal seams or gas outburst emissions. Sensory perceptions and disturbances in judgment result from the lack of oxygen and elevated CO$_2$ levels.

Nitrogen dioxide (NO$_2$) is a severe respiratory irritant. Lung problems such as bronchitis, emphysema, and pulmonary edema can result with excessive exposure and can occur immediately or follow after several days or weeks.

Irritant gases such as nitric oxide, aldehydes, and sulfur oxides irritate the mucous membranes of the body such as parts of the eye, nasal passages, throat, and lungs. The ambient gas concentrations and individual sensitivity influence the degree of irritation experienced.

The health effects, ACGIH's TLVs, and MSHA's permissible exposure limits for diesel gaseous pollutants are summarized in Table 22.5.

Measurement

The sampling strategy for measuring diesel exhaust emissions includes ambient and personal sampling to determine the gaseous and particulate concentrations in the raw exhaust and the in-mine work environment. Raw exhaust from diesel engines is measured in terms of volume and gas content (CO, nitric oxide [NO], and NO$_2$). Electronic equipment can be used to accurately measure gaseous component levels.

Ambient airborne concentration of diesel emissions and its constituent gaseous and particulate components can be taken at fixed locations in the work environment.

TABLE 22.5   Health effects, TLVs, and MSHA's permissible exposure limits for diesel gaseous pollutants

Pollutant	Health Effects (ACGIH)*	ACGIH TLVs* (ppm)	MSHA PELs† Coal (ppm)	MSHA PELs† Noncoal (ppm)
Carbon monoxide	Anoxia, central vascular system, central nervous system, reproductive	25	50	50
Carbon dioxide	Asphyxiation	5,000 30,000‡	5,000	5,000
Nitric oxide	Anoxia, irritation, cyanosis	25	25	25
Nitrogen dioxide	Irritation, pulmonary edema	3 5‡	5§	5§
Sulfur dioxide	Irritation	2 5‡	2	5
Formaldehyde	Irritation, cancer (nasal)	0.3§	2§	2§

* Source: ACGIH 1998
† Source: 30 CFR
‡ Short-Term Exposure Limit (STEL)
§ Ceiling (C)

Sampling methodologies for gases and DPM are subject to a variety of advantages and technical limitations. The following describes some of the common methodologies and their associated limitations (Williams et al. 1987).

Detector Tubes for Measuring Gaseous Pollutants   Detector tubes, such as stain tubes and passive sampler tubes, are simple measurement devices that are available for the gaseous pollutants–CO, CO_2, NO, and NO_2–and for sulfur dioxide (SO_2). Detector tubes are simple and cost effective and may be useful for characterizing air quality. However, they do not provide sufficient accuracy as a measurement technique if accuracy greater than • 25% is required.

Electrochemical Instrumentation for Measuring Gaseous Pollutants   More sophisticated and expensive instrumentation, based on electrochemical cells, is available for detecting and measuring gas concentrations. This instrumentation is intrinsically safe for mine atmospheres, can be calibrated, has a typical accuracy of • 2%, and provides quick response times.

Personal Diesel Particulate Sampling and Analysis   Equipment and analytical methods to accurately measure DPM levels are not yet available. The presence of carbon particles–such as carbonaceous ores, coal dust, explosives, rubber tires, cigarette smoke, and oil mist–may confound accurate measurements of diesel particulates.

Currently, a size-selective sampler that measures the mass concentration of diesel aerosol in mines is used. The technique is based on the premise that 90% of the diesel portion of the aerosol is predominantly in the submicrometer range and that the mineral dust portion is greater than 1 µm in size. The sampler has three stages: a preclassifier stage to select for respirable aerosol, an inertial impaction stage to collect mineral dust, and a final filtration stage to collect the diesel fraction of the sample (Cantrell and Rubow 1992). The sample should be collected on a preweighed 5.0-pin-pore-size vinyl Metricel® filter for gravimetric analysis. About 80% to 85% of the DPM mass is total carbon, which is composed of elemental and organic carbon. A thermal/optical reflectance elemental carbon analytical method (NIOSH Method 5040), which is a chemical analysis, is used to determine DPM if the submicrometer mass is less than 0.3 mg. The method can be used to distinguish between the elemental carbon core, the absorbed organic carbon, and the very fine coal dust in the submicron mass. For the chemical analysis, a preconditioned quartz fiber filter that has been heated in air at 400°C for 1 hour should be used (MSHA 1997). These monitoring techniques are research tools and required considerable technical skills to obtain satisfactory exposure results with acceptable accuracy (Joint Coal Board [JCB] 1999).

Risk Management

Recent advances in new engine technology and higher quality fuel for over-the-road diesel equipment have spillover benefits for the mining community. Nonetheless, diesel engine manufacturers still consider mining as a niche market. It is expected that new emission regulations and in-mine air quality standards will force the technology for the mining industry, revolutionizing conventional mining equipment.

In the interim, mining operators can adopt an integrated approach to managing workplace exposures to diesel exhaust emissions. Management commitment is fundamental to this approach. Management must be willing to allocate sufficient resources for managing diesel equipment, educating and training the workforce education and training on diesel emissions, and identifying and controlling diesel emission risks.

A suite of options is available for managing diesel emission risks. As a minimum, operators need to establish low baseline emissions by specifying and selecting clean engines and machines, using high quality diesel fuel and applying efficient aftertreatment devices.

Key factors in the reduction of particulates during diesel operation are prestart checks, routine maintenance, start-up procedures, driving and shut-down procedures, and adequate ventilation (Broken Hill Properties [BHP] Limited 1999).

Table 22.6 summarizes the control options available to reduce diesel emissions (NSW Minerals Council 1999).

Engine Design and Selection   Engine manufacturers are producing low emission, electronically controlled engines that continually optimize the fuel-injection timing and rate to match each power requirement. The control logic determines the timing and duration of fueling and results in

TABLE 22.6   Diesel emissions control options

Risk Control Measure	Effect/Advantages	Disadvantages/Penalty
Engine Selection		
More efficient engines and electronic engine control systems	Produces less emissions	Initial cost and/or replacement costs. Retrofit and reengineering costs
Totally enclosed operator compartment with filtered air	Significantly reduces operator exposure	Initial cost. Increased ongoing maintenance
Engine Maintenance		
Improved tuning, oil cleanliness	Optimizes efficiency and lowers total emissions	None. Cost-effective
Chemical decoking of engines	Reduces particulates, may increase power. The effects of decoking may be less for newer designed engines or engines operating on low emission fuels.	When decoking engines underground, exhaust emissions immediately following decoking need to be effectively managed
Diesel test station (controlled airflow over vehicle while testing engine exhaust gases)	Reduces confounding influences. Eliminates detector tubes. Better engine monitoring. Improves fleet availability	Initial cost
Fuel Quality		
Use low emission fuels (less than 0.05% sulfur)	Reduces particulates, carbon monoxide, and hydrocarbons. Reduces odors.	Requires engine retuning to maintain power. Mixing of different fuels may have adverse effects. This may be a problem with hired equipment that has been used across a range of sites. Some low emission fuels may freeze in winter. Cost premium.
Engineering Controls		
Filters	Reduces particulate emissions by up to 85%	Ongoing cost. Back pressure may become excessive if maintenance/replacement intervals are not strictly followed. Excessive back pressure may increase emissions, reduce engine life, and lower water-based conditioner (scrubber) water levels.
Exhaust post-treatment (e.g., catalytic converters, catalyzed filters, precipitation)	Lowers emissions in some situations	Cost penalty.
Advanced engine control systems	Reduces emissions if properly used.	Reliability may be an issue. May require retraining of maintenance personnel.
Ventilation		
	Currently the major method used to manage the exposure of personnel to emissions.	Not well understood. May not be adequate when multiple vehicles in use.
Work Practices		
Vehicle control systems	Has been shown to lower exposure to emissions in conjunction with adequate ventilation.	May limit the most cost effective and flexible use of equipment.
Road maintenance		
Driving procedures		

Source: NSW Minerals Council 1999

precise fuel delivery, as well as improved fuel economy and engine performance, all of which result in a cleaner burning engine. A corollary benefit is the marked reduction in the emissions of oxides of nitrogen and particulates from these types of diesel engines. However, a number of engines in the existing fleet of diesel mining equipment do not have this state-of-the-art technology. For these engines, maintenance and the application of other risk control options become critically more important for reducing miners' exposures to diesel emissions.

Engine Maintenance   Engine maintenance has an important role in the reduction of reducing diesel emissions, maximizing the service life of the engine and its components, and enhancing the reliability of engine performance. A diesel engine management program makes use of the manufacturer's specification procedures, onboard diagnostic readings to monitor engine condition, and trend analyses of emission tests. Other tools that assist in reducing diesel emissions and prevent burning off the dirty or excess hydrocarbons are chemical decoking of engines, use of high quality oil, and enhanced filtering of lubricating oil.

Fuel Quality Specifications   Fuel properties, such as cetane number, density, viscosity, volatility, and sulfur content, affect diesel emissions. The fuel quality greatly affects the sulfate particulates and the fuel aromatics on the particulates and the oxides of nitrogen. Increased cetane number and volatility can reduce hydrocarbon and carbon monoxide emissions. Whereas low sulfur fuel (0.05% sulfur) emits less sulfur dioxide and sulfate particulates, reformulated fuel has lower sulfur, a lower distillation range, a higher cetane number, and lower aromatics, and generates generally lower levels of particulates, carbon monoxide, hydrocarbons, and oxides of nitrogen. However, problems may arise in mining applications with logistics, supply, engine redesign, economics, and safety concerns for flammability, storage, handling, and other toxic emissions.

Engineering Controls   Advances have been made in recent years in engineering controls for diesel engines; however, there are technological limitations in their effectiveness of lowering diesel emissions for a range of mining equipment (NSW Minerals Council 1996; Waytulonis 1992). These engineering controls include:

Water scrubbers—The primary purpose of water scrubbers is to perform evaporative cooling on exhaust gases and to act as a flame trap. Although water scrubbers are able to reduce soot by 10% to 30%, there are no reductions in gaseous emissions. As a control technology, their applications are limited.

Dry systems technology (DST)—This alternative allows indirect cooling of exhaust gases via a tube or shell water-cooled heat exchanger. To reduce emissions, the DST includes a waterjacketed oxidation catalytic converter. Spark and flamer arrest are provided via mechanical means.

Exhaust aftertreatment devices—Exhaust aftertreatment devices must control solid (carbon), liquid (the organic fraction, such as unburned and partially burned fuel and lubrication oils) and gas-phase mixtures. Oxidation catalytic converters and filters are included in this category.

Oxidation catalytic converters—Oxidation catalytic converters are able to reduce emissions of carbon monoxide (80% to 95%), hydrocarbons (85% to 90%), and total particulates (25% to 35%) with very good reliability, durability, and odor control (Thakur and Hamilton 1998).

Filters—High-temperature and low-temperature filters are available, nonetheless, there are some limitations in their applications and costs, as well as some problems resulting from regeneration constraints. Ceramic (wall-flow) filters have questionable reliability and durability, are costly, and have two functional drawbacks: the ceramic filter element deteriorates with mechanical and thermal shock, and regeneration (self-cleaning) is dependent on exhaust temperatures greater than 400°C (752°F). Low-cost disposable filters are commercially available for mining equipment with water scrubbers and have been found to be safe and efficient. New filtration technology for mining machines is currently being developed.

Ventilation   Ventilation systems have served as the primary and supplementary sources of control for reducing miners' underground exposures to toxic air pollutants. Dilution ventilation supplemented with other types of controls should be used to reduce exposure to diesel emissions. As a minimum, ventilation rates must meet statutory and regulatory requirements for underground mines.

Work Practices   An additional method for controlling diesel emission exposures is to monitor and manage established work practices documented in procedures for operating diesels, vehicle control, road design and maintenance, and driving. Shift scheduling, in particular, altered shift work, has an impact on miners' overall exposures to diesel emissions.

Future Research Needs

Continued research efforts are necessary to reduce miners' exposures to diesel emissions to the lowest achievable levels. Among other topics, research needs to be focused on control technology, with particular attention paid to the development of cleaner engines, alternative engine and power sources, alternative sulfur-free fuels, and more efficient aftertreatment devices like ceramic systems and enhanced paper-filter-based systems.

SOLVENTS

A solvent is "a substance that dissolves another substance, most commonly water but often an organic compound" (DiNardi 1998). Solvents have many applications, ranging from pesticides to dry-cleaning chemicals. In the mining environment, solvents are used as paint thinners, parts cleaners, metal extraction chemicals, and laboratory reagents.

The toxicological effects and target organs vary according to the type of solvent. Some act as systemic poisons, anesthetics and narcotics, simple and chemical asphyxiates, and/or irritants. Although inhalation of vapors and mists is the primary route of entry for acute and chronic toxicity, oral ingestion and skin absorption can also contribute to solvent overexposures. When exposures occur above threshold levels, harmful effects can impair a person's health and functioning. These impairments can be reversible, irreversible, or deadly. Factors that complicate the solvents' effects are individual susceptibility because of age and health, the resultant effect of the different solvents in a mixture, the duration of exposure and the concentration.

Moreover, it is not sufficient to determine the hazard potential of a solvent based on toxicological effects alone. Other components to consider in evaluating potential hazard are vapor pressure, flammability, ventilation, handling procedures, volume, and air concentration. Other factors that contribute to exposure through skin contact and absorption include handling procedures and the type of clothing worn. There are also safety considerations such as the potential for ignition, flammability, and explosion that contribute to the hazard potential.

Concepts about Physical Properties of Gases and Vapors

For the purposes of this section, it is important to understand several concepts about the physical properties of gases and vapors.

- A gas (e.g., oxygen or nitrogen) is a material in a gaseous state at room temperature.
- A vapor (e.g., water, gasoline, mercury, or naphthalene) is the gaseous phase of a substance that ordinarily exists as a liquid or a solid at room temperature.
- A mist (e.g., sulfuric acid mist) is a liquid suspension in air or a material that ordinarily exists as a liquid at room temperature.

The partial pressure of gases indicates the amount of gas present in a mixture and is reflected in a ratio present at any one time even though the total pressure may change as a result of elevation changes.

The vapor pressure is the pressure characteristic, at any given temperature, of a vapor in equilibrium with its liquid or solid form.

Temperature affects the vapor pressure of a gas and not its partial pressure. Therefore, the higher the temperature, the higher the volatility or vapor pressure, which increases the potential worker exposure, especially through inhalation.

There is equilibrium in the blood between the gas concentration and the liquid in contact (i.e., the air and blood within the alveoli of the lungs). Equilibrium also exists between the atmospheric and blood concentration, which is described as the distribution coefficient (i.e., the milligram of solvent per liter of blood divided by the milligram of solvent per liter of air).

The lower the coefficient, the more rapid the saturation of the blood and distribution in the body. The differences result from differences in solubility and reactivity within the body.

Health Effects

Major Solvent Classification and Health Effects (McFee 1988; Cornish 1975)   Aqueous and organic systems are used to describe the types of solvents.

Aqueous systems are based on water and may contain acids, alkalis, detergents, and other chemicals. Aqueous systems tend to have lower systemic toxicity and lower vapor pressures than organic solvents, thus, they present lower potential inhalation hazards. Prolonged exposures to excessive levels of mists from heating, agitation, and/or spraying can potentially lead to irritant effects, contact dermatitis, throat irritation, and bronchitis.

Organic systems are based on solvents containing carbon compounds and include naphtha, mineral spirits, turpentine, benzene, carbon tetrachloride, and trichloroethylene. Organic solvents typically have higher vapor pressures than aqueous solvents. Organic solvents affect the central nervous system as either a depressant or anesthetic, and effects can range from mild narcosis to respiratory arrest and death. The following are 11 categories of organic solvents with examples and their respective TLVs (ACGIH 1998).

Aliphatic Hydrocarbons   Aliphatic hydrocarbons are straight or branched chains of carbon and hydrogen. These include alkanes, alkenes, cycloalkanes, acetylenes, and arenes. Generally, aliphatic hydrocarbons, with the exception of hexane, exhibit toxic health effects at high concentrations. Unsaturated aliphatic hydrocarbons, alkenes and alkynes, are similarly inert in the body. Examples of aliphatic hydrocarbons and their 8-hour time-weighted average TLVs are n-hexane (50 ppm), hexane (500 ppm), and octane (300 ppm).

Cyclic Hydrocarbons   Cyclic hydrocarbons are saturated and unsaturated ring structures. These solvents have physical properties similar to those of aliphatics, although they are typically more toxic. Examples of cyclic hydrocarbons and their TLVs are cyclohexane (300 ppm) and turpentine (100 ppm).

Aromatic Hydrocarbons   Aromatic hydrocarbons are characterized by one or more six-carbon ring structures with one hydrogen atom per carbon atom. The name "aromatic" comes from the solvent's aroma. On the whole, aromatic hydrocarbons are local irritants and vasodilators that cause severe pulmonary and vascular injury when absorbed into the body in sufficient concentrations. They can cause dermatitis and can be potent narcotics, with effects on the central nervous system. Of this group, benzene—with its link to leukemia—is strongly regulated and appears to be the most toxic aromatic hydrocarbon. Examples of aromatic hydrocarbons and their respective TLVs are benzene (0.5 ppm), toluene (50 ppm), and xylene (100 ppm).

Halogenated Hydrocarbons   In halogenated hydrocarbons, halogen atoms replace one or more hydrogen atoms on the backbone or branched carbon structure. Five halide elements—fluorine, chlorine, bromine, iodine, and astatine—are noted for their stability, nonflammability, and wide range of solvency. The toxicity of these compounds is related to their metabolic fate within the body. Of the halogenated hydrocarbons, carbon tetrachloride is acutely toxic to the kidney (nephrotoxic), liver (hepatotoxic), central nervous system (neurotoxic), and the gastrointestinal tract. It is suspected of causing liver cancer. Examples of halogenated hydrocarbons are tetrachloromethane (5 ppm), 1,1,1 trichloroethane (350 ppm), and trichlorofluoroethane (1,000 ppm).

Nitrohydrocarbons   Nitrohydrocarbons contain an NO_2 group and their toxicity is related to the hydrocarbon structure, aliphatic (also referred to as a paraffin) or aromatic.

Nitroparaffins are irritants and cause nausea. Acute exposures affect the central nervous system and liver. Nitroaromatics are much more acutely hazardous; they cause the formation of methemoglobin and affect the central nervous system, liver, and other organs. Examples of nitrohydrocarbons with their respective TLVs are 2-nitropropane (a suspected carcinogen; 10 ppm); nitroethane (100 ppm); and nitrobenzene (cyanosis, anoxia, liver, neurotoxicity, irritation, dermatitis; 1 ppm).

Esters   Esters and the remaining class of hydrocarbons (alcohols, aldehydes, ketones, carboxylic acids, and anhydrides) contain an oxygen in a functional group attached to a chain or ring carbon. Esters are formed by the interaction of an organic acid with an alcohol. Their toxic effects include irritation of the skin and the respiratory tract. They can also affect the central nervous system and become potent anesthetics. Examples of esters and their respective TLVs are ethyl acetate (400 ppm) and amyl acetate (100 ppm).

Ketones   Ketones contain the double-bonded carbonyl group, C=O, with two hydrocarbon groups attached to the carbon. Ketones are stable solvents with high dilution ratios compared to other hydrocarbon solvents. They have a narcotic type action and are irritating to the eyes, nose, and throat. At high concentrations, the irritant effects cannot be tolerated. At lower concentrations, impairments to judgment can result in secondary hazards. Methyl n-butyl ketone (5 ppm) causes neuropathy and peripheral neuritis.

Alcohols   Alcohols contain a single-OH group. Methanol (200 ppm) slowly produces toxic metabolites and has been associated with fatalities and injuries, vision impairment, and optic nerve injury. Ethanol (1,000 ppm) is quickly metabolized and converted to CO_2; it is the least toxic of the alcohols. Propanol (200 ppm), metabolized to toxic by-products, is more toxic than ethanol, but less toxic than other alcohols. Alcohol has a depressant, not a stimulant effect on the central nervous system. Alcohols reduce brain and spinal cord activity. Exposures to extremely high doses can result in death by involuntary ceasing of the respiratory system. The liver can also be a vulnerable target organ for alcohols.

Ethers   Ethers contain the C-O-C linkage and are made of two hydrocarbon groups held together by an oxygen atom. Ethers are characterized by their greater volatility, lower solubility in water, and higher solvent power for fats, oils, and greases. Ethers are anesthetic, irritating to the mucous membranes, and have the potential to form explosive peroxides. Halogenated ethers are highly toxic. Examples of ethers and their respective TLVs are ethyl ether (400 ppm) and isopropyl ether (250 ppm).

Glycols   Glycols are polyhydric alcohols that contain the double-OH groups. They present little exposure hazard because of their low volatility and low vapor pressure. Although mists and vapors can be irritating, inhalation exposures are not likely unless the material is heated or sprayed. Overexposures can affect the brain, the blood, and the kidneys. Examples of glycols are ethylene glycol (100 mg/m^3 ceiling) and 2-ethoxyethanol (5 ppm).

Aldehydes   Aldehydes contain the double-bonded carbonyl group, C=O, with only one hydrocarbon group on the carbon. Aldehydes irritate the skin and mucosa, act on the central nervous system, have sensitizing properties, and can cause dermatitis and allergic responses. An example of an aldehyde is acetaldehyde with a ceiling limit of 25 ppm because of its irritant properties.

Measurement

Solvents are measured with various techniques and instrumentation. A brief overview of the direct-reading field instrumentation and other sampling techniques for solvents and their laboratory analyses follows (McFee 1988).

Direct Reading Field Instrumentation   Direct reading field instrumentation includes:

Detector tubes—used for grab samples; accuracy of • 25% to 50%.

Diffusion badges—used without pumps or batteries. Badges rely on solvent diffusion and results can be read directly in the field or via laboratory analysis.

Combustible gas meter—useful for flammable solvents with high TLVs, although, they are not sufficiently accurate below 100 ppm. The meter requires calibration, is not specific, and its response is dependent on the oxygen and other gas concentrations present in the test atmosphere.

Halide meter—useful for direct measurement of halogenated hydrocarbons; however, it lacks specificity for distinguishing the different halogenated hydrocarbons.

Portable flame ionization meter—useful, highly versatile, and extremely sensitive with highly reproducible results. Measures levels less than 1 ppm but requires calibration for accurate results.

Portable infrared meter—more specific than the flame ionization meter but requires careful calibration for accurate measurements of a wide range of solvents.

Photoionization meter—more specific with increased sensitivity (on the order of a magnitude lower than the flame ionization meter).

Other Sampling Methodology   Other sampling methodologies include:

Grab samples—Devices such as evacuated flasks or plastic bags (saran, Mylar, or tedlar) can be used to collect samples that can be analyzed in the laboratory.

TWA samples—Air is drawn through a tube containing a collecting solution or solid adsorbent like silica gel, charcoal, or a molecular sieve.

Solid adsorbents—Charcoal sampling tubes collect solvent vapors and are then analyzed in the laboratory.

Diffusion badges—These can be used to confirm nondetectable levels.

Certain types of laboratory instrumentation are particularly useful for distinguishing and analyzing the concentrations of specific solvents, including:

Gas chromatograph (GC)—separates the closely related solvent components.

UV spectrophotometer—can analyze aromatic hydrocarbons when it is known that concentrations are low IR spectrophotometer—particularly useful in identifying solvents by certain functional chemical groups and with greater specificity.

Mass spectrophotometer (MS)—good for identifying unknowns. When coupled with the GC, the MS-GC can separate and quantify solvent components.

Risk Management

Because of the toxicity of most solvents, special attention needs to be paid to risk identification and management of solvent exposures. A number of risk management actions can be taken in the mining environment to prevent overexposures to solvents.

Substitution   Where feasible, less toxic solvents should be substituted for highly toxic solvents. As discussed earlier, aqueous systems are the least toxic and are nonflammable. Water with safe additives may be effective; however, if water has insufficient solvent power, "safety solvents," such as aliphatic hydrocarbons and fluorinated hydrocarbons should be considered before the more toxic solvents, such as toluene, ethylene dichloride, and trichloroethylene. When the more toxic solvents must be used, control measures such as local exhaust ventilation systems should be employed to remove volatile vapors and mists at the source. A review system should be in place to identify highly toxic solvents such as benzene, carbon tetrachloride, and gasoline and to ensure that appropriate substitutions are considered and/or controls are in place to address potential hazards.

Enclosure and Ventilation   Inhalation of volatile solvents can be controlled by using enclosures. Closed systems or enclosures can also reduce the potential for exposure by minimizing the propensity for spills and leaks. If a closed system is not feasible, properly engineered local exhaust ventilation is the next most effective control measure.

Respirators   As a secondary measure of control, air-purifying respirators with the appropriate cartridges or canisters can be effective if properly fitted on the worker. The proper selection, fitting, testing, and maintenance of respirators should be administered by a trained professional through a respiratory protection program.

Personal Protective Clothing   In a typical work environment, significant organic solvent exposure can occur through skin contact. Under certain circumstances, this can pose a serious health risk, especially when the skin has been compromised by cuts, abrasions, or dermatitis. Proper gloves, face shields, and impervious clothing should be worn to prevent skin contact and absorption. Selection of glove and clothing material should be based on the contact frequency, the duration of contact, and the solvent's characteristics. Manufacturer information should be obtained to ensure that the gloves and clothing selected will provide adequate protection. In addition, workers should be trained in replacing or discarding defective PPE.

Exposure Monitoring   Exposure monitoring is a critical risk management tool. Additionally, it assures the evaluation of enclosures and ventilation systems for proper design and efficient operation. If exposure monitoring results indicate a potential or existing problem, immediate actions should be taken to correct or mitigate the problem.

Training and Education   Workers should be provided with comprehensive training and education about the health effects of solvents, the symptoms associated with overexposure, monitoring, engineering controls, work practices, proper use of PPE, good hygiene, and reporting system failures.

SULFURIC ACID

Sulfuric acid is one of the most widely used chemicals and has recently been used in large quantities in hydrometallurgical processes. This process has gained prominence in the recovery of metals from low-grade ore. It has been most successful for extracting copper, uranium, gold, silver, potash, and sodium chloride (Malouf 1990). In this process, the metal oxide ore is leached with a solution through a heap or pad. The leach solution used in leaching copper and zinc minerals is commonly the raffinate from the solvent extraction process adjusted to a specified pH (1 to 2) with sulfuric acid. The leachate is an acidic solution of zinc or copper sulfate. In cells containing this sulfate solution, current is passed between electrodes that force the metal to plate onto the cathode. The cells, which number from a few to several hundred, are contained in an open building, typically called a tank house. Throughout the process, sulfuric acid exposure may occur on or around the leach pads and in harvesting the cathodes in the tank house.

Health Effects

Sulfuric acid is corrosive to living tissues. In a concentrated form, it produces charring rather than acid burns. Sulfuric acid mist is a skin, eye, and respiratory irritant. Erosion of teeth has been observed in workers exposed to the acid in the storage battery industry (Malcolm et al. 1961). In 1991, IARC evaluated the carcinogenic risk of strong acid mists containing sulfuric acid to humans and published their conclusion in a monograph in 1992 (IARC 1992). The mixture was categorized as a Group 1 for they believed that there was sufficient evidence of carcinogenicity in humans. The IARC conclusion remains controversial. Although it did not specifically evaluate sulfuric acid, the implications of the conclusion are far reaching in increased scrutiny and perhaps promulgation of sulfuric acid regulations. Critics of the IARC classification claim that, among other problems with the studies evaluated, the confounding factors such as smoking, alcohol, and exposure to known/suspected carcinogens were not controlled adequately.

Measurements

The OSHA and MSHA permissible exposure limits for sulfuric acid is 1 mg/m^3 as an 8-hour TWA. NIOSH and OSHA have developed several sampling methods for sulfuric acid. They are, however, based on the analysis of total sulfates. These methods create a problem in assessing sulfuric acid mist exposure considering the presence of several metal sulfates throughout the hydrometallurgical process. A new method appears to be promising in determining sulfuric acid in the presence of other sulfates (Hethmon 1997).

Risk Management

Throughout the hydrometallurgical process, the greatest potential for sulfuric acid mist exposure is in the tank house above the cells that contain the sulfate solution. The mist generation in the tank house depends on many variables. They include ambient temperature and relative humidity, barometric pressure, current efficiency and density, cell temperature, and the concentration of sulfuric acid in the solution. The acid mist is created when bubbles rupture at the surface of the solution. Therefore, the workers at greatest risk of inhaling sulfuric acid mist are those that harvest the cathodes from above the cells. Studies to control the mist are continuing and include surfactants that affect bubble generation and devices to coalesce rising bubbles (Kaliva-Papachristodoulou 1983). Surfactants appear to lower the concentration of acid mist; nonetheless, additional controls or a combination of controls may be required if exposure limits are reduced. Engineering controls—such as ventilation—are problematic especially for tank houses that are large and require the use of overhead cranes to mechanically lift the heavy cathodes above the cells.

CYANIDES

Cyanide salts, more commonly known as sodium cyanide (NaCN), are used in mining to extract metals from the ore, primarily the precious metals gold and silver. The salts are used in typically two processes, hydrometallurgical and flotation. In a hydrometallurgical process, a solution of cyanide in water may be sprayed over an ore pile, also known as a heap-leaching, and as the solution seeps through the heap, it forms a metal cyanide solution, such as $Au(CN)_2$, for example. The solution is then collected in a storage pond or tank. Further recovery of the precious metal from the solution requires the electrowinning or zinc precipitation process.

In the flotation process, cyanide is used to treat the surface of mineral particles for processing in flotation machines. In general, the cyanide solution is used as a depressing agent for pyrite and sphalerite and occasionally for copper sulfides. The cyanide portion of the process constitutes only a small part of the total. Toxic cyanide concentrations can exist from the point of preparation of the solution to its addition into the actual milling process. Once in the milling process, cyanide is reacted and diluted to low concentrations, to about 1/1000th of its original concentration (McAlexander et al. 1981).

In mining, potential exposure to cyanide can occur when dust is generated during handling of the cyanide salt. Another could be through improper handling and mixing so that the cyanide salts come into contact with acid. This mistake could result in the formation of hydrogen cyanide gas. The pH of a cyanide solution can indicate the potential generation of hydrogen cyanide gas. Adjustments to maintain a pH above the critical point, believed to be about 10, are generally made by adding lime, caustic soda, or soda ash. The cyanide gas evolution also depends on solution temperature and concentration.

Health Effects

Low concentrations of cyanide can be found in human blood; it has been estimated that "normal" blood cyanide levels can be 0.4 mg/L blood (Ellenhorn and Barceloux 1988). A nonoccupational source of cyanide is smoking. Smokers tend to have higher thiocyanate, a metabolite of cyanide, concentrations in their urine and plasma than nonsmokers (Hartung 1991).

The toxicity of cyanide compounds is associated with its ability to dissociate and release CN^- ions. The simple salts of hydrogen cyanide such as sodium, potassium, calcium, and ammonium cyanide readily dissociate. Hydrogen cyanide (HCN) and these simple salts are the most rapidly acting poisons. Inhalation of high concentrations may be followed by almost immediate collapse and halt in respiration. Table 22.7 presents the effects of various concentrations of HCN (Hartung 1991). Ingestion by humans of 50 to 100 mg of sodium or potassium cyanide, described in the literature as the weight of a standard paper clip, may also be fatal. At lower dosages, the initial symptoms may be weakness, headache, confusion, and possibly nausea and vomiting. It is thought that chronic exposure to cyanides can interfere with iodine uptake by the thyroid gland and can lead to thyroid enlargement.

Cyanide binds with metal ions that are biological constituents of several enzymes. Most important of these is the Fe^{3+} in cytochrome oxidase. The cell requires this enzyme to utilize oxygen and cyanide will inhibit its function and ultimately result in cell death (Dixon and Webb 1958). It will also inhibit methemoglobin that competes with cytochrome oxidase for the cyanide ion. This competition is the basis for the first-aid procedures established for cyanide poisoning.

If death does not occur from exposure, the cyanide ion is metabolized to thiocyanate and the ion is excreted in urine. The process on conversion to thiocyanate involves the enzyme rhodanese in the presence of thiosulfate (Hartung 1991). This process also brought about another procedure and is used in conjunction with methemoglobin production therapy to counteract cyanide poisoning.

Measurement

The MSHA exposure limit for cyanide is 5 mg/m^3, as an 8-hour TWA. Airborne cyanide can be measured with NIOSH sampling method 7904 (NIOSH 1994). The sampling media consists of a 37-mm, 0.8-µm PVC (polyvinyl chloride) membrane filter followed by a glass midget bubbler containing 15 mL of 0.1 KOH (potassium hydroxide). The sampling pump is calibrated and set at a flow rate between 0.5 and 1 L/min. The cyanide aerosol (e.g., salt) adheres to the filter while the bubbler traps the cyanide gas. Both the filter and the bubbler solution are analyzed to determine total airborne cyanide. For hydrogen cyanide gas alone, a solid sorbent tube can be used NIOSH Method 6010 (NIOSH 1994). Another method, although less accurate, is the stain-developing detector tubes. Interpretation of results from all three methods, though, must take into consideration the potential interference of various compounds associated with each method.

Risk Management

Storage Cyanide salts should be stored in a dry, weather-tight, ventilated enclosure that is adequately controlled to prevent unauthorized entry. They should be separated from areas/containers where acid vapors, acid salts, could be generated. Furthermore, they should not be stored near oxidizing

TABLE 22.7   Effects of hydrogen cyanide gas at various concentrations

Concentration	Effect
270 ppm	Immediately fatal
181 ppm	Fatal after 10 minutes
135 ppm	Fatal after 30 minutes
110 ppm	Fatal in 1 hour

Source: NIOSH 1978

agents such as nitrates, peroxides, or chlorates. These materials may be found in blasting agents, other mill reagents, or laboratory chemicals. Inadvertent contact of oxidizing agents with cyanide can result in the formation of toxic, dangerous, or highly irritating gases, fires, and/or explosions.

Ventilation   Storage enclosures should be ventilated to remove hydrogen cyanide or acetylene gas that may be liberated if the cyanide salt becomes wet. Furthermore, ventilation for the storage area, the mix tank, and other areas where workers' tasks require handling the cyanide salt or solution should be designed and constructed to include mechanical ventilation. These designs can prevent dust or gas from entering the operator's breathing zone.

PPE   In addition to cyanide toxicity, the cyanide solution can be highly alkaline (pH > 10) and, therefore, can be corrosive to human tissue. Anyone who handles cyanide salts, solutions, or open containers during normal mixing, maintenance, and leaching procedures should wear protective equipment—including goggles, waterproof clothing, face shields, gloves, and rubber boots—to prevent eye and skin contact. Respirators should be worn when there is a potential for inhalation exposure and the type worn should efficiently remove cyanide dust and gas. Hand wash and emergency eye-wash and shower facilities should be provided throughout the area, especially in the mixing area.

Work Practices   Although a common safe work practice, prohibiting eating, drinking, and smoking is especially important in the mixing area where cyanide dust could easily contaminate surface areas. To reduce possible contamination of areas within the immediate work area, workers should be cautioned to avoid splashing and spills during the mixing process and to properly clean all spills immediately. Contamination outside the work area can be prevented if workers remove contaminated clothing and wash thoroughly (especially their hands and face) before entering lunchrooms, and shower before leaving the workplace. Shower rooms should be designed similar to those described in the metals section of this chapter.

The pipelines or equipment carrying water and cyanide solutions should be clearly identified by color coding or other means to prevent misconnection and improper mixing. Procedures should be established for maintenance, inspection, and repair of tanks and equipment that contain or may have contained solutions of cyanide salts. Employees that conduct these activities should be well trained on these procedures.

Fire extinguishers in the area should not contain carbon dioxide as an extinguishing agent. Carbon dioxide as a gas or in solution is a mild acid and hydrogen cyanide gas could be liberated upon contact with cyanide salts or solution.

Medical Surveillance   Preplacement and periodic evaluations should include a complete history with emphasis on the history of fainting spells that may be a result of a cardiovascular or a nervous disorder and also notations of those conditions that may create a susceptibility to the effects of anoxia or anemia. Physical examinations should emphasize the cardiovascular, nervous, and upper respiratory systems, along with the thyroid. Because cyanide is a defatting agent and can cause dermatitis on prolonged exposure, the skin should also be examined during these evaluations.

Poison Treatment   As discussed previously, methemoglobin binds well and competes with cytochrome oxidase for cyanide ions. Consequently, the antidote developed for cyanide poisoning involves increasing the formation of methemoglobin in the blood, by inhalation of amyl nitrate vapor (Chen 1952). Antidote kits contain amyl nitrate ampoules. To administer the antidote, the ampoule is broken in a cloth such as a handkerchief and held close to the victim's nose while artificial respiration is being conducted. Resuscitation by mouth is not recommended; a mechanical resuscitator should be used instead. If the victim does not respond to the amyl nitrate treatment, a medical professional would then increase the methemoglobin production by intravenous injection of sodium nitrate followed by administration of thiosulfate to increase the activity of the rhodanese enzyme.

Physicians and nurses along with first responders must be thoroughly familiar with the toxic effects of cyanide, first aid procedures. and medical therapy. All personnel who may come in contact with cyanide should be properly trained in the effects of cyanide, specific artificial respiration procedures, the locations of cyanide first-aid kits, and the use of amyl nitrate ampoules. These kits should be conveniently located throughout the areas where cyanides, whether salt or solution, are handled. Additionally, first aid emergency procedures should be posted and visible throughout the same area.

THERMAL STRESSORS

The human body regulates itself to maintain a core body temperature of 96.8°F (36°C), although it is able to tolerate fluctuations within a very narrow, protected range of internal body temperatures. Deviations from this range can greatly affect thermal comfort and are influenced by many variables including ambient air temperatures, seasons of the year, humidity, acclimatization, cultural practices and habits, and work (physical activity). The body's thermoregulatory system can be stressed when exposed to cold or heat.

The body's thermal equilibrium can be expressed in the following equation:

$$M \bullet R \bullet C \bullet K - E = 0 \qquad \text{(EQ 22.1)}$$

where

M = metabolic heat
R = radiant heat
C = convective heat
K = conductive heat
E = evaporative heat.

In hot environments, heat can be stored and expressed as, $M \bullet R \bullet C \bullet K > E$. In cold environments, heat is lost and expressed as $M \bullet R \bullet C \bullet K < E$.

Cold Stress

"A cold environment is defined by conditions that cause greater than normal body heat losses" (Holmer 1998). As a practical matter, temperatures less than 18° to 20°C would be considered cold. For miners, work in the cold outside environment can create cold stress and result in an imbalance in whole-body heat or in the heat of local tissue extremities (skin and lungs). Prolonged imbalance can result in cold stress and ultimately death.

Temperature Regulation in the Cold   Human thermoregulatory response to reduce heat loss in cold environments includes decreasing blood flow to the skin, or skin vasoconstriction. Skin vasoconstriction works to better insulate the body. Shivering is an involuntary contraction of muscle fibers that serves to generate heat, to offset heat loss. Although cold perception, cold tolerance, and thermal comfort are highly individualistic, the amount of subcutaneous fat can affect the speed by which shivering will occur when exposed to a cold environment.

Cold stress, that is cooling the whole body or parts of the body, results in discomfort, sensory impairments, neuromuscular impairments, and cold injury. Table 22.8 shows the physiological and psychological reactions to core body temperatures of 37° to 25°C.

Cold Injuries   Cold disorders can result when the body's thermoregulator fails to maintain adequate control of normal body heat losses. These disorders can either be localized in the tissue extremities or generalized throughout the body. The main factors contributing to cold injury are exposure to cold, humidity and high winds, contact with metal or wetness, inadequate clothing, age, and general health. The following injuries and disorders are associated with excessive heat loss (Alpaugh 1988).

- Hypothermia is the condition of reduced temperatures. Most cases of hypothermia develop when air temperatures are between 2° and 10°C (30° to 50°F). Uncontrollable shivering and the sensation of cold lead to decreased and/or irregular heartbeats, cool skin, impaired judgment and mental functioning, low blood pressure, and fatigue. Severe hypothermia can result in death.

- Blood vessel abnormalities can be associated with increased cold sensitivity.

TABLE 22.8   Human response to cooling

Phase	Core Temperature (°C)	Physiological Reactions	Psychological Reactions
Normal	37	Normal body temperature	Thermoneutral sensation
	36	Vasoconstriction, cold hands and feet	Discomfort
Mild hypothermia	35	Intense shivering, reduced work capacity	Impaired judgment, disorientation, apathy
	34	Fatigue	Conscious and responsive
	33	Fumbling and stumbling	
Moderate hypothermia	32	Muscle rigidity	Progressive unconsciousness, hallucinations
	31	Faint breathing	Consciousness clouds
	30		Stuporous
	29	No nerve reflexes, heart rate slow and almost undetectable	
Severe hypothermia	28	Heart dysrhythmias (atrial and/or ventricular)	
	27	Pupils nonreactive to light, deep tendon and superficial reflexes absent	
	25	Death caused by ventricular fibrillation or asystole	

Source: Holmer (ILO 1998)

- Raynaud's phenomenon is the abnormal constriction of the blood vessels in the fingers upon exposure to cold temperature.
- Acrocyanosis is a relatively benign condition that results in a bluish tinge to the hands and/or feet caused by the reduction of hemoglobin in the blood.
- Thromboangitis obliterans is arterial blockage caused by the inflammation and fibrosis of the connective tissue that surrounds the medium-sized arteries and veins.
- Frostbite is a localized cold disorder. It occurs when extremities do not receive sufficient heat from the central body stores because of inadequate circulation and/or insulation. Frostbite, which can cause damage and tissue loss, results in the freezing of fluids around the tissue cells. Vulnerable body parts include the nose, cheeks, ears, fingers, and toes.
- Trench foot is a condition caused by long, continuous exposure to cold without freezing in combination with persistent dampness or actual immersion in water. Blistering, skin tissue death, and ulceration follow after swelling, tingling, itching, and severe pain.
- Chilblains is similar to trench foot except that it affects other parts of the body.
- Frostnip occurs when the skin of the face or the extremities turns white as a result of exposure to cold wind.

Table 22.9 describes various factors that can affect work in cold environments.

Measurement and Control   The TLVs for cold stress and the windchill index can be used to evaluate the cold environment. The windchill index expresses the cooling power of wind on exposed skin as an equivalent temperature. The human body senses "cold" as a result of both air temperature and wind velocity.

The windchill factor is the cooling effect from any of the combination of temperature and wind velocity or air movement. Cooling of exposed flesh increases rapidly as the wind velocity goes up. Frostbite can occur at relatively mild temperatures if wind penetrates the body insulation. For example, when the air temperature is 4.4°C (40°F) and wind velocity is 48 km/h (30 mph), the exposed skin perceives an equivalent still air temperature of −11°C (13°F).

The ACGIH TLV booklet describes in detail the evaluation and control measures necessary to protect cold disorders. Unless the skin is protected, continuous exposure should not be permitted when the equivalent windchill temperature of −32°C (−25.6°F) occurs. Refer to the TLV booklet for

TABLE 22.9   Recommended cold health control program components

Factor	Outdoor Work	Arctic and Subarctic Work
Infectious Diseases (Endemic diseases occurring in the arctic and subarctic regions)	**	***
Cardiovascular Diseases (Cold raises cardiac output and heart rate)	***	***
Metabolic Diseases (For example, diabetes mellitus, which makes work in cold impossible because of peripheral arteriosclerosis)	**	***
Musculoskeletal Problems (Work outdoors in cold is demanding on the muscles, tendons, joints, and spine because of the high workload	***	***
Cryopathies (Hypersensitivity to cold)	**	**
Psychological Stress (Cold exposure in combination with other cold-related factors and remoteness increase psychological stress)	***	***
Smoking and Snuffing (Nicotine increases peripheral vasoconstriction, reduces dexterity, and raises cold injury risk)	**	**
Alcohol (Gives false sense of warmth and bravado and impairs judgment)	***	***
Pregnancy (Sensitivity to cold is diminished because metabolism is raised)	**	***
Medication (May impair defense mechanisms and awareness of cold exposure and hazards)	**	***

** = Important factor to consider

*** = Very important factor to consider

Source: Holmer (ILO 1998)

recommendations on properly clothing workers for periods of effort at below freezing temperatures (ACGIH 1998).

Prevention of Cold Stress   Cold disorders arising from cold stress can be minimized or avoided with adequate preventive measures, including:

Adaptation—Human adaptation results with repeated exposures to cold conditions and can lead to improved judgment and awareness.

Training and education—Appropriate behavior to cold exposures and precautions can be reinforced with training and education, knowledge, experience, motivation, and personal requirements for thermal comfort. Survival training in cold environments should not be neglected.

Acclimatization—Although subject to individual variation, acclimatization can result from long-term cold exposure, leading to increased tissue insulation, hypothermic reaction of "controlled" drop in core temperature, and increased metabolism.

Diet and water balance—Adjustments in diet to meet the energy demands of cold work activities include increased caloric intake (carbohydrates and fat) to compensate for the body's energy demands. Water deficits contribute to dehydration and increased risk to cold injuries. Efforts should be made to avoid water loss and maintain an adequate water balance.

Conditioning—Worker training, education, and practice allow human adaptation to occur.

Workers should be made aware of specific problems related to cold exposure: physiological and psychological reactions, health risks and controls, and sufficient and appropriate protective clothing. Special precautions need to be taken for older workers or workers with circulatory problems.

Other Control Measures   Engineering controls can be used to reduce cold stress in the mining environment. These include general or spot heating to increase workplace temperatures; warm air jets, radiant heat, or contact with warm plates to keep hands warm; work area shielding from air velocity; thermal insulating material for metal tool handles at temperatures below −1°C (30°F); use of power tools, hoists, and cranes to reduce metabolic load; and heated warming shelters when work is performed continuously in equivalent chill temperatures of −7°C (20°F).

Work practice and administrative controls can also minimize the risks associated with cold stress. For example, by adopting a work-warming regimen, workers can use heated warming shelters, change into dry clothing, and drink warm, caffeine-free, sweet drinks and soups for caloric and fluid intake. Resting periodically and working more slowly are important to reduce heat loss and the peak of cold stress.

PPE and Clothing   PPE, as well as the proper clothing, is essential for working in cold environments. The proper equipment will protect the head, face, hands, feet, and other exposed skin. To retain heat, the clothing should be layered to preserve the air space between the body and the outer layer of clothing. However, it is important to note that cold weather gear, including boots and headgear, can easily add bulkiness and load (3 to 6 kg). This will result in the need for more space to perform the tasks and the need to compensate for the additional workload or energy output.

Heat Stress

Extremely high temperatures in the workplace have the potential to affect the miner's health and ability to function. Miners exposed to heat as a result of elevated indoor and outdoor air temperatures, radiant heat sources, high humidity, contact with hot objects, and strenuous work can add to their overall metabolic load. Work in deep underground mines, that performed in hot weather, and around furnaces are some examples.

Heat stress is the total heat load imposed on the body by environmental and physical work factors. Environmental factors that affect heat load are ambient air temperature, radiant heat, air movement, conduction, and relative humidity. Physical work contributes to heat stress by producing metabolic heat in the body proportional to the work intensity. PPE and protective clothing can significantly increase the risk of heat stress, especially in hot environments where miners may be required to wear semipermeable or permeable protective clothing and respirators to perform moderate or strenuous work.

Health Effects   Heat strain is the range of physiological responses to heat stress. The body's protective mechanisms come into play when workers are exposed to extreme heat. The hypothalamus of the brain acts like a thermostat to establish a set point temperature and to control the central nervous system's cooling and heating mechanisms. When exposed to heat, the body's core temperature is cooled as the blood vessels near the skin surface dilate and sweating increases to dissipate excessive heat and control body temperature. Although sweating is an important natural mechanism, it is critical that water and electrolyte balance be maintained. Working in extreme heat can produce 6 to 8 quarts of sweat loss per day, losses that must be replaced with fluids. Progressive loss of water can result in lower sweat production and increased body temperature, leading to the onset of serious heat disorders.

A variety of factors can affect a person's sensitivity and tolerance to heat, such as age, gender, ethnicity, body dimensions, weight, physical fitness, acclimatization, metabolism, alcohol or drug use, and medical conditions such as obesity, hypertension, and history or predisposition to heat injuries. Individuals with degenerative cardiovascular system diseases, diabetes, and/or malnutrition are at increased risk when exposed to heat and when stress is placed on the cardiovascular system (Ogawa 1998; NIOSH 1986).

Various clinical manifestations in response to heat stress range from fainting to complications resulting from heat stroke. Common features of all heat disorders are elevated body temperature and a corresponding loss of body water.

NIOSH's *Criteria for a Recommended Standard ... Occupational Exposure to Hot Environments,* (1986) gives five classifications of heat disorders:

- Temperature regulation—heatstroke
- Circulatory hypostasis—heat syncope

- Water and/or salt depletion—heat exhaustion, heat cramps
- Skin eruptions—heat rash (prickly heat, miliaria rubra), heat exhaustion (miliaria profunda)
- Behavioral disorders—transient and chronic heat fatigue.

Heatstroke is a serious medical emergency that can result in death. It occurs when the sweating function ceases, the body temperature rises rapidly, and the skin becomes dry and flushed. Unconsciousness sometimes follows quickly. Of all heat disorders, heatstroke is the most serious. Heatstroke is defined by three criteria: severe hyperthermia with a core body temperature usually exceeding 42°C; disturbances of the central nervous system; and hot, dry skin with the cessation of sweating.

Heat syncope, or heat collapse, is fainting caused by the reduction of cerebral blood flow and circulation. Often, the fainting is preceded by skin pallor, vision blurring, dizziness, and nausea. Mild dehydration contributes to heat syncope.

Heat exhaustion is the most common heat disorder and results from severe dehydration and water and/or salt depletion. It occurs when the heart rate decreases and the body temperature remains low. The victim presents with skin pallor and profuse sweating upon heavy exertion.

Heat cramps occur when there the body loses moisture over a long period of time; with heavy exertion, muscles can cramp because of salt depletion and water loss. Painful spasms develop in the limbs and abdominal muscles subjected to intensive work and fatigue. However, the body temperature hardly rises. The term "Miner's cramps" was coined to describe heat cramps in normally fit individuals who could perform sustained physical activity yet suffered heat cramps upon dehydration.

Heat rash, or miliaria, is associated with heat load. It occurs when the body is unable to sweat because the sweat ducts are blocked. Anhidrosis, which is the inability to release sweat, can predispose an individual to heatstroke. Miliaria can be classified into three types depending on the depth of the sweat retention.

Table 22.10 presents classifications, medical aspects, and methods for prevention of heat illness and is an adaptation of NIOSH's revised criteria table (DHHS-NIOSH 1986).

Measurement and Evaluation

The heat stress TLVs established by ACGIH (1998) refer to

> ... heat stress conditions under which it is believed that nearly all workers may be repeatedly exposed without adverse health effects. These TLVs are based on the assumption that nearly all acclimatized, fully clothed (e.g., lightweight pants and shirt) workers with adequate water and salt intake should be able to function effectively under the given working conditions without exceeding a deep body temperature of 38°C (100.4°F).

Although measurement of a worker's deep body temperature is more accurate, it is impractical in the workplace setting. The wet-bulb globe temperature (WBGT) index is the simplest technique currently available for measuring environmental factors resulting from the net effect of dry air temperature, radiant heat transfer, and humidity. The TLVs are calculated using a formula based on a dry-bulb thermometer, a natural static wet-bulb thermometer, and a black globe thermometer. Specific measurement techniques are detailed further in the ACGIH TLV booklet.

WBGT values are calculated for:

Outdoors with solar load

$$WBGT = 0.7\ NWB + 0.2\ GT + 0.1\ DB \qquad \text{(EQ 22.2)}$$

Indoors or outdoors with no solar load

$$WBGT = 0.7\ NWB + 0.3\ GT \qquad \text{(EQ 22.3)}$$

where
- WBGT = web-bulb globe temperature index
- NWBT = natural wet-bulb temperature
- DBT = dry-bulb temperature
- GT = globe temperature.

TABLE 22.10   Classification, medical aspects, and prevention of heat illness

Category and Clinical Features	Predisposing Factors	Treatment	Prevention
1. Temperature Regulation			
Heatstroke: (1) hot, dry skin usually red, mottled or cyanotic; (2) rectal temperature 40.5°C (104°F) and higher; (3) confusion, loss of consciousness, convulsions, rectal temperature continues to rise; fatal if treatment delayed.	(1) Sustained exertion in heat by unacclimatized workers; (2) lack of physical fitness and obesity; (3) recent alcohol intake; (4) dehydration; (5) individual susceptibility; and (6) chronic cardiovascular disease.	Immediate and rapid cooling by immersion in chilled water with massage or by wrapping in wet sheet with vigorous fanning with cool, dry air, avoid overcooling, treat shock if present.	Medical screening of workers, selection based on health and physical fitness, acclimatization for 5–7 days by graded work and heat exposure, monitoring workers during sustained work in severe heat.
2. Circulatory Hypostasis			
Heat syncope: fainting while standing erect and immobile in heat.	Lack of acclimatization	Remove to cooler area, rest recumbent position, recovery prompt and complete.	Acclimatization, intermittent activity to assist venous return to heart.
3. Water and/or Salt Depletion			
(a) Heat exhaustion: (1) fatigue, nausea, headache, giddiness; (2) skin clammy and moist, complexion pale, muddy, or hectic flush; (3) may faint on standing with rapid thready pulse and low blood pressure; (4) oral temperature normal or low but rectal temperature usually elevated (37.5°–38.5°C) (99.5°–101.3° F); water restriction type: urine volume small, highly concentrated; salt restriction type: urine less concentrated. Chlorides less than 3 g/L.	(1) Sustained exertion in heat; (2) lack of acclimatization; and (3) failure to replace water lost in sweat	Remove to cooler environment, rest recumbent position, administer fluids by mouth, keep at rest until urine volume indicates that water balances have been restored.	Acclimatize workers using a breaking-in schedule for 5 days, supplement dietary salt only during acclimatization, ample drinking water to be available at all times and to be taken frequently during work day.
(b) Heat cramps: painful spasms of muscles used during work (arms, legs, or abdominal); onset during or after work hours	(1) Heavy sweating during hot work; (2) drinking large volumes of water without replacing salt loss	Salted liquids by mouth, or more prompt relief by IV infusion.	Adequate salt intake with meals, in unacclimatized workers supplement salt intake at meals.
4. Skin Eruptions			
(a) Heat rash (miliaria rubra; "prickly heat"): profuse tiny raised red vesicles (blister-like) on affected areas pricking sensations during heat exposure.	Unrelieved exposure to humid heat with skin continuously wet with unevaporated sweat.	Mild drying lotions, skin cleanliness to prevent infection.	Cool sleeping quarters to allow skin to dry between heat exposures.

Continues next page

TABLE 22.10 Classification, medical aspects, and prevention of heat illness (continued)

Category and Clinical Features	Predisposing Factors	Treatment	Prevention
4. Skin Eruptions (continued)			
(b) Andriotic heat exhaustion (miliaria profunda): extensive areas of skin that do not sweat on heat exposure, but present gooseflesh appearance, which subsides with cool environments; associated with incapacitation in heat	Weeks or months of constant exposure to climatic heat with previous history of extensive heat rash and sunburn.	No effective treatment available for anhidriotic areas of skin, recovery of sweating occurs gradually on return to cooler climate.	Treat heat rash and avoid further skin trauma by sunburn, periodic relief from sustained heat.
5. Behavioral Disorders			
(a) Heat fatigue—transient: impaired performance of skilled sensorimotor, mental or vigilance tasks, in heat	Performance decrement greater in acclimatized and unskilled worker.	Not indicated unless accompanied by other heat illness.	Acclimatization and training for work in the heat.
(b) Heat fatigue—chronic: reduced performance capacity, lowering of self-imposed standards of social behavior (e.g., alcohol overindulgence), inability to concentrate	Workers at risk come from temperate climates, for long residence in tropical latitudes.	Medical treatment for serious cases, speedy relief of symptoms on returning home.	Orientation on life in hot regions (customs, climate, living conditions)

Source: Adaptation of NIOSH 1986

Table 22.11 provides the TLV WBGT values in °C and °F.

Although the WBGT index considers the portion of heat stress that results from the net effects of dry air temperature, radiant heat transfer, and humidity, it does not sufficiently reflect the air movement effects on convective heat transfer, heat loss, or heat produced by physical work, all major contributors to heat strain.

These values are based on the assumption that the WBGT value of the resting place is the same or very close to that of the workplace and that the thermometers are placed so that the readings are representative of the worker exposure. As the workload increases, the heat stress on an unacclimated worker is exacerbated. A correction, or reduction of 2.5°C, is made to the permissible heat exposure TLV for unacclimated workers performing at a moderate level.

A portable heat stress meter or monitor may also be used to integrate and calculate the WBGT information. Combined with information on the work being performed, the heat stress meter can determine the duration for which an individual can work safely in a hot environment.

Other thermal stress indices are available; however, like the WBGT, they also have their advantages and disadvantages.

Risk Management

The incidence and severity of heat disorders can be prevented using a variety of techniques (Nunneley 1998; NIOSH 1986). Maximizing individual heat tolerance is key to preventing heat stress. As mentioned previously, individual disposition and tolerance to heat depend on a variety of factors. Factors affecting adaptation are body dimensions, gender, ethnicity, age, physical fitness, heat acclimation, obesity, medical conditions, and other stresses. Medical screening can identify individuals who are unable to tolerate heat.

TABLE 22.11   Permissible heat exposure TLVs

Work–Rest Regimen	Workload		
	Light	Moderate	Heavy
Continuous work	30.0°C (86°F)	26.7°C (80°F)	25.0°C (77°F)
75% work—25% rest, each hour	30.6°C (87°F)	28.0°C (82°F)	25.9°C (78°F)
50% work—50% rest, each hour	31.4°C (89°F)	29.4°C (85°F)	27.9°C (82°F)
25% work—75% rest, each hour	32.2°C (90°F)	31.1°C (88°F)	30.0°C (86°F)

Source: ACGIH 1998

TABLE 22.12   Checklist for controlling heat stress

Item	Actions for Consideration
Controls	
M, Body heat production of task	Reduce physical demands of the work; powered assistance for heavy tasks.
R, Radiative heat	Interpose line-of-sight barrier; furnace wall insulation, metallic reflecting screen, heat reflective clothing, cover exposed parts of body.
C, Convective heat	If air temperature is above 35°C (95°F): reduce air temperature, reduce air speed across skin, wear clothing.
	If air temperature is below 35°C (95°F): increase air speed across skin and reduce clothing.
E_{MAX}, Maximum evaporative cooling by sweating	Increase by: decreasing humidity, increasing air speed
	Decrease clothing
Work Practices	Shorten duration of each exposure; more frequent short exposures better than fewer long exposures.
	Schedule very hot jobs in cooler part of the day when possible.
Exposure limit	Self-limiting, based on formal indoctrination of workers and supervisors on signs and symptoms of overstrain.
Recovery	Air-conditioned space nearby.
Personal Protection	
R, C, and E_{MAX}	Cooled air, cooled fluid, or ice cooled conditioned clothing
	Reflective clothing or aprons
Other Considerations	Determine by medical evaluation, primarily of cardiovascular status
	Careful break-in of unacclimatized workers
	Water intake at frequent intervals
	Fatigue or mild illness not related to job may temporarily contraindicate exposure (e.g. low-grade infection, diarrhea, sleepless nights, alcohol ingestion).
Heat Wave	Introduce heat alert program

Source: NIOSH 1986

Heat Acclimation   Heat acclimation is a series of physiological and psychological adjustments that occur in an individual during the first week of exposure to a hot environment. Following the acclimation period, the individual is less likely to suffer from heat stress. A properly designed and applied acclimation program decreases the risk of heat-related disorders and illnesses.

Table 22.12 is a checklist for controlling heat stress. Because of the many factors that influence the risk of heat stress, a number of actions can be taken to control the various contributors to heat load resulting from metabolic load, convective and radiant heat sources, and evaporative cooling.

Workplace Controls

Efforts should be taken to keep workers within the body's narrow window of thermoregulation. Heat disorders can be prevented by keeping the core temperature within the normal range. Methods that can be employed (DHHS/NIOSH 1986) include:

Engineering controls—Reduce the heat source by moving it away from workers or lowering the temperature (although not always practical). Control convective heat by modifying air temperature and air movement such as ventilation and control radiant heat using reflective shield between the radiant source and the worker and/or reducing surface temperature. Control evaporative heat by increasing air movement and decreasing water vapor pressure via air conditioning and fans.

Fluid replacement—Ready access to water or other rehydration drinks will replace water and electrolytes. Workers should be encouraged to replace sweat loss with at least 1 cup (150 mL) every 15 to 20 minutes. The water should be kept reasonably cool (10°C to 15°C) and conveniently placed. During the hot season or upon exposure to artificially generated heat, salting of food and/or drinking water is recommended, especially for unacclimated workers.

Modified administrative and work practices—Establish adequate work-rest regimens relative to work load physical demands. Exposure time and/or temperature can be limited by scheduling hot jobs for cooler times of the day and year. Cool areas can be provided to encourage cooling and rest. Heat acclimation programs assist in enhancing heat tolerance and keep workers physically fit. Having relief workers available, worker pacing, assigning extra workers, and/or limiting worker occupancy can also assist in reducing heat generated from excessive workload.

Climate control—Where feasible and practical, use air-conditioning and ventilation to avoid heat stress.

Protective clothing—Commercially available garb includes reflective clothing such as aprons, jackets, or suits for limiting radiant heat

Auxiliary body cooling—Air-cooled clothing can provide evaporative cooling to the body through a connection to an air source. By directing compressed air around the body from a supplied air system, both convective and evaporative cooling are highly effective; however, the complicated systems can limit worker mobility.

Auxiliary body cooling—Liquid-cooled protective clothing (e.g., ice vests) are usually filled with water, carbon dioxide, or dry ice as a coolant. Other liquid-cooled protective garments circulate a water-antifreeze mixture through a network of channels or small tubes. Liquid cooling provides greater cooling potential than air systems; however, both types of cooling devices add weight and bulk to the body and can interfere with the ability to move freely while working. Auxiliary body cooling and protective clothing should be used if it is impossible to modify the work or environment, and if heat stress is still above limits.

Medical Evaluation   Before workers are placed in high-risk heat-stress activities, they should be evaluated by a physician to ensure that conditions that limit an individual's ability to cope with heat are identified. Special emphasis should be placed on the skin, along with the cardiovascular, renal, hepatic, endocrine, and respiratory systems. The evaluation should also include a complete medical history with specific emphasis on previous heat-related disorders or illnesses. First-aid responders should be available and trained to recognize the signs and symptoms of heat illness and disorders.

Training   Employee education and training should comprise comprehensive information of good work practices and heat stress hazards. NIOSH (DHHS/NIOSH 1986) recommends that a good heat-stress training program should include these topics:

- Knowledge of the hazards of heat stress
- Recognition of the predisposing factors, danger signs, and symptoms
- Awareness of first-aid procedures for heat stroke and other heat disorders
- Employee responsibilities in avoiding heat stress
- Dangers of illegal and therapeutic drug use and alcohol in hot work environments
- Use of protective clothing and equipment
- Importance of environmental and medical surveillance programs and worker participation
- Information on fluid and electrolyte replacement
- Caution that should be exercised in situations where employees are exposed to toxic agents and/or other stressful physical agents in hot work environments.

WORK AT HIGH ALTITUDES

Work at high altitudes poses unique challenges and health risks to miners. High altitude is considered to be 2,438 m (8,000 ft) or more above sea level and very high altitude is more than 4,270 m (14,000 ft) above sea level. As ascents higher and higher above sea level are made, both the total air pressure (barometric pressure) and the amount of oxygen in the atmosphere fall progressively. As a result, this not only decreases the amount of oxygen reaching the body's tissues, but also negatively affects the amount of work that can be accomplished (Reeves and Weil 1998).

Maintaining an adequate supply of oxygen to tissues is fundamental to work performance at high altitudes. Increased breathing, or ventilatory acclimation, is the body's main response to low oxygen states. This response is an attempt to maintain the oxygen pressure in arterial blood and its importance increases progressively with higher altitude.

Acclimation to high altitudes with reduced oxygen levels occurs when the body can maintain an adequate supply of oxygen to meet the metabolic demands of work. Those most sensitive to reduced barometric pressure risks are individuals who are either not sufficiently acclimatized to oxygen-deficient atmospheres or suffer from medical conditions that may be aggravated at altitude. Rapid ascents to high altitudes in unacclimated individuals can result in death.

For a more extensive background on the physical and physiological aspects of reduced barometric pressures, sources are available through the International Labor Organization (ILO 1998), the National Safety Council (NSC 1988), and the American Industrial Hygiene Association (AIHA 1997).

Health Effects

Work at high altitudes can bring on headaches, increased muscular fatigue, marked mental function deterioration (i.e., memory and computation), impairments in decision making and judgment, and poor sleep quality. These symptoms result from reduced barometric pressure and oxygen intake.

Altitude-related illnesses and disorders are serious and should be considered life threatening. Acute cases can be rapidly reversed by descending or by administering oxygen, but the failure to diagnose a disorder early, with the inability to descend or relocate to sea level, or the lack of alternative treatments, can lead to death. Some altitude-related illnesses are listed below (Heath 1981; Berger and Rom 1998).

Hypoxia   Hypoxia is a lowered oxygen state that affects the central nervous system. It is demonstrated by a reduction in response time and vision disruption. Symptoms of hypoxia include headaches, confusion, drowsiness, and loss of coordination. Hypoxia reportedly induces a state of euphoria. Although acute hypoxia can be resolved rapidly with oxygen administration or descent to lower altitudes or sea level, it can result in death if not addressed.

Acute Mountain Sickness   Acute mountain sickness (AMS) is the most common disorder at high-altitude environments. But with proper acclimation, it is preventable. The most common symptoms are headache (more pronounced at night), loss of appetite with or without nausea and vomiting, sleep disturbances, and fatigue. Often AMS is accompanied by shortness of breath, cough, memory loss, and visual and auditory disturbances. Fluid retention may be an early sign that may lead to the development of edema or swelling in the interstitial spaces of the lungs. More severe cases can lead to pulmonary or cerebral edema. Descent is the most effective treatment, but oxygen may be administered when descents to lower altitudes are not possible. Drugs such as acetazolamide and dexamethasone can improve the symptoms of AMS.

High-Altitude Pulmonary Edema   High-altitude pulmonary edema is the most common cause of death encountered at high elevations, with a mortality rate of 11%. The symptoms develop from 6 to 96 hours after ascent and include those described for AMS, accompanied by decreased exercise tolerance, increased recovery time, shortness of breath on exertion, and persistent, dry cough. Moreover, as the patient's condition worsens, high-altitude pulmonary edema can bring on shortness of breath at rest, lung congestion, and cyanosis in the nails and lips. Prevention methods are similar to those for AMS; however, limitations in physical exertion are key to counteracting high-altitude pulmonary edema. Treatments include assisted evacuations to a lower altitude. If descents are not possible, oxygen therapy can be useful.

High-Altitude Cerebral Edema   This form of edema represents an extreme form of AMS that progresses to generalized brain dysfunction. Early symptoms and prevention methods are identical to those of AMS. However, with the progression of cerebral edema, other neurological symptoms arise such as severe irritability, insomnia, twitchy muscles (ataxia), hallucinations, paralysis, seizures, and eventually coma. Although descent is the preferred treatment, oxygen therapy and diuretic administration may be necessary.

Retinal Hemorrhages   Although usually asymptomatic, retinal hemorrhages caused by arterial hypoxia are common at high altitudes. Spontaneous resolution can occur within 2 weeks.

Chronic Mountain Sickness   This disease affects long-term inhabitants of high altitudes. Symptoms of chronic mountain sickness include a feeling of fullness (plethora), blue-tinged tissues (cyanosis), and (as a result of elevated red blood cell mass) neurological effects such as headaches, dizziness, lethargy, and memory impairment. Right heart failure (cor pulmonale) can also develop. By relocating the patient to sea level and administering alternative treatments, these symptoms can be eliminated.

Measurement

Special Industrial Hygiene Monitoring Considerations at High Altitudes   Determining workplace exposures at high altitudes requires special industrial hygiene considerations (Dummer 1998; Berger and Rom 1998). High-altitude conditions (i.e., reduced barometric pressure) influence the accuracy of sampling instrumentation that is calibrated at lower altitudes. Although instrument calibrations are best performed at altitude, corrections for barometric pressure can be made for altitude changes. Measurements used to determine part per million concentrations should be volumetric because volume at higher altitudes contains a smaller mass, which gives a lower reading in parts per million. Because they are not volumetric and measure in parts per million, then, the accuracy of colorimetric tubes will be affected. Barometric corrections will need to be made by taking the reading, multiplying by the barometric pressure at sea level, and dividing the result by the barometric pressure at the sampling site and using the same units (such as torr or mbar) for both pressures.

High altitude also increases respiratory ventilation with acclimation and increases total dosages of inhaled occupational air contaminants. Therefore, workers may be excessively exposed compared to workers at sea level, even when measurements are below the exposure limits. Exposure limits should be reduced proportionately to the barometric pressure at the workplace when expressed as milligrams per cubic meter. For exposure limits expressed as parts per million, no *barometric adjustment is necessary because the proportion of millimoles of contaminant per mole of oxygen required by a worker stay approximately constant at different altitudes.*

The exposure limits or TLVs for extended shifts (>8 hours per workday and >40 hours per work week) require a barometric pressure correction for altitude to account for possible accumulation of toxic substances in the body as a result of increased exposure and reduction in detoxification time. For cumulative hazards where detoxification does not occur (e.g., silica), extended work shift correction should be proportional to the actual hours worked exceeding the usual 2,000 hours per year.

Risk Management

Because of the risk of altitude-related illnesses and disorders for unacclimated individuals at high altitude, preventive risk management is critical. In "Health Considerations for Managing Work at High Altitudes" (1998), J.B. West recommends the following management concepts.

Pre-Employment Examination   In addition to the standard preemployment examination protocol, special attention should be given to the cardiopulmonary system. Work at high altitudes places greater demands on the circulatory and respiratory systems. For example, medical conditions such as early chronic obstructive pulmonary disease and asthma are more disabling at altitude. Workers with blood disorders (such as sickle cell anemia, anemia, or polycythemia) will find working at high altitudes much more difficult. Medical professionals should be consulted to establish the appropriate medical protocols for the preemployment examinations.

Worker Selection   A segment of the workforce population will be unable or unwilling to tolerate living and working at high altitudes. One possible preventive measure is to screen for such workers. Predictors of tolerance include previous work history at high altitudes, testing for ventilatory response to hypoxia, and work capacity testing during acute hypoxia at sea level.

Preventive Measures   Because altitude-related illnesses and disorders are preventable in the majority of the population, efforts should be taken to prevent and reduce symptoms. The following highlights some of these recommendations (BHP 1997).

- Make a slow ascent. Travel by road rather than by air is recommended. If possible, it is best to avoid going directly from sea level to the high-altitude location in 1 day. The best prevention is slow ascent of not more than 300 m (1,000 ft) per day once above 2,400 m (approximately 8,000 ft).
- Upon arrival at altitude, avoid strenuous activity until acclimated.
- Sleep at the lowest possible level. Even at high altitudes, sleep low.
- Take medication, such as 250 mg of Diamox (acetozolamide) the evening before you travel and twice the following 2 days (morning and evening). This will ease the symptoms. It is best to check with a physician before taking any medication.
- Eat light meals for the first few days. The efficiency of the digestive system is impaired at high altitudes.
- Drink plenty of fluids, but avoid alcoholic beverages.
- Do not smoke.
- Do not take sleeping pills for insomnia; they can worsen respiratory depression, even causing death.
- Request oxygen if you experience any of the following while at altitude: headache, nausea, unusual fatigue while walking, resting pulse over 110, rapid breathing at rest, loss of appetite, or sleep disturbances.
- Immediately descend to lower altitude if you develop a cough, difficulty breathing, vomiting, confusion, or drowsiness. Call the medical officer in the event of these medical problems.
- If you have existing health problems associated with the cardiovascular or respiratory system, check with the physician to obtain a travel release.
- Immunize as recommended before traveling. Food and water precautions should be exercised while on site since dehydration from other factors, such as fever and/or diarrhea, can have a more severe effect in combination with physiological changes at high altitudes.

Scheduling Between High Altitudes and Sea Level   Acclimation studies have indicated that people who develop AMS after ascent to high altitudes feel better after several days. Additional findings indicate that the ventilatory response to hypoxia takes 7 to 10 days to reach a steady state; "therefore it is reasonable to recommend that the working period at high altitude be at least ten days ... whatever schedule is used, it is highly advantageous if the workers can sleep at a lower altitude than the workplace ... setting up sleeping quarters at this lower altitude (several hundred meters lower) will improve sleep quality, workers' comfort and sense of well-being, and productivity" (West 1998).

Oxygen Enrichment   To reduce high-altitude hypoxia, adding oxygen to normal room ventilation or the air conditioning system may be feasible in locations where decision making is conducted (such as in offices), as well as in worker sleeping quarters. Every 1% increase in oxygen concentration reduces the equivalent altitude by 300 m. Give consideration to the normal precautions for handling pure or nearly pure oxygen in the workplace.

Emergency Treatment   Descent, oxygen therapy, and rest are the three most effective and practical treatments for AMS, high-altitude pulmonary edema, and high-altitude cerebral edema. Management must allow adequate resources for providing emergency treatment in the event of altitude-related illnesses and disorders.

BIOHAZARDS

Among the range of mining-related health hazards, biohazards garner little attention. However, bio-hazards, especially bloodborne pathogens, can pose a health risk in a number of potential situations. Here, we briefly outline the health effects associated with selected biological agents and the recommended prevention and risk management options.

According to the AIHA Biohazards Committee, "a biohazardous agent is one that is biological in nature, capable of self-replication and has the capacity to produce deleterious effects upon other biological organisms, particularly humans" (AIHA 1986). The four broad classes of microorganisms that can interact with humans are bacteria, fungi, viruses, and protozoan parasites.

The three most common sources of these biohazards are: (1) those rising from microbial decomposition, (2) those associated with certain environments (water-borne, food-borne), and (3) those present in individuals infected with the pathogen.

The most common routes of exposure are oral, respiratory, skin puncture, penetration through unbroken skin, and penetration through eye tissue (conjuctival).

Health Effects

For an exhaustive compilation of diseases associated with biological agents, organizations such as the U.S. Centers for Disease Control and the World Health Organization provide extensive information and advice. The scope of diseases that can be prevented by immunization, transmitted by contaminated water, food or other insects, and communicable through humans is presented below. Included is a brief description of the disease and prevention methods for some diseases endemic to North America or in regions abroad where U.S. mining companies tend to operate (BHP Intranet Web site 1999; BHP 1994).

Diseases Prevented by Immunization   Routine immunizations provide protection against preventable diseases such as tetanus and diphtheria (effective for 10 years), as well as measles, mumps, and rubella (boosters recommended for those with birth dates after 1956). Vaccinations are imperative, especially for travel to risky areas.

Hepatitis—Four types of hepatitis viruses cause liver inflammation with symptoms ranging from mild and flu-like to fatal (liver failure). Because all hepatitis strains are serious, efforts should be taken to avoid exposure. Get immunized and avoid unsafe behaviors and risky sources of food and drink.

Hepatitis A, the most common type, is spread through food and water contaminated with feces under poor sanitary conditions. Symptoms include rash, fatigue, loss of appetite, jaundice, dark urine, fever, abdominal pain, and aching joints.

Hepatitis B is highly infectious, transmitted directly by exposure to infected blood and body fluids and indirectly through contact with contaminated equipment. Potential severe complications such as cirrhosis, liver cancer, and chronic hepatitis can develop. Hepatitis B can be fatal.

Hepatitis C is usually transmitted by unsafe sex practices, contaminated needles, or unscreened blood transfusions.

Hepatitis E is usually spread by drinking water contaminated with sewage. Pregnant women who contract this form of hepatitis have an unusually high mortality rate.

Under an approach to infection control known as "universal precautions," all human blood and certain human body fluids are treated as if infected with bloodborne pathogens such as hepatitis and human immunodeficiency virus (HIV). Universal precautions should be taken because certain strains of hepatitis are contagious from person to person via the transfer of body fluids—in sexual intercourse, blood transfusion, injection with unsterilized needles, childbirth, inadequately sterilized medical/dental equipment, tattooing, electrolysis, or IV drug use. Immunization offers protection against certain strains of hepatitis.

Typhoid fever—This serious and sometimes life-threatening disease is caused by the *Salmonella typhi* bacteria. Spread through the consumption of food and/or water that has been contaminated by feces or urine from patients or carriers, it is often spread through food handlers.

Meningococcal meningitis—This is an acute bacterial infection that causes the inflammation of the linings of the brain and spinal cord. It can be fatal if left untreated.

Bubonic plague—Bubonic plague is transmitted to humans through bites of infected animals, usually by rodents or rabbits. The pneumonic form of plague is transmitted directly from an infected person through coughing. Because plague can be fatal, full medical treatment is required.

Rabies—Rabies is spread through bites or licks from infected mammals on an open wound. It can also be picked up by eating rabies-infected meat. Medical attention and treatment is necessary if an individual is exposed.

Diseases Transmitted by Contaminated Food and Water   The best disease prevention is awareness of potential sources of food and drink contamination. Proper food handling and water purification precautions can be taken to prevent illnesses caused by bacteria, viruses, and parasites. The goal is to prevent disease by avoiding bacteria such as *Salmonella* and others that cause cholera, typhoid, and dysentery; viruses that cause hepatitis and polio; and parasites such as tapeworms, hookworms, or *Giardia* cysts.

Diarrhea—Bacteria, viruses, or parasites can cause diarrhea, which depletes the body of nutrients and fluids. Loose watery stools are accompanied by nausea, abdominal cramps, and vomiting. Oral rehydration treatment acts to replenish fluid loss and rectify electrolyte imbalances. Different types of diarrhea include "travelers diarrhea," normally caused by *Escherichia coli;* bacterial dysentery (shigellosis), an acute bacterial infection of the large intestine; amoebic dysentery, where cysts of infecting organisms are transmitted through food and water; and giardiasis, caused by parasites that infect the small intestine.

Giardiasis—Giardiasis is a common parasitic disorder that is contracted either by direct contact with animal or human feces, or by drinking feces-contaminated water. The disease may be self-limiting or become chronic.

Cholera—Cholera is caused by a bacterium and is spread through sewage-contaminated food and water. Although it can be life threatening, it is preventable and easily treated through fluid replacement therapy.

Legionnaires' disease (LD)—LD is an acute respiratory infection caused by the bacterium *Legionella pneumophila,* which is transmitted through the air. Recent cases have documented bacteria contamination of cooling tower water and the spread of aerosols through air-handling systems. LD manifests as a form of pneumonia and has a 15% fatality rate. Susceptible populations include people with reduced immunologic capacity, risk factors such as cigarette smoking and alcohol abuse, and exposure to high concentrations of the bacteria. Good maintenance, water sterilization, and procedures to control bacterial growth are fundamental to the prevention of LD.

Trichinosis—This disease is caused by parasites found mainly in pigs and bear meat. All meat should be thoroughly cooked. Salting, drying, and smoking procedures will not kill the parasitic larvae, but freezing will.

Scromboid poisoning—Spoilage bacteria from improperly preserved fish produce histamine and other toxic by-products that can induce a toxic response when eating this fish.

Insect-Borne Diseases   The "four way approach" can assist with the successful avoidance of insect bites. The approach includes using DEET-containing insect repellents on skin and clothing, wearing clothing with long sleeves and tucking long pants into socks, using bed nets treated with permethrin, and applying knock-down sprays containing pyrethroids and permethrin.

Malaria—Travelers to all tropical regions are susceptible to this parasitic disease, which is spread by the night-biting *Anopheles* mosquito infected by one of four varieties of malarial parasites. After the bite, the parasites invade the liver and multiply. To avoid infection, take active measures to avoid mosquito bites and use prophylactic medication (USDHHS NCID 1995).

Lyme disease—Lyme disease is a tick-borne disease that can cause severe arthritis, neurological disorders, and/or heart problems if left unrecognized and undiagnosed. The bite of infected deer ticks in the adult or nymph stage transmits the disease to humans.

Rocky Mountain spotted fever—This rare disease is caused by rickettsia-parasite-infected wood or dog tick bites. If untreated with antibiotics, this disease can be fatal.

Hantavirus Pulmonary Syndrome (HPS)—HPS is a fairly uncommon, newly recognized, and potentially deadly disease found in North America. Once its nonspecific "flu-like" symptoms appear, immediate intensive care is essential. Hantaviruses are carried by rodents, especially the deer mouse, and can infect humans who are exposed to mouse droppings.

Other Diseases

Leptospirosis—This is an acute occupational illness for field workers and miners who are in contact—either directly through an open wound, or through the mucous membranes of the eyes, nose, or mouth—with water or soil contaminated with animal urine. Rats frequently spread the disease. Efforts should be taken to avoid swimming or bathing in stagnant pools or sluggish streams, to be aware of the dangers of urine contamination, and to carefully wash (or avoid) fresh vegetables grown in soil with suspected contamination.

Histoplasmosis—Serious fungal infections (mycosis) can result from inhaling high concentrations of fungal spores from bat or bird droppings. Old mine workings and caves may present a health risk to those who enter and are exposed to fungal spores and droppings from large populations of bats or birds. Dust masks or respirators should be worn to minimize exposure to airborne spores. Clothing worn to enter these old mine workings or caves should be discarded or thoroughly cleaned before the next use.

Tuberculosis (TB)—TB is a bacterial disease that—despite advances in medical science—is still prevalent around the world. Infections are transmitted by prolonged contact with a diseased person who has an active case of TB. The bacillus, spread through aerosol droplets in the air or saliva, can remain dormant for years. However, when the disease is active, it causes cavitation in the lungs, coughing (during which blood may be present, depending on the stage of the disease), fever, and weight loss. Active cases must be treated with a strict regimen of antibiotics that lasts 9 months and with periodic screening using chest x-rays as well as sputum smears and cultures.

AIDS—Acquired Immune Deficiency Syndrome is caused by the family of viruses called HIV. The predominant strains affecting humans are HIV 1 and HIV 2. The virus attacks the immune system and the central nervous system, causing susceptibilities to unusual infections, tumors, and mental conditions, leading to death. There is no cure and no vaccine. Because the virus can be transmitted from person to person via the transfer of body fluids through sexual intercourse, blood transfusion, injection with unsterilized needles, childbirth, inadequately sterilized medical/dental equipment, tattooing, electrolysis, or IV drug use, universal precautions should be taken.

REFERENCES

Alpaugh, E.L., revised by T.J. Hogan. 1988. Temperature extremes. In *Fundamentals of Industrial Hygiene.* Edited by B.A. Plog. Itasca, IL: NSC.

ACGIH. 1998. 1998 TLVs• and BEIs•, *Threshold Limit Values for Chemical Substances and Physical Agents, Biological Exposure Indices.* Cincinnati: ACGIH Worldwide.

AIHA. 1986. *Biohazards Reference Manual.* Akron, OH: AIHA.

——. 1997. *The Occupational Environment—Its Evaluation and Control.* Edited by S.R. DiNardi. Fairfax, VA: AIHA.

AWS. 1973. *The Welding Environment.* Miami: AWS.

Baker, E.L. 1990. Role of medical screening in the prevention of occupational disease. *Journal of Occupational and Environmental Medicine* 32(9): 788.

Berger, K.I., and W.N. Rom. 1998. Physiological effects of reduced barometric pressure. In *Encyclopaedia of Occupational Safety and Health.* Geneva: ILO Publications.

BHP. 1994. *BHP Exploration Department Safety Manual.*

——. 1997. *High Altitude Travel.*

——. 1999. *Diesel Emissions Awareness.*

BHP Intranet Web site. 1999. *Medical Disease Risk.*

Bouchet, J.P., H. Roels, and A. Bernard, et al. 1980. Assessment of renal function of workers exposed to inorganic lead, cadmium or mercury vapor. *Journal of Occupational and Environmental Medicine* 22: 741–751.

Bureau of Mines Information Circular 9324. 1992. Washington, DC: U.S. Department of Interior, Bureau of Mines.

Cantrell, B.K., and K.L. Rubow. 1992. Measurement of diesel exhaust aerosol in underground coal mines. In *Diesels in Underground Mines: Measurement and Control of Particulate Emissions. Proceedings: Bureau of Mines Information and Technology Transfer Seminar.* Minneapolis. September 29–30.

Carlson, A.J., and A. Woelfel. 1913. The solubility of lead salts in human gastric juice, and its bearing on the hygiene of lead industries. *Journal of the American Medical Association* 61: 181–184.

Chen, K.K., and C.L. Rose. 1952. Nitrite and thiosulfate therapy in cyanide poisoning. *Journal of the American Medical Association* 149: 113–119.

Cornish, H.H. 1975. Solvents and vapors. In *Toxicology—The Basic Science of Poisons.* 4th ed. Edited by L.J. Casarett, and J. Doull. New York: Pergamon Press.

Dixon, M., and E.C. Webb. 1958. *Enzymes.* New York: Academic Press.

Dummer, W. 1998. Prevention of occupational hazards at high altitude. In *Encyclopaedia of Occupational Health and Safety.* Geneva: ILO Publications.

Ellenhom, M.J., and D.J. Barceloux. 1988. *Medical Toxicology.* New York: Elsevier.

Elinder, C.G., T. Kjellstrom, B. Lind, L. Linnman, M. Piscator, and K. Sundstedt. 1983. Cadmium exposure from smoking cigarettes. Variations with time and country where purchased. *Environmental Research* 32: 220–227.

Finkel, A.J. 1983. *Hamilton and Hardy's Industrial Toxicology.* 4th ed. Boston: John Wright & Sons.

Goyer, R. 1991. Toxic effects of metals. In *Casarett and Doull's Toxicology, The Basic Science of Poisons.* Edited by J. Doull, C.D. Klaasen, and M.O. Amdur. New York: Pergamon Press.

Hartung, R. 1991. Cyanides and nitriles. In *Patty's Industrial Hygiene and Toxicology.* 4th ed. Edited by G.D. Clayton and F.E. Clayton. New York: John Wiley & Sons.

Hathaway, G.J., N.H. Proctor, and J.P. Hughes. 1996. *Procotor and Hughes' Chemical Hazards of the Workplace.* 4th ed. New York: Van Nostrand Reinhold.

Heath, D., and D.R. Williams. 1981. *Man at High Altitude.* Edinburgh. Churchill: Livingstone.

HEI (Health Effects Institute). 1999. *Diesel Emissions and Lung Cancer: Epidemiology and Quantitative Risk Assessment.* Cambridge, MA: Health Effects Institute.

Hethmon, T., and S. Ludlow. 1997. Air sampling methodologies for sulfuric acid mist in copper electrowinning: field evaluations and development of a new method. *Applied Occupational and Environmental Hygiene* 12(12): 1041–1046.

Holmer, I. 1998. Cold indices and standards. In *Encyclopaedia of Occupational Health and Safety.* Geneva: ILO Publications.

IARC. 1987. *Monographs on the Evaluations of Carcinogenicity: An Update of IARC Monographs.* 1–42(7). Lyon, France: IARC Press.

——. 1989. *IARC Monographs on the Evaluation of Carcinogenic Risks to Humans; Diesel and Gasoline Engine Exhausts and Some Nitroarenes* 46. Lyon, France: IARC Press.

——. 1992. *IARC Monographs on the Evaluation of Carcinogenic Risk to Humans: Occupational Exposure to Mists and Vapours from Strong Inorganic Acids; and Other Industrial Chemicals* 54. Lyon, France: IARC Press.

JCB. 1999. *Diesel Particulate in Coal Mines—Questions and Answers.* 1st ed. Sydney, Australia: JCB. See http://www.jcb.org.au/dieselbook4.pdf.

Kaliva-Papachristodoulou, A. 1983. *A study of the acidic aerosol resulting from zinc electrowinning operations.* Ph.D. thesis. University of Toronto.

Kneip, T.J., M. Eisenbud, C.D. Strehlow, and P.C. Freudenthal. 1970. Airborne particulates in New York City. *Journal of the Air Pollution Control Association* 20: 144–149.

Lancrajan, I., H.I. Popescu, O. Gavanescu, I. Klepsch, and M. Servanescu. 1975. Reproductive ability of workmen occupationally exposed to lead. *Archives of Environmental Health* 30: 396–401.

Levin, M., J. Jacobs, and P.G. Polos. 1988. Acute mercury poisoning and mercurial pneumonitis from gold ore purification. *Chest* 94: 554–556.

Lillis, R., A. Miller, and Y. Leman. 1985. Acute mercury poisoning with severe chronic pulmonary manifestation. *Chest* 82: 306–309.

McAlexander, R.M., R. Lewis, G.A. Tweedy and R.L. Fields. 1981. *Cyanide Mill Reagents.* Washington, DC: U.S. Department of Labor.

McFee, D.R., and P. Zavon. 1988. Solvents. In *Fundamentals of Industrial Hygiene.* Edited by B.A. Plog. Itasca, IL: NSC.

Malcolm D., and E. Paul. 1961. Erosion of teeth due to sulphuric acid in the battery industry. *British Journal of Industrial Medicine* 18: 63–69.

Malouf, E.E. 1990. Open pit rock mechanics. In *Surface Mining.* 2nd ed. Edited by B.A. Kennedy. Baltimore: Society for Mining, Metallurgy, and Exploration.

Marsden, J., and I. House. 1992. *The Chemistry of Gold Extraction.* Chichester, West Sussex, England: Ellis Horwood Limited.

MSHA. 1999. *Draft Guidelines for Medical Surveillance & Biological Monitoring for Miners Exposed to Arsenic, Cadmium, Lead and Mercury.* MSHA Internet home page. See http://www.msha.gov/ S&HINFO/TOOLBOX/METALEXP/METALEXP.PDF.

———. 1998. In *Code of Federal Regulations.* Title 30–Mineral Resources. Parts 30 CFR Part 56, 58, 72.

———. 1997. *Practical Ways to Reduce Exposure to Diesel Exhaust in Mining–A Toolbox.* See http://www.gov/5%26hinfo/toolbox/tbcover.html.

Mody, V., and R. Jakhete. 1988. *Dust Control Handbook.* Park Ridge, NJ: Noyes Data Corporation.

NIOSH. 1978. *Occupational Health Guideline for Cyanide.* Washington, DC: U.S. Department of Health and Human Services, Public Health Service, Centers for Disease Control.

———. 1979. *Current 32: Arsine (Arsenic Hydride) Poisoning in the Workplace.* Washington, DC: U.S. Department of Health and Human Services, Public Health Service, Centers for Disease Control.

———. 1986. *Occupational Exposures to Hot Environments.* Washington, DC: U.S. Department of Health and Human Services, Public Health Service, Centers for Disease Control.

———. 1988. *Carcinogenic Effects of Exposure to Diesel Exhaust.* Current Intelligence Bulletin 50. Washington, DC: U.S. Department of Health and Human Services, Public Health Service, Centers for Disease Control.

———. 1988. *Criteria for a Recommended Standard–Welding, Brazing, and Thermal Cutting.* Washington, DC: U.S. Department of Health and Human Services, Public Health Service, Centers for Disease Control.

———. 1994. Elements by ICP: Method 7300. In *NIOSH Manual of Analytical Methods (NMAM).* 4th ed. Washington, DC: U.S. Department of Health and Human Services, Public Health Service, Centers for Disease Control.

———. 1994. Arsenic trioxide as As: Method 7901. In *NIOSH Manual of Analytical Methods (NMAM).* 4th ed. Washington, DC: U.S. Department of Health and Human Services, Public Health Service, Centers for Disease Control.

———. 1994. Arsine: Method 6001. In *NIOSH Manual of Analytical Methods (NMAM).* 4th ed. Washington, DC: U.S. Department of Health and Human Services, Public Health Service, Centers for Disease Control.

———. 1994. Cyanides, aerosol and gas: Method 7904. In *NIOSH Manual of Analytical Methods (NMAM).* 4th ed. Washington, DC: U.S. Department of Health and Human Services, Public Health Service, Centers for Disease Control.

———. 1994. Hydrogen cyanide: Method 6010. In *NIOSH Manual of Analytical Methods (NMAM).* 4th ed. Washington, DC: U.S. Department of Health and Human Services, Public Health Service, Centers for Disease Control.

———. Elemental Carbon: Method 5040. *NIOSH Manual of Analytical Methods.* Washington, DC: U.S. Department of Health and Human Services, Public Health Service, Centers for Disease Control.

NSC. 1988. *Fundamentals of Industrial Hygiene.* Edited by B.A. Plog. Itasca, IL: NSC.

NTP (National Toxicology Program). 1998. *Report on Carcinogens. Background Document for Diesel Exhaust Particulates.* Research Triangle Park, NC: U.S. Department of Health and Human Services.

Nelson, K. 1983. Industrial sources. In *Arsenic: Industrial, Biomedical, Environmental Perspectives.* Edited by W.H. Lederer, and R.J. Fensterheim. New York: Van Nostrand Reinhold.

NSW Minerals Council. Revised Draft 1999. *Diesel Emissions in Underground Mines Management and Control.* Sydney, Australia.

———. 1996. *Guidelines for Minimising Exposure to Diesel Emissions in Underground Mines.* Sydney, Australia.

Nordberg, G.F. 1972. Cadmium metabolism and toxicity. *Environmental Physiology and Biochemistry* 2: 7–36.

Nunneley, S.A. 1998. Prevention of heat stress. In *Encyclopaedia of Occupational Health and Safety.* Geneva: ILO Publications.

OEHHA (Office of Environmental Health Hazard Assessment). 1998. *Health Risk Assessment for Diesel Exhaust.* Sacramento: California Environmental Protection Agency.

Ogawa, T. 1998. Heat disorders. In *Encyclopaedia of Occupational Health and Safety.* Geneva: ILO Publications.

Platcow, P.A., and G.S. Lyndon. 1998. Welding and thermal cutting. In *Encyclopaedia of Occupational Health and Safety.* Geneva: ILO Publications.

Reeves, J.T., and J.V. Weil. 1998. Ventilatory acclimatization to high altitude. In *Encyclopaedia of Occupational Health and Safety.* Geneva: ILO Publications.

Thakur, P.C., and C.R. Hamilton. 1998. "An Integrated Approach to Control Diesel Particulate Matter in Underground Coal Mines." Presentation to the West Virginia Diesel Equipment Commission.

U.S. EPA. 1998. *Health Assessment Document for Diesel Emissions: SAB Review Draft.* Washington, DC: Office of Research and Development.

U.S. Department of Health and Human Services, Public Health Service, Centers for Disease Control/ National Center for Infectious Diseases. 1995. *Preventing Malaria in Travelers.* Washington, DC: U.S. Department of Health and Human Services.

Vogt, J.J. Heat and cold. 1998. In *Encyclopaedia of Occupational Health and Safety.* Geneva: ILO Publications.

Wang, Z., and T.G. Rossman. 1996. The carcinogenicity of arsenic. In *Toxicology of Metals.* Edited by L. Chang. Boca Raton, FL: CRC Press.

Watts, W.E. 1992. Health risks associated with the use of diesel equipment underground. In *Diesels in Underground Mines: Measurement and Control of Particulate Emissions. Proceedings: Bureau of Mines Information and Technology Transfer Seminar.* Minneapolis, MN. September 29–30. Bureau of Mines Information Circular 9324. Washington, DC: U.S. Department of Interior, Bureau of Mines.

Watts, W.E. 1987. Industrial hygiene issues arising from the use of diesel equipment in underground mines. In *Diesels in Underground Mines Proceedings: Bureau of Mines Technology Transfer Seminar* (Louisville, KY, April 21, and Denver, CO, April 23). Bureau of Mines Information Circular 9141. Washington, DC: U.S. Department of Interior, Bureau of Mines.

Waytulonis. R.W. 1992. Modern diesel emission control. In *Diesels in Underground Mines: Measurement and Control of Particulate Emissions. Proceedings: Bureau of Mines Information and Technology Transfer Seminar.* Minneapolis, MN. September 29–30. Bureau of Mines Information Circular 9324. Washington, DC: U.S. Department of Interior, Bureau of Mines.

West, J.B. 1998. Health considerations for managing work at high altitudes. In *Encyclopaedia of Occupational Health and Safety.* Geneva: ILO Publications.

Williams, K.L., J.E. Chilton, D.P. Tuchman, and A.F. Cohen. 1987. Measuring gaseous pollutants from diesel exhaust in underground mines. In *Diesels in Underground Mines Proceedings: Bureau of Mines Technology Transfer Seminar* (Louisville, KY, April 21, and Denver, CO, April 23). Bureau of Mines Information Circular 9141. Washington, DC: U.S. Department of Interior, Bureau of Mines.

World Health Organization (WHO). 1996. *Diesel Fuel and Exhaust Emissions: International Programme on Chemical Safety.* Geneva: WHO.

CHAPTER 23

Ground Control Issues for Safety Professionals

Christopher Mark, Ph.D.
Rock Mechanics Section Chief

Anthony T. Iannacchione, Ph.D.
Deputy Director
National Institute for Occupational Safety and Health (NIOSH), Pittsburgh, Pennsylvania

INTRODUCTION

Falls of ground continue to be one of the most serious causes of injury to U.S. miners. Of the 256 fatal injuries that occurred in mining between 1996 and 1998, 59 (23%) were caused by falls of ground (Table 23.1). Falls of ground affect some sectors of the mining industry more severely than others. For instance, nearly 40% of the 98 coal mine fatalities between 1996 and 1998 were caused by falls of ground. Underground miners are at much greater risk than surface miners. Nearly half (45 out of 101) of underground mine fatalities were attributed to roof, rib, and face falls, while only 6% of the 155 surface fatalities were caused by falls of highwalls or slopes.

The goal of this chapter is to provide guidance to safety professionals tasked with preventing ground fall injuries. This chapter combines an analysis of the Mine Safety and Health Administration's (MSHA) accident and injury data with a survey of industry "best practices" to safeguard miners from ground falls. Ultimately, this approach can help to form the basis of a sound, proactive ground control program for the mining industry.

SOURCES OF DATA

All the injury data examined in this study were derived from MSHA's fatal investigation reports and the MSHA accident database. Because falls of ground often result in serious injury, MSHA "Fatalgrams" and fatal investigation reports provide a useful snapshot of ground control issues in the mining industry. These reports are available to the public (on the MSHA Web site at www.msha.gov). Fatalgrams are one-page summaries that are usually published within a month of an accident. They contain very basic information about the accident with a graphic and a short section on relevant best practices. Fatal investigation reports are the official accident investigation reports filed by MSHA personnel. These reports contain general information about the mine, a description of the accident, physical factors involved in the accident, a conclusion, and enforcement actions. Enforcement actions typically identify citations and discuss violations to the Federal Mining Law.

MSHA also maintains comprehensive statistical data on the mining industry's accident and injury record. The law requires that mines file a report on every reportable accident that occurs, containing information on the accident's location, severity, classification, activity, and nature of injury. A short narrative is generally included as well. Accident reports can be searched by many of the above fields.

TABLE 23.1 Fatalities from 1996 to 1998 by commodity for both falls of ground and other mining classifications

	1996		1997		1998		Total	
	Under-ground	Surface and Prep Plants	Under-ground	Surface and Prep Plants	Under-ground	Surface and Prep Plants	Under-ground	Surface and Prep Plants
Coal falls of ground	13	1	9	0	14	1	36	2
Coal total	**33**	**6**	**22**	**8**	**22**	**7**	**77**	**21**
Metal falls of ground	1	0	2	1	3	0	6	8
Metal total	**5**	**3**	**7**	**5**	**5**	**5**	**17**	**13**
Nonmetal falls of ground	0	0	0	0	0	0	0	0
Nonmetal total	**0**	**1**	**1**	**2**	**2**	**4**	**3**	**7**
Stone falls of ground	2	2	1	1	0	1	3	4
Stone total	**2**	**25**	**2**	**26**	**0**	**23**	**4**	**74**
Sand/gravel falls of ground	0	0	0	0	0	0	0	0
Sand/gravel total	**0**	**11**	**0**	**17**	**0**	**12**	**0**	**40**
Total falls of ground	**16**	**3**	**12**	**2**	**17**	**2**	**45**	**7**
Total mining	**40**	**46**	**32**	**58**	**29**	**51**	**101**	**155**

From 1996 to 1998, U.S. miners suffered a total of 55,096 injuries, which ranged in severity from death (degree 1) to injuries with no days away from work or restricted duty (degree 6). Six percent of the total injuries were from falls of ground, including machine accidents where caving rock was coded as the source. As the data in Table 23.2 indicate, 98% of all nonfatal fall of ground injuries occurred in underground mines, with underground coal mines accounting for 83% of the total.

Table 23.2 also shows the distribution nonfatal fall of ground injuries by severity and commodity. The injuries are classified into lost time injuries that resulted in permanent disability (degree 2) or days off work (degrees 3–4), and injuries without lost time that resulted in no more than restricted duty (degree 5–6). Overall, groundfall injuries appear to be more serious than other types of mining injuries. Sixty-five percent of all ground fall injuries resulted in lost time, compared to 54% of all types of mining injuries.

Analysis of the accident database allows safety professionals to learn from the experience of the entire industry. The factors responsible for many ground fall injuries emerge from this analysis, and possible solutions can be identified as well. It also allows for the timely recognition of trends, both from a standpoint of identifying successful interventions as well as focusing on emerging issues.

LEGAL FRAMEWORK

Laws governing mining in the United States are listed in the *Code of Federal Regulations* (CFR) under Title 30—Mineral Resources. Laws pertaining to the control of ground in surface and underground mines are covered in four parts, characterized by surface coal mining (Part 77), underground coal mining (Part 75), metal/nonmetal surface mining (Part 56), and metal/nonmetal underground mining (Part 57). The U.S. Mining Law contains both specific and sweeping statements, and its generalized

TABLE 23.2   Nonfatal fall of ground injuries from 1996 to 1998

Severity	Commodity	Underground	All Other	Total
Lost time injuries (degree 2 to 4)	Coal	1807	23	1830
	Metal	140	5	145
	Nonmetal	15	0	15
	Stone	14	9	23
	Subtotal	**1976**	**37**	**2013**
Injuries without lost time (degrees 5 and 6)	Coal	777	9	786
	Metal	269	3	272
	Nonmetal	23	1	24
	Stone	16	7	23
	Subtotal	**1085**	**20**	**1105**
All nonfatal injuries	Coal	2584	32	2616
	Metal	409	8	417
	Nonmetal	38	1	39
	Stone	30	16	46
	Total	**3061**	**57**	**3118**

TABLE 23.3   Violations of Part 75 from fall of ground fatal investigation reports, 1996–1998

Subsection Violated	Title	Number
75.202	Protection from falls of roof, face, and ribs	18
75.203	Mining method	1
75.204	Roof bolting	0
75.205	Installation of roof support using mining machine with integral bolter	0
75.206	Conventional roof support	0
75.207	Pillar recovery	0
75.208	Warning devices	0
75.209	Automated temporary roof support systems	1
75.210	Manual installation of temporary support	0
75.211	Roof testing and scaling	0
75.212	Rehabilitation of areas with unsupported roof	1
75.213	Roof support removal	3
75.214	Supplemental support materials, equipment, and tools	0
75.215	Longwall mining systems	0
75.220	Roof control plan	6
75.221	Roof control plan information	0
75.222	Roof control plan—approval criteria	0
75.223	Evaluation and revision of roof control plan	0

language promotes flexibility and innovation. For example, in coal mining, each mine is required to submit its own roof control plan, which contains, in many cases, many details as to how the mine will comply with ground control aspects of the law.

Underground coal mining roof control is covered in 18 subsections within Part 75. Although each of these sections outlines an important step in controlling falls of ground, some sections are cited more frequently in fatal investigation reports. Between 1996 and 1998, a total of 30 citations were given to mines following fatal accidents, citing 6 of the 18 sections (Table 23.3). The most frequently cited subsection was 75.202–protection from falls of roof, face, and rib. Section 75.202 requires that ground support must protect persons from hazards related to falls of the roof, face, or ribs and coal or rock bursts in areas where they work or travel. It also states that no person may work or travel under an unsupported roof unless in accordance with special procedures. Another common citation listed was violation of the roof control plan. The language also states that additional measures shall be taken to protect persons if unusual hazards are encountered.

Underground metal/nonmetal mining roof control is covered in nine subsections within Part 57. Between 1996 and 1998, the most frequently cited subsection following fatalities was 57.3200, which requires that hazardous ground conditions be taken down or supported before other work or travel is permitted (Table 23.4). The law also requires that the affected area be posted with a warning against entry and, when left unattended, that a barrier be installed to impede unauthorized entry. Many of the fatal investigation reports reveal that geologic structures contributed to the conditions referred to in subsection language. In four of the reports, inadequate examination of ground conditions was cited.

Surface mining ground control is covered in 9 subsections within Part 56 for metal/nonmetal mines and 15 subsections within Part 77 for coal mines. Several violations cited subsection 56.3200, which requires hazardous ground conditions to be taken down or supported before work or travel is permitted. The directive states that until corrective work is completed, the area shall be posted with a warning against entry and, when left unattended, a barrier shall be installed to impede unauthorized entry.

ROOF CONTROL PLANS

Each coal mine operator is expected to develop and follow a roof control plan, approved by the MSHA district manager, that is suitable to the prevailing geological conditions and the mining system to be used at the mine. The law also outlines what should be contained within the plan (75.221), how the plan will be approved (75.222), and how revisions to the plan will be evaluated (75.223). The data discussed above suggest that violations to the plan can result in serious injury to the miner. Management *must* communicate and enforce the specifics of the roof control plan to the workforce. Additionally, the plan cannot be viewed as a static document. As conditions of mining change, the plan must be updated and resubmitted to the local MSHA district manager for approval. Safety professionals may have no greater tool at their disposal for addressing ground control issues than the roof control plan.

The mine operator is also responsible for taking any necessary measures to protect persons if unusual hazards are encountered. When new support materials, devices, or systems are used as the only means of roof support, the MSHA district manager may require that their effectiveness be demonstrated by experimental installations as part of a test plan.

Roof control plan implementation begins by instructing all persons who are affected by its provisions. The approved plan and any revisions must be available to the miners and their representatives and must be posted on a mine bulletin board.

Subsection 75.221 lists the information that must be included in the roof control plan. Some of the most important issues include:

- Specifications of all supports that may be used, including the length, diameter, grade, type of anchorage, drill hole size, and bolt torque or tension ranges for roof bolts
- Installation procedures for supports, including spacing and sequence of roof bolts
- Maximum automated temporary roof support (ATRS) distance beyond the last row of permanent support
- Entry width, size of pillars, method of pillar recovery, and the sequence of mining pillars
- Frequency of test holes to be drilled at least 12 in. above the roof bolt anchorage horizon
- Special support and mining systems, such as for mine entries within 45 m (150 ft) of an outcrop.

The roof control plan sets forth minimum requirements, specifically in areas such as bolt length and bolt spacing. Additional support measures must be used to adequately support local adverse conditions. When conditions indicate that the plan is not suitable for controlling falls of ground, the operator must propose revisions of the roof control plan (Sec. 75.223). Conversely, when the accident and injury experience at the mine indicates the plan is inadequate, MSHA will generally require changes to the plan. MSHA reviews the roof control plan at each mine every six months. To assist with the review, all unplanned roof falls, rib falls, and coal or rock bursts that occur in the active workings must be plotted on a mine map.

TABLE 23.4 Violations from Part 57 from fall of ground fatal investigation reports, 1996–1998

Subsection Violated	Title	Number
57.3200	Correction of hazardous conditions	6
57.3201	Location for performing scaling	1
57.3202	Scaling tools	1
57.3203	Rock fixtures	0
57.3360	Ground support use	0
57.3400	Secondary breakage	0
57.3401	Examination of ground conditions	4
57.3460	Maintenance between machinery or equipment and ribs	0
57.3461	Rock bursts	0

GROUNDFALL HAZARDS AND BEST PRACTICES TO CONTROL THEM

The 51 fatal investigation reports from 1996 to 1998 provide a window on the most significant groundfall hazards facing today's miners. Some of these hazards, such as geologic features, affect all miners to one degree or another. Others are specific to the commodity or mining method. Many are the subject of recent or ongoing NIOSH research and are addressed in papers available at www.cdc.gov/niosh/pit. Best practices can also be obtained from MSHA literature, including the "cards" available at www.msha.gov/s&hinfo/prop/prophome.htm.

Geologic Discontinuities

Mines are unique structures because they are not constructed of manmade materials, such as steel or concrete, but are built of rock, just as nature made them. Thus, integrity of a mine structure is greatly affected by the natural weaknesses or discontinuities that disrupt the continuity of the roof and rib. Geologic discontinuities can originate while the material is being deposited by sedimentary or intrusive processes, or later when it is being subjected to tectonic forces. Depositional discontinuities include slips, clastic dikes, fossil remains, bedding planes, and transition zones. Structural discontinuities include faults, joints, and igneous dikes. Some of the most important discontinuities that affect mine safety are described below.

- *Slips* are breaks or cracks in the roof, and they are the features most often cited in underground coal mine fatality reports. When slips are more than several feet long and are steeply dipping, they form a ready-made failure surface. Their surfaces are usually *slickensided*–i.e., smooth, highly polished, and striated. Two slips that intersect form an unsupported wedge that is commonly called a *horseback*. Undetected slips that do not fail during development have a tendency to pop out when subjected to abutment pressures generated during pillar recovery operations. Longer or angled bolts may be used to support slips, and straps or truss bolts can be even more effective.

- *Joints* are fractures commonly found in hard rocks. They occur in sets with similar orientation. Often several sets of joints occur at angles to each other, creating unstable blocks that must be supported by roof bolts.

- *Fossil remains* are the remnants of plants and animals that lived during the time when the sediments that later became rocks were being deposited. For example, kettlebottoms are fossil trees that grew in ancient peat swamps (Figure 23.1). They occur in every U.S. coal basin, but are especially abundant in southern West Virginia and eastern Kentucky. Dinosaur footprints are another fossil remain found in the roof rocks of coal mines in Utah, Wyoming, and Colorado. Fossil remains can fall without warning and should always be carefully supported (Chase 1992). Roof boltholes should never be drilled directly in fossil remains, because the vibrations could cause them to be dislodged.

- *Bedding planes* are typically found in sedimentary rocks and can extend great lateral distances. Bedding planes represent sharp changes in deposition (e.g., limestone to clay, or sandstone to coal). These planes can separate readily and are frequently involved in roof falls.

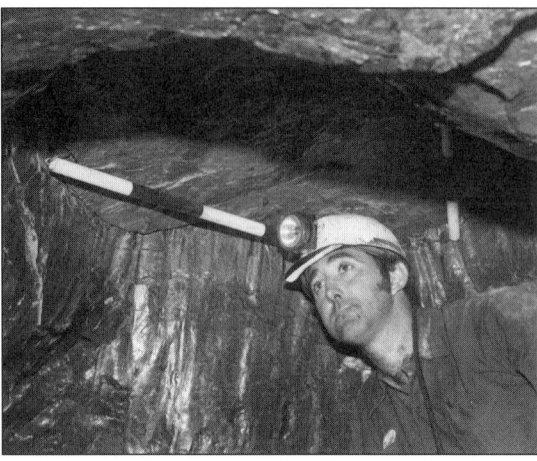

FIGURE 23.1   Large kettle bottom in an underground coal mine (photo by F. Chase)

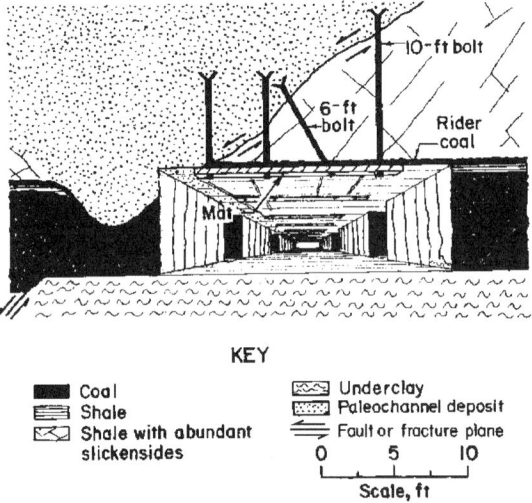

FIGURE 23.2   Suggested roof support for a stream channel transition zone (Chase 1992)

- *Transition zones* occur in many types of strata but are particularly common in sedimentary rocks. A transition zone occurs when some change in deposition causes a change in sedimentation. Different types of sediments compact at different rates. Discontinuities are abundant in the transition zones between distinct strata. For example, where ancient streambeds eroded the adjacent sediments, remnants of the stream channel disrupt the continuity of the normal roof beds, resulting in large slip planes (Figure 23.2).

- *Faults* are structural displacements within the rock. Tectonic forces can cause rocks to break and slip. Faults often contain weak *gouge* material, and the country rock around them can be distorted, fractured, and hazardous (Figure 23.3). Faults are often cited as contributing to surface mine highwall failures.

Discontinuities occur in many shapes and sizes and are generally difficult to recognize in advance of mining. They often contribute to fatal accidents, frequently in combination with other factors. Miners, and particularly roof bolt operators and face drillers, need to be trained to recognize geologic discontinuities as soon as they are exposed by mining. They must also be aware of the proper support techniques and have the necessary support materials available.

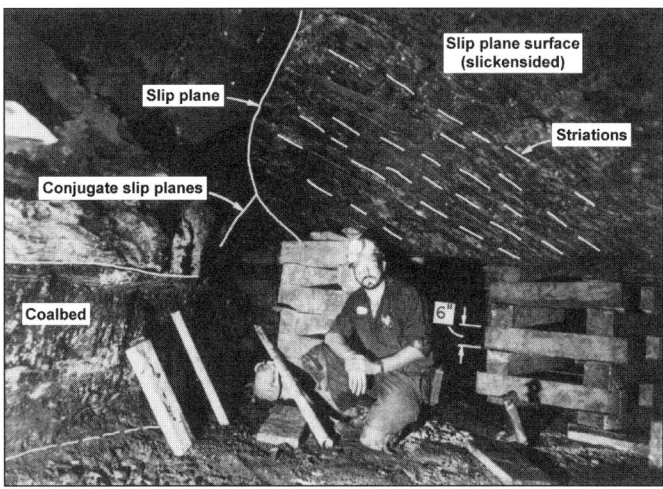

FIGURE 23.3   Fault in an underground coal mine (photo by G. Molinda)

TABLE 23.5   Factors in underground coal mine fall of ground fatalities

Factor	1996	1997	1998	Total
Pillar extraction	4	4	5	13
Inby roof support	4	0	5	9
Intersections	1	3	2	6
Geology	1	4	1	6
Rib	2	3	0	5
Construction	1	0	3	4
Skin control	1	0	2	3
Longwall face	1	1	0	2

Underground Coal Mine Hazards

Between 1996 and 1998, 36 underground coal miners were killed in 33 separate incidents. Table 23.5 lists the hazards that contributed to these incidents and their frequency. In some cases, more than one hazard was involved. For example, 13 fatalities occurred during pillar extraction, with 3 of the accidents resulting from premature intersection collapses.

Unsupported Roof

Roof bolts and the ATRS are the first lines of defense against roof falls in underground coal mines. When miners go under unsupported roof, they are completely unprotected. Between 1996 and 1998, approximately 25% of coal mine roof and rib fatalities occurred when miners were beyond roof supports. While there are no grounds for complacency, the recent record does represent an improvement from a decade ago, when nearly 50% of ground fall fatalities occurred beneath unsupported roof (Peters 1992). The improvement was achieved through new equipment, enforcement and a persistent educational campaign.

By definition, roof support activities take place very close to unsupported roof. Therefore it is not surprising that most of the fatal accidents involved roof bolt operators or other miners engaged in roof support. Based on the accident record, single-head roof bolt machines appear to be a risk factor. Roof control plans carefully specify the sequence of bolt installation with single-head machines to avoid placing the operator inby support. If these guidelines are not followed, the roof bolt operator can be at risk.

During the early 1990s, the U.S. Bureau of Mines (USBM) conducted an extensive series of interviews with miners to determine why they might go out under unsupported roof (Peters 1992). The most common response was that they had unintentionally walked out beyond the supports. The most effective countermeasure, then, is to ensure that all areas of unsupported roof are clearly posted with highly visible warning devices. Other activities that were associated with going inby supports included:

- Operating a continuous miner or scoop
- Hanging or extending ventilation tube or curtain
- Retrieving items left lying on the ground
- Repairing or restoring power to a continuous miner
- Marking the roof for bolt installation.

Relatively simple procedures or technologies can be implemented to reduce the temptation for workers to intentionally go beyond support. However, training is essential. Mallett and colleagues (1992) argue that verbal admonitions and threats of discipline are less effective than training that graphically imparts the severe consequences of roof falls. A series of three videos was prepared that shows actual miners being interviewed about roof fall accidents that they experienced. The videos also emphasize the impact that roof fall accidents have on people other than the one caught in the fall. These highly effective videos, together with training manuals, are available from the MSHA Academy in Beckley.

Finally, the prevalence of dangerous behavior depends greatly on the miner's perception of the company's policy concerning going under unsupported roof, on how that policy is enforced, and on the attitude and behavior of his supervisor and coworkers. The best prevention programs involve high-level managers who directly communicate their commitment to the goal of keeping people away from unsupported roof.

Roof Bolter Safety

Roof bolt operators are on the front line in the fight against ground falls. They are continually exposed to roof and rib hazards, and historically they have experienced more groundfall-related injuries than any other occupation in mining. Although large roof and rib falls have been responsible for several fatalities, most injuries are caused by relatively small pieces of rock.

A detailed study of the hazards associated with roof bolting was conducted in West Virginia (Klishis et al. 1992; Grayson et al. 1992). The average time for bolting a place was 26.9 minutes, and that time was spent engaged in four primary activities:

- General face preparation
- Tramming, positioning, and setting ATRS
- Drilling holes
- Installing bolts.

The most hazardous face preparation activity was scaling and barring roof. Thick coal seams where the roof is high posed particular hazards. Having a long scaling bar available was essential.

The most severe injuries (with an average of 45 days lost) were associated with setting the ATRS. Pressurizing the ATRS against the top can disturb the roof, and large pieces may rotate and actually fall underneath the support. It is particularly important, then, that other miners stand back while the ATRS is being set.

The greatest number of injuries occurred during the drilling process, which also involved the greatest amount of the total cycle time. Drilling also disturbs the rock, causing pieces to fall. Analysis of the injury data found that operators placed themselves at risk whenever a part of the body left the protective coverage of the canopy. Placing hands around the drill steel or across the drill head also resulted in a number of injuries.

Bolt installation required only 17% of the cycle time but was associated with 25% of the injuries. Miners sometimes went out from under the canopy during installation, particularly in high top. Accidents appeared to be more frequent during the installation of the last row of bolts in a place, because of face falls and a tendency to overextend the ATRS.

The roof bolt machine, with its ATRS and canopy, is the critical piece of safety equipment. It should always be in proper operating condition before it is used. The proper bolting sequence, as defined in the roof control plan, must always be followed. Several fatalities have resulted when operators of single-boom machines installed bolts out of sequence and placed themselves under unsupported roof.

Rehabilitation of roof falls and construction of overcasts and boom holes present special hazards. In many such areas the roof is unusually high, and often the ATRS cannot effectively contact it. If the ATRS cannot be set against the top, it is necessary to set jacks for temporary support or use a manufacturer's approved ATRS extension. Two roof bolt operators have been killed in recent years while bolting high top during mine construction activities.

Roof bolt operators are also responsible for protecting the entire crew with high-quality bolt installations. Poorly installed roof bolts can be worse than none at all, because they provide a false sense of security. Manufacturers' recommendations regarding resin spin and hold times must always be followed. Holes must be drilled to the proper length (not more than one-inch deeper than the bolt's length). The torque on tensioned roof bolts must be checked as required by CFR 75.204(f).

A wide variety of roof bolts are now available, and installation problems may be caused by geologic changes, incorrect practices, or malfunctioning supports. To help identify and resolve problems with roof supports, an extremely valuable *Trouble Shooting Guide* is available (Mazzoni et al. 1996).

If there are any indications of adverse conditions, additional test holes should be drilled and additional support installed. Roof conditions detected during drilling should be communicated to coworkers and management.

Skin Failures of Roof and Rib

Skin failures are those that do not involve failure of the roof support elements, but result from rock spalling from between roof bolts, around ATRS systems, or from ribs. They are of particular concern because they cause injuries and fatalities to workers who should have been protected by supports. In 1997, 98% of the 810 roof and rib injuries suffered by mine workers were attributed to skin failures (Bauer et al. 1999).

Roof skin failures almost always involve pieces of rock that are less than 0.6 m (2 ft) thick. About 40% of the 669 roof skin injuries in 1997 involved roof bolt operators and occurred beneath the ATRS. The other roof skin injuries occurred beneath permanent support and involved workers in a wide variety of activities. Common roof skin control techniques include oversized plates, header boards, wood planks, steel straps, meshing, and (in rare instances) spray coatings (sealants).

Between 1996 and 1998, rib failures resulted in 6 fatalities in underground coal mines. Only one of these fatal injuries was to a face worker, the other five were all mechanics and electricians performing their duties well outby the face. Nearly 80% of the 128 rib injuries that occurred in 1997 took place beneath permanently supported roof. Nonfatal rib injuries resulted in an average of 43 lost workdays each, versus 25 days for the average roof skin injury.

The seam height is the single greatest factor contributing to rib failures (Figure 23.4). The seam height was greater than 2.5 m (8 ft) in all six of the fatalities and was greater than 3 m (10 ft) in three of them. The incidence of rib injuries increases dramatically once the seam height reaches 2.2 m (7 ft). Interestingly, mines with the very thickest seams see lower rib injury rates, probably because

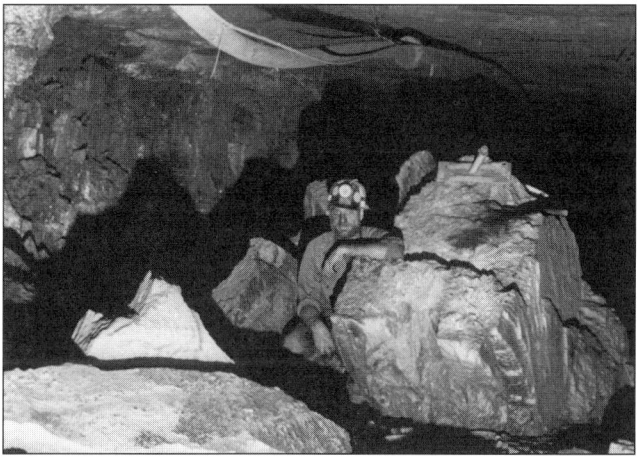

FIGURE 23.4   Large rib failure in a thick coal mine seam (photo by Chase)

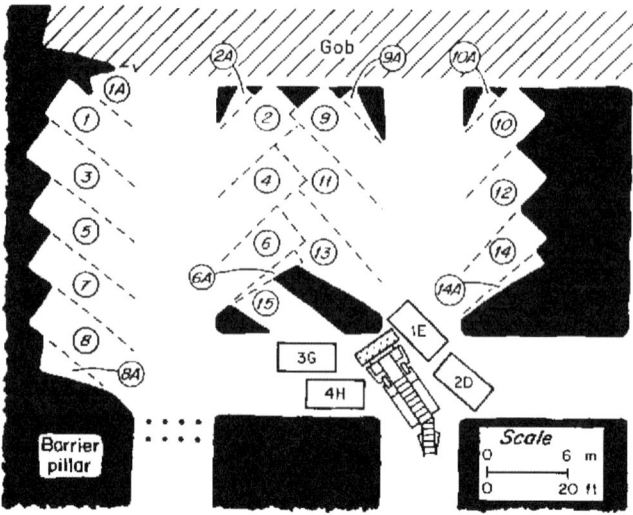

FIGURE 23.5   Christmas tree pillaring plan (Chase et al. 1997)

most of them routinely use rib support. No rib support was used in any of the six fatal accidents, however. Rib failure is often associated with rock partings and/or discontinuities within the pillar, or with overhanging brows created by roof drawrock. The most effective rib supports employ full planks or mesh held in place by roof bolts.

Pillar Recovery

Pillar recovery has always been an integral part of U.S. underground coal mining. It can be a less capital-intensive, more flexible alternative to longwall mining for small, irregular reserves. A recent study estimated that pillar recovery accounts for about 10% of the coal mined underground (Mark et al. 1997).

The process of pillar recovery removes the main support for the overburden and allows the ground to cave. As a result, the pillar line is an extremely dynamic and highly stressed environment. Safety depends on controlling the caving through proper extraction sequencing and roof support. Historically, retreat mining has accounted for a disproportionate number of roof fall fatalities, including 13 between 1996 and 1998. Three of the accidents during this period resulted in double fatalities.

A wide variety of pillar recovery techniques are used. "Partial pillaring" methods include pillar splitting, split-and-tee, three-cuts, and many others. These plans leave a substantial amount of coal in the remnant fenders and therefore postpone the caving action of the roof. When "full pillaring" is practiced, roof caving normally occurs soon after mining is completed. Popular full-pillaring techniques include the outside lift and the Christmas tree (Figure 23.5).

Today, most pillar recovery plans employ 9 to 12 m (30 to 40 ft) extended cuts. The pillars are usually sized so that no roof bolting is required during second mining. One apparent consequence is that because roof bolting accidents are eliminated, nonfatal roof/rib accident rates at pillar recovery mines are actually lower than at other room-and-pillar mines (Mark et al. 1997).

Traditional roof control plans require that numerous timber posts be set during each stage of pillar recovery (Figure 23.6). Recently, mobile roof supports (MRS) have become available that replace many of the timbers (Figure 23.7). MRS resemble longwall shields mounted on bulldozer tracks. They can have many safety advantages over timbers. In particular, they are more effective as roof supports, they do not require workers to approach the mined-out gob area to set them, and they reduce the potential for materials handling injuries (Chase et al. 1997).

Following the roof control plan is absolutely critical to safe pillar recovery operations. Fatality investigations have frequently found that lifts were too wide, too deep, or out of sequence. The plan may also specify the minimum dimensions of the remnant coal left in place called *stumps* and *fenders*. However, the roof control plan is a minimum plan, and additional supports should be used at any indication of bad roof.

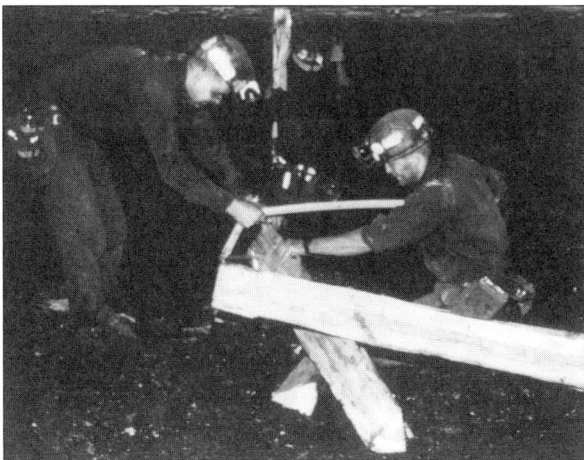

FIGURE 23.6   Timber support being set on a retreat mining section

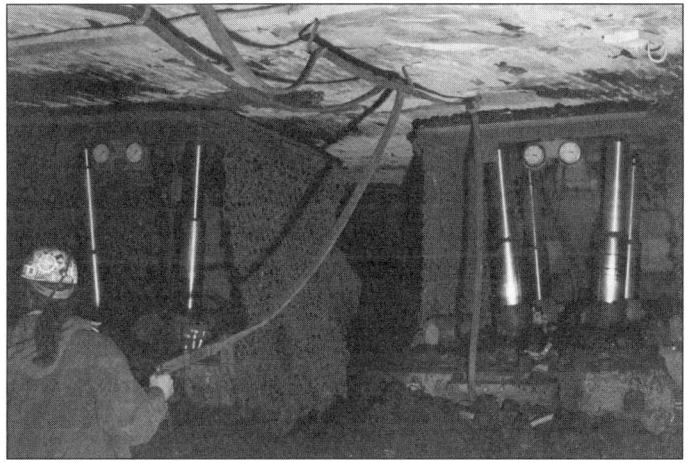

FIGURE 23.7   Mobile roof support (MRS) for retreat mining (photo by Chase 1992)

The recovery of the final stump, or pushout, is the most hazardous aspect of pillar recovery operations. During the past 20 years, nearly half of all fatalities during retreat mining have occurred while the pushout was being mined. The pushout should never be mined if conditions do not look safe or if adverse conditions arise during mining. All unnecessary personnel should remain outby the intersection at all times during pillar recovery, but especially while the pushout is being mined.

Many fatal investigation reports cite geologic features, especially slips, as contributing to the accident. Geologic features should be carefully supported and observed during retreat mining. Special precautions need to be taken near the outcrop, where the presence of groundwater and weathered joints (sometimes called "hill seams") can reduce roof competence. In general, pillar recovery should not be conducted when the distance to the outcrop is less than 45 m (150 ft).

Pillar recovery can also be difficult under deep cover. Between 1996 and 1998, nearly half of the pillar recovery fatalities occurred where the depth of cover exceeded 200 m (650 ft). Under deep cover, barrier pillars and special mining sequences may be required.

Extended Cuts and Remote Control Mining

Extended (deep) cut mining is where the continuous mining machine advances the face more than 6 m (20 ft) beyond the last row of permanent supports. The development of remote control for continuous miners (Figure 23.8), spray fan systems, and flooded-bed scrubbers has provided the technology to

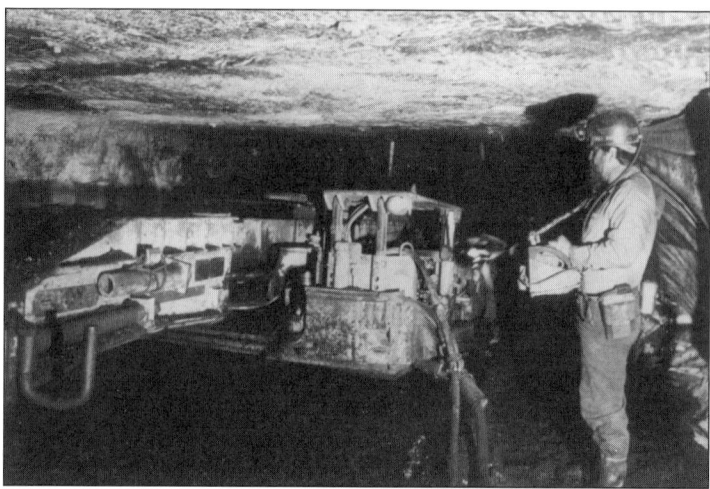

FIGURE 23.8   Miner operating a continuous mining machine by remote control (photo by E.R. Bauer)

enable deep cuts. By 1997, about 75% of all underground labor hours were worked at mines with extended cut permits. However, extended cuts raise a number of ventilation, ground control, and human factor issues. Between 1988 and 1995, extended cuts may have been a factor in 26% of all roof fall fatalities in underground coal mines (Bauer et al. 1997).

In practice, many mines with permits only take extended cuts when conditions allow for them. Where the roof is competent, extended cuts are routine. At the other extreme, when the roof is poor, miners may not even be able to complete a 6-m (20-ft) cut before the roof collapses. A premature roof collapse can trap the continuous miner or endanger the crew, or it can create uneven and hazardous conditions for the roof bolters. Where premature collapses are likely, additional roof supports (extra bolts, planks, mesh, or straps) should be used within the last two rows of supports to prevent the fall from overriding these supports.

A study conducted at 36 mines found that in 50% of all underground coal operations, extended cuts were routinely used nearly all the time (Mark 1999). In 22% of the mines, extended cuts were rarely feasible. In the remaining mines, extended cuts were sometimes stable, sometimes not. The prevailing conditions were found to be determined by the roof quality, the entry width, and depth of cover. Another study found that extended cut mines were no more prone to roof falls after bolting than non-extended cut mines (Bauer et al. 1997).

Remote control mining allows the operator to stay further back from the unsupported roof, but it also removes him from the protection provided by the canopy. The freedom of movement, combined with a lack of visibility, can tempt the operator to stray into dangerous locations. Several fatalities have occurred during the mining of the first cut in a 90-degree crosscut to operators who had gone inby permanent supports (Figure 23.9). In response, some companies have limited the length of the initial cuts in a crosscut to 20 ft, and others have angled the crosscuts to provide better visibility.

Training is an essential element in safe deep cut mining. Other workers on the section should know not to go in by the continuous miner operator unless they are operating coal haulage equipment at the face. If the continuous miner breaks down inby permanent roof support, the roof must be properly supported before repairs are made. Finally, all crosscuts must be supported before a cut is taken inby or the opposite crosscut is started.

Intersection Stability

In underground coal mines, tens of thousands of intersections are driven each year. Intersections create diagonal spans of 8 to 12 m (25 to 40 ft), well over the normal width of an entry. The hazards of wide spans can be increased when pillar corners are rounded for machine travel (turnouts), or when rib spalling increases the span.

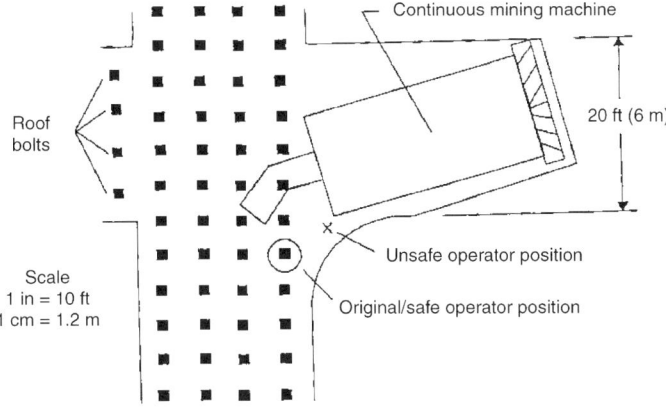

FIGURE 23.9   Unsafe location for a continuous mining machine operator while mining a crosscut (Bauer et al. 1997)

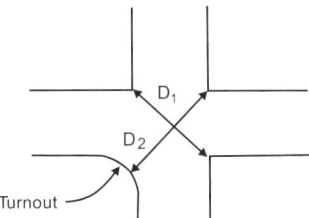

FIGURE 23.10   Sum-of-the-diagonals for intersection span measurement (G. Molinda et al. 1998)

Subsection 50.20-5 requires every roof fall in the active workings that occurs above the roof bolt anchorage, impairs ventilation, or impedes passage be reported. In 1996, there were 2,105 noninjury reportable roof falls. More than 71% of these occurred in intersections, despite the fact that intersections probably account for less than 25% of all drivage underground.

Intersection spans are often measured as the sum of the diagonals (Figure 23.10). Because the rock load increases in proportion to the cube of the span, even a small increase in the span can greatly reduce the stability of an intersection. For example, widening the entry from 5.5 to 6 m (18 to 20 ft) increases the rock load from 82 to 120 tonnes (96 to 132 tons)! A study conducted at one mine in western Pennsylvania found that 83% of the roof falls occurred in 13% of the intersections where the sum of the diagonals exceeded 22 m (70 ft) (Molinda et al. 1998).

Many roof control plans specify the maximum spans that are allowed. Mining sequences can also be designed to limit the number, location, and size of turnouts, and to restrict turnouts to specific entries. Extra primary support, such as longer roof bolts, installed within intersections can also be very effective in reducing the likelihood of roof falls. On the other hand, replacing four-way intersections with three-ways may be not an effective control technique. Three-way intersections are more stable, but since it normally takes two three-ways to replace one four-way, the total number of falls is likely to increase (Molinda et al. 1998).

Hazards in Underground Metal and Nonmetal Mines

Between 1996 and 1998, nine fatal fall of ground injuries from eight different accidents occurred in underground metal and nonmetal mines (Table 23.6). Two major contributing factors were the failure to conduct proper roof and rib examinations and problems with removing loose rock. Both of these activities are more difficult in large mine openings. Overall, metal and nonmetal underground mines have lower ground fall injury rates than coal mines. For example, a study by Iannacchione et al.

TABLE 23.6   Factors associated with nine metal/nonmetal underground fatalities, 1996–1998

Date	Commodity	Factor	State	Type of Fall	Job	Mining Height (m)
11/4/98	Metal	Inadequate examination/failure to remove loose ground	CO	Rib	Driller	3
3/4/98	Metal	Failure to remove loose ground	AZ	Roof	Installing support	Not applicable
1/19/98	Metal	Failure to support or remove loose ground	MO	Roof	Surveying	4.9
4/1/97	Stone	Inadequate examination/geology	TN	Rib	Driller	7.6
2/5/97	Metal	Unsafe location	NV	Roof	Scaling	2.4
2/3/97	Metal	Large span/geology	TN	Roof	Driller	5.5
7/24/97	Metal	Unsafe practice/loose ground	NV	Rib	Driller	12.2
5/10/96 (double fatal)	Stone	Failure to support loose ground	MO	Roof	Blasters	7.6

(1999) found that 92 falls of ground injuries from 1990 to 1996 were reported from the underground stone mining industry, which employs approximately 2,000 miners. This high groundfall rate is certainly related to the large size of the openings in stone mines, and to the problems of scaling them.

Large Openings

Many metal/nonmetal mines have large openings, especially nonmetal stone and salt mines and metal mines with stopes. Large mine openings have roof or back greater than 5 m (16 ft) high, with spans greater than 10 m (30 ft) wide. When the back is high, a miner's ability to observe the ground conditions is greatly reduced. Additionally, many metal/nonmetal mines use roof bolts on an infrequent basis. Ventilation of large openings is sometimes poorly controlled, promoting dramatic fluctuations in humidity, and sometimes fog. High humidity can cause even strong rocks to split and crack, creating hazards for miners. Because of these factors and others, mines with large openings rely on mining both a stable roof beam and a stable roof line to reduce ground control hazards (Iannacchione and Prosser 1998).

A stable roof beam is generally massive, strong, thick, and persistent. Additionally, a persistent, smooth roof profile at the bottom of the stable roof beam is very helpful in creating a stable roof. Natural laminations, bedding planes, or interfaces between rock layers often providing the best roof lines (Figure 23.11). Too many bedding planes or rock layer interfaces can allow the roof to separate with time into many thin layers that are inherently unstable. Thicker roof beams sag less than thinner beams and therefore are less likely to fail (Figure 23.12). A meter or more of competent rock has been observed to form a stable beam in rooms up to 15 m (50 ft) wide.

However, as more joints intersect the roof beam or the associated room is widened, the chances for instabilities increase.

If a natural smooth roof plane does not exist, special blasting procedures like presplitting or smooth blasting can be used to produce an artificial smooth roof plane. Pre-splitting requires additional drill holes along the roof and rib line. Postsplitting or trimblasting is another technique used to produce an even, stable roof line. Conversely, poor blasting practices often have a negative influence on roof and rib stability. Overbreak can damage the roof and rib rock, while bootlegs (poor rock breakage at the end of a blasthole as a result of inadequate explosive burn) can leave broken rock along uneven rib and face surfaces.

Scaling

Scaling is necessary to remove loose rock from the sidewalls (rib) and hanging walls (roof) of mine openings. It is particularly important when the rock and ore is removed by blasting, as in most underground metal and nonmetal mines.

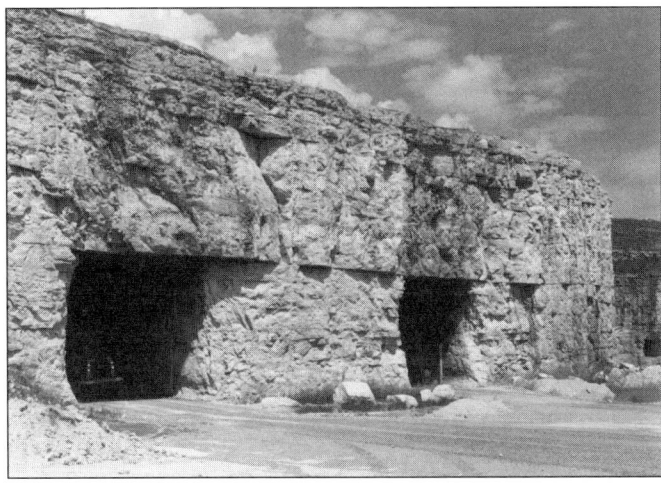

FIGURE 23.11   Smooth roof line produced by a persistent bedding plane lamination within the roof rock beam

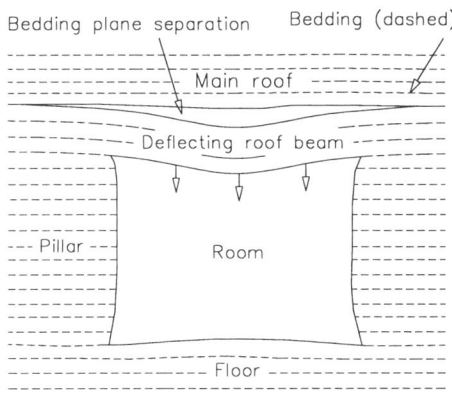

FIGURE 23.12   A common mode of roof rock failure in underground stone mines

Scaling may be conducted either with a hand-held pry bar or with mechanical equipment. Mechanical scalers usually remove the greatest portion of the loose rock, using an assortment of prying, hammering, or scraping attachments. Hand scaling is often conducted by a worker mounted in a lift basket in high openings. It can be the primary means of scaling or it can be done on an as-needed basis before any mining operation (drilling, blasting, mucking, haulage, etc.). Periodic reexamination of working areas is essential to identify new loose rock.

A study of accidents in underground stone mines between 1985 and 1994 found that nearly one-third of the ground control injuries involved scaling (Grau and Prosser 1997). More than 90% of these involved hand scaling. Mechanical scaling generally affords greater protection, because the miner is positioned in a protective cab at a greater distance from the loose rock. The data from this study also showed that the extremities and limbs were the body parts most often injured during scaling. Arm and leg padding, such as worn by athletes, may be one way to cushion the blow from falling rock and may also lessen the severity of an accident.

Although nearly two-thirds of the scaling accidents were caused by a direct hit from falling rock, many are related to loss of balance of the worker because of machine movement or a loss of bar control. Scaling bars that are too short can put workers in danger, but longer bars can be too heavy. A scaling bar experiment in 1988 indicated that a counterbalanced bar might be a better ergonomic design. At one coal mine, workers welded a 0.6-m (2-ft) end piece of a scaling bar to the end of an 2.4 m (8-ft) metal pipe, creating a bar that was relatively lightweight and strong (Klishis et al. 1992).

Training is a basic consideration for reducing scaling accidents. The stone mine data cited above indicated that nearly two-thirds of the accidents occurred to miners with less than two years of scaling experience (Grau and Prosser 1997). Workers should stand under supported top whenever it is available. To prevent hand injuries when using a scaling bar, one method suggested by MSHA is to slip a piece of water hose about half way down the bar. If the material being pried away slides down the bar, it will then be deflected away from the hands. Finally, miners should always pry *up* when scaling, so that if they lose their balance they do not fall underneath the loose rock.

Global Safety Strategies

Best practices, as discussed in the previous section, generally address ground control safety in the immediate vicinity of the miner. Creating a stable mine environment begins much earlier, however, during the process of mine design. Ground monitoring can also be central to the creation of a ground control safety culture at a mine.

Safe Mine Design

Mine design includes pillar sizing, layout of drifts and entries, dimensions of openings, and artificial support. Mine planners seek optimum designs that balance the competing goals of ground control, ventilation, equipment size, production requirements, and costs. In recent years, a number of design aids have been made available to assist with the ground control aspects of design.

The role of pillars is to support the great weight of the overburden above the mine. No manmade supports (except filled stopes in metal mines) have anything near the tremendous load-carrying capability of mine pillars. The tributary area concept is often used to estimate the loads applied to pillars. Mine designers must consider all of the loads the pillars may be required to carry during their service lives, however. Longwall panel extraction, pillar recovery, and multiple seam operations can all increase pillar loads, and benching can reduce pillar strength. Design aids for coal mines include the Analysis of Longwall Pillar Stability (ALPS), the Analysis of Retreat Mining Pillar Stability (ARMPS), and LAMODEL (Mark 1999b; Heasley and Chekan 1999). Guidelines for sizing limestone pillars were recently published (Iannacchione 1999).

Mining layout can often be used to minimize the effects of geologic hazards. Traditionally, features such as joints, cleats, and faults have been considered in design. More recently, horizontal stress has become an important concern. Global plate tectonics are the primary source of horizontal stress in mines, and measurements have shown that horizontal stresses are often three times as great as vertical overburden stresses. Horizontal stresses have caused roof potting, cutter roof, and roof falls in coal and limestone mines (Mark and Mucho 1994; Iannacchione et al. 1998). Their destructive effects can be reduced by orienting the mine so that most of the drivage parallels the direction of the maximum horizontal stress.

The maximum stable size of mine openings depends greatly on the geology. The back in some stone and salt mines is so competent that it can routinely maintain spans of 15 m (45 ft), while 5-m (15-ft) spans may be unstable in the weak, fractured ground found in some coal and hard rock mines. Rock mass classification systems can be especially helpful in estimating the safe span. In hard rock mines, examples include the RMR system, the Q system, the MBR system, and the Stability Graph System (Hoek et al. 1995). The Coal Mine Roof Rating System is increasingly used for many aspects of coal mine design (Molinda and Mark 1994).

U.S. mines use more than 100 million roof bolts every year. Only mines with exceptionally competent country rock can do without pattern roof bolting, and even they require some spot bolting. A wide variety of rock bolts are available, but matching the proper bolt type and pattern with the ground conditions remains as much an art as a science (Peng 1999).

Controlling Catastrophic Failures in Underground Mines

One of the most difficult and longstanding ground control issues is the catastrophic failure of mine structures. Catastrophic failures that create hazards for miners in coal, metal, and nonmetal underground mines include coal mine bumps, hard rock bursts, large collapses, and outbursts. The driving mechanisms include both excessive stresses from geologic forces like faults or from mining induced situations. Catastrophic failures of mine structures range in size from small pieces of ribs or roofs to entire mining sections. When gases under elevated pressures are present in the strata, outbursts of rock and gas can occur. Hazards to miners range from injuries associated with flying rocks to complete burial in ejected rock. Pressure waves from large collapses can throw miners into natural and manmade structures. When large quantities of gas are instantaneously released, gas ignition or asphyxiation can occur.

"Coal mine bumps" have presented serious mining problems since the early 1900s. Iannacchione and Zelanko (1995) compiled a coal bump database that included 172 specific events. The database was constructed from USBM and MSHA coal bump accident and incident reports written between 1936 and 1993. A total of 87 fatalities and 163 injuries were identified. The 1980s witnessed the greatest outbreak of bumps, accounting for 31% of the total. In 1996, three miners were killed in two different bump events. Two Kentucky miners were fatally injured when six pillars suddenly failed violently during pillar recovery operations. The second event claimed the life of a Utah miner when coal along a longwall face violently ejected into the shields. Both of these events occurred in characteristic settings for coal bumps, with elevated overburden, proximity to a gob area, and a strong hanging roof.

Many recommendations have been proposed to mitigate bump hazards. Special mining techniques like the Olga pillar extraction technique and U.S. Steel's thin-pillar method have the ability to reduce stresses around pillar extraction areas. Longwall mines can use techniques like abutment and yielding pillars. Finally as a last resort, several destressing techniques, such as shot firing, auger drilling, water infusion, hydraulic fracturing, and partial pillaring, have proven useful in combating the most hazardous conditions.

"Hard rock bursts" have been occurring in deep metal mines for as long as records have been kept (White et al. 1995). Federal regulations have been developed mainly in the form of administrative controls (Subsection 57.3461). When a rock burst causes miners to withdraw, impairs ventilation or impedes passage, MSHA must be notified. A rock burst control plan should then be developed and implemented. This plan is required to reduce the occurrence of rock bursts through monitoring and minimizing exposure. Monitoring can range from simple deformation measurements to mine-wide microseismic monitoring systems. Minimizing exposure can range from administrative controls to the use of remote controlled equipment.

A "pillar collapse" is a sudden, violent event that can pose a serious hazard in a room and pillar mine. A collapse occurs when one pillar in a mining layout fails, transferring its load to neighboring pillars, causing them to fail, and so on in a domino fashion. A pillar collapse can induce a devastating airblast that can disrupt the ventilation system and send flying debris that can injure or kill miners. In recent years, at least 13 coal mines and 6 metal/nonmetal mines in the United States have experienced pillar collapses. Fortunately, only one fatality has resulted, following a collapse of hundreds of pillars at a Wyoming trona mine (Zipf and Mark 1997).

The mechanics of pillar collapses are very different from either coal bumps or the more common slow pillar failure. Collapses occur when the pillars are so thin that they cannot carry any weight once they fail. Pillar collapses can be *prevented* by increasing the stability factor of the pillar design, or *contained* by conducting high extraction in localized compartments that are protected by barrier pillars.

"Outbursts" of gas and rock have occurred mainly in evaporite and to a lesser degree coal mines. With the occurrence of the multiple fatal explosion at the Belle Isle Salt Mine in 1981, domal salt mines in Louisiana and Texas were recognized as potential locations for large outbursts. Modifications to mining regulations were made in 1984 creating special levels of gassy metal/nonmetal mines (Subcategory II-A and II-B, 57.22003). Each advance in the gassy level requires additional operational safeguards. Outbursts in Canadian bedded salt and New Mexico potash mines have periodically created serious safety hazards. Outbursts in coal have been relatively rare, occurring most frequently along the grand hogback of Colorado. However, the most deadly outbursts in the recent U.S. history occurred in 1981 at the Dutch Creek No. 1 Mine in Colorado where 16 miners were killed. It is commonly felt that outbursts will become much more prevalent as average mining depths increase below 600 m (2,000 ft).

Roof Monitoring

Roof falls seldom occur entirely without warning. Often, however, miners are not aware of the warning signals until it is too late. Most underground mines use observational techniques, primarily visual inspection, as a means of determining roof stability. Traditionally, miners have sounded the rock, listening

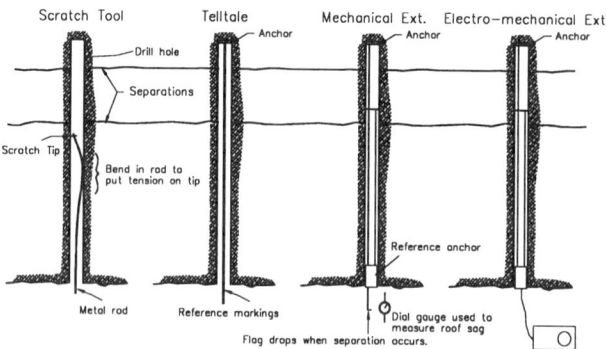

FIGURE 23.13   Four types of mechanical tools

for the drummy sounds that signal loose rock. Also, the act of drilling exploration roof bolt or blast holes can provide much information about the rock. During drilling, blasting, and scaling operations, additional knowledge related to roof conditions can be gained. For example, a driller preparing to bolt may notice a sudden increase in the penetration rate, and then realize that possibly a gap or clay seam was encountered. Much of this "hands-on" information provides an overview of the general conditions related to roof stability. Observational techniques can be extended by monitoring the movement of the mine roof in boreholes using mechanical tools (Figure 23.13). Four types are available (Iannacchione et al. 1999):

- *Scratch tools* can detect separations and provide an indication of loose rock layers or roof beam deflection. Information on the location and size of the separation can be marked on the roof and used to assess potential future roof degradation.

- *Telltales* are rigid bars, possibly just a roof bolt, anchored into the roof. A small section of rod protruding from the borehole is covered with three bands of reflective tape. The portion of the bar closest to the roof is generally green, followed downward by yellow and then red. As the roof deflects downward, the roof line can easily be seen to move through the green, yellow, and finally red tape zones. Telltales are required by law in British and Canadian coal mines (Altounyan et al. 1997).

- *Mechanical extensometers* consist of a top and bottom anchor, steel wire or rigid tubing, and some kind of micrometer or dial gauge. These devices have been used for decades in metal mines in Michigan, Missouri, and Idaho. The most common commercially available mechanical extensometer monitoring devices are the Miners Helper and the Guardian Angel. These monitors generally have one or two anchor points that measure the overall separation of rock layers in the immediate roof. If roof deflection is detected, a reflecting flag drops from the roof line, signaling the potential for imminent roof failure. In some cases, this information has been used to indicate a need to add roof support, remove roof rock, or mark off affected areas.

- *Electromechanical extensometers* include sonic probes that allow for up to 20 permanent anchors up to a 6-m (20-ft) height. The probes have the added benefit of being remotely read by portable devices or by connection to a data acquisition system. Recently, NIOSH introduced an easy to fabricate and install extensometer called the Remote Monitoring Safety System (RMSS). This instrument can be read remotely with a multimeter or can be connected directly to a data acquisition system.

A comprehensive ground control plan not only includes the basic observational, visual, and hands-on components, but also uses supplemental observational and monitoring techniques and regularly reads, analyzes, and displays information gained from these efforts. When this type of information is logged or mapped, it provides a documented history of ground conditions. Data from monitoring can be analyzed and prepared either by consulting firms or with in-house expertise. The information is extremely useful in deciding a course of action or alteration of the mining plan at the time of a major groundfall or when unstable geologic conditions are encountered. Mines that follow these practices and promote open communication and participation from everyone at the site are the mines with the most proactive approaches towards ground control safety.

SURFACE HIGHWALLS AND SLOPES

Surface mines have relatively few serious falls of ground, with six fatalities in the period from 1996 to 1998. However, six additional fatal falls of highwalls and slopes fatalities occurred in the first half of 1999. Two of these six were initially classified as powered haulage, but they were actually caused by slope failure beneath haulage equipment. The large jump in fatalities in 1999 is hopefully an aberration, but it may signal a new safety issue caused by a change in mining method or equipment, different enforcement practices, or a social issue such as the experience level of the mining workforce.

Most highwall injuries occur when loose pieces of rock fall on workers located below. Small pieces of rock can be dangerous when they fall from great height; even a fist-sized rock caused one recent fatality. At the other extreme, an entire section of a highwall or spoil pile may collapse, endangering miners working either on or beneath it.

Good basic design is essential to highwall safety. The height should be limited for stability and to allow scaling. Where the pit is deep, benches should be used to limit the slope height. Angling the highwall back from vertical also increases stability. Good blasting practices make for a smoother wall and reduce the need to scale. Drainage ditches should be used to divert springs and groundwater away from slopes.

Geologic features have contributed to many rockfall injuries from highwalls. Faults or "hill-seams" (weathered joints) can create wedges of unstable ground that can slide into the pit. In dipping strata, the rock can also be prone to slide along bedding planes. Freeze-thaw action acts to loosen rocks, and has been cited in several fatality reports. A review of accident records indicates that highwall accidents are twice as likely to occur in December and January than they are in the summer months. The presence of abandoned underground mine openings in the highwall has contributed to three of the recent fatalities.

Rock faces should be monitored frequently to check for loose rocks, and scaling should be conducted as needed. As highwalls age, weathering may cause additional loosening. The surface at the top of the highwall should also be checked for tension cracks that could indicate pending massive slope failure. In very large pits, various kinds of electronic surveying and monitoring systems are in use to provide early warning.

Good work practices can also help reduce rockfall hazards. Workers should not position themselves beneath highwalls except when absolutely necessary to perform their duties. Where possible, equipment cabs should be designed for object protection, and equipment should be positioned with the cab away from the highwall.

The stability of spoil piles can be reduced by extra surface loads ("surcharges") or by removing the bottom ("toe") of the slope. One recent fatality occurred when an uncompacted spoil pile gave way beneath the weight of a loaded truck. Another miner was killed when he excavated material at the base of the slope to widen a road, causing the pile to collapse.

CONCLUSION

This chapter has presented an overview of the most significant ground control hazards facing today's mineworkers. Underground miners, particularly in coal mines, are at the greatest risk from ground falls. The six highwall and slope fatalities that occurred in the first half of 1999 show that surface miners are at risk as well.

The analysis of recent fatality investigations and accident statistics identified certain job categories, mining techniques, and geologic environments that appear to pose the greatest hazards. Best practices have been developed through experience and research to reduce these risks. They combine engineering design, roof support, equipment, mining methods, and human factors to create safer workplaces and work practices. The roof control plan is another valuable tool in this effort.

Unfortunately, recent trends indicate that ground fall injury rates have stopped decreasing, and may even be on the increase. A renewed effort by the entire mining community will be necessary to finally eradicate the groundfall hazard.

REFERENCES

Altounyan, P.F.R., D.N. Bigby, K.G. Hurt, and H.V. Peake. 1997. Instrumentation and procedures for routine monitoring of reinforced mine roadways to prevent falls of ground. Paper presented at the 27th International Conference of Safety in Mines Research Institute. New Delhi, India. 759–766.

Bauer, E.R., D.M. Pappas, D.R. Dolinar, F.E. McCall, and D.R. Babich. 1999. Skin failure of roof and rib in underground coal mines. In *Proceedings 18th International Conference on Ground Control in Mining*. West Virginia University, Morgantown, WV. 108–114.

Bauer, E.R., G.J. Chekan, and L.J. Steiner. 1997. Stability evaluation of extended cut mining in underground coal mines. *International Journal of Rock Mechanics and Mining Science* 34(3-4): Paper No. 302.

Chase, F.E. 1992. Geologic structures that affect Appalachian coal mines. In *Preventing Coal Mine Groundfall Accidents: How to Identify and Respond to Geologic Hazards and Prevent Unsafe Worker Behavior*. USBM IC 9332. 3–14.

Chase, F.E., A. McComas, C. Mark, and C.D. Goble. 1997. Retreat mining with mobile roof supports. In *New Technology for Ground Control in Retreat Mining: Proceedings of the NIOSH Technology Transfer Seminar*. NIOSH IC 9446. 74–88.

Grau, R.H. III, and L.J. Prosser. 1997. Scaling accidents in underground stone mines. *Rock Products* 1: 39–41.

Grayson, R.L., L.A. Layne, R.C. Althouse, and M.J. Klishis. 1992. Risk indices for roof bolter injuries. *Mining Engineering* 44(2): 164–166.

Heasley, K.A., and G.J. Chekan. 1999. Practical boundary element modeling for mine planning. In *Proceedings of the Second International Workshop on Coal Pillar Mechanics and Design*. Vail, CO. NIOSH IC 9448. 73–88.

Hoek, E., P.K. Kaiser, and W.E. Bawden. 1995. *Support of Underground Excavations in Hard Rock*. Rotterdam, Netherlands: Balkema.

Iannacchione, A.T., and J.C. Zelanko. 1995. Occurrence and remediation of coal mine bumps: a historical review. In *Proceedings: Mechanics and Mitigation of Violent Failure in Coal and Hard-Rock Mines*. USBM Special Publication 01-95. 27–67.

Iannacchione, A.T., and L.J. Prosser. 1998. Roof and rib hazards assessment for underground stone mines. *Mining Engineering* 50(2): 76–80.

Iannacchione, A.T., D.R. Dolinar, L.J. Prosser, T.E. Marshall, D.C. Oyler, and C.S. Compton. 1998. Controlling roof beam failures from high horizontal stress in underground stone mines. In *Proceedings of the 17th Conference on Ground Control in Mining*. West Virginia University, Morgantown, WV. August 4–6. 102–112.

Iannacchione, A.T., L.J. Prosser, R. Grau, D.C. Oyler, D.R. Dolinar, T.E. Marshall, and C.S. Compton. 1999. "Preventing Injuries Caused by Unrecognized Stone Mine Roof Beam Failures with a Proactive Roof Control Plan." Presented at the Society of Mining Engineering Annual Meeting Preprint 99-87. Denver, CO. March 1–3.

Iannacchione, A.T. 1999. Pillar design issues for underground stone mines. In *Proceedings of the 18th Conference on Ground Control in Mining*. West Virginia University, Morgantown, WV. 271–281.

Klishis, M.J., R.C. Althouse, L.A. Layne, and G.M. Lies. 1992. Increasing roof bolter awareness to risks of falling roof material during the bolting cycle. In *Preventing Coal Mine Groundfall Accidents: How to Identify and Respond to Geologic Hazards and Prevent Unsafe Worker Behavior*. USBM IC 9332. 69–78.

Mallett, L.G., C. Vaught, and R.H. Peters. 1992. Training that Encourages Miners to Avoid Unsupported Roof. In *Preventing Coal Mine Groundfall Accidents: How to Identify and Respond to Geologic Hazards and Prevent Unsafe Worker Behavior*. USBM IC 9332. 32–45.

Mark, C. 1999. Application of the coal mine roof rating (CMRR) to extended cuts. *Mining Engineering* 4: 52–56.

——. 1999. Empirical methods for coal pillar design. In *Proceedings of the Second International Workshop on Coal Pillar Mechanics and Design*. NIOSH IC 9448, 45–154.

Mark, C., F.E. McCall, and D.M. Pappas. 1997. A statistical overview of retreat mining of coal pillars in the U.S. In the *Proceedings of the 16th International Conference on Ground Control in Mining*. West Virginia University, Morgantown, WV. 204–210.

Mark, C. and T.P. Mucho. 1994. Longwall mine design for control of horizontal stress. In *New Technology for Longwall Ground Control: Proceedings of the USBM Technology Transfer Seminar.* USBM SP 94-01. 53–76.

Mazzoni, R.A., G.J. Karabin, and J.A. Cybulski. 1996. *A Trouble Shooting Guide for Roof Support Systems.* MSHA IR 1237. 101 pp.

MSHA. Best Practices. Series of cards available on the Internet at www.msha.gov/s&hinfo/prop/prophome.htm.

Molinda, G., and C. Mark. 1994. *The Coal Mine Roof Rating (CMRR)–A Practical Rock Mass Classification for Coal Mines.* USBM IC 9387. 83 pp.

Molinda, G., C. Mark, E. Bauer, D. Babich, and D. Pappas. 1998. Factors influencing intersection stability in U.S. coal mines. In *Proceedings 17th International Conference on Ground Control.* West Virginia University, Morgantown, WV. 267–275.

Peng, S.S. 1999. Roof bolting adds stability to weak strata. *Coal Age* 12: 32–38.

Peters, R.H. 1992. Miners' views on how to prevent people from going under unsupported roof. In *Preventing Coal Mine Groundfall Accidents: How to Identify and Respond to Geologic Hazards and Prevent Unsafe Worker Behavior.* USBM IC 9332. 25–31.

White, B.G., J.K. Whyatt, and D.F. Scott. 1995. Geologic factors in rock bursts in the Coeur d'Alene mining district. In *Proceedings Mechanics and Mitigation of Violent Failure in Coal and Hard Rock Mines.* USBM SP 01-95. 217–230.

Zipf, R.K., and C. Mark. 1997. Design methods to control violent pillar failures in room-and-pillar mines. *Transactions of the Institution of Mining and Metallurgy* 106 (September–December): A124–A132.

CHAPTER 24

Mine Fires and Explosions

BASIC CONCEPTS

Ian Loomis
Senior Ventilation Engineer, Mine Ventilation Service, Inc., Fresno, California

CONTROL OF FIRES AND EXPLOSIONS

John W. Stevenson, Jack Tisdale, Don Mitchell (deceased), and Bill Marston
Hoover, Alabama; Chesapeake, Virginia; McCalla, Alabama

BASIC CONCEPTS

Fires and explosions require fuel, oxygen, and heat, the intuitive fire triangle. This two-dimensional figure excludes the combustion process, a self-sustained chemical reaction, which lifts the fire triangle into a three-dimensional state. A fire can be extinguished by removing any of the three elements or by interrupting the reaction process.

Fires and explosions can be separated into two categories of energy release. A general segregation between a fire and an explosion is intuitive for most. For the sake of discussion in this chapter, a fire will refer to a relatively slow combustion process without substantial pressure developments, whereas an explosion will refer to a very rapid combustion process accompanied by a severe pressure gradient. In other words the fire grows/advances at a rate less than the speed of sound, and an explosion advances at the speed of sound or faster.

Fires

A general treatment of fires in mines must deal with the general scenarios under which they are likely to occur. The origin of fires may be a diverse field, but the basic manifestations can be limited to a few variables. The first of these will be the consideration of the basic fire presentation. Next will be the state of the fire with respect to the combustion chemistry. The method of ignition will be considered also, particularly in respect to self-ignition. Finally, some discussion is warranted with respect to the general behavior of fire-related phenomena.

Open Versus Concealed   Open fires, as the name suggests, occur where they are visible, such as entries of the active mine ventilation system. During the preliminary stages, these fires can be attacked directly and at relatively close quarters. As an open fire grows in size and strength the only means of direct attack may be from the upstream side. At a very advanced stage of fire growth, direct attack may not be possible from any angle. These fires may be classified as open, but the underground mine environment presents severe limitations on access to a developed fire.

Concealed fires, on the other hand, are those that occur in otherwise access restricted locations, such as gob areas, abandoned sections, within coal pillars, and so forth. These fires are more likely to go unnoticed, at least in the early stages. Methods of attacking a concealed fire may include inert gas flooding, sealing of the affected area, and excavation of the burning material.

Oxygen-Rich versus Fuel-Rich Fires   The distinction between an oxygen-rich or fuel-rich fire is used to describe the state of the fire relative to a nominal or stoichiometric combustion process. In the oxygen-rich state there is sufficient oxygen to allow for, theoretically, complete combustion of the available fuel. Remember that the combustion process is a series of competitive equilibrium chemical reactions; therefore, it is fair to assume that not all of the intermediate products will be fully converted in the reaction chain. Growth of a fire in the oxygen-rich state is marked by direct heat transfer from the flame to the additional fuel supply. The exhaust gases mix readily with available fresh air and are cooled and diluted.

As the fire becomes fuel-rich, growth begins to occur without direct contact of the flame. There is no longer sufficient excess air to cool and dilute the products of combustion. The resulting hot gases cause liberation of excess fuel into the exhaust stream. At advanced stages of growth the exhaust from a fuel-rich fire may contain virtually no oxygen and very high levels of both carbon dioxide and carbon monoxide. Because they are not diluted by excess air, the exhaust gases leave the location at nearly the same temperature as the flame.

A convenient method of assessing the state, and hence the expected behavior, of the fire is based on the oxygen (O_2) concentration in the products of combustion immediately downstream of the fire. Research conducted by Roberts and Clough (1967) in the late 1960s suggests that a fire involving wood lagging tends to behave in a fuel-rich manner as the products of combustion oxygen concentration fall below 15%. Recent research by Loomis and McPherson (Loomis 1995; Loomis and McPherson 1995) finds a similar number, approximately 12%, in small-scale wind tunnel tests using coal as the fuel. In these recent tests, the rate of carbon dioxide increase downstream of the fire makes a marked acceleration as the level of oxygen falls below that 12% to 15% range. The concentration of carbon dioxide then begins to fall as the oxygen concentration is depleted, moving toward zero. At this point, a truly fuel-rich condition exists.

Spontaneous Combustion   In conditions of just the right air movement, just the right fuel, and just the right material, the heat generated by natural oxidation will not be fully removed by the combined processes of convection and conduction. The result is a self-heating process that leads to combustion of the fuel, commonly called spontaneous combustion. Factors that appear to have an influence on the development of a spontaneous combustion event include, but are not limited to, sulfur content, humidity, and coal rank.

The development of the natural slow oxidation process into an accelerated, typically concealed, fire condition occurs under a fairly well understood set of conditions. Sufficient air must be made available to the process for a self-sustaining reaction to develop, but not so much that excess heat is carried away in the air. In other words, for a material that exhibits the tendency to undergo spontaneous combustion, it is possible to starve the material of oxygen, thus preventing the development of a fire; or it is possible to flood the material with air, so that the excess heat is carried away rather than accumulating.

Fire Phenomena   Fires in underground mine environments can quickly begin to govern the behavior of airflow in the immediate vicinity of the fire, and possibly the entire mine. The influence of the fire on the ventilation system arises from the same source as natural ventilation, the conversion of heat energy to mechanical work. In the case of fire-induced effects, the magnitude can be rather exaggerated. Effects of interest include stratification, rollback, and throttling.

Stratification occurs as a response to the differences in density between the warmer, lighter gases heated by the fire and the cooler, heavier ambient air. In areas of low velocity flow stratification may be evident and pronounced for quite some distance downstream of a fire. As the average airflow velocity increases, turbulent mixing will disperse the stratified layer into the main body of flow.

Rollback may be visualized as an extreme form of stratification, in which the rising plume has sufficient energy and velocity to spread out against the main body flow. Hence the development of a stratified layer flowing counter-current to the main airflow. This condition may also be seen in inclined airways with normally downward airflow. The highly buoyant heated air may take on upward flow, against the normal air movement.

Throttling of the airflow to a section of the affected mine, or even to the entire mine, begins as the conversion of heat energy to mechanical work becomes significant in relationship to the work being done on the system by the fans.

Explosions

Explosions may or may not be associated with a mine fire. In other words, an explosion may simply be an event in the mine, or it may occur as a result of an ongoing fire, or it may even lead to the development of a fire. A distinguishing characteristic of the explosion is the very rapid conversion of chemical energy to heat and mechanical work. Even a relatively small explosion has the capability to blow out stoppings, bulkheads, and structural steel, and to displace heavy machinery.

In a typical description of an explosion, a shock wave expands out from the source of ignition. This shock wave travels away from the source at the speed of sound or faster. A methane, coal dust, and air mixture can produce a shock wave that travels as much as 6 times the speed of sound through the mine workings. Confinement is a physical factor to consider in the development of the explosion. The shock wave begins to occur as the expanding gases accelerate into the ambient air. This can be exacerbated in the mining environment because the paths of release are limited (i.e., the mine opening dimensions are restricted).

Although a number of explosion scenarios could be identified as plausible in an underground mining environment, the discussion here will be limited to two generalized cases—that of methane and air, and that of methane, coal dust, and air.

Methane and air explosions occur in the well-known mixture range of 5% to 15% methane in air. The most energetic mixture, occurring at approximately 10% methane in air, may produce as much as 5,200 kJ/kg of mixture. An explosion under these conditions may result in a shock wave traveling on the order of twice the speed of sound in the ambient air. In these conditions, the shock wave precedes the flame front, acting to thoroughly mix the methane and air, or, even worse, to entrain dust into the mixture (McPherson 1993).

Methane, coal dust, and air typically occur following an initial methane air ignition. The shock wave generated by the ignition draws from the surrounding surfaces and mixes it with the air before the arrival of the flame front. The energy available to be released from the methane, coal dust, and air mixture is significantly greater than methane and air alone. Explosive mixtures may contain a range of 50 to 5,000 grams of coal dust per cubic meter. Once coal dust has become involved in the explosion, the rate of advance can quickly accelerate to the order of six times the speed of sound in the ambient air (McPherson 1993).

The prudent, judicious, and liberal use of stone dust greatly minimizes the likelihood of a coal-dust-based explosion by acting to break down the path of the combustion process between the dust particles, which are the fuel elements.

CONTROL OF FIRES AND EXPLOSIONS

The relevant published literature offers a comprehensive review of the subject of mine fires and explosions. As a result, this section will concentrate on practical concepts and aspects that mine managers and engineers will find most useful in combating these hazards. It is most important to remember the warning of Woods Talman, an internationally renowned expert on explosions and fires, "When you have a fire in your mine, TIME IS NOT YOUR FRIEND."

Failure to take quick and proper action invariably leads to weeks, if not months, of imposed closure and the expenditure of many times the cost of an effective fire prevention, detection, and fighting program. When personnel are withdrawn from the mine and it is sealed at the surface, there is little chance of getting back into the mine within a reasonable amount of time.

Consider that firefighters left the mine because of a safety consideration, usually a methane accumulation that someone fears will come in contact with heated material and cause an explosion. Once personnel are out of the mine, the conditions inside become unknown. How does one know that the potential for an explosion has not worsened? For that matter, what, if anything, is known about conditions inside of the mine? Unless it can be demonstrated that conditions are safe and no explosions can result, personnel will remain on the outside looking in.

How can conditions in the mine be determined? Usually this is accomplished with boreholes from the surface. A sampling tube inserted through the borehole can be used to draw samples for analysis. How many boreholes will be necessary to make a determination for everyone's satisfaction? This is hard to say, and it may take several at strategic locations. How will the samples be analyzed? In fortunate instances, the Mine Safety and Health Administration (MSHA) will have its apparatus at the site and be able to provide prompt analytical information. If not, where is the nearest laboratory that can do the work and provide accurate analysis? MSHA will be taking samples and mailing them for analysis, if analytical equipment is not at the mine site. Waiting for these results by mail can delay operations.

As part of the planning process for mine emergencies, one should ponder these questions. Consider a fire at a particular location and go through the thought process. One might consider installing sampling lines as people retreat from the mine, if there is time. The mine-wide monitoring system, if installed, usually cannot be depended on—it may not be possible to leave it on, and it usually does not give sufficient information about particular gases present.

Emergency management personnel must be able and ready to make timely decisions based on facts, knowledge, and experience. Delays in decision making can be worse than wrong decisions. They can be dangerous because the plan you are evaluating was or should have been based on the facts and knowledge that existed at the time the plan was made and submitted. Real fires are dynamic, unstable beasts. What was true an hour ago is seldom true now.

Fortunately, most fires are controlled. There is a "rule-of-thumb," a rule you can bet on, that almost always proves true: A fire that is not controlled within 8 hours will have to be sealed. The act of sealing has grave implications. First of all, where can seals be built? That depends on many factors, discussed in the sections that follow.

The Size of the Fire

The larger the fire, the farther from it the seals must be built. If too close, it will be difficult to cool and dilute the heat, smoke, and gases enough to build seals. Invariably, sealing operations reduce the flow of air through the fire, causing the formation of ignitable bodies of gases, leading to explosions. Not too many years ago in England, miners were stacking sandbags to form a seal; the fire behind the seal ignited accumulating gases; and pressures from the resulting explosion sent the sandbags flying, which resulted in three fatalities. These and other problems are detailed in the chapter "Sealing," in the book *Mine Fires* by Don Mitchell.

Stability

Another critical factor is the need to build seals where ribs, roof, and floor can be expected to remain stable. What good comes from building seals where ground movements will crush them or where the coal breaks loose leaving gaps between the seal and ribs?

Position of the Mining Equipment

Following a fire in a Western mine a few years ago, seals were built in the mains 4,000 feet from the fire. Behind those seals are 900 feet of longwall shields, the shearer, the stage loader, three continuous mining machines, and three roof bolters, as well as 40 million tons of reserves.

It took the mine operator 4 months to get enough equipment to begin a new section. The company had to buy coal to meet the demands of contracts with power plants. The coal cost $12 per ton more than it had before the fire. Obviously, the operator suffered, and continued to do so for many months. His suffering, however, was minor compared to that of the 300 miners who were out of work for at least 5 months. The mine is in the Rocky Mountains; the nearest other source for jobs is more than 100 miles away; and what about the people in the town who depended on these miners and their families to buy food, get haircuts, rent videos, and pay taxes?

What caused the fire? Rock was breaking at the tailgate end of the longwall. To put in a shield that would prevent rock from rolling onto the face, exposed roof bolts were cut. Instead of using a bolt cutter, they lit a cutting torch, which in turn ignited methane. It is almost impossible to extinguish flames in methane streaming out from roof strata.

The importance of training and preparation cannot be overemphasized. The planning should start with "what-ifs." Assume a fire started at a particular location in the mine. What materials will be needed, in what quantities, to fight the fire, and how soon? Where are those materials, and how long will it take to get them to the site? Are the water lines sufficient? Are the minimum fire hoses and nozzles required by the regulations sufficient? If sealing is required, where would they be built? How will samples be taken to determine the products from the fire or the concentrations of fire gases in the sealed area?

That introduces a subject of great importance. For more than 20 years, we have been advocating the development of fire brigades—teams of miners on each shift who:

- Can reach the fire within 20 minutes
- Have all—and we emphasize **all**—the equipment needed to fight any kind of fire likely to develop in the mine
- Are expert in the use of that equipment
- Have received continuous hands-on training.

This concept has finally begun to take hold. Fire brigades are being formed, and their successes have been so outstanding that many people who were not supportive have begun to reconsider. Two excellent works are available from the National Mine Rescue Association on the subject of fire brigades: *Planning for What You Hope Never Happens* and *Mine Rescue Teams, Fire Brigades, and Control of Their Ventilation*.

Fires in mines can be caused by many factors but one of the major causes is spontaneous combustion ("spon com"). Spon com occurs when air is allowed to percolate through organic materials, including coal. Through a progressive series of adsorptive, absorptive, and chemical processes, heat is produced, which causes the temperature of the material to rise. As we discussed in the introduction to this chapter, fires occur when the temperature of the material reaches its minimum self-heating temperature, where a continuous exothermic reaction is sustained and the material goes into thermal runaway.

The best means for controlling spon com is to develop a zero-pressure differential across the fire zone. Dr. Frances at the French research station CERCHAR and Dr. Both at the German station in Essen developed this technique in 1972. Our first opportunity to try it was in 1985 at a fire that had been burning for three weeks in the gob of a mine in Craig, Colorado. On Friday and Saturday, we made pressure differential measurements around the area and built the stoppings and checks needed to get these to equal zero. Saturday night the fire quit spreading; Sunday morning all fire indicators were down; and on Monday production resumed. The chapter "Concealed Fires" in *Mine Fires* (Mitchell 1996) describes several techniques for obtaining a zero-pressure differential. It is best to test these and to train fire brigades in using them long before the need arises. As too many experiences have shown, following that advice might save your company millions of dollars.

Many experts emphasize spon com control by incubation time—that is, get in and out before the coal begins to self-heat. Incubation time is generally determined by laboratory studies. It has been the basis for design of some mines in Europe, the United States, Australia, and China. This technique was developed in the 1920s. Today, we believe it to be a dangerous, wasteful basis for decisions—dangerous because fires have broken out in shorter periods of time—and because these unexpected fires have ignited methane and initiated explosions. A few years ago, 11 miners were killed when this happened in a mine in Australia.

The technique is wasteful because there have been too many instances when no heating developed long after the incubation time had lapsed. The panel designed for too short a period leads to high mining costs.

It is, however, important to be aware of incubation times. In addition, remember that incubation times depend on many factors other than those simulated in a laboratory or experienced in another mining area.

Fires are ventilation-controlled; therefore, control ventilation rather than base mine designs on incubation time. Where there is a potential for spon com, make every effort to minimize pressure differentials across the gob, and maintain ventilation controls that prevent air from getting behind the shields and chocks. Equally important is constant monitoring of the atmosphere flowing into and out of the gob. Remember, in the analysis of those data, specific numbers are not relevant; follow trends only. This too is discussed in the book *Mine Fires*, particularly on pages 31 and 32. The procedures described have never yet failed.

When the mine ventilation, methane, and dust control plan is up for a 6-month review, all coal mines should determine satisfactory locations on the main entries for temporary seal locations. Furthermore, they should provide doors between intakes and return air courses where the ventilating air current could be short-circuited under emergency fire or explosion conditions. When a coal mine is operating in a seam that has a history of spon com, it is important to take actions to reduce the personal, physical, and financial disaster that can result from the phenomenon. High velocities result in high ventilating pressure losses. Therefore, reduce high velocities by increasing cross-sectional area, possibly by increasing the number of entries. Other techniques could include all methods of degasification, which result in decreased air quantities for methane dilution. Spraying sealants on ribs or side walls to reduce leakage from intake to return air courses decreases the possibility of spon com. All of these precautions reduce the quantity of air migrating through the gob and reduce the potential for spon com. But the possibility of heatings that result in fires and explosions lingers.

Mine ventilation is the most important factor in fighting mine fires. In past years it was thought that ventilation should be immediately reduced across a mine fire. This has been taught to the extent that some advocate opening doors to the return immediately upwind of the fire so as to reduce the amount of air over the fire. We have learned that can be a bad mistake. Never reduce the ventilation without giving thought to the possible results. The heat and smoke created by the fire tends to establish a ventilation system of its own. It can cause air reversals, disrupt the conditions in the immediate fire area, and cause a condition known as "smoke rollback." Smoke rollback happens when heat from the fire creates an up-draft of air. The rising air hits the mine roof and rolls out in all directions. Some of the air will roll forward even against the air stream. Reducing the ventilation can allow smoke and heat rollback that is so intense that the fire cannot be approached. In that situation there is no chance that the fire can be fought directly. You might think that by decreasing the ventilation one might be able to go around the fire and head it off. But the reduction in ventilation may allow the fire to develop to a fuel-rich stage, where incomplete combustion occurs in the fire proper and the gases produced are still combustible, but do not have enough oxygen to burn. Opening a ventilation door on the return of such a fire will introduce oxygen, and if the fire gases have not cooled, flame can erupt at that point.

Slowing the ventilation, then reestablishing it can create a hazard. Fire gases can be moved back over the flames, and cause an explosion. This is more of a hazard in highly volatile coal seams such as the Pittsburgh seam.

It is generally best not to disturb the ventilation until fire-fighting activities are under way and sufficient information points are set to provide feedback on the effects of changes as they are made.

In the United States there has been a most exciting change in the mine-fire incidence. In 1970, the regulations of the Federal Coal Mine Health and Safety Act of 1969 were implemented. Many regulations were related to fire, but the most important, in our opinion, were those that:

- Led to the use of alternating rather than direct current electrical power for mining machines
- Mandated the use of flame-resistant conveyor belts with slippage and sequence switches
- Required dedicated escape ways.

The results were immediate. Before that law, there were typically 200 or more fires each year, causing many deaths and serious injuries. From 1970 to 1990, the number of fires averaged 15 per year, and the current average is 6. We believe that increased use of carbon monoxide and smoke detectors, which permit detection of developing rather than active fires, coupled with the quick response of fire brigades, can be credited for much of that improvement.

Case Study of a Mine Fire

On December 19, 1984, fire swept through Emery Mining Corporation's Wilberg Mine in Orangeville, Utah. As horrible as it was, this fire was interesting and much can be learned from it. The MSHA report states that it started in an air compressor in a crosscut between the main intake and return. No one had used that compressor for days, but it was running. Some weeks before, a mechanic removed the defective heat-sensing and cutoff switches. He "RED" tagged the compressor to let others know the machine should not be used. The oil overheated and hoses ruptured. Flaming oil thrown into the intake entry ignited coal. The air from this fire went directly into the intake entry of 5 Right, which was a longwall panel. The headgate consisted of an intake and a belt entry. Air went up the intake, some returning down the belt but most going across the face. This was the second shift for that day. Production was so great on the first shift that management decided it had a chance to go for a record. To achieve this goal, the company's vice president of Operations, the mine foreman, the chief mechanic, and all other key officials were on the face to make sure nothing went wrong. Shortly before someone smelled smoke, the supply man came on the section. He had parked his diesel-powered supply truck in the intake entry. Because the air was cold, he left the engine running. Everyone agreed that the smoke they smelled was from that diesel exhaust. After a while, however, the smoke became so heavy that the chief mechanic went into the intake to see what was the matter. He saw dense smoke, grabbed an oxygen self-rescuer, went back and gave the warning, and started down the belt entry. He was the only person who found his way out of the section.

In the meantime, others reached the fire in the Mains and applied water. No one, however, went downstream to get water flowing into the path of the advancing fire. It didn't matter, though, because someone outside decided to cut off the power. You might cut the power in the event of an explosion, and perhaps that person was trained to do that. But in this case, the water flow stopped when the power went off because the pump supplying the water was also on that electrical circuit. Eventually, the power was restored as was the flow of water. No one, however, did anything to try to stop the fire from spreading down the returns. It is more important to get water into the path of the fire than it is to put it on the fire—it's useless to try to extinguish a fire at its source as it spreads unimpeded down the return and into adjoining entries (there is much about that in *Mine Fires*). The next day, a mine rescue team 3,000 feet down from the fire was poised to inject high expansion foam into the return. When they opened the door in the stopping into the return they saw a pitch black flow, and within seconds it burst into flame. This was the only known instance of a fuel-rich fire in a mine. Certainly there have been others, but none has actually been observed. We can see in this story that fuel-rich fires should be of particular concern to miners. As explained earlier, they result when there is an inadequate flow of air through the fire. The gases and tars pulled out from downstream coals become so hot and concentrated that they ignite themselves whenever sufficient oxygen is added—that's what happened when they opened the door in the stopping. The fire could not be controlled and the mine was sealed. Recovery operations made history. Two openings on the far left of the mine had been free of signs of fire, although they did contain hot, toxic gases. Carbon dioxide, which was chosen because it could be injected at zero degrees, was injected into the mouth of one. Teams could go where temperatures were below $80°$F and the carbon monoxide concentration was less than 750 parts per million. The teams recovered these two entries by air locking and sealing the openings into the adjoining fire area. As a result, reserves, which today form one of the most profitable producers in the United States, were saved. Few, however, would be willing to adsorb the costs—more than $67 million.

Abandoned Mine Fires

Fires in abandoned mines are causing increased concern and receiving additional attention now. Unfortunately, there are many mines for which the original owners claim no responsibility, and fire rage in many of these. Some fires resulted from spon com; some from people burning garbage in unprotected openings into the mine; and some from forest fires blowing burning leaves into those openings. One such fire destroyed the town of Centralia, Pennsylvania. Another almost destroyed the city of Shamokin, Pennsylvania. Others spew toxic gases into the air while leaving hidden holes into which people and animals can fall. All make it impossible to develop the overlying land for homes, farms, and industry.

After fighting a mine fire, almost everyone experiences (or should experience) humility. Fighting a mine fire pits Man against Nature and, as the old truism teaches, "You can't fool Mother Nature." So instead, work with her and ask her questions—the sooner the better. When fighting a fire, don't have all the answers, be an errand boy—ask the fire! She gives good answers if you ask the right questions.

Be careful, though. Correct questions and answers are nonexistent; bad ones are worse than none at all; and the most common—the obstinate, ignorant ones—are dangerous. Two questions you must constantly ask are, "What am I doing?" and then, "Why am I doing this?" If you don't know what you are doing and why—DON'T. A mine fire can be unforgiving of errors. Don't, however, just stand there and wring your hands. Do something, but only one small thing at a time. If it doesn't work, you can stop, remove what you have done, and start over again. Remember, plans don't have to be perfect. Think of them as a wire rope, strong enough to carry the load, yet flexible enough to stretch a little.

Four Immutable Fire Laws

Law 1   Heat rises and because it is stopped by the mine roof, it generates forces. (Unfortunately, miners can't do what other firefighters do. To reduce forces, firefighters break windows in the upper floors and chop holes in the roof of buildings.)

Law 2   Every force creates an equal and OPPOSITE FORCE (this leads to smoke and fire rollback and methane layers).

Law 3   The Universal Gas Law–pressure and volume are directly related to temperature.[1] The hotter the fire, the higher the pressure it develops. Confining the pressure (like in a dead end or in a roof cavity) increases the pressure and leads to explosions. The only difference between a FIRE and an EXPLOSION is how HEAT IS CONFINED.

Law 4   The Fan Law–air always flows from the point of high to low pressure. While fighting a fire think of it as a fan. Fans produce pressure. Generally, the larger the fan, the higher the pressure. The greater the difference in pressure between two or more points, the greater the quantity of air–or, in a fire, the more heat and products of combustion that can be pushed back against the ventilating air toward you and the other firefighters.

Your Fire Laws

Just as fires obey immutable laws, so must you.

1. Never stop asking, "What am I doing?" and "Why am I doing this?"
2. Always be able to take one step back to safety.[2]
3. Control the ventilation.[3] If you don't, the fire will. This does not mean you should reduce the quantity or velocity[4] of the air flowing into the fire. NEVER do so without good compelling reasons.
4. Remove FUEL[5] downstream from the fire.
5. Fight the fire by removing the HEAT.
6. Know when and how to quit. This requires competent monitoring and interpretation of the atmosphere flowing into and through the fire. Easy to write, difficult to do. We suggest that all readers who need to monitor and interpret these atmospheres study the works and practical advice of noted experts, especially Mike Zabetakis, E.A.C. Chamberline, and Ivan Graham.

In conclusion, it is critical to understand that fires are fuel- and ventilation-controlled. The fuel in coal mines and in heavily timbered areas can be inexhaustible; therefore, if YOU don't control the ventilation, the fire will.

---

1. PV = nRT where P is pressure, V is volume, n is amount of gas, R is a gas constant, and T is temperature.
2. The more smoke that rolls back, the less the chance the fire can be fought safely and effectively. The rollback is often hot enough to weaken roof strata and loosen resin-anchored bolts–conditions that make travel under such questionable if not wrong, particularly if the smoke limits visibility. The rollback not only contains heat and smoke, it contains fire gases that can act like a wick, bringing flame from the fire back into firefighters.
3. If airflows are too low, fire gases can recirculate and envelope firefighters. When selecting nozzles, remember that they will be like fans and, if too large, will recirculate fire gases. A 1.5-in. diameter nozzle can introduce as much as 6,500 cfm of air, and a 2.5 in. nozzle almost 9,000 cfm. Fire gases will recirculate should the flow of air into the fire be less. For example, assume 10,000 cfm of air are flowing through the fire and miners are applying water from four hoses with 1.5-in. nozzles:

   4 nozzles × 6,500 cfm/nozzle = 26,000 cfm of air induced

   26,000 cfm − 10,000 cfm of air inflow = 16,000 cfm of recirculated fire gases

   Also remember that fog and spray, although more effective than a solid stream, can change into large volumes of steam when fighting a hot fire in a confined place–such as in the face or near a box check.
4. To mitigate against smoke rollback (not prevent) the minimum velocity should >100 $H^{1/2}$ where H is entry height. In a typical entry this might be >24,000 cfm, an unlikely quantity in many sections. Therefore, section crews need to know how and where to get such flows before they need them. Among the other hazards of inadequate quantities are the probabilities for recirculating fire gases, leading to an explosion or to a fuel-rich fire, the worst of all kinds. Even worse is hot smoke in a confined place turning fog and fine sprays into steam, enveloping and burning the firefighters.
5. Don't forget, the fuel is the gases and tars being pulled out of the coal and wood by the heated air; therefore, to remove FUEL, cool the air. This might require adding more air; best of all is to spray water, preferably as fog, downstream from and into the paths of the fire.

REFERENCES

Hartman, H.L., J.M. Mutmansky, R.V. Ramani, and Y.J. Wang. 1997. *Mine Ventilation and Air Conditioning.* 3rd ed. New York: Wiley Interscience.

Huntley, D.W., R.J. Painter, J.K. Oakes, D.R. Cavanaugh, and W.G. Denning. 1984. *Underground Coal Mine Fire, Wilberg Mine, Emery Mining Corporation, Report of Investigation.* U.S. Department of Labor, MSHA, Report #204,858.

Loomis, I.M. 1995. *Application of water mist to fuel-rich fires in model coal mine entries.* Master's thesis. Blacksburg, VA: Virginia Polytechnic Institute and State University.

Loomis, I.M., and M.J. McPherson. 1995. Application of water mist for the control of fuel-rich fires in model coal mine entries. *Proceedings 7th U.S. Mine Ventilation Symposium.* Lexington, KY: Society for Mining, Metallurgy, and Exploration.

McPherson, M.J. 1993. *Subsurface Ventilation and Environmental Engineering.* London: Chapman and Hall. 904 pp.

Mitchell, D.W. 1996. *Mine Fires: Prevention, Detection, Fighting.* Chicago: Intertec Publishing.

Roberts, A.F., and G. Clough. 1967. The propagation of fires in passages lined with flammable materials. *Combustion and Flame* 11: 365ff.

CHAPTER 25

Mining with Explosives:
Safety First

Susan J.P. Flanagan
Counsel
Institute of Makers of Explosives, Washington, D.C.

Lon Santis
Manager, Technical Services
Institute of Makers of Explosives, Washington, D.C.

INTRODUCTION

The importance of safety awareness in the handling and use of explosive materials cannot be overstated. A well-trained and experienced blaster[1] appreciates the awesome power of explosive materials and knows that each blast must be carefully and thoughtfully planned using proper materials and equipment. In the hands of an inadequately trained or inexperienced individual, this powerful tool has the potential for disastrous misuse. Individuals who mishandle or misuse explosives—whether out of ignorance or negligence—run the risk of causing significant property damage, serious injury, and death. Clearly, such risks should never be tolerated.

In this chapter, we outline methods for the safe handling and use of explosives in mining operations. The information is general in nature and is not intended to be applicable to every situation that may be encountered in the field. Moreover, this chapter is not intended to be a comprehensive safety course for anyone who handles explosive materials.

Every situation that requires the handling and/or use of explosives must be evaluated on a case-by-case basis taking into consideration the unique physical, geological, and meteorological conditions characterizing the area where explosive materials are to be used. In addition, safety always is a key consideration in every blasting operation and will influence the blaster's selection of materials and the design of the blasting sequence.

Each individual involved in the process of handling and using explosive materials must be knowledgeable about the characteristics of the particular products being used and the proper procedures for handling and use. All members of the blasting crew must be adequately trained in the principles of explosives technology, safety, handling, and use. The blasting crew should be experienced in handling explosives on a day-to-day basis. Assembling a blasting crew of "part time" blasters with limited experience should always be avoided.

The qualified "blaster in charge" directing a blasting operation should be fully informed regarding the appropriateness of the product(s) to the intended use and the conditions under which the product(s) should and should not be used. The blaster-in-charge also should be responsible for supervising the blasting crew and the blasting operation and should ensure that all applicable safety precautions, regulatory requirements, and proper handling procedures are observed.

The actual destructive capacity of modern-day explosives may not be fully appreciated by those unfamiliar with explosives or by those who witness only the controlled energy of a well-planned and executed blast. As stated by the International Society of Explosives Engineers (ISEE) in that organization's *Blasters' Handbook*:

> *Consider that a single 2 × 8" cartridge of 80% gelatin that weighs less than a pound may produce nearly 1.4 million foot pounds (454 kcal) of energy in less than 0.00004 seconds; such energy release corresponds to 76 million horsepower. This energy and power is multiplied many thousand times in a surface mine blast or a large construction shot. However, even to a casual observer, a well-designed blast is marked not by the violence of detonation, but by the orderly progression of the rock movement and the muffled sound.*[2]

The relative safety and stability of contemporary explosive products and the ability of the experienced blaster to effectively harness and direct their tremendous power must never be allowed to engender complacency when working with or around explosives. An acute awareness of the potential consequences of mishandling explosives products should drive the actions of all those working with the materials.

ELEMENTARY BLASTING MECHANICS

An exhaustive technical explanation of blasting mechanics is well beyond the scope of this chapter, but the following is a very simplified description of the physical effects generated by a detonation.

Explosives are a tool designed to function by rapidly producing a large quantity of energy in the form of shock compression waves that are transmitted to the surrounding rock. Within a certain distance of the charge, this tremendous transference of energy succeeds in pulverizing and/or plasticizing the rock. As the compression waves progress through the rock formation and/or are reflected back into the rock, additional fragmentation and fracturing of the formation occurs. Fissures or cracks created by the shock wave fill almost instantaneously with expanding gases that further move the broken pieces of rock. As would be expected, the amplitude and energy of the shock compression waves decrease with distance from the borehole, producing a correspondingly lesser degree of impact on the surrounding material.[3]

Three essential properties characterize high explosives: (1) high explosives are chemical compounds or mixtures that are initiated by heat, shock, impact, friction, or a combination of the above; (2) when initiated by a detonator or booster, high explosives decompose rapidly in a detonation; and (3) detonation produces a rapid release of heat and large quantities of high-pressure gases, which, in turn, rapidly expand with sufficient force to overcome confining forces such as a surrounding rock formation.[4]

High explosives also are susceptible to deflagration (i.e., burning). If confined, the resulting pressure can cause the chemical reaction to progress from deflagration to detonation. This transition is referred to as the Deflagration to Detonation Transition, or DDT, and can occur even in the absence of ambient oxygen.[5]

REGULATION AND CLASSIFICATION OF EXPLOSIVE MATERIALS

The manufacturing, transportation, storage, distribution, and use of explosives are comprehensively regulated on the local, state, and federal level.

Federal Regulations

Federal regulations with the greatest impact on the mining industry are those promulgated (i.e., published) by the Mine Safety and Health Administration (MSHA), the Office of Surface Mining Reclamation and Enforcement (OSM), the Bureau of Alcohol, Tobacco, and Firearms (ATF), the Department of Transportation (DOT), and the Environmental Protection Agency (EPA).[6]

MSHA   MSHA is part of the U.S. Department of Labor and is responsible for administering the Federal Mine Safety and Health Act of 1977. Among other things, this responsibility includes developing and enforcing mandatory safety and health standards applicable to explosives. MSHA regulations covering explosives are included in the *Code of Federal Regulations* (CFR) at the following locations.

- 30 CFR Part 48–Training and Re-Training of Miners[7]
- 30 CFR Part 56 (§§56.6000–56.6905)–Surface Metal and Nonmetal Mines

- 30 CFR Part 57 (§§57.6000–57.6960)–Underground Metal and Nonmetal Mines
- 30 CFR Part 75 (§§75.1300–75.1328)–Underground Coal Mines
- 30 CFR Part 77 (§§77.1300–77.1304)–Surface Coal Mines and Surface Work Areas of Underground Coal Mines.

These regulations are quite detailed and cover issues as diverse as storage in underground and surface magazines, multiple shot blasting, loading boreholes, stemming boreholes, firing procedures, misfires, the proper handling of damaged or deteriorated explosives, and requirements for "qualified persons" authorized to use explosives. MSHA regulations also govern the transportation of explosive materials on mine property.

OSM   OSM is part of the Department of the Interior (DOI) and is responsible for administering portions of the Federal Surface Mining Control and Reclamation Act of 1977 (SMCRA). OSM regulations governing use of explosives at surface coal mining operations are set out at 30 CFR §816.61–816.68. SMCRA authorizes DOI to delegate administration of SMCRA to qualified state agencies. Most states with significant surface coal mining activity have been granted this authority.

ATF   ATF is a federal law enforcement organization within the U.S. Department of the Treasury. ATF regulates the importation, manufacture, distribution, and storage[8] of explosive materials and administers and enforces the Federal Explosives Law.[9] ATF regulations are found at 27 CFR Part 55. These regulations impose licensing and permitting, magazine construction, and record keeping requirements. ATF prescribes three classes of explosives for storage purposes:

High explosives–explosive materials that can be caused to detonate by means of a No. 8 Test Detonator. Typical examples include dynamites, cast boosters, and certain emulsions, water gels, and slurries.

Low explosives–explosive materials that can be caused to deflagrate when confined. Typical examples include black powder, propellants, safety fuse, igniters, and fuse igniters.

Blasting agents–explosive materials that cannot be initiated by a No. 8 Test Detonator when unconfined, but which will detonate with a stronger stimulus. Typical examples include ammonium nitrate/fuel oil (ANFO), blends, and certain emulsions, water gels, and slurries.[10]

DOT   The classification of explosives and the transportation of explosive materials over public highways are regulated by DOT. DOT regulations are set out in 49 CFR §§390–399.

Classification

For purposes of transportation, explosives are regulated as DOT Class 1 materials. This class is further divided into six divisions corresponding to the hazardous properties of the materials.

Division 1.1–explosives that have a mass explosion hazard. Typical examples are: dynamite, detonator (cap) sensitive emulsions, slurries, water gels, cast boosters, and mass detonating detonators.

Division 1.2–explosives that have a projection hazard but not a mass explosion hazard. Typical examples include: certain types of ammunition, mines, and grenades.

Division 1.3–explosives that have a fire hazard and either a minor blast hazard or a minor projection hazard or both, but not a mass explosion hazard. Typical examples include: certain types of fireworks, propellants, and pyrotechnics.

Division 1.4–explosives that present a minor explosion hazard, do not have a mass explosion hazard, and explosion is largely confined to the package. Typical examples are: safety fuse and certain electric and nonelectric detonators.

Division 1.5–explosives that are very insensitive. Division 1.5 explosives have a mass explosion hazard but are very unlikely to initiate or detonate from burning under normal transportation conditions. Typical examples include: blasting agents, ANFO, non cap-sensitive emulsions, blends, slurries, water gels, and other explosives that require a booster for initiation.

Division 1.6–extremely insensitive explosives which do not have a mass explosion hazard. Commercial explosives generally do not fall into this division.[11]

Transportation over Public Highways. DOT regulations governing explosives carriers cover (among other things) vehicle placarding, shipping papers specifications, driver qualification requirements, vehicle inspections, vehicle loading and unloading, accidents and accident reporting, vehicle attendance and parking requirements, insurance, controlled substance testing, registration, and training.[12]

Properties of Explosives; Types of Commercial Explosive Materials. According to the National Mining Association (NMA), some form of mining is conducted in all 50 of the United States.[13] This geographic diversity, coupled with the myriad metals, minerals, and fuels that are produced by the mining industry, has necessitated the development of a similar diversity of explosive materials. Although all explosives have certain physical characteristics in common, each explosive product is designed with specific, unique properties. It is this differentiation that allows the qualified blaster to select or engineer the most appropriate product for the job at hand.

This section gives a broad overview of commercial explosives products commonly used by the mining and/or minerals/fuels exploration industries. This overview is not intended to suggest the appropriateness of any type of explosive product to a particular blasting situation. Such an evaluation must be performed on a case-by-case basis by a qualified blaster experienced in blast design.

In elementary terms, the process of blast design involves prediction and measurement of explosive performance: (1) a determination of the amount of energy needed to achieve the desired level of rock fragmentation and/or displacement; (2) selection of the most appropriate type of explosive products to achieve the intended result; and (3) a determination of how explosives will be distributed within the blast area to maximize energy efficiency (both in space and time), obtain the necessary degree of fragmentation, avoid waste, and safeguard the surrounding environment, property, and human health and safety. In general, a detonation will produce certain predictable results: (1) rock fragmentation, (2) rock displacement, (3) ground vibration, (4) airblast, and (5) fumes associated with the explosive chemical reaction.[14]

The blaster will have an in-depth understanding of the chemical and physical properties of explosives in general and will have a working familiarity with or understanding of specific explosives products. This base of knowledge will allow the blaster to design a blast that is tailored to achieving a desired result. By applying his or her knowledge of detonation velocity (including factors such as explosive type, confinement, temperature, charge diameter, and priming), packing density, detonation pressure, borehole pressure, energy, sensitivity, water resistance, and flammability, the blaster can design a sequence of blasts that will successfully displace even the most stubborn of rock formations.

MSHA Permissibles

Before we launch into a general discussion of commercial explosive materials, a few words about "permissible explosives." The term "permissible" is defined in MSHA regulations as "[a]ny substance, compound or mixture which is approved by MSHA and whose primary purpose is to function by explosion."[15] Permissible explosives included on MSHA's Active List of Permissible/Sheathed Explosives are the ONLY explosives that may be used in underground coal mining operations and in certain underground metal and nonmetal "gassy" mines.[16]

Specifically, permissible explosives are those explosive materials (certain dynamites, water gels, or emulsions) that have been approved by MSHA after satisfying technical performance criteria in a battery of tests prescribed in MSHA regulations.[17] These tests are performed by the National Institute for Occupational Safety and Health (NIOSH).[18] Permissible explosives are designed to produce a small-volume, low-temperature flame of short duration and are approved for use in conditions where the presence of dust or gases creates a potentially explosive atmosphere. Permissible explosives are identified by the markings "MSHA Approved Explosive" on the explosive cartridges.

Commercial Explosive Materials

Dynamite Alfred Nobel was credited with the invention of dynamite when, on May 26, 1868, he patented his formula of three parts nitroglycerin to one part kieselguhr (kieselguhr is an inert base more commonly known as diatomaceous earth). Historically, dynamites have been the most widely used and recognizable of all commercial explosive materials. Dynamite still is used today, but its use is declining. However, it is still available in a variety of strengths and detonation velocities that allow the material to be used in various conditions. The five principal types of dynamites currently available are:

- Straight dynamite
- Extra or ammonia dynamite
- Gelatin dynamite
- Extra or ammonia gelatin dynamite
- Semigelatin dynamite.

In simplistic terms, the types of dynamites are differentiated by the use (or lack) of the ingredient "nitrocotton." Nitrocotton is a cellulose nitrate that, combined with nitroglycerin, creates a gelatinous product. Straight dynamite and extra dynamite do not contain nitrocotton and are often referred to as "granular dynamites" because of their grainy composition.

Dynamite products are available in a number of different sized "packages," or cylindrical cartridges for special applications. Diameters of $7/8$ in. to 8 in. (22 mm to 244 mm) are considered standard.[19] Large diameter cartridges (4 in. diameter and greater) normally are shipped uncased or bundled and may weigh anywhere from 10 to 60 lb (4.5 kg to 27.2 kg) depending on the size. Smaller diameter products often will be shipped in fiberboard cases weighing approximately 50 lb (22.7 kg). Dynamite products axe available in a number of shells or overwraps that influence a product's resistance to moisture and its fume production potential. A product's packaging also will determine the proper procedures to be followed in loading and tamping the boreholes.

The blaster will consider a number of factors to determine whether a dynamite product is appropriate for use in a particular blast. Such factors may include the physical characteristics of the rock itself (i.e., density, hardness, and friability); the degree of fragmentation to be achieved by the shot; the moisture content in the boreholes; the possible presence of combustible gases or dust; and the availability of adequate ventilation in underground mining operations.[20]

Certain general rules of safe practice are applicable to the storage of dynamites: (1) storage must be in a container or magazine that meets all federal, state, and local requirements; (2) inventories of dynamites should correspond to the rate of use (i.e., storage of excess quantities of dynamites should be avoided, and may be expressly prohibited under certain circumstances); (3) dynamite products should be used according to age—older stocks should be used first;[21] and (4) dynamite products that are found to be deteriorated (e.g., if nitroglycerin is determined to be leaking into the overwrap) or that have exceeded their recommended shelf life should be destroyed by a qualified person(s) in accordance with applicable federal, state, and/or local requirements.

Unpleasant effects caused by nitroglycerin vapors (e.g., "NG" headaches) usually demand enhanced ventilation of the magazine and/or limited exposure to workers inside the magazine. The storage of permissible dynamites should be monitored particularly closely. The low velocity grades of many permissibles are susceptible to a more rapid deterioration process because of their greater tendency to absorb moisture. Inventories of permissibles should be carefully maintained and storage time minimized. Excess quantities of permissible dynamites should not be transported underground. Current MSHA regulations prohibit the underground storage of more permissibles than are required for a 48-hour period of use.[22]

It is vitally important to be familiar with the properties of any commercial explosive product identified for disposal or destruction. Both the Institute of Makers of Explosives (IME) and ISEE recommend that the manufacturer or distributor be consulted regarding the proper identification, handling, and disposal of a deteriorated or overage product.[23] In addition, a number of explosives manufacturers and distributors offer removal and disposal services.

Water Gels and Slurries   IME defines water gel explosives as "[a]n explosive material containing substantial portions of water, oxidizers and fuel, plus a cross-linking agent."[24] A slurry explosive is defined, in turn, as "[a]n explosive material containing substantial portions of a liquid, oxidizers and fuel, plus a thickener."[25]

The chemical composition of water gels and slurries renders these explosives less sensitive to accidental detonation than nitroglycerin-containing dynamites.[26] In other words, water gels and slurry explosives are less likely to detonate when exposed to accidental shock, impact, and fire. This decreased sensitivity, coupled with improved handling characteristics, has led to the widespread development and use of water gels and slurries since the original water gel was patented in 1960.

The fact that water gels and slurries are less sensitive than other explosive materials does not, however, mean that accidental detonation cannot occur. The relative sensitivity of an explosive material is determined under controlled test conditions. Although these tests provide some degree of predictability in assessing how an explosive will react to stresses in the field, the tests are not intended to be all encompassing. The sensitivity of a particular product can be affected by (among other things) the ambient ground and air temperature, product temperature, degree of confinement, and the priming method being used. Sensitivity test results should not—under any circumstances—be the sole factor used in determining proper handling procedures or the appropriate response to a potential accident scenario. Reduced sensitivity does not mean "accident-proof," and, unfortunately, there are documented cases of fatalities resulting from the accidental detonation of water-based explosives.

In addition to their reduced sensitivity, water gels and slurries have other properties that make these products appealing for a wide variety of applications. These properties include, but are not limited to, the following:[27]

Because of the aqueous consistency of the products, borehole density can be increased (i.e., controlled) by slitting the cartridge packaging and tamping the loaded product, which allows the material to substantially fill out the borehole diameter.[28] Bulk loading of water gels and slurries offers another option for increasing borehole density. Further density control options can be provided by combining water gels or slurries with ANFO in the borehole.

Water gels and slurries can be delivered premixed and packaged or can be mixed on site as the product is loaded into the borehole. Premixed formulations also can be delivered to the blast site via pump truck.[29] Various packaging options are available for special blasting operations or conditions. Underground loading or the loading of small boreholes typically is accomplished using pressure pot-type loaders equipped with holding tanks that are filled using bulk or large packaged material.[30]

Water gels and slurries are substantially water-resistant and can be formulated for use in conditions where water is present in the boreholes being loaded.

The products can be formulated to be cap-sensitive or cap-insensitive, depending on the particular application.[31]

Use of water gels and slurries may reduce the potential for hole-to-hole propagation and eliminate NG headaches.

Water gels and slurries that are packaged in cartridge form can generally be stored in appropriate storage magazines for 1 year or longer. Because of the considerable number of products available today, however, it is advisable to consult the manufacturer of each product to ensure that proper storage practices axe being observed.[32]

Emulsions IME defines an emulsion explosive as "[a]n explosive material containing substantial amounts of oxidizer dissolved in water droplets, surrounded by an immiscible fuel, or droplets of an immiscible fuel surrounded by water containing substantial amounts of oxidizer."[33]

Emulsions are typically described as having two "phases." Emulsion explosives consist of microscopic droplets of an oxidizing salt solution (water/oxidizer solution phase) surrounded by a continuous external oil phase. An emulsifying agent is added to stabilize the material. Slight modifications in the formulation result in a range of products including those with a putty-like consistency to fluid, high viscosity, pumpable products. Because of their physical structure, emulsion explosives have a very high velocity of detonation (VOD) and accompanying detonation pressure. The ISEE notes that these properties make emulsion explosives "particularly well-suited for improving fragmentation in hard massive rock, for breaking hard bottom rock, and for use as a booster for ANFO mixtures and other blasting agents."[34]

Because emulsion explosives are "water-in-oil" emulsions, they have excellent water resistance properties. In addition, if the materials are spilled, they retain a discrete physical form and can be easily recovered and used as originally intended. By adding other constituents such as aluminum or ANFO to emulsion explosives, the detonation characteristics of the material can be substantially adjusted.[35] Emulsion explosives are available in both sensitized and desensitized forms, which allows the blaster to select products best suited to a particular blasting operation. The relative sensitivity of emulsion products can be varied by the manufacturer and can range from DOT oxidizer 5.1, to blasting agent

1.513 (requiring booster initiation), to a sensitivity level equivalent to a high explosive (initiation by No. 8 Test Detonator or lower).[36]

Emulsions appear to have even a greater margin of safety than water gels and slurry explosives in impact sensitivity tests. When subjected to burning tests, emulsions generally do not detonate.[37] As in the case of all explosives, however, results obtained from tests performed under controlled conditions do not guarantee that a given product will behave in a like manner in the field. Emulsion explosives must be handled and used with the same attention to safety afforded any explosive material.

Emulsion products are available in a variety of packaged forms (e.g., paper and/or plastic cartridges). Emulsion products can also be manufactured to be pumped or augered. Particular care must be taken when using pumped emulsions (or any pumped water-based explosive) to avoid accidental detonation. Despite the fact that emulsions retain their stability over a wide temperature range, friction caused by allowing a pump to run dry (i.e., "deadheading"), or operating a pump when the discharge is substantially blocked or closed off, can raise the temperature of the material beyond the point where ammonium nitrate is destabilized.[38] At this point, there is a significant potential for accidental detonation.[39] At least one major accident has been attributed to pump blockage.[40]

ANFO—Ammonium Nitrate/Fuel Oil   Statistics gathered by IME indicate that nearly 6 billion pounds of blasting agents were consumed in the United States in 1997 (more than 2 million metric tons).[41] Blasting grade ammonium nitrate (AN) represents a significant percentage of this total amount. In turn, the predominant use of blasting grade AN is as ANFO—AN mixed with fuel oil.

ANFO is classified by DOT as a blasting agent (Division 1.5) because of its extreme insensitivity.[42] In its most common form, ANFO is a mixture of ammonium nitrate "prills," and No. 2 diesel fuel oil.[43] Because of its relatively low density (0.8–1 g/cc, depending on the packaging and loading technique used) and water solubility, ANFO is unsuitable for use in wet borehole conditions. ANFO often is blended or mixed with water-based or oxidizer explosive matrices. These materials are known as "blends," or, in some cases, as "heavy ANFO."[44] Blends are discussed more fully in the following section.

ANFO is available as a premixed product, or it can be delivered in bulk and mixed on site immediately before loading. Manufacturers often deliver the product in combination tank trucks that are equipped to mix the AN and fuel oil as they are loaded into the borehole via pump or auger. In addition, it is common for open pit operators to receive AN in bulk and prepare the ANFO mixture themselves.

The standard ANFO formulation used is 94% AN prills and 6% No. 2 diesel fuel oil. The percentage of fuel oil used impacts on the energy, detonation velocity, sensitivity, and fume generation potential of the ANFO. For wet conditions, ANFO can be crushed, mixed with fuel oil, and packaged in water resistant cartridges. Used in this form, ANFO will perform well provided that "water conditions are not too severe, exposure time is not excessive, cartridges are loaded and remain intact, and the column of cartridges is adequately primed, [coupled,] and boostered."[45] Cartridged products intended for use in wet conditions also may contain additives to increase density and sensitivity thus enhancing the energy and detonability of the material. Although ANFO is relatively insensitive, temperature cycling can increase its sensitivity. Repetitive cycling from warm temperatures in the day to cold temperatures at night can destroy the structural integrity of AN prills. This can result in an AN/fuel mixture containing very small particles of AN. Testing has shown that unconfined mixtures of fine particle size AN and fuel can be detonated with a blasting cap.

MSHA regulations at 30 CFR §57.6100–6205 govern the storage and transportation of blasting agents, including ANFO, at surface and underground metal and nonmetal mine sites. MSHA regulations covering the use of blasting agents at surface coal mines are set out at 30 CFR §77.1304. At the current time, there are no MSHA permissible blasting agents. Accordingly, blasting agents of any type are prohibited from use in underground coal mining operations and/or in other mine environments where gassy or dusty conditions pose a potential hazard.

Blends   IME defines an explosive "blend" as "[a] mixture consisting of (a) a water-based explosive material matrix and ammonium nitrate or ANFO; or (b) a water-based oxidizer matrix and ammonium nitrate or ANFO" (IME SLP 12).[46] The "blending" of AN or ANFO with water-based explosives or oxidizers frequently is done to increase the explosive energy of the AN/ANFO or to provide other desirable performance characteristics to the planned shot. Water-based explosives or oxidizers can be added to give the final mix (among other things), increased density, improved resistance to wet conditions, appropriate viscosity and sensitivity, and better energy efficiency.

A blended explosive product can be mixed to virtually any percentage specification. Although most blends are not cap-sensitive (i.e., blasting agents, Division 1.5), some manufacturers do produce blends classified as Division 1.1 explosives (e.g., products sensitized by the addition of glass microspheres). These products must be managed and stored accordingly.

An explosive blend normally is prepared in bulk form. Many mine operators prepare bulk blends at a stationary field location where the various products used in blending are kept in designated storage tanks. Blends also may be prepared directly at the borehole where the mix is specifically tailored to accommodate the conditions existing at the time that blasting is scheduled. A blending operation that takes place at the borehole often is accomplished using a mobile blend truck equipped with various product tanks, blending/mixing equipment, and a pump or auger for borehole loading.[47]

Cast Boosters   The increasing use of less sensitive water-based and AN blasting agents has necessitated the development of cast booster products. IME describes a booster as "[a]n explosive charge, usually of high detonation velocity and detonation pressure, designed to be used in the explosive initiation sequence between an initiator or primer and the main charge" (IME SLP 12).[48] Explosives manufacturers make a fairly wide range of boosters. A detailed description of booster products is, however, beyond the scope of this chapter. Accordingly, this section primarily focuses on cast booster products.

Cast boosters are generally a 50/50 mix of TNT and PETN or RDX. The mixture is melted in a steam kettle and poured into molds to harden. Speaking strictly from a performance standpoint, cast boosters are often preferred over other booster products because of their high detonation pressures, insensitivity, water resistance, and ease of priming.

In designing a blast or series of blasts that require a cast booster, the blaster will select the cast booster product most appropriate to the type of explosive being used, the surrounding conditions, and the design of the blast sequence. In addition, the blaster will ensure that the initiator being used is compatible with the cast booster. Not all cast boosters and initiating systems are designed to be used together. It is very important to verify the compatibility of the cast booster and initiation products before using them. This type of information is easily obtained from the product manufacturers.

Initiating Devices   In this chapter, we use the term "initiating device" to mean the various types of detonators[49] and detonating cords that are used to initiate the downstream detonation of explosive materials. The term "initiation system" commonly refers to a detonator, the particular device(s) used to transmit an initiation signal, and a power source.[50] By choosing the appropriate initiation devices/system, the blaster can design an instantaneous blast or a blast sequence with a controlled, predetermined delay **pattern** that maximizes rock fragmentation with minimal ground vibration and flyrock.

Initiation devices contain extremely sensitive explosive materials and are very sensitive to external influences such as flame, heat, friction, shock, and (in the case of electric detonators) stray current or other sources of electricity.[51] Initiation devices should be treated like any explosive material and be properly handled and managed. Obviously, initiation devices should be used only as intended and should never be tampered with or altered.

All initiation devices manufactured in North America are imprinted with a safety warning: "EXPLOSIVE-EXPLOSIF-DANGER-DÉTONATEUR-BLASTING CAP." Initiating devices typically are made of brightly colored plastic materials or wire insulation that may make them especially appealing to children. In addition, initiation devices are quite small and can easily be concealed in a pocket or other small space. For these reasons it is particularly important to carefully maintain an accurate inventory of all initiation devices and to store them in appropriate, locked magazines separate from other explosives.

MSHA has promulgated regulations that specifically address the storage and management of initiating devices. For example, MSHA regulations for all types of mines prohibit detonators from being stored in the same magazine with other explosives (see for example, 30 CFR §57.6100). Similarly, certain of the regulations restrict the underground transportation of detonators on the same vehicle with other explosives except under certain conditions meeting standards set by IME (see, e.g., 30 CFR §57.6201). Other regulations applicable to all mining situations provide that primers must be made up only at the time of use and as close as possible to the blast area (see, e.g., 30 CFR §57.6303), and that initiation systems be used in accordance with the manufacturer's instructions.

MSHA regulations governing the handling and use of initiating devices at underground mining operations prohibit aluminum-cased detonators, aluminum alloy-cased detonators, detonators with aluminum leg wires, and safety fuses. In addition, at the current time, nonelectric systems are prohibited from use in underground coal mines. Accordingly, before beginning any work involving explosive materials, it is essential that the correct, applicable MSHA regulations (and any other applicable federal, state, and local regulations) be reviewed.

Explosives manufacturers produce myriad initiating devices and initiation systems that are suitable for a host of diverse applications. This product diversity allows the blaster to select the most effective and safest means of initiating a blast. Always remember—it is the responsibility of the blaster in charge to ensure that all explosives products selected for a particular job, including primary explosives, boosters, initiation systems, and accessory equipment, are mutually compatible and will function properly and safely when used together.[52]

Blasting Machines and Accessory Equipment

A blasting machine is used to deliver electrical energy to the detonators. Specifically, IME defines a blasting machine as "[a]n electrical or electromechanical device which provides electrical energy for the purpose of energizing detonators in an electric blasting circuit. [The term is] also used in reference to certain nonelectric systems."[53] Two types of blasting machines are commonly used: (1) generator machines, which do not have a self-contained energy source and are operated by pushing a rack bar or twisting a handle; and (2) capacitor discharge machines, which contain storage capacitors charged by batteries or a manual generator. Capacitor machines are operated by a firing switch.

Blasting machines are sophisticated pieces of electrical equipment that are capable of transmitting high voltages. Accordingly, before using the machine the blaster should ensure that the equipment is properly charged and equipped with the correct power source, that the rated voltage is being produced, and that the machine is compatible with other items in the initiation system (e.g., the blaster will ensure that the machine is rated to handle the number of detonators that will be used in the blast). In addition, the blaster must observe proper procedures for calibrating the machine and attaching the lead lines. A malfunctioning blasting machine should be returned to the manufacturer for repair or replacement. The blaster must never attempt to repair the machine.

In terms of safety, it is vitally important to maintain all blasting equipment and accessories in optimum condition. Regular inspection and periodic testing of all systems and equipment is strongly advised. Under no circumstances should equipment be used if any malfunction is identified or suspected. Likewise, the equipment must not be used if any parts or connections are in disrepair. Moreover, testing of equipment must always be performed using the appropriate testing apparatus. Before performing any test on blasting equipment, the blaster will always confirm that the correct test equipment is being used.[54] A variety of testing equipment is available to test blasting equipment, to detect stray voltage and/or extraneous ground currents, and to identify the possible presence of electrical storms in the area of the blast.

Testing of equipment and circuits also must be performed during use. The qualified blaster will incorporate a number of safety checks and tests into the procedure for setting up the shot. In most cases, federal regulations require that safety procedures be followed and that specific checks be performed at various stages of blast preparation and initiation system hookup.[55]

As an additional safety precaution, access to the blasting machine or other initiating power source should be strictly limited to the blaster in charge. The power source should be locked at all times and the key or other means of unlocking the system kept exclusively within the control or possession of the blaster in charge.[56] Lead wires connecting the initiation system also should remain unattached until the blaster in charge has completed all preblast inspection procedures, cleared the area of all nonessential personnel, and performed all necessary safety checks on the system and circuitry.

Ground Vibration, Airblast, and Flyrock

Ground Vibration   Ground vibration is an inevitable result of blasting. One of the goals of the blaster when designing the blast is to minimize the intensity of residual ground vibration. In general terms, ground vibration is a form of kinetic energy resulting from the conversion of the potential energy in an explosive upon detonation. Vibration occurs as the seismic wave generated by detonation propagates through the ground away from the borehole.

To some extent, good blast design can significantly reduce the occurrence of ground vibration. Reduction of potential ground vibration is particularly important in populated areas where there may be nearby residential, commercial, or industrial structures and/or activity. Special precautions also must be observed in areas where underground mining activity is being conducted. Regulations governing allowable limits for ground vibration have been promulgated on the federal, state, and local level.[57] A complete description of the factors potentially affecting the generation of ground vibration and the methods that the blaster can use to predict and control vibration are beyond the scope of this chapter. For more detailed information, consult the ISEE *Blasters' Handbook*.

Airblast   Airblast, or air overpressure, is another residual effect of blasting that blasters should seek to minimize. Airblast is the "airborne shock wave or acoustic transient generated by an explosion."[58] In the vast majority of cases involving normal blasting operations, airblast is unlikely to cause any actual structural damage to surrounding buildings or facilities. The occurrence of airblast (and vibration) can, however, be an annoyance to people in the immediate area. Consequently, when designing a blast, the blaster should include consideration of the factors tending to affect generation of airblast (e.g., geological and physical characteristics of the site, stemming, initiation system, blast delay pattern, temperature gradient, wind, and other atmospheric conditions). Technical mitigation measures for reducing the potential for airblast are included in ISEE's *Blasters' Handbook*.[59]

More than one mining company has faced the prospect of litigation resulting from real or imagined property damage associated with ground vibration and airblast. To better defend against such claims, IME and ISEE offer a number of recommendations: (1) establish good public relations with residential and commercial neighbors and clearly communicate the precautions that are taken to control vibration and airblast within allowable limits; (2) schedule blasting at appropriate times during the day and notify neighbors when blasting is scheduled; (3) record and promptly investigate all complaints; (4) if possible, arrange an inspection of nearby structures before the blasting project begins and document any preexisting damage; and (5) maintain a complete and accurate blasting log that records vibration and airblast.[60] In a suit for damages, the chances of being held liable increase dramatically where a company is unable to produce complete and accurate records of blasting activity.

Flyrock   The potential for generating flyrock from an explosion is always real and must always be carefully considered when planning a blast. The term "flyrock" is used to describe the situation where rocks are propelled from the blast area by the force of an explosion. A recent blasting mishap in Salem, Massachusetts, in which more than 40 condominiums and 30 vehicles were damaged by flyrock, underscores the importance of containing the effects of a blast within a designated impact area. Fortunately, the Massachusetts incident did not result in any injuries, but the potential for injury in the affected residential neighborhood was, nevertheless, considerable.

Excessive flyrock can be caused by a number of factors, including (but not limited to) overcalculation of the amount of explosives needed, inadequate or improper stemming, overconfinement of the explosives, inconsistent burden in the borehole (e.g., gaps or mud seams), boreholes drilled too close to a free face or too shallow for the amount of burden, and improper sequencing of detonator delay timing. In setting up a blast, the blaster in charge should work closely with the driller and should examine the drilling logs for each borehole. Examination of the drilling logs will assist the blaster in estimating the actual amount of burden to be moved and will alert him/her to any abnormalities encountered down hole (e.g., mud seams or voids). The blaster then will be able to make adjustments to accommodate actual conditions. In areas where the potential damage from flyrock is significant, a blasting mat or other protective measures should be employed.

General Safety Precautions for Blasting Effects

Certain precautions should always be taken to safeguard workers and the public from detrimental blasting effects. Several such precautions are specified in OSM regulations at 30 CFR §816.66. These regulations specify that:

- A blasting schedule must be prepared and disseminated to the public by posting it in a local newspaper 30 days prior to initiating the blasting program.
- Changes in the schedule and/or blasting location must be published at least 10 days prior to blasting.

- The blasting schedule must contain specific information, including (but not limited to) contact information on the operator, identification of the areas covered by the blasting, timing of blasting, methods to be used to control access to the blasting area, and type and patterns of audible warning and all-clear signals.

- Blasting warning signs must be posted near all avenues of public access such as public roads and/or highways and at all entrances to the blasting area accessible by public roads.

- Warning signals must be audible within a range of a half mile from the blast.

- Access within the blasting area must be controlled to prevent the presence of livestock or unauthorized persons during blasting and until an authorized representative of the operator has determined that no unusual hazards exist at the site and that access to and travel within the site can safely be resumed.

Although OSM regulations are generally enforced only at surface coal mines, the rules can serve as useful guidance/reference in planning a blasting project. At the very least, as the scheduled time for blasting approaches, the blaster in charge should use audible warnings to clear the site of all unnecessary personnel and equipment. Workers should be instructed to remain in a safe location until blasting is completed and the blaster in charge indicates that it is safe to reenter the area. The safety precautions used at any site should be communicated to workers as part of a training program well before blasting actually begins. It is essential that all employees working at a site where explosives are used be adequately trained to recognize warning and all-clear signals and to know where to retreat to a safe location. Ideally, this information will be incorporated into a comprehensive training program developed by the mine operator. The generation of flyrock and the encroachment of personnel on the restricted blast area are by far the most common causes of blasting accidents.

Metal and Nonmetal Mining

Explosives are used extensively in metal/nonmetal surface or "open pit" mining operations. The use of explosives in open pit mining is regulated by MSHA in 30 CFR §§56.6000–56.6905. These regulations are quite detailed and govern virtually every aspect of explosives handling and use including (but not limited to) storage and magazine construction; transportation to and within blast site areas; separation of transported explosive materials; vehicle specifications; loading, blasting, and security; initiation systems; fuel oil requirements for ANFO; specific requirements for electric and nonelectric detonating systems; detection and control of extraneous electricity; management of damaged or deteriorated explosive material; and restrictions on the use of black powder.

Most of the above requirements are directed specifically at the blasting crew. Certain of the rules, however, should be made clear to all personnel working at the mine site. In particular, once the loading of explosives begins, the only activities permitted within the blast site are those activities directly relating to the blasting operation. The blasting area is required to be posted and barricaded against unauthorized entry, and only persons trained and experienced in the handling of explosives (or trainees working under the direct supervision of experienced personnel) are permitted on the blasting site.[61]

In addition, before connecting the electric power source or nonelectric initiating device, all personnel are required to leave the blast area except for those in a blasting shelter or other location that affords adequate protection from blasting effects such as air overpressure and flyrock. Work is not permitted to resume in the blast area until a postblast inspection has been conducted by a qualified member(s) of the blasting crew. Blasting is required to take place as soon as possible after loading is completed. Delays exceeding 72 hours must be reported to the district MSHA office.[62]

IME and ISEE also have developed recommendations and/or guidelines for blast design at open pit mines. These guidelines are relatively technical in nature and are most useful to the driller, the blaster-in-charge, and members of the blast crew. Safety considerations include design of the drill patterns to achieve desired fragmentation and avoid flyrock; diameter, depth, and water content of the boreholes; loading procedures (e.g., primers should be made up at the borehole and lowered—never dropped—into the borehole); proper materials for stemming the boreholes (e.g., large stones and combustible materials should not be used to stem boreholes); and other general recommendations (e.g., primer cartridges are never split or tamped).[63]

MSHA also regulates explosives use in metal/nonmetal underground mining. The regulations are set out at 30 CFR Part 57, Subpart E.[64] Most of the requirements are identical to those described above governing surface mines. General requirements applicable specifically to underground operations are set out at 30 CFR §57.6960. These rules prohibit the mixing of bulk explosives below ground unless approved by MSHA. MSHA approval will be granted or denied after consideration of the mine's storage practices, the sensitivity of the product, transportation and use of the product, and any other factor deemed relevant to safety. Storage facilities for any explosive ingredients to be mixed must provide leak and spill drainage leading away from the facilities.

Surface Coal Mining   Surface coal mining is regulated by OSM and MSHA. OSM regulations are set out at 30 CFR §816.61–816.68. Many of the regulatory requirements already have been discussed in the section on blasting effects and will not be repeated here. By way of reference, OSM regulations cover the following matters: (1) preparation and dissemination of a preblast survey; (2) preparation of the blasting schedule; (3) use of blasting signs, warnings, and access control; (4) control of adverse effects (i.e., airblast limits, monitoring); and (5) maintenance of records of blasting operations.

Most of the foregoing requirements typically must be completed and/or planned and documentation submitted to OSM before a blasting permit will be issued. In addition, OSM regulations provide that any person living or owning a structure within a half mile of the permit area may request that a preblast survey be completed. This survey should be conducted by a professional and should note all preexisting damage to structures within the area.

Underground Coal Mining (Permissible Blasting)   MSHA regulates the use of explosives in underground coal mining. The regulations are set out at 30 CFR Part 75, Subpart N. As was previously noted, only MSHA-approved "permissible" explosives and associated equipment may be used in underground coal operations. In addition, the regulations govern borehole drilling, loading, and stemming. All explosives used underground must be placed in boreholes. Two exceptions are permitted: (1) the use of permissible "sheathed" or other approved explosives and (2) shots fired in anthracite mines for battery starting or blasting coal overhangs.[65] The regulations also cover (among other things) transportation and storage of explosives underground, loaded explosive weight limits in bituminous and lignite mines, wiring of blasting circuits, post-blasting examination, and management of deteriorated or damaged explosives.

Although a complete recitation of the Subpart N MSHA safety requirements is beyond the scope of this chapter, several safety rules do warrant particular mention. These safety precautions are somewhat general in nature, and all persons working in an area where explosives are used should be familiar with the various requirements: (1) explosives may be loaded only by a qualified blaster or by a person under the direct supervision of a qualified blaster;[66] (2) workers may not be transported in the same vehicle with explosives except those workers needed to operate the transportation equipment or accompany the explosives; (3) at the time boreholes are loaded, no work other than that necessary to protect workers may be performed in the blasting area; (4) immediately before each shot is fired, measurements of methane levels must be taken (explosives may not be fired if methane levels meet or exceed 1.0 volume percent); (5) before blasting, all persons must leave the blasting area and each adjacent work area, to an area that is around at least one corner from the blasting area; (6) the qualified person is responsible for determining that all personnel have moved a safe distance from the blasting area; (7) a preblast warning must be given and adequate time allowed for personnel to respond and retreat to a safe location, (8) reentry to the blasting area is authorized only after smoke and dust have cleared; and (9) immediately following blasting, the area must be inspected by a qualified person. The inspection will cover potential misfires, partial detonation, methane levels, and any other potentially hazardous conditions.

A number of additional safety measures relevant to personnel actually designing blasts and working directly with explosives are included in the regulations and in the IME Safety Library Publications.

Stemming, Misfires, and Fumes

Stemming   Requirements for stemming loaded boreholes and handling misfire situations are set out in MSHA and OSM regulations applicable to each type of mining activity (e.g., underground coal or surface metal/nonmetal).

Stemming describes the process of placing inert material in a loaded borehole on top of or between separate charges of explosive material. In general, stemming a borehole confines explosive energy in the rock. Thus, proper stemming helps to control flyrock and minimize airblast. Stemming also is used to separate explosive charges within the same borehole to facilitate decking (i.e., to limit the quantity of explosives detonating within a specific time frame and/or to accommodate zones of geological weakness identified in the drilling log).

Various materials may be used by a blaster to stem a borehole depending on the type of explosives being used, the type of mining operation, and the size and condition (i.e., wet or dry) of the borehole. Such materials may include clean, crushed stone; drill cuttings; or packaged stemming material. IME recommends that combustible materials and large rocks not be used for stemming. Large rocks in particular can pose a flyrock problem.[67] It is the responsibility of the blaster to select the appropriate stemming material for each shot. The blaster also must determine the appropriate depth for stemming in each borehole and must ensure that all regulatory requirements are met. In addition, the blaster must take care that initiating devices and associated connections are not damaged during the stemming and tamping process.

Misfires   Although all blasts are carefully designed to avoid misfires, a blaster must be prepared to respond appropriately in the event a misfire does occur.[68] A misfire poses a very serious safety threat and only those individuals who have the requisite training and experience in the management of explosives should attempt to handle a misfire situation. Only those whose expertise is absolutely essential to the handling of a misfire should be permitted to respond. The area around the misfire should be secured, and no other persons allowed access.

The potential for a misfire is present in every blasting situation. Because misfires can be caused by a number of conditions, each occurrence must be evaluated individually and a proper course of action determined on a case-by-case basis. Depending on the situation, many misfires can be refired by removing stemming material and repriming the hole. In cases where refiring is not possible, the blaster in charge may elect to wash the charge out of the borehole or otherwise remove the charge. On rare occasions where neither of the above options is available, a misfire may be handled by recovering the misfired charge or by drilling and blasting holes near the misfired charge. This latter method is intended to generate sympathetic detonation or displacement of the unfired material.[69] IME cautions that both of the latter methods "can be extremely hazardous and should be attempted only by experienced, qualified persons."[70]

IME recommends a waiting period of 30 minutes for misfires involving fuse detonators, and 15 minutes for electric and nonelectric detonator misfires. Where the product manufacturer or government regulation prescribes a longer waiting period, the longer period should be observed.

The occurrence of a misfire also may result in a situation where some explosive material fails to detonate, but does ignite and burn or "deflagrate." This situation is commonly termed a "hangfire," and may escalate to a detonation. In responding to a misfire, an experienced blaster should always check for the possible presence of a hangfire. If a hangfire is detected or even suspected, no one should be allowed near the blast area until the burning is determined to have ceased.

Federal regulations that govern the various types of mining operations all prescribe procedures for dealing with misfires. Personnel working with explosives should be thoroughly familiar with the applicable regulations. At a minimum, all regulations require that misfires be reported to the mine management. In some jurisdictions, misfires also must be reported to regulatory authorities.

Fumes   The generation of reaction product gases is an unavoidable result of detonation. Although most of these gaseous substances are relatively innocuous, others, such as carbon monoxide and oxides of nitrogen, are considered toxic and are classified as "fumes."[71] Fortunately, these fumes or "noxious gases" are generated in very small amounts and rarely pose a hazard in wellventilated or open environments. Nevertheless, personnel working with or around explosive materials should observe certain safety precautions to avoid exposure to any fumes produced by a detonation. Most importantly, mandatory postblast waiting periods should be strictly observed. All workers should be made aware that toxic fumes may be odorless and colorless. Accordingly, the dissipation of smoke and dust from the blast area does not mean that potentially hazardous fumes have similarly been dispersed.

IME has established fume classifications for nonpermissible products, and MSHA has defined classifications for permissible explosives. In areas where the presence of fumes may present a problem, the blaster will consider the fume classifications of available products as part of the blast design process. The generation of fumes is influenced by the product itself and the conditions characterizing the blast site (e.g., ventilation, the amount of explosive used, and the presence of wet conditions). The generation of fumes can be minimized by selecting products with a low fume classification, by carefully evaluating the blast site, and by following proper procedures in setting up the blast (e.g., adequate product confinement and priming).

Safety and Storage; Effective Security Measures

All explosives products must be stored in a manner that ensures safety and security. Most explosives will be stored in a magazine that must comply with certain federal, state, and/or local requirements. IME also publishes a guide for the construction of storage magazines.[72] Depending on the type of mining operation and relevant regulations, bulk blasting agents may be stored in locked bins or tanks.

ATF has promulgated magazine construction, storage, and location regulations. On mine site property, ATF and MSHA share jurisdiction for administering and enforcing these requirements is shared between.[73] Accordingly, MSHA regulations also include requirements applicable to magazines. In 1980, ATF and MSHA entered into a revised Memorandum of Understanding (MOU) addressing their dual jurisdiction. The MOU provides that MSHA "agrees to perform on behalf of ATF inspections of explosives storage facilities and records required at the storage site of all mines subject to MSHA jurisdiction."[74] However, ATF remains responsible for conducting inspections of the storage facilities of applicants for explosives licenses and permits.[75]

MSHA regulations governing explosives storage are substantively similar for operations at surface coal and metal/nonmetal mines. Separate regulations govern underground magazines.[76] The regulations are designed to prevent unauthorized access to stored explosive materials. IME storage guidelines also are intended to enhance security in and around storage magazines. Specifically, both IME guidelines and MSHA rules provide that magazines be kept locked at all times other than when explosives are being moved in and out, or during inspections and inventories. Access to storage magazines should be restricted to an absolute minimum number of workers. Mine operators also should rigorously maintain an inventory of all explosive materials located in on-site magazines, bins, or tanks. In addition, the mine operator should conduct regular inspections of all storage facilities. The amount of explosives removed from a magazine should be limited to that quantity necessary for a planned blast. Any excess material should be returned to the magazine or removed to a safe, attended location and must never be allowed to remain at or near the blast area.

In underground operations, powder chests or "day boxes" often are used to transport explosives from the magazine to the blasting area. These boxes should always be locked or attended by authorized personnel. At the end of each shift, all unused materials in the day box must be returned to the storage magazine.

Transportation of explosives to and from the magazine should be direct (i.e., no delays or detours) and should be performed only by authorized personnel using dedicated transportation equipment. Once removed from a magazine, explosives should *never* be left unattended. Deteriorated or damaged explosives should never be stored with unused explosive materials and should be managed and disposed of in strict accordance with all federal, state, and/or local requirements.

No storage magazine, bin, or tank can ever be guaranteed to be "theft-proof." However, by following the above procedures and all applicable regulatory requirements, mine operators can effectively minimize opportunities for theft and quickly determine whether a theft or loss of explosive materials has occurred and take appropriate measures.

1. As used herein, the terms "blaster," "blaster in charge," and "qualified blaster" have the following meanings unless otherwise indicated: (1) a "blaster" is a person who works with explosives; (2) the "blaster in charge" is the person with the highest authority over blasting operations; (3) a "qualified blaster" is a person who meets certain regulatory requirements. Many federal, state, and/or local authorities require that personnel handling and using explosives be certified and licensed as "qualified blasters." This certification typically is granted after the explosives user has successfully completed a comprehensive training program and has logged a requisite amount of actual "hands-on" experience. ISEE offers a blaster certification program that is accepted by a number of state authorities.

2. ISEE. 1998. *Blasters' Handbook.* 17th ed. Cleveland: ISEE. 5.

3. For a detailed discussion of detonation mechanics, see Persson, Per-Anders, Roger Holmberg, and Jaimin Lee. 1994. *Rock Blasting and Explosives Engineering.* Boca Raton: CRC Press.

4. *Blasters' Handbook.* 31.

5. *Blasters' Handbook.* 31.

6. Explosives manufacturers are subject to regulations promulgated by the EPA and OSHA. Mine operators disposing of waste explosive materials and explosives-contaminated packaging also may be subject to EPA and OSHA regulatory requirements. Increasingly, EPA and state environmental regulatory agencies are seeking to control emissions of oxides of nitrogen and other chemicals that may be associated with blasting activities. Prior to initiating any operation involving use of explosives, the mine operator should confirm that all necessary governmental permits and approvals have been obtained.

7. At the time of this writing, MSHA has proposed new rules on training and retraining of miners employed at sand, gravel, surface stone, surface clay, colloidal phosphate, and surface limestone mines. 64 *Federal Register* 18497. 1999.

8. As noted above, MSHA regulates storage of explosives at the mine site. OSHA governs the storage of explosives at general industry and construction sites. Many states also have promulgated regulations controlling the construction, location, and permitting of explosives magazines. It is important to consult all potentially applicable local, state, and federal requirements prior to locating or building a storage magazine.

9. 18 USC 841. Organized Crime Control Act of 1970, Title XI.

10. IME. 1996. *Safety in the Transportation, Storage, Handling and Use of Explosive Materials.* Vol. 17 of *IME Safety Library Publications.* Washington, DC: IME. 7.

11. *Safety in the Transportation, Storage, Handling and Use of Explosive Materials.* 5–6.

12. As previously noted, the transportation of explosives cargo on mine property is governed by MSHA. As in the case of explosives storage, state and local transportation requirements also must be reviewed prior to transporting explosives on-site and/or off of mine property.

13. See www.nma.org.

14. *Safety in the Transportation, Storage, Handling and Use of Explosive Materials.* 7.

15. 30 CFR §75.1300.

16. 30 CFR §15.1.

17. 30 CFR Part 15.

18. NIOSH assumed the responsibilities of the U.S. Bureau of Mines (USBM), which was abolished by Congress in 1996.

19. *Safety in the Transportation, Storage, Handling and Use of Explosive Materials.* 10.

20. *Blasters' Handbook.* 63.

21. MSHA regulations require this particular storage practice to be implemented at most mines. See, for example, 30 CFR §57.6102(a)(1).

22. 30 CFR §75.1312.

23. IME. 1996. Policy: destruction of commercial explosive materials. In *Blasters' Handbook.* Washington, DC: IME. 64.

24. IME. 1996. *Glossary of Commercial Explosives Industry Terms,* Vol. 12 of *IME Safety Library Publications.* Washington, DC: IME. 30.

25. *Glossary of Commercial Explosives Industry Terms.* 27.

26. For more detailed information regarding the chemical formulation of water gel and slurry explosives, see *Blasters' Handbook.* 69–76.

27. A number of the properties listed below are more fully described in the *Blasters' Handbook,* 71–76.

28. It is important to note that permissible water gel explosives used in underground mining must NEVER be slit or tamped. Additional, specific safety precautions regarding the use of explosives in particular mining applications are discussed later in this chapter. At the time of this writing, no bulk, water-based explosives (including water gels, slurries, and emulsions) have been approved by MSHA as permissible explosives.

29. IME. 1998. *Guidelines for the Pumping of Bulk, Water-Based Explosives.* Washington, DC: IME.

30. *Safety in the Transportation, Storage, Handling and Use of Explosive Materials,* Vol. 17, *IME Safety Library Publications.* 11. But see, note 28, supra, regarding permissible explosives.

31. A cap-sensitive explosive material is one that will detonate with an IME No. 8 Test Detonator when the material is unconfined. *Glossary of Commercial Explosives Industry Terms.* 7.

32. See IME. 1988. Policy: *Shelf Life of Explosive Materials*. Washington, DC: IME. IME notes in this policy paper that current regulations governing the storage and handling of explosive materials were promulgated before the development of modern explosive materials. Accordingly, the regulations often fail to account for the inherent stability of today's explosive products. IME policy advises:

    Due to the diversity of the products manufactured by its member companies, IME does not feel that any one shelf life standard can, or should be applied, to all explosive materials. In keeping with current practices, IME recommends "Always store explosive materials so that corresponding grades, brands, sizes and 'Date-Plant-Shift' codes are together and rotate stocks so the oldest material in the magazine is used first. Consult with the manufacturer to assure that accepted practices for the use and storage of explosive materials are being followed."

    (Unanimously approved at the 1988 Annual Meeting of the IME Board of Governors, December 7, 1988, Washington, D.C.).

    (Emphasis in original.)

33. *Glossary of Commercial Explosives Industry Terms*. 13.

34. *Blasters' Handbook*. 82.

35. For a more in-depth discussion of the physical and chemical characteristics of emulsion explosives, see *Blasters' Handbook*, 77–84; and Bampfield, Howard A. and John Cooper. 1988. Emulsion explosives. Chapter 7 in *Encyclopedia of Emulsion Technology*. New York and Basel: Marcel Dekker. Mixtures consisting of a water-based explosive material matrix or an oxidizer matrix, and ammonium nitrate or ANFO, may also be referred to as "blended explosives," "blends," or heavy ANFO.

36. Because of the unique two-phase physical structure of emulsion explosives, the sensitivity of emulsion products can be heightened simply by reducing the product's density. In simplistic terms, the lower the density of an emulsion explosive, the greater its sensitivity and the more easily it is detonable. For this reason, it is not always necessary to use high explosives or chemicals to sensitize emulsions. A number of emulsion products are sensitized by the addition of metals such as aluminum, or the addition of expanded plastic, AN grills, perlite, chemical gassing agents, and/or microscopic glass "air bubbles" or "microballoons." See *Blasters' Handbook*. 82; *Safety in the Transportation, Storage, Handling and Use of Explosive Materials*. 10.

37. *Rock Blasting and Explosives Engineering*. 76.

38. The internal, water/oxidizer solution phase of emulsion products contains ammonium nitrate.

39. IME publishes a comprehensive guide to pumping water-based explosives. IME. 1998. *Guidelines for the Pumping of Bulk, Water-Based Explosives*. Washington, DC: IME.

40. See *Rock Blasting and Explosives Engineering*, 75. The accident referenced involved the pumping of a water gel explosive.

41. IME. 1997. *Tonnage Report*. Washington, DC: IME.

42. See 49 CFR Part 300; (ANFO cannot be initiated unconfined by a No. 8 test detonator).

43. A prill is a small, porous pellet of ammonium nitrate formed by a series of chemical and physical processes. Prilled ammonium nitrate used in blasting operations is referred to as "explosives grade," "low density," or "industrial grade" ammonium nitrate.

44. "Heavy ANFO" generally refers to combinations where less than 50% of the mixture is a water-based or oxidizer matrix.

45. *Safety in the Transportation, Storage, Handling and Use of Explosive Materials*. 12.

46. *Glossary of Commercial Explosives Industry Terms*. 5.

47. More detailed information regarding available blend trucks, pumps, augers, and other blending equipment is available from the *Guidelines for the Pumping of Bulk, Water-Based Explosives* and the *Blasters' Handbook*, 95–97.

48. *Glossary of Commercial Explosives Industry Terms*. 12.

49. The term "blasting cap" was frequently used to describe such devices in the past, but is now considered somewhat outdated.

50. For example, fuse detonators may be initiated by safety fuse that is "crimped" to the detonator (IME recommends that a minimum of 3 ft (0.9 m) of safety fuse be used with each detonator). *Safety in the Transportation, Storage, Handling and Use of Explosive Materials* 14. Electric detonators are triggered by electric current carried through wires. The power source for nonelectric detonators can be conveyed by detonating cord, detonable gas (infrequently used in North America), and/or shock tube.

51. Electric detonators manufactured in North America are equipped with shunts that protect the detonator leg wires from contacting and transmitting stray or extraneous current to the internal detonator mechanism. In areas that are prone to exposure to extraneous current and/or radio frequencies, a blaster may prefer to use detonating cord or other nonelectric initiation system. It is important to understand, however, that even nonelectric systems are susceptible to premature detonation caused by lightning strikes, heat, and impact stresses.

    Other sources of extraneous electrical current may include; stray current from inadequately insulated and grounded electrical equipment, induced currents from high-voltage transmission lines, static electricity, and galvanic currents. These various sources of extraneous current can be measured using appropriate measuring devices. IME maintains that the maximum "safe" current allowed to flow through an electric detonator without presenting an initiation hazard is 1/5th of the minimum firing current for the detonator. This recommendation provides a safety factor of five. Tables of recommended distances for blasting near radio frequency sources are included in IME SLP 20. IME. 1988. *Safety Guide for the Prevention of Radio Frequency Radiation Hazards in the Use of Commercial Electric Detonators (Blasting Caps)*. Vol. 20 of *IME Safety Library Publications*. Washington, DC: IME.

52. For a more detailed description of the mechanisms used in initiation devices and initiation systems, consult the *Blasters' Handbook* and *Safety in the Transportation, Storage, Handling and Use of Explosive Materials*.

53. *Glossary of Commercial Explosives Industry Terms*. 5.

54. IME advises particular caution when testing electric-type blasting equipment: "CAUTION: Use only those meters specifically designed for testing electric detonators and blasting circuits. Some meters look like blasting test meters but they utilize test currents that may be capable of firing an electric detonator." *Safety in the Transportation, Storage, Handling and Use of Explosive Materials.* 17. Likewise, ISEE cautions that; "[I]t is imperative that only instruments designed for circuits containing electric detonators be used. Many serious injuries and fatalities have occurred when an ordinary volt-ohmmeter or electrician's meters were used in a blasting circuit." *Blasters' Handbook.* 140–141.

55. See, for example, 30 CFR §57.6407 (circuit testing); 30 CFR §57.6404 (separation of blasting circuits from power source); 30 CFR §57.6600 (loading practices; extraneous electricity); and 30 CFR §77.1303 (regulations governing explosives, handling and use).

56. Such practices may be expressly required by federal regulations. See, for example, 30 CFR §56.6405(c), which specifies that only the qualified blaster shall have the key or other control to an electrical firing device.

57. See e.g., OSM regulations governing vibration and airblast at 30 CFR §816.67.

58. *Glossary of Commercial Explosives Industry Terms.* 5.

59. *Blasters' Handbook.* 64243.

60. *Glossary of Commercial Explosives Industry Terms.* 23; *Blasters' Handbook.* 591–592.

61. 30 CFR Subchapter N, Part 56.

62. 30 CFR Subchapter N, Part 56.

63. *Safety in the Transportation, Storage, Handling and Use of Explosive Materials.* 24–29; *Blasters' Handbook.* Chapter 23.

64. Part 57 actually contains regulations applicable to underground and surface metal/nonmetal mining. The surface mining regulations are substantively identical to those set out in 30 CFR Subchapter N, Part 56. Accordingly, most of the regulations applicable to surface operations also govern explosives use in underground metal/nonmetal mines.

65. 30 CFR §75.1315. MSHA defines a "sheathed explosive unit" as "a device consisting of an approved or permissible explosive covered by a sheath encased in a sealed covering and designed to be fired outside the confines of a borehole."

66. 30 CFR §75.1318(a). A "qualified person" or blaster, is defined by MSHA at 30 CFR §75.1301. A qualified person must be certified by a responsible state authority. In states that do not provide certification, to be considered a qualified person, a blaster must have at least one year of experience handling explosives and must demonstrate his/her competency to an MSHA official.

67. *Safety in the Transportation, Storage, Handling and Use of Explosive Materials.* 45.

68. A "misfire" is defined as a blast or specific borehole that fails to detonate as planned, or explosive materials that similarly fail to detonate as planned. *Glossary of Commercial Explosives Industry Terms.* 20. Detonation of only a portion of the explosive material in a borehole should be handled as a misfire.

69. The presence of undetonated explosives can be notoriously difficult to detect. Accordingly, new boreholes should never be drilled near a borehole that has previously been loaded with explosives. An alarming number of preventable accidents have been caused by drilling into a previously loaded hole containing unfired explosive material.

70. *Safety in the Transportation, Storage, Handling and Use of Explosive Materials.* 47.

71. The term "fumes" should be distinguished from the smoke or dust generated by a blast. The word "fume," used in the context of explosives safety, refers specifically to the gaseous, toxic by-products of detonation. The presence of smoke poses its own safety hazards; gases present in smoke may cause headaches or other discomfort. In addition, smoke may obscure other hazardous conditions in the blast area.

72. IME. 1993. *Construction Guide for Storage Magazines*, Vol. 1 of *IME Safety Library Publications*. Washington, DC: IME.

73. ATF is responsible for administering and enforcing the explosives section of the Organized Crime Control Act of 1970. MSHA is responsible for administering and enforcing the Federal Mine Safety and Health Act or 1977, including establishing safety standards for the transportation, storage, and use of explosives in mining operations. MSHA also is required to periodically inspect storage facilities located on mine property.

74. 45 *Federal Register.* 25564. 1980.

75. 45 *Federal Register.* 25564. 1980.

76. See 30 CFR §§56.6100–56.6132 (metal and nonmetal); 30 CFR §77.1301 (surface coal and surface areas of underground coal mines); 30 CFR §§57.6100–57.6160 (underground metal/nonmetal); and 30 CFR §75.1312 (underground coal).

77. MSHA regulations impose similar requirements. See, for example, 30 CFR §75.1313.

CHAPTER 26

Haulage

Ronald R. Backer and C.M.K. Holt

NIOSH Spokane Research Laboratory, Spokane, Washington

INTRODUCTION

In this chapter, we will not attempt to cover all aspects of haulage safety, but we will focus on generic safety and health issues appropriate for all topics related to mine haulage, particularly off-road surface haulage trucks. There are four basic components to haulage safety: the working environment around the machine, the machine itself, the worker, and the work process.

Why focus on surface haulage? Because surface mines yield about 85% of the approximately 3.1 billion metric tons of ore extracted yearly from U.S. mines (Maclean Pub. 1983; Mundell and Schatzel 1992), and surface haulage accidents are a significant component of mining fatalities and injuries. For example, in 1996, more than 50% of the 84 mining fatalities were in surface mining. Out of the approximately 2,800 accidents reported, surface metal/nonmetal mines accounted for 60% and surface coal accounted for 40%. Of the 47 surface mining fatalities, metal/nonmetal mines accounted for 32 and coal accounted for 15.

TYPES OF ACCIDENTS

Powered haulage is not the only issue with surface mines. Materials handling, slips or falls by an individual, machinery, hand tools, and powered haulage accounted for 89% of all nonfatal mining injuries in underground and surface mines, mills, and preparation plants between 1980 and 1988 (Figure 26.1) (Hodous and Layne 1993). With a focus on surface mine haulage, statistical information on accident frequency and severity for five major types of surface mine mobile equipment—haulage trucks, front-end loaders, bulldozers, scrapers, and road graders—was examined for the period between 1989 and 1991 (Figure 26.2). This equipment was responsible for 12% of all accidents and 39% of all fatalities. In 40% of these accidents, the operator was the injured party (Aldinger and Keran 1994).

Haulage equipment can be nonpowered or powered, stationary or moving. Nonpowered haulage refers to smaller pieces of equipment, such as wheelbarrows and pushed mine cars. Accidents and injuries resulting from the use of nonpowered haulage generally involve overexertion and resultant sprains and strains.

Powered haulage includes dozers, motor graders, haulage trucks, front-end loaders, load-haul-dump units (LHDs), train locomotives and rail cars, shuttle cars, forklifts, conveyors, and mine skips. Characteristics of this equipment, such as weight, horsepower, speed, and the ability to travel long distances create tremendous potential and/or kinetic energy. This, in turn, creates environments for serious accidents and injuries.

Haulage trucks were involved in 42% of the accidents and 60% of the fatalities between 1989 and 1991 (Aldinger and Keran 1994), which is not surprising considering that they travel at the greatest speed, have some of the poorest visibility, weigh the most, and travel the longest distances. The

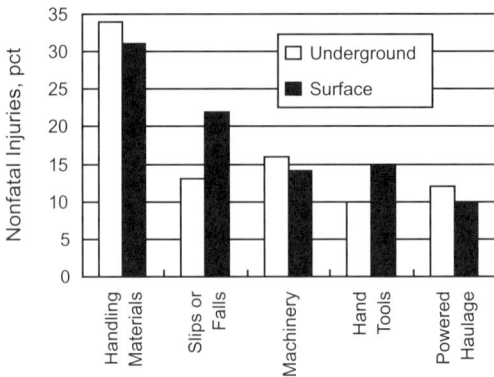

FIGURE 26.1 Leading causes of nonfatal injuries in underground and surface mining, 1985–1991 (after Hodous and Layne 1993)

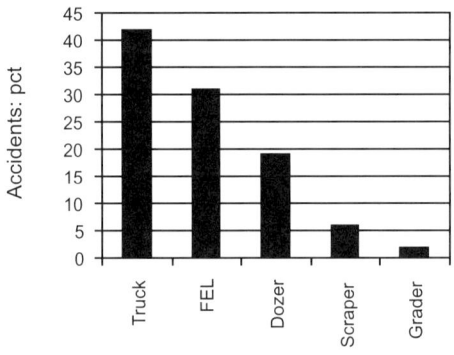

FIGURE 26.2 Surface mine mobile equipment accident frequency by equipment type, 1989–1991 (after Aldinger and Keran 1994)

same factors are involved in accidents with front-end loaders, which have the second highest number and severity of accidents (31% of the accidents and 21% of the fatalities).

In Aldinger and Keran's study (1994), more than 2,800 lost-time injuries involved surface mine mobile equipment. More than 40% of all reported injuries were classified as sprains or strains. About 1,200 of the injuries were received while operating haulage trucks. The leading cause (about 35%) was jarring or jolting of the operator when the vehicle encountered bumps, rocks, or potholes during normal operation, and during dumping or loading. The second major cause of injury (at 16%) and the cause of the most severe injuries was loss of control, which resulted in serious accidents or rollovers. The third most frequent classification (8%) was passive strain caused by repeated shock and vibration. Other unusual events were categorized individually. Of the 28 fatalities involving haulage trucks, 16, or 57% of the total, involved the driver of the mobile equipment. A breakdown of these figures showed that the 16 fatalities resulted from loss of control during dumping, tramming, or parked runaway. "Loss of control" implies driver-only error. However, there are often several factors contributing to these accidents, including system(s) or equipment failure, suboptimal operating visibility or operating surfaces, and slope failure.

An earlier study (Mason 1987) of metal/nonmetal off-highway truck accidents suggested that human error was a significant factor in these accidents, often the result of lack of training, inattention, not following proper operation techniques, or not using required safety equipment such as seat belts. Aldinger and Keran (1994) studied the use or nonuse of seat belts by equipment operators. In 2,720 accidents involving equipment operators, seat belts were discussed for 163 of the incidents, or only about 5%. Of the 163 accidents, seat belts were in use about 55% of the time. In all eight of the fatalities in which it could be determined whether a seat belt was being worn or not, the operator did not have the belt engaged. There were about 31 lost workdays for each lost-time accident for belted operators and an average of 41 lost workdays for operators without belts.

The lack of training Mason mentioned was reinforced by the Aldinger and Keran report, which showed that about one-third of the accidents involved operators with 1 year or less of experience. In a 1993 report of acute injuries in underground bituminous coal mines, Lee and colleagues (1993) noted that total mining experience was inversely related to fatal and nonfatal injuries and, in general, inexperience was related more to high injury rates than age. In another study (Hunting and Weeks 1993) that focused on transport-related injuries in coal mines, the authors concluded that inexperienced miners were at higher risk for injury and that workers in small mines had less experience than workers at large mines.

SAFETY ISSUES FOR MAJOR TYPES OF POWERED HAULAGE

Currently, most large mining companies have standard operating procedures (SOPs) in place within mine, mill, and preparation plant sites to encourage safe work practices. The SOPs cover safety indoctrination, road design and maintenance, traffic control standards, accepted or best practices for conducting various operations, regular maintenance schedules for equipment, conveyor guards and crossovers, task safety analysis and training, communications systems, dispatchers, and safety personnel. Many smaller operations have fewer full-time safety professionals and standardized procedures and thus may be less prepared to deal with conditions that contribute to accidents. The Mine Safety and Health Administration (MSHA) trains miners, inspects mines, and issues citations for violations of safety regulations. MSHA is also involved in development of training materials, such as safety videos, best-practices pamphlets, and on- and off-site miner training. These activities encourage safety, but are not the total answer for safe operations at mines.

Safety and health on the job require support from owners, managers, and workers. Owner-operators and managers must believe in and support the safety program for such a program to work. Without "walking the talk," any program will generate cynicism and failure among workers. The safety message must be followed through with safety actions. Effective and proactive training is one way to follow through. Many sources of specific training materials can be used to focus on safety topics. Mixing training formats such as video, toolbox, interactive discussion groups, and self-paced modules are available. These materials can be found through commercial sources or from state and federal government agencies such as the Occupational Safety and Health Administration (OSHA), MSHA, and the National Institute for Occupational Safety and Health (NIOSH). Industry and worker associations such as the National Mining Association (NMA) and the United Mine Workers of America (UMWA) also provide training and information support.

How mine management deals with near misses is another example of how management-supported follow-through can affect a safety program. For instance, near incidents and near misses, as well as accidents, can be used as topics for discussion and analysis in future training to improve safety programs. Optimally, a case can serve to initiate discussion among drivers and support personnel on how to improve work processes and environments, as well as to alter operator attitudes and behaviors to avoid similar scenarios.

Some mines authorize (and commonly require) any on-site personnel to shut down production if they observe unsafe practices or conditions. These problems are then reported to maintain and promote safety on the worksite. Empowering field personnel to recognize and stop production when they observe unsafe acts or conditions is one means of emphasizing the importance and ownership of safety in the workplace.

At various mining or industrial health and safety conferences, one of the main issues is employee behavior and how behavior contributes to accidents. This usually brings up the benefits of "behavior-based" training. Employee complacency, lack of work ethic, risk-taking behaviors, degrees of alertness and wellness, and drug abuse are often cited as significant factors in accidents. Some in the industry believe that accidents can no longer be reduced by engineering design of equipment or physical surroundings, but by changing human behavior. This topic was covered in chapter 5 of this volume.

Other issues of concern for haulage safety include production and perceptions of efficiency and production. Economic and production pressures (and even the perception of these pressures) can induce miners to act unsafely or take shortcuts. Examples of activities that may compromise safety are extended work shifts, rotating shifts, production optimization practices such as end-dumping over a berm when short-dumping and dozing over a berm would be safer, regrading slumps near a failed berm where slope instabilities might be concealed, extreme weather that creates slippery conditions or visibility problems, poorly designed intersections on haul routes, servicing moving conveyors, and ignoring maintenance needs until shift change.

Miners have a high incident rate of hearing loss resulting from exposures to noisy environments. It is estimated that 90% of all coal miners will have a hearing impairment by age 52 (compared to 9% of the general population), and 70% of all male metal/nonmetal miners will experience a hearing impairment by age 60 (NIOSH 1999).

However, noise is one of the most widespread physical exposures in mining (NIOSH 1996) and is an issue that may contribute to injuries as well as long-term health of operators and workers around haulage equipment. Miners may not be able to hear an alarm or may fail to respond to warnings or sense danger. Mobile equipment, such as haulage trucks, front-end loaders, and forklifts, are equipped with automatic backup alarms. Startup alarms are sounded on stationary haulage equipment, such as conveyors. While being able to hear the alarms above usual mining noises is important to warn nearby workers, studies have shown that constant alarms tend to desensitize workers, who may no longer recognize the alarms (Johnson et al. 1986). Ignoring an alarm can be just as serious as not hearing it at all.

In a study by the U.S. Bureau of Mines (USBM), slips and falls were the most frequently cited causes of injuries and deaths related to accidents around surface coal mine mobile equipment between 1989 and 1991 (Aldinger et al. 1995). More than 70% of the slip or fall accidents occurred as the operator was mounting or dismounting the equipment. Awkward body positioning, bent and swinging ladders, elevated work platforms, and icy or muddy conditions contributed to the hazard. Improved steps from the ground to the truck bumper have been designed that reduce the "swingout" of the step and increase tread cohesion (Long 1983), and alternative safety steps are on the commercial market.

Caution must be taken to prevent oversimplifying an accident cause and attributing it to only one source. Many conditions and factors usually contribute to an incident or accident. However, often only one factor is reported. For example, a truck driver slips as she dismounts a truck, wrenches her back, and stays home recuperating for 2 days. The reportable incident is recorded as a slip and fall. However, of greatest benefit to workers and supervisors is to recognize the events leading up to the slip. For example, (1) the driver got off the truck for the fourth time during the shift to check on unusual noises from the tires (poor equipment maintenance); (2) the first step of the truck was made of angle iron and cable, causing it to swing under (poor equipment design); (3) the side of the road where the driver stopped to get off the truck was littered with loose rocks, which caused her to lose her balance (poor roadway maintenance); and (4) the driver was carrying a thermos and sack of garbage as she climbed down the ladder (poor training and behavior). By examining all the factors contributing to an incident, much could be learned to prevent future injuries.

Safety must be considered an integral part of production. Continuous maintenance of equipment and proper repairs to guards, roadways, and berms must be a priority. Work processes designed to reduce cycle times and increase daily production will be failures if a worker is severely injured or killed. A study conducted in 1981 in which the direct cost of injuries to the company was quantified indicated average costs of $12,400 per accident and $674,000 per fatality (Dicanio 1983). Present-day costs would be much higher. However, no costs can be set high enough to compensate for a lost parent, spouse, or friend. Avoiding accidents and injuries adds value to the workers' quality of life as well as the company's bottom line.

Off-Highway Haulage Trucks

Between 1986 and 1995, approximately 120 fatalities and more 5,500 lost-time injuries resulted from operating haulage trucks (Randolph and Boldt 1997). This activity accounted for the most deaths and lost-time injuries in this 10-year period. In 1995, powered haulage was the factor most frequently cited as a major contributor to the 100 fatalities in surface mines. Loss of control was the primary reason given for these accidents, followed by collisions. Fesak and coauthors (1996) summarized surface haulage accidents between 1990 and 1996 and provided recommendations to reduce such injuries and fatalities.

There are many reasons why accidents involving mobile equipment are so severe. Haul trucks have been getting larger. In the 1980s, a 240-st-capacity truck was considered the flagship. In the 1990s, the 320-st truck has replaced it. The size of the equipment and the multitude of blind spots around haulage trucks are contributing factors to the accidents (Figure 26.3). These trucks can weigh more than a million pounds, with dimensions up to 9 m (30 ft) wide, 15 m (50 ft) long, and 7 m (25 ft) high (Figure 26.4) (Fiscor 1998; Zaburunov 1990). Operational speeds of up to 64 km/h (40 mph)

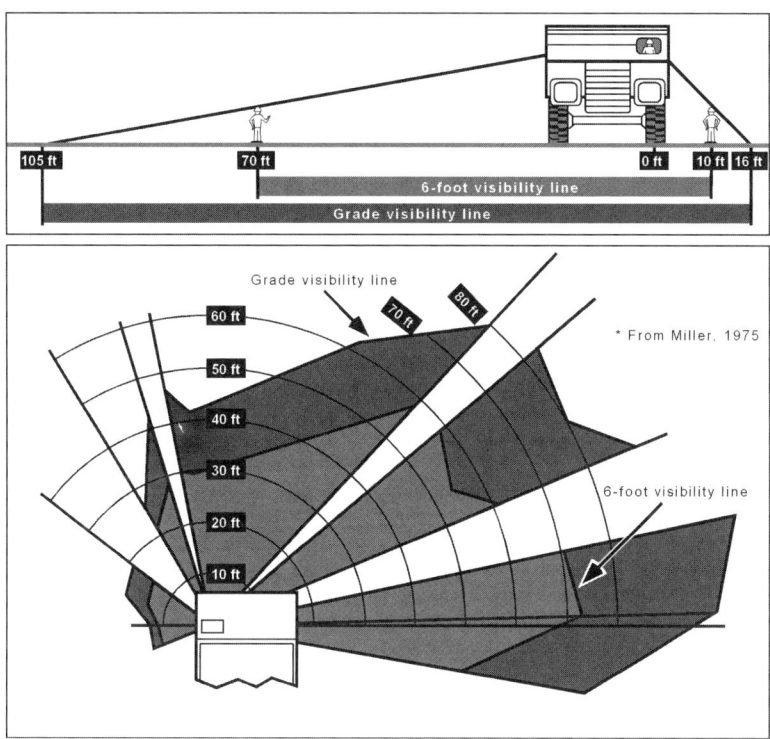

FIGURE 26.3 Side (top) and plan (bottom) views of vision limitations looking to the rear from cab of 150-st dump truck

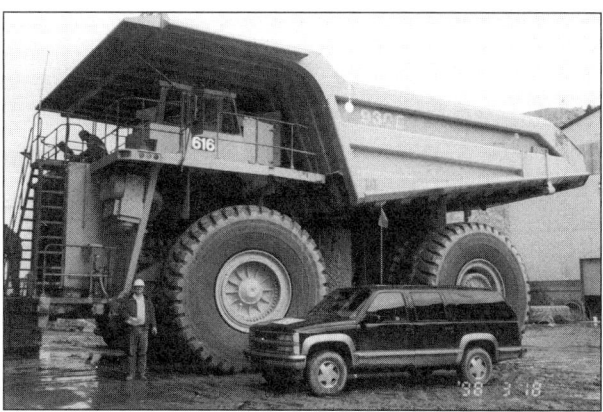

FIGURE 26.4 First truck in the 320-st class to challenge 240-st trucks. As of this writing, manufacturers are offering 340- and 360-st trucks

increase the potential for fatalities and severe accidents, particularly in the rugged terrain and variable road surfaces common in surface mines. In surface mining, haulage trucks do specific repetitive tasks, such as backing, stopping, loading, hauling, and dumping. These activities are often performed 24 hours a day and in all types of weather. The dynamics of the mine environment, a truck's proximity to other pieces of moving equipment, the driver's reaction to hazards such as obstacles, mechanical malfunctions, and severe weather all contribute to the safety of the operation.

In the beginning of the chapter, we presented the four major components that affect safety: the work environment, the machine itself, the worker, and the work process. In relation to off-highway haulage trucks:

- The *work environment* includes mine site characteristics, such as road design and maintenance, weather and climate, and time of day. Road widths, road alignments, lines of sight, intersections, grades, and curves must be designed with consideration to the largest trucks using the system. Berms and guardrails must be installed and built around hazardous areas, such as along roadways and at dumping points. Roadbeds must be able to withstand the weight of the trucks. Road maintenance means constant grading-out of potholes and spilled materials, keeping drainage areas and runaway truck ramps clear and functioning, and reducing roadway dust with water and chemical additives.

- *Equipment* is, in a sense, also part of the work environment. Keeping trucks in optimum operating conditions means that they will perform within expected ranges. Truck systems and tires must be properly maintained. Truck cabs must be kept free of loose items, such as cleaning rags, rolling coffee thermoses, or empty oil cans that create distractions and footing hazards. Truck decks must be kept clean of slippery oils, tools, and spilled muck. Truck accessories, such as radios, mirrors, and safety strobes, must be kept in proper working order.

- The *driver* is the third vital component of truck safety. Truck operators and workers around trucks must be given the tools and skills required to complete tasks safely and efficiently. This requires training focused on understanding the controls, gauges, and miscellaneous systems unique to the truck. It also requires operational and safety training on the vehicle. Unfortunately, the total training effort is often insufficient.

Training also must include knowledge of a truck's mechanical system and that system's safe operating ranges, how to conduct a thorough preoperation inspection, and how to get on and off the equipment. Many of the sprains and strains involving large equipment operators result from slipping and/or falling while getting on or off a machine. Swinging ladders, ice or mud, and holding on to a lunch box while climbing onto the truck can all contribute to slips and falls.

An employee's role in and responsibility for ensuring safety must be continually reinforced and built upon through safety meetings and preshift inspections of equipment. Maintaining good physical condition is much like maintaining a haul truck. It is a lifestyle commitment that cannot be achieved only in the workplace. It is also not limited to eliminating alcohol and drugs in the workplace. The workplace is not an isolated portion of a person's life—what a person does on and off the job has a direct impact on wellness.

Using seat belts is an important truck operator behavior that should be fostered. Drivers should understand the value of seat belts when an accident occurs (especially during rollovers or loss of control of the vehicle). Data indicate that drivers have been killed when they tried to jump clear of a runaway truck. Seat belts also reduce jolting and jarring injuries during normal loading or hauling activities.

- *Work processes*—how the work gets done—are the fourth component vital to truck safety. Components of work processes are management commitment, equipment maintenance, organizational structure, chains of responsibility, shift length, and rotation and traffic patterns.

Traffic pattern studies have suggested rationales for right-hand or left-hand traffic while on mine property. Most mines use left-hand traffic, meaning that the driver's side of a vehicle is on the outside edge of the roadway. The advantages of left-hand traffic are that drivers have a clearer line of sight to hazards at the edge of the roadway, they are able to see another vehicle while passing, and they are better protected during head-on collisions by being positioned on the outside edge of colliding vehicles. The major disadvantage is that left-hand traffic runs counter to highway driving in the United States, making the shift from highway to mine roadway driving somewhat difficult. Regardless of how traffic patterns are designed, traffic management is extremely important to mining safety. Right-of-way at intersections, although it is defined, cannot be always guaranteed. MSHA's *Guidelines for Traffic Control at Surface Mines and Installations* (1997) summarizes applicable regulations, planning and placement, and sign design.

Being able to see without obstruction is another part of traffic control. Lack of visibility because of dust, poor weather, obstructed views, and low or glaring light conditions may compromise a driver's ability to recognize other vehicles in the area. Visibility issues include proper illumination. The USBM assessed illumination needs at 22 surface mines, particularly among different age groups and operators of mobile equipment (Mayton 1987). The agency computed the amount of illumination needed for 25-year-old workers and 50-year-old workers. Fifty-year-old truck drivers needed roughly twice the amount of light as 25-year-old drivers for such tasks as seeing the rear edge of the loading shovel or the sloped waste pile at the base of a bench highwall. The two ages are particularly relevant for mining safety because the average age of a miner is between 45 and 50 years. Extended shifts and rotating shifts may compromise driver alertness and may contribute to errors in judgment and slower response times. Lighting and traffic control signs may need to be reviewed for effectiveness, depending on whether the operation is conducted during the day or at night.

Contractors and other visitors on site may act in unexpected ways and must be made aware of the hazards associated with being on the site. The work process must address how to safely handle the comings and goings of workers who are not part of the normal work group.

Many of these components are organized into training materials that mine companies can use to begin haul truck safety discussions among employees. For example, MSHA has published a series of best-practice cards for truck driver training (MSHA 1998). These cards are easily carried in shirt pockets and feature concise reviews of safety topics, such as truck inspection, driver training checklist, cab inspection, dumping procedures, roll-over protection, protection from falling objects, and steering and braking. Although they are not an exhaustive compendium of information, the cards are meant to stimulate discussion, learning, and implementation of site-specific safe work practices.

Conveyors

Conveyors are a subset of MSHA's category of "Powered Haulage" as a source of accidents, injuries, and illnesses. The MSHA accident and injury database attributes more than 7,000 accidents between 1986 and 1995 to conveyors (1996). Many of these accidents were caused in "pinch points," such as the head or tail pulleys, or return idler. Every year, MSHA's "Fatalgram Bulletin" has included a fatality resulting from a worker being drawn into a running conveyor (Figure 26.5). Working around conveyors requires basic safe work processes, such as powering down the system, lockout and tag-out of the power source, and blocking belts from sudden movement. Walking around or passing over or under moving conveyors can be hazardous because loose clothing, hair, and tools can catch in pinch

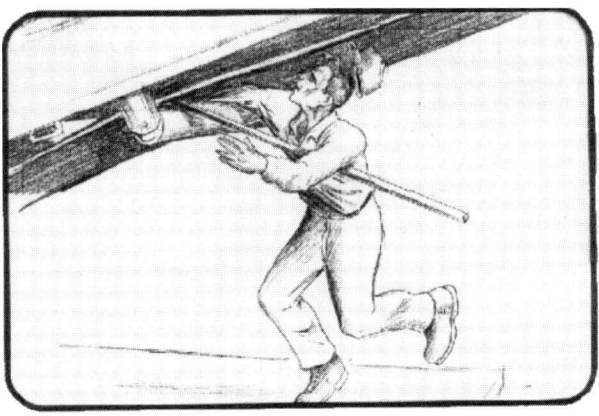

FIGURE 26.5   The dangers of working around powered conveyors. Based on a 1999 MSHA publication, this illustration shows a worker being drawn into a conveyor return idler while attempting to scrape mud off the equipment

points. Slips and falls around or onto a moving conveyor are other major causes of accidents. Stop-start switches, guardrails, toe-boards, and stop cords are all required and should be installed around conveyors to minimize the potential for accidents and injuries. Proper maintenance and regulated work practices define accepted, safe procedures for conducting tasks such as manually cleaning the conveyor, applying belt dressing, and lubricating the belt (*Code of Federal Regulations* [CFR] 30 1998).

Machine guards are another significant safety concern. Generally, guarding regulations are performance oriented; that is, the performance of a guard is mandated, not its design, manufacture, or installation. MSHA requires guards to protect people from any moving machine or conveyor part, including gears, chains, drive, pulleys, fan blades, and so forth. Examples of guard designs and work processes around machines and conveyors are published in an MSHA guidebook entitled *MSHA's Guide to Equipment Guarding for Metal and Nonmetal Mining* (1992).

Specific safety regulations are associated with underground conveyors. MSHA defines regulations for underground coal mines that mandate fire-resistant conveyor belts and specific electrical requirements. Underground coal conveyors are occasionally used to transport both workers and materials in confined spaces. Such working conditions are regulated by CFR 30 Part 75.1403-5. Safe work practices include stopping the belt during loading and unloading workers, limiting belt speed, and examining the belt before a man-trip after materials have been hauled.

Underground Haulage Equipment

LHDs are trackless machines capable of loading, tramming, and dumping material and are used primarily in underground mines. Most surface haulage issues are also safety issues pertaining to LHDs and other underground mobile equipment. However, additional constraints are imposed by limited visibility (darkness and confined spaces) and more restricted operating areas. Other problems include mine opening configurations, blind intersections, air quality, noise, and falls of rock.

The hazards associated with continuous haulage systems underground have been described by el-Bassioni (1996) in an article that documents fatalities, injuries, safety issues, and safe work procedures. Continuous haulage systems, also known as bridge conveyors, are used with continuous miners. Concerns unique to continuous haulage systems include lack of communication between a miner and haulage operators, the lack of space around the systems, and limited visibility. Figure 26.6 illustrates an actual fatality in a coal mine. The operator was killed when his shuttle car bumped into the rib, and he was crushed between the rib and the car.

SOURCES OF INFORMATION ABOUT HAULAGE SAFETY

The Internet is the most recent (and expanding) source of mining-related occupational safety and health information. All federal agencies maintain Web pages and many contain downloadable publications and hyperlinks to government regulations, as well as other links. Agencies that are concerned with mining safety and health include NIOSH, OSHA, and MSHA. The value of contacting these agencies through the Internet is that the information posted is up to date. This is especially useful when investigating regulatory standards. In addition, most Internet sites have, or will have, on-line interaction. For example, MSHA allows electronic filing of 7000-2 forms for Quarterly Mine Employment and Coal Production reporting, as well as downloadable forms, such as the 7000-1, Mine, Injury and Illness Report, and the 5000-23, Certificate of Training. NIOSH maintains safety and health information, such as the *Certified Equipment List*, which includes respirator data, and the *Pocket Guide to Chemical Hazards*.

Most state governments have Web sites that may make navigating the bureaucratic structure easier, and some states provide on-line training materials and up-to-date state labor statistics. As the Internet matures, the information and knowledge gained through its use will expand. Most mining industry associations, such as the NMA, the National Stone Association, and the Canadian-based Mines and Aggregates Safety and Health Association, maintain Web pages. Occupational associations, such as the American Society of Safety Engineers (ASSE) and the National Safety Council (NSC), also have Web sites.

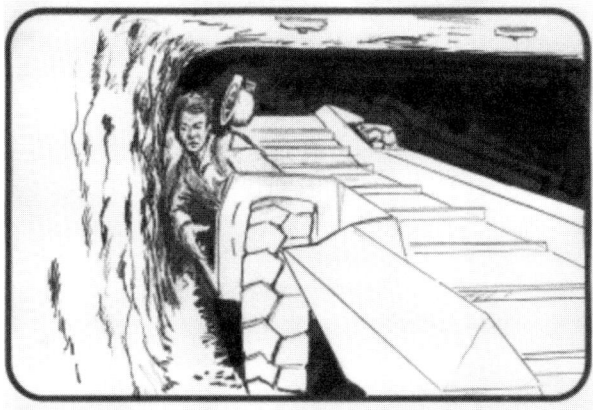

FIGURE 26.6   The hazards of underground haulage conditions are exacerbated by limited visibility and confined spaces, as shown in this illustration of a 1999 accident in which an underground shuttle driver was killed when he was crushed between the car and the coal rib (MSHA Fatalgram 1999)

International Internet support should also be considered when looking for safety and health information. For example, the Institute of Occupational Safety Engineering at the Tampere University of Technology in Finland maintains a Web page index that includes major occupational safety and health links. Although not strictly mining-oriented, many of the occupational topics are relevant to mining issues. The Department of Minerals and Energy in western Australia maintains information about safety and health in the Australian mining industry in a system called EXIS. Incident reports and safety bulletins are downloadable from this site. This site and the one maintained by MSHA are excellent sources of case studies that can be used to illustrate unsafe acts, processes, and equipment, as well as how to correct unsafe situations.

RESEARCH AND EMERGING TECHNOLOGIES TO REDUCE ACCIDENTS

One of the most effective ways to reduce injuries is through training to create habits of safe work practices. Safety training for operators of mobile haulage vehicles can be enhanced by incorporating driving simulators. Driving simulators are currently on the market for drivers of emergency vehicles, and a large driving simulator called the North American Driving Simulator is under construction in Iowa City, Iowa. These systems have specific vehicle operation stations (i.e., cabs) mounted on them and provide dynamic feedback through motion tables, sound systems, and vision systems coupled to computers. This can provide "situational training," such as slippery roads, vehicle systems failures, and hazardous driver behaviors, that cannot safely be introduced outside of the simulator. Exposure to unexpected events can demonstrate the consequences of actions, so the trainee can get a chance to improve response by continued exposure to a variety of situations. Simulators can introduce operators to various vehicle control layouts, the feel and response of a vehicle, job function, and vision deficiencies and aids, etc. Thus, operators can safely operate a variety of types of equipment and get "hours" of experience before actually going on the road in real equipment.

Another technology currently being investigated is virtual reality. Virtual reality is used to allow students to go into areas or situations where hazards exist so they can evaluate how they should act in them. Investigators can also use these systems to visualize and analyze accidents. Research is being conducted to produce and evaluate computer-based programs to reconstruct accidents for focused training as well as to train miners in mine evacuation and hazard recognition (Filigenzi et al. 1999). By using off-the-shelf software programs on which to construct the mining environment and desktop personal computers to run the training modules, costs are minimized and the flexibility to take the modules to the workers is greatly enhanced.

For mobile haulage equipment, specific devices have been and continue to be developed to improve visibility so that drivers can detect obstacles and hazardous situations. Mirrors, video cameras, and backup alarms are continually being upgraded and added to equipment as technology

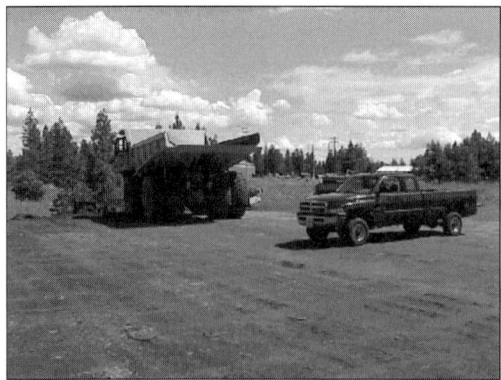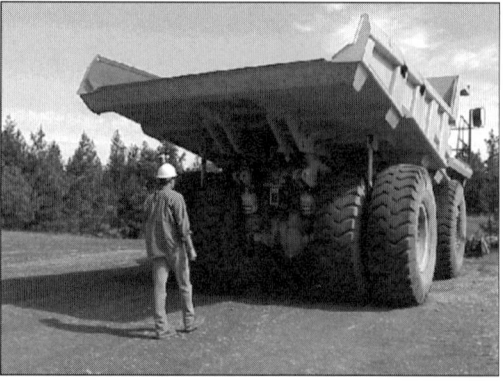

FIGURE 26.7 Determining the effective working range of various blind-area warning systems. A radar system mounted on the rear of a 50-st truck is being tested to evaluate its sensitivity to a pickup truck (left) and a person (right) directly behind it

improves. Hazard detection, proximity warning systems, and tracking systems include, but are not limited to, radio-frequency identification (RFID), radar, and global positioning systems. Some of these technologies have been tested over the years (USBM 1983; Utt 1995; Boldt and Backer 1997). Figure 26.7 shows recent tests being conducted to document the performance of an RFID-based proximity alarm around the blind areas of a 50-st, off-road haulage truck. RFID technology requires that personnel and smaller vehicles are each outfitted with a tag that has a unique identification (ID) code. Each piece of large equipment has a tag detector or reader that "listens" for the unique transmitted frequency and ID of a tag in the equipment's blind spots within a defined radius. If any tag is detected, an alarm alerts the equipment operator (Ruff and Hession-Kunz 1998). Several other detector technologies, such as sonar, laser, and infrared, have been evaluated and discarded because the systems lacked the ability to contend with specific conditions or requirements. This is not to say that these technologies might not be useful in the future as advances are made. For example, in a study done by the USBM, infrared beam detectors did not perform well in mining environments (Johnson et al. 1986). However, in 1999, infrared technology is being used for intelligent traffic sensing between highway vehicles and shows great promise in withstanding environmental and physical demands.

Another technology currently being used on more recently constructed haulage units is one that continually monitors all on-board systems capable of causing equipment failure. This information is transmitted to a central computer center. Any operating parameters falling outside normal operating ranges, such as temperature and load, initiate an alarm to stop the unit so the problem can be investigated.

In addition to monitoring the equipment, sensors can also monitor the driver. Just as instruments have advanced to the point where a driver's breath can be analyzed for alcohol content prior to allowing a vehicle to be started, so can they monitor a driver's eyes, breathing, heart rate, and other vital functions that indicate alertness and set off alarms to make others aware of the driver's ability to continue operating the vehicle.

SUMMARY

Powered haulage is a significant element in mining safety and health. Off-road haulage trucks, conveyors, front-end loaders, forklifts, and underground shuttle cars are examples of powered haulage. Although mining injuries and fatalities have steadily decreased over the years, powered haulage continues to be a major factor in these incidents. Haulage equipment has extensive blind areas, requires operator experience and skills, and is operated in harsh working environments. In addition, their mobility and their potential to do harm are often overlooked.

To continue to improve haulage safety, many organizations and agencies have turned to the Internet for distributing safety and health information in a timely manner. Emerging technologies and advanced training methods are also continuing to improve haulage safety. Only by continuing to focus on the entire package—the environment, the machine, the worker, and the work process—will accident frequency and severity decrease.

REFERENCES

Aldinger, J.A., J. Kenney, and C. Keran. 1995. *Mobile Equipment Accidents in Surface Coal Mines.* USBM IC 9428. 51 pp.

Aldinger, J.A., and C. Keran. 1994. A review of accidents during surface mine mobile equipment operation. In *Proceedings: 25th Annual Institute on Mining Health, Safety and Research.* Blacksburg, VA: Department of Mining and Minerals Engineering, Virginia Polytechnic Institute and State University. 99–108.

Boldt, C.M.K., and R.R. Backer. 1997. Surface mine truck haul safety–where are we? In *Proceedings: 28th Annual Institute on Mining Health, Safety and Research.* Blacksburg, VA: Department of Mining and Minerals Engineering, Virginia Polytechnic Institute and State University. 89–95.

Dicanio, D.G. 1984. *Analysis of Economic Impact of Fatal/Nonfatal Accidents in Surface Coal and Metal/Nonmetal Mines.* USBM Contract No. J0113005. SRI International. 145 pp.

el-Bassioni, S. 1996. Continuous haulage systems. *Holmes Safety Association Bulletin* (May–June): 10–11.

Fesak, G.M., R.M. Breland, and J. Spadaro. 1996. Analysis of surface powered haulage accidents, January 1990 to July 1996. *Holmes Safety Association Bulletin* (September): 10 pp.

Filigenzi, M.T., T.J. Orr, and T.M. Ruff. 1998. Computerized accident reconstruction and training for metal/nonmetal mines. In *Proceedings: 7th Joint Science Symposium on Occupational Safety and Health.* Hidden Valley, PA. October 26–29. *American Journal of Industrial Medicine*, in press.

Fiscor, S. 1998. Ultra-class haul trucks. *Coal Age* 103(10): 37–41.

Hodous, T.K., and L.A. Layne. 1993. Injuries in the mining industry. *Occupational Medicine: State-of-the-Art Review* 8(1): 171–184.

Hunting, K.L., and J.L. Weeks. 1993. Transport injuries in small coal mines: an exploratory analysis. *American Journal of Industrial Medicine* 22(3): 391–406.

Johnson, G.A., R.E. Griffin, and L.W. Laage. 1986. *Improved Backup Alarm Technology for Mobile Mining Equipment.* USBM IC 9079. 19 pp.

Lee, T., C. Anderson, and J. Kraus. 1993. Acute traumatic injuries in underground bituminous coal miners. *American Journal of Industrial Medicine* 23(3): 407–415.

Long, D.A. 1983. Solving the problem of getting on and off large surface mining equipment. Safety in the use and maintenance of large mobile surface mining equipment. In *Proceedings. Bureau of Mines Technology Transfer Seminars* (Tucson, AZ, August 16; Denver, CO, August 18; St. Louis, MO, August 23). USBM IC 8947. 3–16.

Maclean Hunter Publishing. 1983. *Keystone Coal Industry Manual.* Chicago: Maclean Hunter Publishing, Mining and Construction Group. 370 pp.

Mason, W.A. 1987. *Metal/Nonmetal Off-Highway Truck Accidents Related to Seat Belts, 1982–1984.* MSHA PC 7016. 4 pp.

Mayton, A.G. 1987. *Assessment and Determination of Illumination Needs for Operators of Mobile Surface Mining Equipment.* USBM IC 9153. 37 pp.

Miller, W.K. 1975. *Analysis of Haulage Truck Visibility Hazards at Metal and Nonmetal Surface Mines-1975.* MESA Information Report 1038. 19 pp.

MSHA. Revised 1992. *MSHA's Guide to Equipment Guarding for Metal and Nonmetal Mining.* 32 pp.

——. 1996. *Metal-Nonmetal Monitor* 1(8): 1 p.

——. 1997. *Guidelines for Traffic Control at Surface Mines and Installations.* OT-26. 14 pp.

——. 1998. *Best Practices Developed by the Surface Haulage Safety Task Force in Cooperation with MSHA.* MSHA BP Cards No. 1–12.

Mundell, R.L., and S.J. Schatzel. 1992. Mining and quarrying trends in the metals and industrial minerals industries. In *Minerals Yearbook, 1990 Annual Report.* USBM. 39 pp.

NIOSH fact sheet obtained at www.cdc.gov/niosh/hpdocs.html. July 13, 1999.

——. 1996. *Results from the National Occupational Health Survey of Mining.* U.S. Department of Health and Human Services, Public Health Service, Centers for Disease Control and Prevention, National Institute for Occupational Safety and Health, DHHS (NIOSH) Pub. 96-136. 209 pp.

Randolph, R.F., and C.M.K. Boldt. 1997. Safety analysis of surface haulage accidents–part 1. *Holmes Safety Association Bulletin* May–June: 1–7.

——. 1997. Safety analysis of surface haulage accidents–part 2. *Holmes Safety Association Bulletin* July: 6–7.

Ruff, T.M., and D. Hession-Kunz. 1998. Application of radio frequency identification systems to collision avoidance in metal/nonmetal mines. In *Proceedings: 23rd Industry Applications Conference*, St. Louis, MO, October 12–15, 1998. New York: IEEE. 6 pp. Available from IEEE on CD-ROM.

USBM. 1983. Safety in the use and maintenance of large mobile surface mining equipment. *Proceedings: Bureau of Mines Technology Transfer Seminars* (Tucson, AZ, August 16; Denver, CO, August 18; and St. Louis, MO, August 23). Information Circular 8947. 97 pp.

Utt, W.K. 1995. *Radar Positioning System Accuracy Test*. USBM RI 9602. 25 pp.

Zaburunov, S.A. 1990. Trends in surface mining equipment: bigger, better, brighter machines cut costs. *Engineering & Mining Journal* October: 22–27.

CHAPTER 27

Electrical Safety

Joseph Sottile, Jr., Ph.D.
Associate Professor, Mining Engineering
University of Kentucky, Lexington, Kentucky

Thomas Novak, Ph.D., P.E.
Head, Dept. of Mining and Minerals Engineering, Virginia Polytechnic Institute and State University
Blacksburg, Virginia

INTRODUCTION

Although tremendous strides have been made in improving worker safety, mining, by its nature, remains a dangerous occupation. Historically, roof falls and explosions receive the most notoriety because of their catastrophic potential. However, other factors, such as electric shock, result in numerous accidents and some fatalities each year. Mine electrical distribution and utilization circuits have evolved into complex systems that must conform to numerous regulations set by government agencies. In most industries, power systems are located in stationary, permanent facilities and are not subjected to harsh operating conditions. In the mining industry, however, this is not the case. Mining equipment is usually mobile and self-propelled, powered by portable cables. With the extraction of the mineral or rock, the electrically driven machines must advance, followed by their source of power. Each move puts stress on both equipment and cables as they are dragged over rough surfaces. The environmental conditions of the mine, such as dirt, dust, and water, detrimentally affect the insulating properties of equipment and increase the possibility of electrical faults. Because of these circumstances, the safe and reliable operation of a mine power system requires elaborate grounding and protection schemes.

Another critical factor that affects the design and construction of mine electrical systems is the ever-present potential for explosion, particularly in underground coal mines. Coal and other carbonaceous rock formations can store large amounts of methane, which are liberated during the mining process. A methane-air mixture in the proper proportions will explode if an ignition source, such as an electric arc, is present. Thus, in some areas of coal and other gassy mines, electrical equipment must be built with explosion-proof (or flameproof) enclosures. For some very-low-power applications, such as monitoring, control, and some types of lighting, intrinsically safe circuits are used. These circuits limit the amount of energy to a level below that required to ignite an explosive methane-air mixture.

A final factor, the physical size of the mine openings, places constraints on electrical equipment. Low seam heights in underground mines, sometimes less than 1 m, severely limit the physical size of electrical equipment. The design of low-profile equipment, which can fit and be safely maintained within these confined spaces, is very challenging.

Safe designs, proper maintenance, and effective training can improve safety and reduce electrical accidents in the mining industry. This chapter is not designed to comprehensively address all aspects of electrical safety in mines. Instead, we provide a general overview of many of the important aspects. We briefly discuss the federal regulations that apply to mine electrical safety. These regulations define a minimum level of protection and play a significant role in the design of mine electrical systems. To familiarize the reader with basic equipment and component, we describe a simple, but typical, mine power system. Next, we cover common electrical hazards and discuss the physiological response to electric shock to enhance the reader's awareness of the human body's sensitivity to electric current. Because the concept of grounding is fundamental to electrical safety, it receives significant treatment in this chapter. We describe the importance of grounding conductors and the devices used to monitor their integrity. The various types of grounding systems, along with their advantages and disadvantages, are presented. We briefly describe the types, design, and construction of ground beds. The chapter concludes with a brief discussion of electrical safety programs.

FEDERAL REGULATIONS

The application of electrical equipment in the mining industry is heavily regulated by Title 30, Mineral Resources, of the *Code of Federal Regulations* (CFR). This level of regulation is understandable when we consider the conditions under which the equipment must operate. For example, electric mining machinery is generally cable-connected and many of the mining machines are mobile. This equipment must operate safely in extreme conditions, including very cold or very hot ambient temperatures, wet conditions, and explosive atmospheres. These operating conditions, coupled with a workforce that, in many cases, is unfamiliar with electrical engineering fundamentals, makes it essential that the mine electrical system and electrical equipment be designed to safeguard employees during both normal and faulted conditions. Indeed, much of the designs and practices used in the industry today are a direct result of regulations developed to make using electricity in mining as safe as is possible.

Part 18 of Title 30 addresses the approval of electrically operated machines and accessories that are intended to be used in gassy mines, the certification of components intended to be used on or with approved machines, the permission needed to modify the design of an approved machine, the authorization required to use experimental machines in gassy mines, and the acceptance of flame-resistant cables (as well as conveyor belts and hoses). Also included are procedures for applying for approval, certification, and acceptance, and construction and design requirements are covered in detail. Some of the specific items addressed include limitations on the maximum surface temperature of external surfaces, requirements for preventing static electricity, maximum length and minimum diameter requirements for portable cables, voltage limitations for equipment, explosion-proof enclosures, and so forth. Part 18 also addresses tests and inspections of components.

CFR Part 56, Subpart K and Part 57, Subpart K address the use of electricity at surface metal and nonmetal mines and underground metal and nonmetal mines, respectively. These subparts address adequacy of cable conductors, circuit and trailing cable overload protection, performance of work on electric equipment and electric power circuits, grounding system requirements and testing of grounding systems, handheld electric tools, fuse removal and replacement, protection of trailing cables from physical damage, installation of trolley wires and track, isolation of communication circuits from power circuits, and so forth.

Part 75, Mandatory Safety Standards, Underground Coal Mines contains six subparts that address the use of electric power in underground coal mines. Subpart F, Electric Equipment–General, deals primarily with requirements for permissibility, map requirements for the electrical system, conditions under which work on electric circuits can be performed and the personnel permitted to conduct such work, frequency of examination and testing, installation and insulation requirements for power wires and cables, and requirements for disconnecting switches. Subpart G addresses trailing cables and includes requirements for cable protection, allowable circuit breaker settings, and type and number of allowable cable splices. Subpart H addresses grounding and primarily includes approved methods of grounding, approved grounding mediums, and the use of grounding conductors. Subparts I and J address high-voltage distribution and low- and medium-voltage alternating current (AC) circuits, respectively. Subpart K addresses trolley wires and trolley feeder wires.

Part 77, Mandatory Safety Standards, Surface Coal Mines and Surface Work Areas of Underground Coal Mines, contains five subparts that address the use of electric power. Part 77 is organized very similarly to Part 75, except that the regulations govern surface coal mines and the surface area of coal mines and there is no subsection for trolley wires.

OVERVIEW OF MINE POWER SYSTEMS

Numerous power system arrangements exist in the mining industry. However, the radial system shown in Figure 27.1 is typical for an underground coal mine and can be used to represent the important aspects of a mine power system. An underground coal mine power system is used because it is generally more complex than that of most other mines to conform to stringent federal regulations. Figure 27.1 shows a one-line representation for a small portion of an underground room-and-pillar operation. (With a one-line diagram, the three-phase line conductors are illustrated as a single line to simplify the diagram.) Figure 27.1 shows only the underground portion of the power system; surface loads, such as the preparation plant, mine-ventilation fans, and belt conveyors may comprise a combined power requirement larger than that of the underground loads. In addition, some mines utilize direct current (DC) trolley systems, not shown in Figure 27.1, for transporting people and supplies.

Mining companies typically purchase electric power from utility companies; however, in very remote locations, electric power may have to be generated on site. Figure 27.1 shows a utility connection at 115 kV. A three-phase power transformer in the surface substation steps down the utility's transmission voltage of 115 kV to the mine's underground distribution voltage of 13.8 kV. The mine operator or the utility company may own the power transformer—both methods are common. Besides voltage transformation, the surface substation also provides overload and short-circuit protection for the mine distribution circuit by means of a vacuum circuit breaker and its associated protective relaying. (Vacuum circuit breakers are used for high-voltage applications, greater than 1,000 V; molded-case circuit breakers are used for low and medium-voltage applications.) Fuses typically provide protection for the transformer's primary winding. Surge arresters are located on the primary and secondary sides of the transformer to divert transient overvoltages, caused by lightning or switching surges, to ground. Three-phase gang-operated switches provide visible disconnects and are used to isolate portions of the power system for maintenance.

Federal regulations require coal mine power systems to be resistance grounded. (Resistance grounding and other forms of grounding are discussed later in this chapter.) For this reason, the secondary of the power transformer is usually wye-connected to provide a convenient power-system neutral point. The neutral grounding resistor is connected between the transformer's neutral point and the safety ground.

The power system enters the mine by means of a borehole, which is a steel-cased hole drilled from the surface to the mine. The depth of this hole typically varies from 100 m to 700 m for coal mines. At the bottom of the borehole, the power system begins its radial branching to supply various equipment, at numerous locations throughout the mine. Figure 27.1 shows a portable, double-breaker switch house, which allows branching of the radial system. The switch house includes vacuum circuit breakers, disconnect switches, surge arresters, and the associated protective relaying. A metal-clad enclosure, which is usually skid mounted (but can also be tire or rail mounted), houses all the electrical components.

The distribution voltage throughout the mine in Figure 27.1 is 13.8 kV, although 7.2 kV, 12.47 kV, and 13.2 kV are commonly used as well. A portable power center steps down the 13.8-kV distribution voltage to the 995-V utilization voltage. The power center essentially consists of input and output plug/receptacles, a high-voltage disconnect switch, a power transformer with fused primary and surge protection, a neutral-grounding resistor, molded-case circuit breakers for each outgoing circuit, and the associated protective relaying. Similar to the switch house, the power center components are housed in a metal-clad enclosure. For the sake of simplicity, a continuous miner is shown as the only piece of mining equipment in Figure 27.1. However, other electrical equipment associated with a continuous-miner section includes a roof bolting machine, shuttle cars or ram cars, and a feeder/breaker. Other ancillary equipment may include scoop tractors and their battery-charging stations, rock dusters, and pumps. Continuous miners usually operate at 995 V, which is near the maximum extreme of the medium voltage classification (661 V–1,000 V). Federal regulations in the United States only permit low or medium voltage to be used at the working face, without the approval of a petition for modification by the Mine Safety and Health Administration (MSHA). Generally, the remaining electrical equipment on a continuous-miner section typically operates at low voltage (600 V or 480 V).

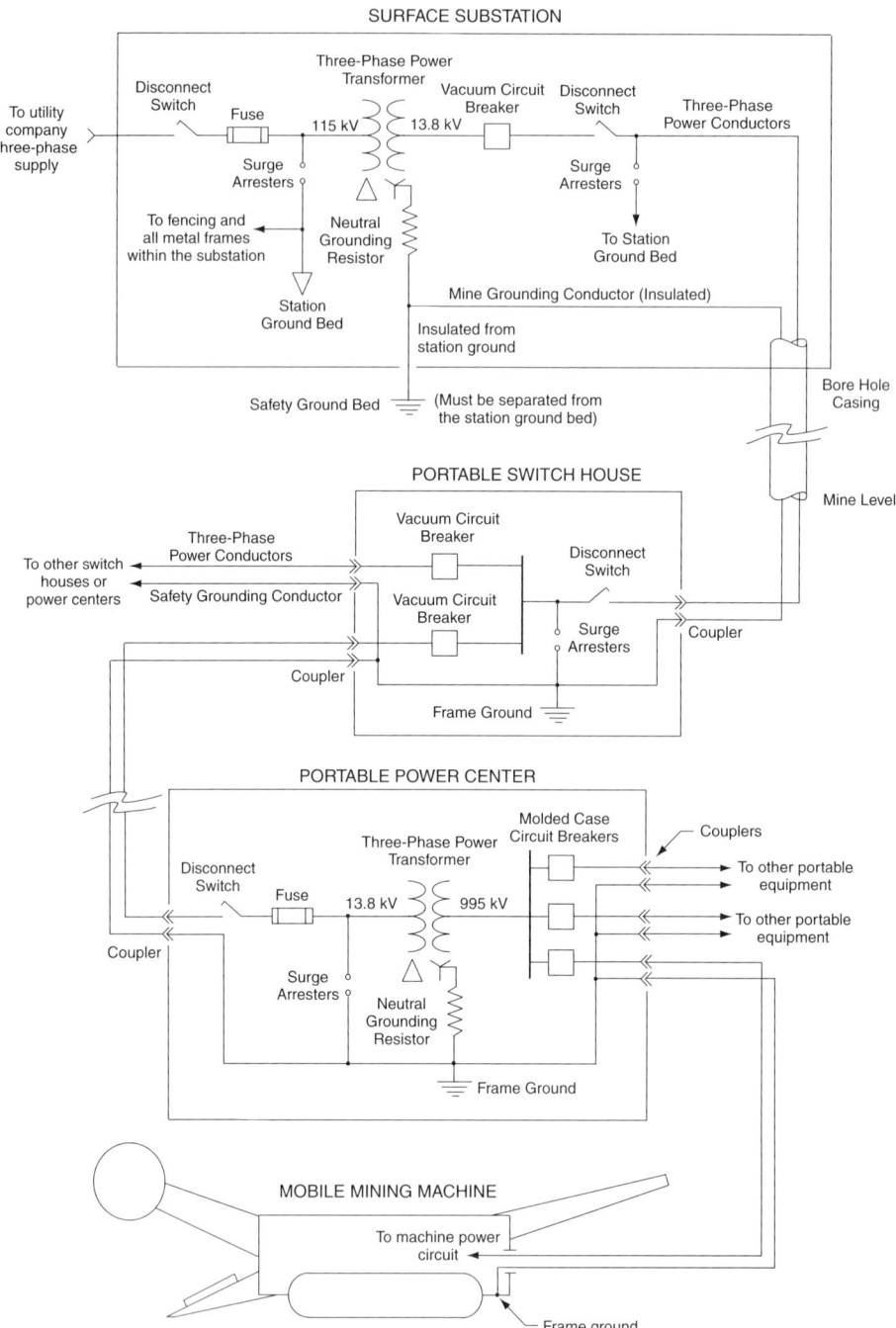

Figure 27.1   Simplified one-line diagram of a mine power system

Proper grounding is essential to the safe and reliable operation of a power system. Well-designed ground beds keep the metal frames of equipment at or near earth potential during normal and abnormal electrical conditions. Figure 27.1 shows two separate ground beds at the surface substation—the station ground bed and the safety ground bed. All metal frames within the substation, along with the metal fence and surge arresters, must be connected to the station ground bed, whereas the frames of all equipment in the mine must be tied to the safety ground bed. Note that the safety grounding conductor in Figure 27.1 extends from the safety ground bed to the metal frames of all equipment in the mine. Federal regulations require the two ground beds to be separated by a minimum of 25 ft. We will discuss the reasons for the two separate beds, and the need to separate them, in subsequent sections.

ELECTRICAL HAZARDS

Most people are familiar with the direct hazards of electricity use, such as being exposed to an electric shock. However, electrical hazards may also be somewhat indirect, for example, when the energy from a fault severely burns an individual or causes a fire. It is imperative for mine personnel to be aware of these hazards and to avoid exposure to them.

Fires, Explosions, and Burns

Under normal operating conditions, electric circuits transmit large quantities of energy to mining equipment in a very safe and efficient manner. However, certain conditions could create excessive heating or arcs that could cause a fire. For example, excessive heating at poorly made cable splices, arcing at fault locations, and excessive heating from severe overloading conditions could generate enough heat to start a fire if they occur near combustible material. In some locations, these heat sources could ignite an air-methane mixture, causing an explosion.

Numerous federal regulations are intended to prevent the conditions that will cause a fire or explosion initiated from an electrical source. These regulations generally address the following broad areas (MSHA 1992; 1999):

- The prevention of overcurrent conditions through overload and short-circuit protection for electric circuits and mining equipment
- Requiring equipment designs to prevent arcing that could cause an explosion during normal operation
- Installation methods and handling procedures for cables to protect conductors from physical damage
- Regular inspection of protective equipment.

With regard to cables, circuit breaker settings are limited to values that will prevent excessive heating of insulation under normal operating conditions. Cable splices are required to be electrically efficient and mechanically strong to prevent excessive heating or failure under normal use. Cables must also have flame-resistant properties. Proper cable handing procedures to prevent damage probably have the most significant impact on **reducing** fire and explosion hazards. Cables must never be run over by mining equipment or subjected to excessive mechanical stress during handling.

Many mining applications require electrical components to be housed inside explosion-proof enclosures. An explosion-proof enclosure is an enclosure that will withstand internal explosions of methane-air mixtures without causing damage or excessive distortion to the enclosure walls or cover. In addition, flames from internal explosions must not propagate to outside the enclosure.

High temperatures resulting from the sources mentioned above can also cause severe burns if mine employees are near the heat sources. For example, the temperature from arcs can be several thousand degrees and will cause severe burns in a very short exposure time.

Shock Hazards—Touch, Step, and Transferred Potentials

Electrical shock hazards to personnel can result from three possible situations: touch, step, and transferred potentials. Touch potentials represent the most obvious situation by which a miner can be exposed to harmful voltages. It occurs when a person comes in direct contact with an object that is at a significantly higher potential than the earth (or floor) that the person is standing on (Institute of Electric and Electronics Engineers [IEEE] Std 80 1986; Cooley and King 1980). To illustrate touch potentials, let us consider the object that the person is touching in Figure 27.2 is a conducting metal tower that has come in contact with a high-voltage line, causing fault current to flow through the tower to the earth. Included in this figure is an equivalent circuit representing the situation. In this circuit, R_V represents the combined body resistance plus any contact resistance of the person's hands and feet, R_1 is the total resistance of the path through the tower and earth between the two points of

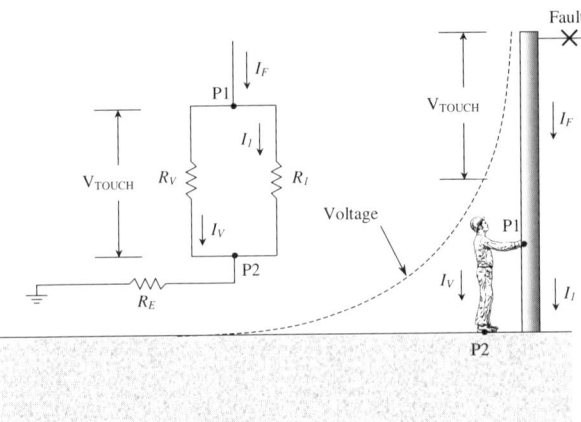

Figure 27.2   Touch potentials near a grounded component

contact, P1 and P2. R_E is the earth resistance between P2 and the point where the effect of the fault is negligible (i.e., infinite earth). With the aid of this circuit model, we observe that the touch potential is equal to I_1R_1.

A good way to visualize the hazards of touch potentials is with a graph of the voltage at points near the fault measured with respect to infinite earth (as shown in Figure 27.2). As illustrated, the most hazardous conditions exist when the voltage gradient is high. It should be noted, however, that this curve is only a representative example; the actual shape depends on many factors, such as, for example, the resistivity of the earth and any buried conductors in the area.

The hazards associated with touch potentials are fairly easy to recognize because a person comes in direct contact with a faulted component. However, the danger associated with step potentials are not as easily recognized. In general, step potential hazards occur when an individual is standing or walking near a faulted component, but is not in direct contact with it (IEEE Std. 80 1986; Cooley and King 1980). The step voltage is produced by the current flow through the earth near the faulted component as shown in Figure 27.3. In the equivalent circuit, R_V again represents body and contact resistance, R_2 represents the earth resistance between the points of contact, and R_E represents the earth resistance from P2 to infinite earth. In this situation, the magnitude of the step potential is the product of the earth resistance and current between the individual's feet. As with touch potentials, a high voltage gradient near the fault creates the most hazardous conditions for step potentials.

Transferred potentials are a special case of touch potentials. Transferred potential hazards occur when someone standing within a faulted area (i.e., the area is at an elevated voltage) comes in contact with a conductor that is grounded at a remote point (IEEE Std. 80 1986). Figure 27.4 illustrates the situation that can cause exposure to transferred potentials and the associated equivalent circuit model. As before, R_V represents the individual's body and contact resistance, R_{E1} represents the earth resistance from the tower to the individual's feet, and R_{E2} represents the earth resistance from the point of contact to infinite earth. (Resistance of the tower and grounded conductor are ignored in this model.) Note that the static wire is only grounded at one point. One characteristic that makes transferred potentials especially dangerous is that the individual is usually exposed to the full voltage rise of the earth at the fault. It should be noted that conditions causing transferred potentials generally occur because of faulty wiring or broken connections.

The hazards created by touch, step, and transferred potentials affect the design and operation of mine power systems, particularly with respect to faults involving ground. In addition, federal regulations mandate specific requirements for the design of substation ground beds, safety ground beds, grounding systems, and monitoring of ground system integrity. Each of these items will be discussed later in this chapter.

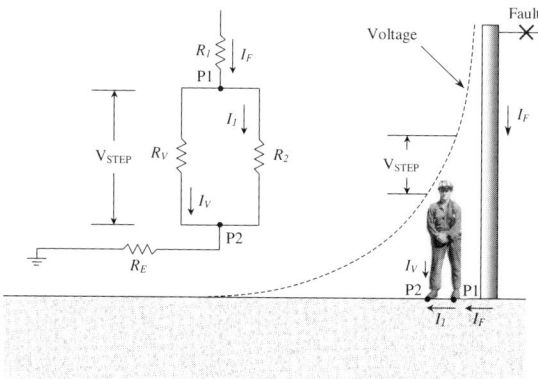

Figure 27.3   Step potentials near a grounded component

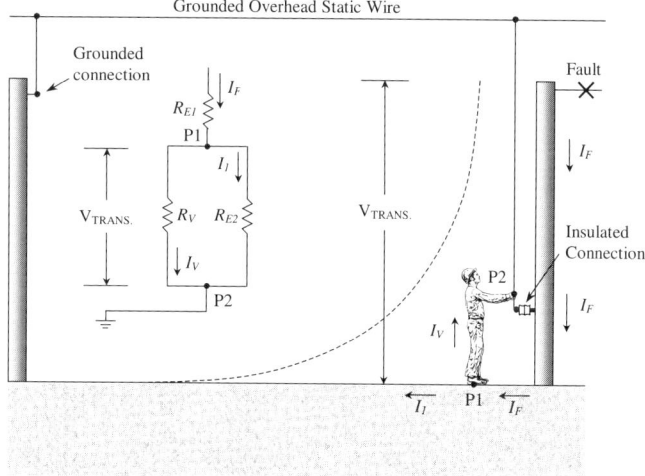

Figure 27.4   Hazards associated with transferred potentials

Physiological Response to Electric Shock

Although a voltage source is usually the cause of electric shock, researchers have quantified shock solely in terms of current. To understand why current is used to define the severity of electric shock, consider a voltage source applied across a person's extremities. With a voltage source, the amount of current through the victim's body depends upon body resistance; and Ohm's Law ($V = IR$) dictates the magnitude of the current. Therefore, body current can vary dramatically for a given voltage, depending on the physical conditions that affect body resistance at the time of the shock. For example, a 120-V source may produce only a mild tingling sensation for a very high body resistance; this same voltage can be fatal when body resistance is very low.

Total body resistance includes the contact resistances between electrical conductors and the skin at points of entrance and exit of current, the resistance of the skin, and the internal resistance of the body (Keesey and Letcher 1970). Skin resistance is the dominant factor because its value is much greater than the combined value of internal body tissues. But skin resistance changes with regard to current density, temperature, sweat-gland secretion, and state of excitement (Jacimovic 1982). Thus, it is impossible to consider body resistance as a constant value. Research indicates that body resistance can vary from 10 kΩ down to 1,000 Ω under various conditions and may even be as low as 200 Ω if skin resistance is lowered by the presence of a small cut. It is obvious that this high degree of variability for body resistance warrants the use of current for defining electric shock. To predict the physical response to a given voltage, an assumption for the value of body resistance must be made. The selection of a value for body resistance should be conservative, yet practical. A value of 1,000 Ω is commonly used for safety analyses, and even the lower value of 500 Ω is used by Underwriters Laboratory (UL) for defining the operating characteristics of single-phase 120-V ground-fault circuit interrupters (GFCIs).

Three physical responses have primarily been used in quantitatively defining electric shock—perception of electric currents, let-go currents (thresholds of currents that result in uncontrollable muscular contractions), and currents that result in death. Large currents (greater than a few amperes), ironically, are less likely to cause immediate death than small currents (less than 1 A), provided the shock duration is not prolonged. The major risk with larger currents is internal heating and burning, whereas the smaller currents disrupt the electrical impulses of the nervous system and can result in ventricular fibrillation. Most of the work on electric shock was performed from 1940 to 1970, and the results of this work continue to be used for safety standards and the design of electrical equipment.

PERCEPTION OF ELECTRIC CURRENT

The threshold of an individual's perception of electrical current varies with the location of the shock and the types of contacts used. Dalziel (1941, 1950, 1954, 1956) determined that the average perception, using wire contacts located on the tip of the tongue, was 0.045 mA of pure DC and the same for 60-Hz AC. More realistic tests with the contacts located on the hand were also conducted. With pure DC, the average threshold was found to be 5.2 mA, as compared with 1.1 mA of AC. Interestingly, the first sensations of DC were those of warmth, in contrast to the tingling sensation of AC. Other tests by Dalziel (1950 and 1954) suggest that the average threshold of perception for women is approximately 66% of that for men. These values, although not dangerous, demonstrate that the human body is extremely sensitive to electric current.

Let-Go Current

Let-go current is defined as the maximum current at which a person is still capable of releasing a conductor by using muscles directly stimulated by that current. Dalziel (1969) performed let-go current tests in which the subjects held and then released a test electrode consisting of No. 6 copper wire. The circuit was completed by placing the other hand or foot on a brass plate, or by clamping a conductive band lined with saline-soaked gauze on the upper arm. The average values of 60-Hz let-go current were determined to be 15.87 mA for men and 10.5 mA for women. Dalziel felt that the average values of let-go currents were interesting but should not be used to define the minimum threshold. Instead, he plotted the let-go values on a probability graph and obtained a straight line for both males and females. To introduce a margin of safety, he decided to use the 0.5 percentile value as the minimum threshold for the general population. As a result, 9 mA for men and 6 mA for women are generally accepted as the safe 60-Hz let-go currents. Let-go current tests were also conducted at sinusoidal frequencies varying from 5 Hz to 10,000 Hz (Dalziel 1956). It is interesting to note that the lowest let-go values lie in the range of 10 Hz to 100 Hz, which encompasses the commercial frequencies of 50 and 60 Hz used throughout the world. An attempt was also made to establish thresholds of DC let-go currents (Dalziel 1956). However, as the DC was gradually increased, internal heating was perceived rather than severe muscular contractions. Sudden changes, such as closing or interrupting the circuit, produced severe muscular contractions and shock. But in all cases, the subjects were capable of releasing the conductor. Each subject held the conductor until his or her limit of pain was reached and then released the conductor. Because the phenomenon of not being able to release the conductor did not exist, Dalziel termed this maximum tolerable DC current as "release current" to distinguish it from the AC let-go current. He established the average DC release current to be 76.1 mA for men and 50.7 mA for women.

The minimum thresholds of AC let-go currents determined by Dalziel have been the primary input for the UL's development of performance standards for GFCIs. The National Electric Code (NEC) requires GFCIs to be installed on all 120-V outdoor and bathroom receptacles of new residences.

Specification UL943 defines the current interruption range of these GFCIs to be 5 mA to 264 mA, with the interruption time based on the following equation:

$$t = \left[\frac{20}{I}\right]^{1.43}$$

(EQ 27.1)

where

t = interruption time (s), and
I = ground-fault current (mA).

Equation 27.1 is graphically illustrated in Figure 27.5. The minimum pickup value is shown as 5 mA, which corresponds to Dalziel's let-go threshold of 6 mA for women. The maximum current in the interruption range is 264 mA. This value is based on the assumption that the minimum body resistance is 500 Ω (Gross 1979). Thus, 264 mA of body current corresponds to a body resistance in contact with a 132-V source (Ohm's Law), which is 10% over the nominal 120-V rating used in the United States.

Lethal Currents

Electric shock can result in death by three different means–respiratory arrest, asphyxiation, and ventricular fibrillation–briefly discussed below.

Respiratory Arrest   It is frequently thought that electric shock stops respiration, which is evidenced by the traditional first aid treatment of artificial respiration. However, experimental work and accident records indicate that such an effect is only produced by electrical current passing through the head, and especially through the respiratory center (Langworthy and Kouwehhoven 1930; Maclachlan 1930). Other tests on small animals have shown that, when current is passed from one forelimb to another forelimb, a shock of up to 1 A does not cause sustained respiratory arrest (Lee and Zoledziowski 1964). Only shocks passing between the head and one of the limbs are likely to cause prolonged arrest of respiration (Lee 1966).

Asphyxiation   As mentioned earlier, if the let-go current is exceeded, the flexor muscles of the forearm contract, which results in the tightening of the grip. This same contraction effect can occur with the chest muscles, which stops respiration and leads to asphyxiation. It is believed that this effect can occur when the chest current reaches approximately 50 mA (Lee 1966). For this situation, consciousness would be lost after a minute or so, followed by death a few minutes later. Since a few minutes of direct contact is required, death by asphyxiation can primarily be attributed to those situations in which the victim is incapable of releasing the source of the shock.

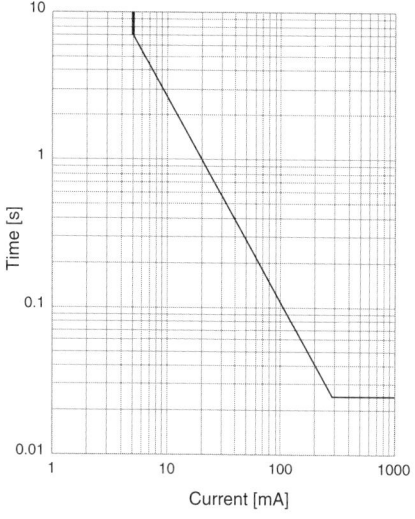

Figure 27.5   Underwriters Laboratory's specification for GFCIs

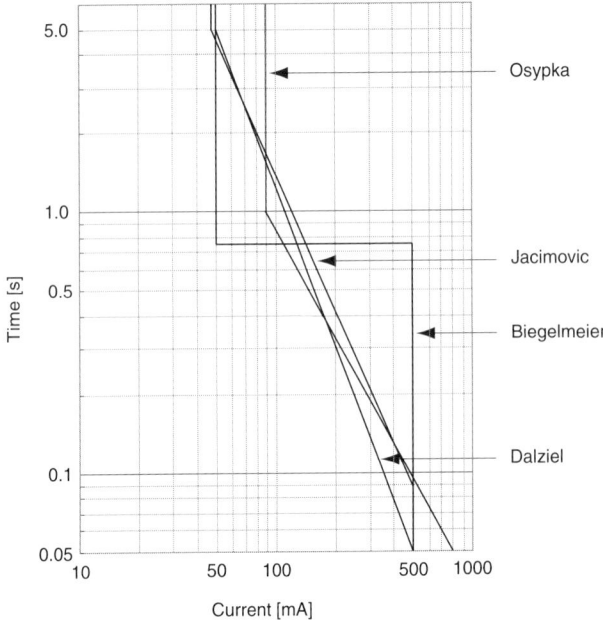

Figure 27.6   Alternating-current ventricular-fibrillation predictions

Ventricular Fibrillation   Because only a small amount of current is required to disrupt the natural rhythm of the heart, ventricular fibrillation is considered the most dangerous electric shock hazard. The shock current needs to pass through the heart during the phase when the ventricles are starting to relax after a contraction (Lee 1966). When fibrillation occurs, the effective pumping action of the heart ceases, the pulse disappears, and death usually occurs within minutes. The lower boundary of the threshold of ventricular fibrillation is generally considered to be 50 mA.

Ventricular Fibrillation Predictions.   The threshold of ventricular fibrillation is not adequately known nor easily determined since experimentation on humans is not realistic; however, approximations have been developed. Researchers have approached this problem by performing shock experiments on animals. The statistical data obtained from these experiments have been fitted to equations for predicting minimum threshold values of fibrillation. Because all of the ventricular-fibrillation predictions are based on tests performed on animals, the threshold equations are open for criticism. However, in an attempt to approach the problem in a realistic sense and because of the lack of opposing scientific data, the fibrillation equations have been widely accepted. Some of the popular predictions will be discussed.

Dalziel's Prediction   Dalziel felt that the three major factors of concern for ventricular fibrillation are body weight, current magnitude, and shock duration. He used the results of animal studies, conducted by Ferris (1936) and Kouwenhoven (1959), to establish an equation for the minimum threshold of fibrillation. Dalziel developed the following equation for predicting the minimum threshold value of fibrillation for a body weight of 50 kg (110 lb):

$$I = \left[\frac{116}{\sqrt{t}}\right](8.3 \text{ ms} \leq t \leq 5.0 \text{ s}) \tag{EQ 27.2}$$

where
I = minimum current (mA, 60 Hz) at which fibrillation occurs for a pathway through major extremities, and
t = duration (s) of the shock.

The equation states that fibrillation current is inversely proportional to the square root of exposure time and is represented graphically in Figure 27.6. According to Dalziel, the area to the left of the line is considered the *safe* area with respect to ventricular fibrillation. As with let-go currents, the equation is based on the 0.5 percentile. In other words, fibrillation should only occur in one out of every 200 people if the fibrillation predictions of the equation are attained.

Jacimovic's Prediction   Dalziel's work is the most widely accepted research in the area of electric shock; however, other researchers also defined minimum fibrillation thresholds for 60-Hz currents. Jacimovic (1982) performed a series of measurements on animals and established the following fibrillation prediction:

$$I = \frac{35}{t^{0.56}}(0.1 \text{ s} \le t \le 5.0 \text{ s}) \tag{EQ 27.3}$$

where

I and *t* are again in milliamperes and seconds, respectively. He concluded that this equation represents maximum nonfibrillation current in the time range of 0.1 to 5 s for 99.5% of the population, independent of weight and sex. Unlike Dalziel, Jacimovic felt that the number of experiments was too small to make a definitive conclusion about the correlation between maximum nonfibrillation current and body weight. However, for the sake of comparison, he applied his equation to a body weight of 50 kg (110 lb) and a time interval from 0.08 s to 5 s and obtained the following equation:

$$I = \frac{122}{t^{0.56}}(0.08 \text{ s} \le t \le 5.0 \text{ s}) \tag{EQ 27.4}$$

with current and time in the same units as before. It is interesting to note that this equation very closely matches Dalziel's prediction (Equation 27.2), as shown in Figure 27.6.

Osypka's Prediction   Using some previously published data and some newly developed results, Osypka suggested that the minimum fibrillation level occurs at approximately 90 mA, as reported by Bridges (1981). Beyond 90 mA, the fibrillation current is proportional to $1/t$. By comparing Osypka's prediction with that of Dalziel in Figure 27.6, it is apparent that Osypka's prediction is generally less conservative.

Biegelmeier's Prediction   A fourth fibrillation-threshold prediction is suggested by Biegelmeier and has been reported by Bridges (1981). Actually, Biegelmeier's interpretation is based on two distinct thresholds, rather than an inverse-time characteristic. The first threshold of 50 mA occurs if the duration of the shock is greater than one heart period (typically 750 ms), as shown in Figure 27.6. The second threshold of 500 mA occurs if the duration is less than one heart period. It is obvious that this prediction is, by far, the most conservative of the predictions for shock duration greater than 750 ms; however, it is the most liberal prediction for a shock duration in the range of 100 to 750 ms.

Ventricular fibrillation can also be caused by DC, but related research has not been nearly as comprehensive when compared with AC. Dalziel (1956) predicted that the fibrillation threshold of DC is approximately five times that for AC.

GROUNDING

Mine workers use electric-powered equipment and tools constantly as an integral part of their jobs. They are well aware of the potential hazards associated with electricity, but rarely give a passing thought about safety in using these electric devices. If asked, "Why is it safe to use a particular electric device?" a typical response may be, "because it is insulated from the electrically energized parts, or the frame is grounded." The concept of insulation is straightforward and easy to comprehend; however, some principles of grounding are less obvious.

Why do we ground electrical systems? According to the NEC, systems and circuit conductors are grounded to:

- Limit voltages resulting from lightning, line surges, or unintentional contact with higher voltage lines
- Stabilize the voltage during normal operation
- Provide a low impedance path for fault current that will facilitate the operation of overcurrent devices under ground-fault conditions.

Although not listed by the NEC, another important purpose of grounding is to reduce electrical noise that can interfere with electronic equipment. Poor grounding practices could affect communication and automation equipment.

Another purpose of grounding, not explicitly stated above, is to maintain all metal equipment frames at, or near, ground potential to minimize shock hazards. If done properly, equipment will also be protected.

Ground Bed

The ground bed, sometimes referred to as a grounding electrode system, establishes the earth as the ground reference. According to IEEE Standard 142 (1991), the resistance of the grounding electrode system consists of:

- Resistance of the metal electrode(s)
- Contact resistance between the electrode(s) and the soil
- Resistance of the soil from the surface of the electrode(s) outward to infinite earth.

The first two resistances can be made very small compared with the third resistance. Resistivity of soil, the most important factor in the ground bed resistance, varies with the depth from the surface, the types and concentrations of soluble chemicals, the moisture content, and the soil temperature.

The connection of the electrode system to earth must have a low resistance if the grounding system is to function effectively. Ground beds of less than 1.5 Ω may be obtained by using a number of individual electrodes connected together, or by using a buried mesh of interconnected bare conductors. A resistance of 5 Ω or less is usually required for mine safety ground beds. Because ground beds are critical to the safety of the electrical system, ground bed functions and design issues will be addressed in additional detail in subsequent sections.

Importance of Grounding Conductors

An example best illustrates the importance of a grounding conductor. Figure 27.7(a) shows a simple power system. A three-phase transformer, with a delta-connected primary and a wye-connected secondary, steps the distribution voltage of 12.47 kV down to the utilization voltage of 480 V. The transformer secondary supplies a tire-mounted vehicle through a molded-case circuit breaker and cable. A tire-mounted vehicle is used in this example because it presents the worst-case shock hazard—the equipment frame is insulated from earth because of the tires. The system shown in Figure 27.7(a) is solidly grounded, which means that the neutral point of the transformer is directly connected to the grounding conductor and the grounding electrodes (ground bed). The grounding conductor connects the equipment frame directly to the grounding electrodes and the neutral point of the transformer.

Figure 27.7(a) shows the proper operation of the grounding system if a ground fault occurs between a line conductor and the frame of the machine. In this case, the grounding conductor provides a low impedance path for the fault current to return to the transformer neutral. The system impedance, which consists of the impedances of the transformers, line conductors, and grounding conductor, solely limits the fault current. Therefore, a very high ground-fault current will flow and initiate instantaneous tripping of the molded-case circuit breaker, thus isolating the fault. The frame of the equipment is only energized for the time it takes the circuit breaker to interrupt the fault current, which is typically one to two cycles (16.7 ms to 33.3 ms) for molded-case breakers. For this short duration, the voltage between the machine frame and ground would be equal to the fault current times the impedance of the grounding conductor. It should be noted that if the ground-fault current could be limited to a lower value, the frame potential would also be lowered proportionally. A means for limiting ground-fault current is discussed in the following section.

Consider now the situation in Figure 27.7(b) with an open grounding conductor. Even with a direct ground-fault between a line conductor and the machine frame, no fault current occurs because there is no return path to the neutral of the transformer. As a result, the circuit breaker will not trip and the system will continue to operate as if no fault existed. Even if the vehicle frame were in direct contact with earth, rather than insulated by the tires, the magnitude of fault current would probably still be insufficient to cause circuit-breaker tripping. In either case, the equipment frame would be elevated to a hazardous potential.

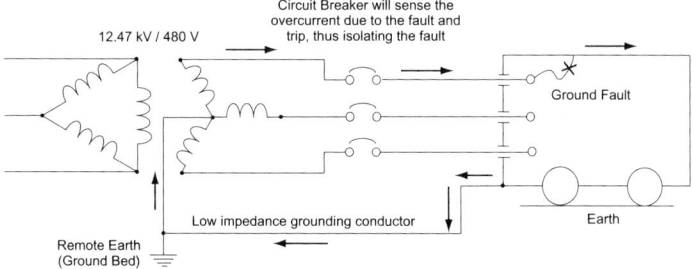

(a) Solidly grounded system with a low impedance grounding conductor.

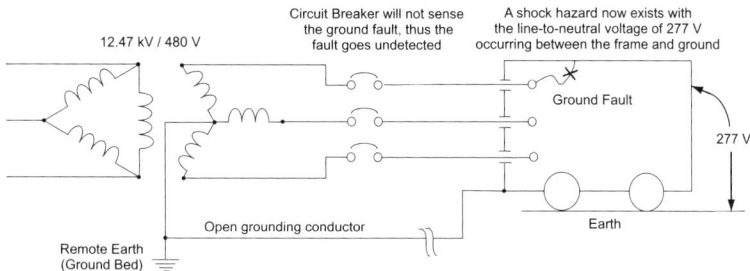

(b) Solidly grounded system with an open grounding conductor.

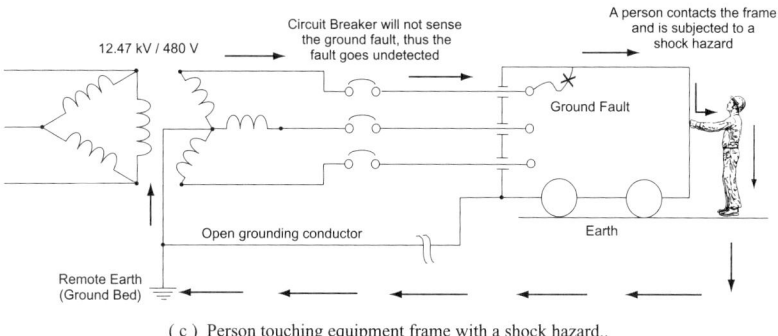

(c) Person touching equipment frame with a shock hazard..

Figure 27.7   Illustration of the importance of a low impedance grounding conductor

Figure 27.7(c) shows a person contacting the energized frame of the equipment. The person's body now completes the circuit, and shock current will flow from the frame, through the body, to the transformer neutral through the earth. The magnitude of the shock current depends upon the contact resistances between the person and the frame and ground, the body resistance of the person, and the resistance of the ground bed. This shock current is far too low to cause circuit-breaker tripping, but may be high enough to result in electrocution.

Because the grounding conductor is critical to the safe operation of power systems, MSHA requires ground-check circuits to continuously monitor the integrity of grounding conductors in coal mine power systems. A monitor must cause its associated circuit breaker to trip if the grounding conductor is broken. Ground-check monitors are divided into two general classifications—impedance types and continuity types.

Impedance monitors require the trailing cable to have a pilot conductor. The pilot is a separate, small conductor, incorporated in the cable construction. The pilot conductor is used to form a continuous loop with the grounding conductor. The monitor is calibrated to the impedance of the loop formed by the pilot and grounding conductors. The device then monitors the change of impedance from the initial calibration. If the impedance of the loop increases beyond a preset value, the monitor trips its associated circuit breaker.

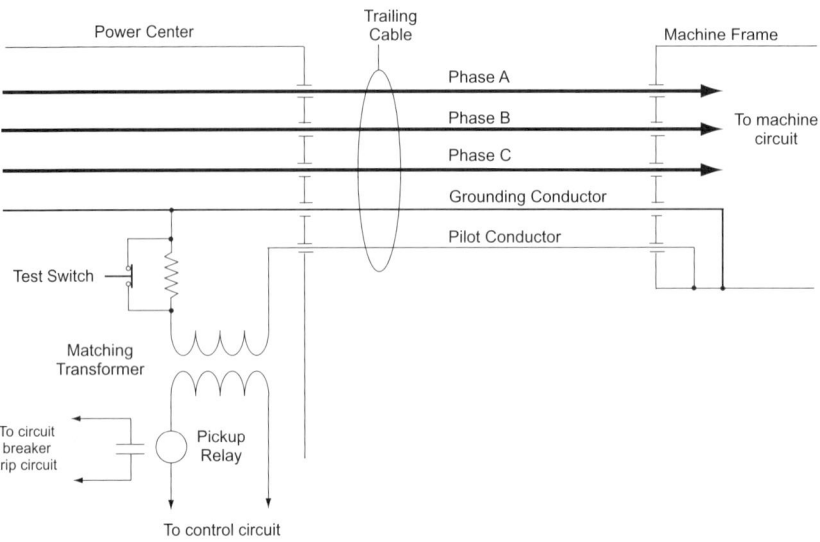

Figure 27.8   Impedance type ground-check monitor

A simplified schematic for an impedance type monitor is shown in Figure 27.8. The circuit in Figure 27.8 uses an impedance-matching transformer to amplify the change of impedance in the pilot and grounding conductor loop. (The primary impedance of the matching transformer equals the secondary impedance times the turns ratio squared.) The monitor also provides a test button, which inserts a resistor into the loop to simulate an increase in impedance. The circuit breaker should trip when the resistor is inserted. A disadvantage of this type of monitor is its susceptibility to parallel return paths through the earth or other grounding conductors.

Continuity monitors do not monitor impedance change, but only the grounding-conductor continuity. They do not require a pilot conductor and are immune to the problems associated with parallel return paths. Figure 27.9(a) shows a block diagram for this type of unit. The monitor generates an audio frequency, which is coupled to the line conductors through the high-pass filter. (The filter allows the audio frequency of the monitor to pass through it, but blocks the low 60-Hz line frequency). The line conductors essentially substitute for a pilot wire. A high-pass filter is also required at the machine to uncouple the audio signal from the line conductors. If the grounding conductor is intact, the receiver coil picks up the audio signal. If the grounding conductor is open, no signal is present in the grounding conductor, and the monitor trips the circuit breaker.

Figure 27.9(b) illustrates another type of ground wire monitor that uses an audio signal to check the continuity of the grounding conductor. Similar to the system just discussed, filters are used to pass the audio signal to the line conductors (alternatively, a pilot wire can be used instead of the line conductors); but the grounding conductor is connected to the grounding system through a ground wire inductor. The purpose of this ground wire inductor can be understood by considering that the grounding conductor shown in Figure 27.9(b) is broken and there is also a parallel path through the earth contact as shown. Without the ground wire inductor, the audio signal could return to the monitor through the parallel path, giving a false indication of an intact grounding conductor. However, because the ground wire inductor exhibits a high impedance to the audio signal, it prevents the audio signal from returning to the monitor through the parallel path, allowing the broken grounding conductor to be detected. (The ground wire inductor exhibits a low impedance to 60 Hz; therefore, the function of the grounding system is not affected.)

Types of Grounding Systems

The major types of grounding in the mining industry include the ungrounded, the solidly grounded, and the resistance-grounded systems. The three systems are shown in Figure 27.10(a), (b), and (c), respectively, and we will discuss their advantages and disadvantages briefly.

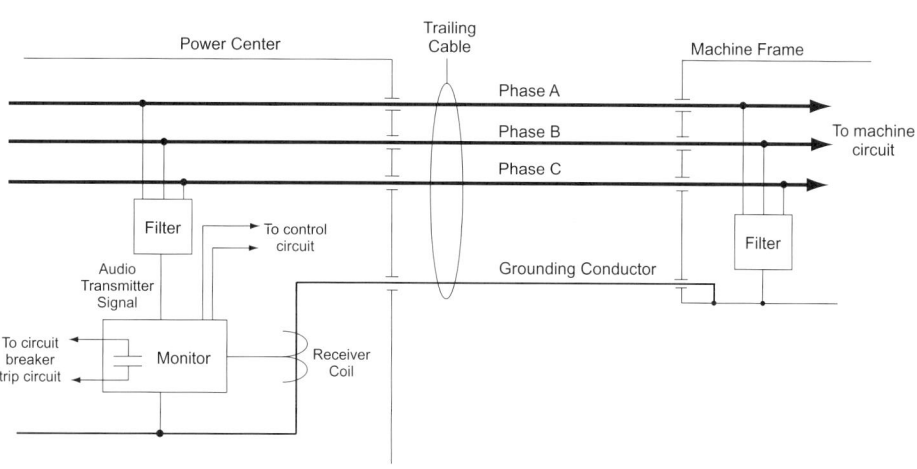

Figure 27.9(a)   Continuity type ground-check monitor

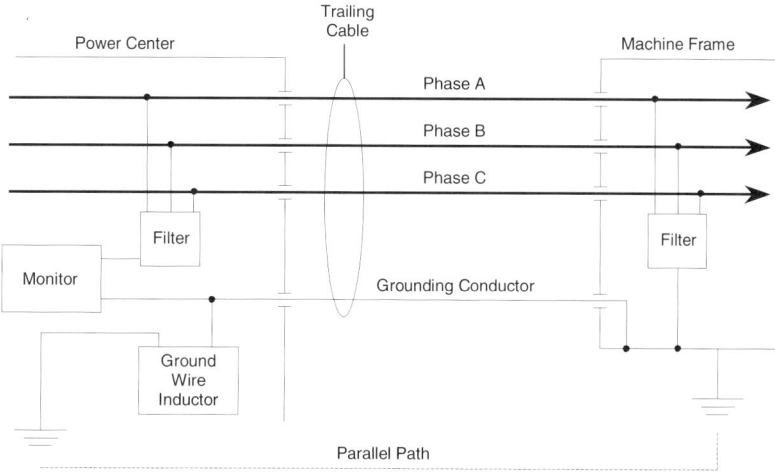

Figure 27.9(b)   Ground wire monitor utilizing a ground wire inductor

Ungrounded System   With an ungrounded system, no intentional connection, except for ground-fault monitoring equipment, exists between any part of the electrical system and ground, as shown in Figure 27.10(a). However, it should be noted that a grounding conductor is still used to tie equipment frames to earth potential. The term ungrounded is somewhat of a misnomer because each line of the system is actually coupled to ground through the inherent per-phase capacitance of transformer windings, motor windings, and cables. Although this capacitance is distributed throughout the entire system, Figure 27.10(a) shows it as lumped capacitors, connected between each line conductor and ground. The magnitude of the system capacitance depends on the size of the power system, particularly the length of cable runs and the type of cable used. For example, shielded type power cables have much more capacitance than unshielded cables. Thus, system capacitance varies considerably from one system to another. Even within a given system, the inherent capacitance changes as branch circuits are connected or disconnected.

The term ungrounded often creates a false sense of security, since a visible return path does not exist for a line-to-ground fault. In fact, some repairmen, who are unaware of this distributed capacitance phenomenon, feel completely safe while working on uninsulated energized components. Figure 27.10(a) shows a line-to-ground fault through a fault impedance. The fault impedance is simply a circuit component used for modeling various types of fault conditions. For example, a direct short-circuit would

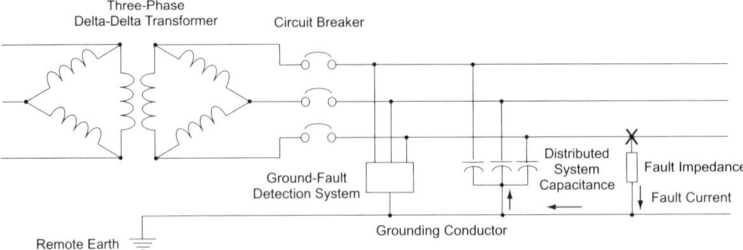

(a) Ungrounded system with a line-to-ground fault.

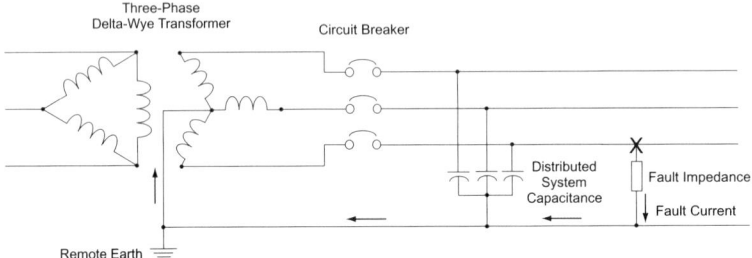

(b) Solidly grounded system with a line-to-ground fault.

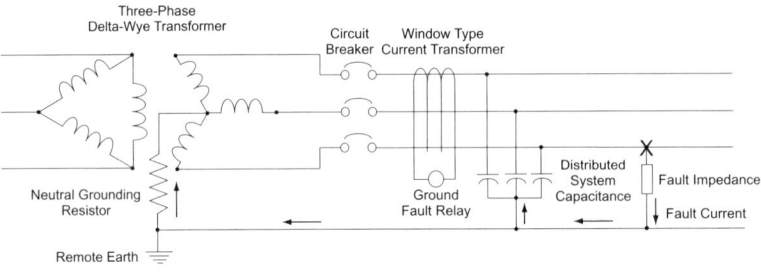

(c) Resistance grounded system with a line-to-ground fault.

Figure 27.10   Various types of grounding systems

be represented by a very low, or even zero, fault impedance. In contrast, deteriorating insulation would be modeled by a very high impedance. The fault impedance could even represent the body resistance of person directly contacting an energized line conductor. Regardless, Figure 27.10(a) shows that ground-fault current, even though it may be very small, will return to its source, the three-phase power transformer, by means of the inherent system capacitance.

The ungrounded system, which is frequently referred to as an isolated system, gained popularity during the early days of the electrification of industrial plants. The initial popularity of the system can be attributed to the fact that the first fault between any line conductor and ground usually causes no interruption of power to any part of the system, so there is no loss of production for a continuous-type process. However, this reason for its popularity can also be considered a disadvantage since no automatic tripping for the first ground-fault occurs, provided a second line-to-ground fault does not occur before the first is cleared. With a single line-to-ground fault, the faulted circuit, therefore, continues to operate with full line-to-line voltage developed between each of the unfaulted lines and ground. If an unsuspecting repairman, particularly one who feels safe with the ungrounded system, contacts one of the ungrounded lines, he will be subjected to the line-to-line voltage of the system.

The ungrounded system is also subjected to insulation failures and increased shock hazards from transient and steady-state overvoltage conditions. Under abnormal conditions, the line-to-ground voltage may rise to many times its rated value. Overvoltages can result from abnormal conditions including physical contact with a higher voltage system, inductive-capacitive resonance effects, intermittent (arcing) ground faults, and switching surges.

Because system capacitance can be very small, distributed throughout the entire system, and highly variable, ground-fault current cannot provide a good indication of a ground-fault condition. Instead, a ground-fault detection scheme that monitors phase imbalance is typically used, which is represented by the box in Figure 27.10(a). The use of an ungrounded system with a ground-fault indicator requires an excellent maintenance program to provide service reliability and continuity equivalent to that found in solidly grounded and resistance-grounded systems.

Solidly Grounded System   The neutral point of the solidly grounded system is connected to ground with no intentional impedance, as shown in Figure 27.10(b). A line-to-ground fault results in a high current, which can easily be detected by a circuit breaker and isolated quickly. Although system capacitance still exists, it does not affect ground-fault current, since the low-impedance path to the transformer's neutral essentially short-circuits the capacitance. With no intentional impedance in the neutral connection, ground-fault current is very high, which can result in significant equipment damage. Even more important, personnel working in the immediate vicinity of the fault are subjected to flash and/or burn hazards. Because of this large ground-fault current, circuit-breaker tripping must be initiated instantaneously, which precludes an orderly shutdown of equipment. Also, equipment frames can be significantly elevated above ground potential during the time it takes the circuit breaker to interrupt the fault current. Conversely, if a high-impedance ground-fault occurs, it is likely to remain undetected unless sensitive ground-fault relaying is used in addition to the normal overcurrent protection provided by a circuit breaker.

A major advantage of the system is that overvoltages are controlled because the system is solidly referenced to ground. Also, the system is designed to provide automatic ground-fault tripping by the same devices used for line-to-line fault tripping. For low-level arcing ground-fault protection, sensitive ground-fault relays can be used.

Resistance Grounded System   Inserting a resistor between the system neutral and the grounding conductor establishes resistance grounding, as shown in Figure 27.10(c). Actually, this method is subdivided into two categories—low-resistance and high-resistance grounding. Although the limits are not well defined, low-resistance grounded systems generally limit the maximum ground-fault current to a range from 100 to 1,000 A. Overvoltages are still controlled because of the ground connection, while ample fault current is available for actuating protective relays. The flash hazard is not as serious as in the solidly grounded system, but a current flow in the specified range can still cause considerable damage.

With high-resistance grounding, which is required in the coal mining industry, ground-fault current is generally limited to 25 A or less. The lower fault current practically eliminates arcing and flashover danger, and the ground connection also serves to limit the amplitude of overvoltages. However, the ground-fault current should not be limited to a value less than the current caused by the system capacitance during a ground fault. If the current limit is set too low, the system could begin to acquire some of the undesirable characteristics of the ungrounded system (Novak 1998; 1999). Some reasons for limiting ground-fault current are to:

- Reduce electric-shock hazards to personnel caused by high frame potentials during a ground fault
- Reduce the arc blast or flash hazard to personnel who may have accidentally caused, or who happen to be in close proximity to, the ground fault
- Reduce burning and melting in faulted electric equipment, such as switchgear, transformers, cables, and rotating machines
- Reduce mechanical stresses in circuits and apparatus carrying fault currents
- Control overvoltages
- Reduce the momentary line-voltage dip occasioned by the occurrence and clearing of a ground fault.

Resistance grounded systems require separate ground-fault relaying because the ground-fault current is limited to a value significantly below the pickup setting of the instantaneous short-circuit protection. Detection of ground-fault current is commonly accomplished with zero-sequence relaying, as shown in Figure 27.10(c). Although other methods of ground-fault protection exist, zero-sequence relaying, also termed balanced flux relaying, is the most reliable first defense against ground faults in the resistance-grounded system. The system basically consists of a single window-type current transformer and ground-trip relay. All three line conductors pass through the core of the current transformer, and the resulting current in the current transformer is the vector sum of the three line currents. Under normal conditions, the three line currents are equal in magnitude and 120° out of phase with each other. Therefore, the vector sum of the currents is zero. However, during a ground fault, a current imbalance occurs and produces a resultant current in the current transformer that activates the ground-trip relay, which in turn trips the circuit breaker.

GROUND BEDS AND GROUND BED DESIGN

Adequate grounding has historically been difficult to achieve in the mining industry. Problems arise because the mine is constantly expanding; therefore, the equipment must be moved frequently. In addition, much of the mining machinery is portable, making it difficult to establish a suitable ground near each machine. This situation is further complicated because mine personnel are required to regularly come in contact with portable machinery, which increases the shock hazards. Because of these shock hazards and the difficulties in trying to establish local ground beds, the U.S. Bureau of Mines (USBM) recommended, in 1916, that the frames of mining equipment be connected to a permanent ground bed located near the main substation.

Resistivity

Probably the most important factor in establishing an adequate ground bed is the soil resistivity. We will briefly review resistivity before discussing ground bed design.

Resistivity, ρ, is a property of a material, rather than a characteristic of a particular specimen of that material. For example, we are much more familiar with resistance, which is a characteristic of a particular specimen of a material. Resistivity is defined as

$$\rho = \frac{E}{j} \tag{EQ 27.5}$$

where

j = current density
E = electric field.

For a conductor of length, l, and a uniform cross-sectional area, A, with a voltage, V, applied across it, the electric field and current density will be constant for all values in the conductor and will be

$$j = \frac{i}{A} \tag{EQ 27.6}$$

$$E = \frac{V}{l} \tag{EQ 27.7}$$

where
i = current.

By substituting (27.6) and (27.7) into (27.5), we obtain the following relationships:

$$\rho = \frac{VA}{i\,l} = R\frac{A}{l} \quad \text{and} \quad R = \rho\frac{l}{A} \tag{EQ 27.8}$$

From these relationships, we see that the resistance of a particular specimen is directly proportional to the resistivity of the material.

Resistivity of a material can be determined by applying a known voltage across a unit cube of the material and measuring the resulting current. The voltage is applied at opposite ends of the cube by conducting plates having the same cross-sectional area as the sides of the cube to maintain a constant current density throughout the material. It is important to recognize, however, that this definition of resistivity and the procedure for determining resistivity assumes a homogeneous material. Unfortunately, soil is rarely homogeneous and it is, therefore, impractical to determine soil resistivity with this procedure. A more practical approach to determining soil resistivity for designing ground beds will be discussed later in this chapter.

Station Ground Bed

Today, the recommended grounding practice for the mining industry (and a requirement in coal mines) is to employ two separate ground beds–the station (or system) ground bed and the safety ground bed. As we will see in this section, each bed has distinctly different functions and design requirements. Our discussion will begin with station ground beds.

The substation ground bed is generally constructed as a horizontal network of wires connected in a grid pattern and buried at a shallow depth directly underneath the mine substation. In some cases, rods are connected at the intersecting points of the grid and driven into the ground to reduce bed resistance. The frame of the substation transformer and all substation switchgear are connected to the station bed. Also connected to the station bed are the substation structure, fence, and static lines of associated overhead lines. Components that cannot be grounded (e.g., the power bus) are enclosed or located such that workers cannot contact them inadvertently.

The primary purpose of the station bed is to protect personnel working within and nearby the substation during normal operating conditions and also during lightning strokes, short-circuits, equipment failures, and situations of human error or carelessness. This protection is achieved by maintaining a low voltage gradient in and around the substation, even during fault conditions. A secondary function of the station ground bed is to limit the electrical stress on insulation by conducting lightning surges to the earth through surge arresters.

One of the most important characteristics of the station bed is the arrangement of the ground mat itself. If the station bed is to achieve its primary purpose, the ground mat be designed to maintain a low voltage gradient in and near the substation during faults so that any individual coming in contact with a faulted component, or working near a faulted component, will not be exposed to hazardous touch and step potentials. Transferred potentials are avoided by proper design and wiring of substation equipment and electrical isolation from the safety bed.

Design Requirements   Adequate performance of the station ground bed can usually be achieved by observing the following guidelines (IEEE Std. 80 1986; Cooley and King 1980).

- The substation must be completely enclosed by a continuous ground wire. To protect individuals outside the substation who may come in contact with the substation fence, this perimeter wire should extend at least 1 m beyond the fence. This perimeter wire should also extend to include the area under gates when they are open as well as when they are closed.

- A rectangular grid of wires should be laid out with a grid spacing of between 1.5 and 5 m. More precise determination of the grid spacing can be found in IEEE Std. 142 (1991).

- A denser grid pattern should be used at corners of the substation where voltage gradients are higher, and in work areas within the substation to provide extra protection where people are most likely to be exposed to shock hazards.

- The grid must be bonded together at all intersecting points. All equipment that is bonded to the station bed should be bonded at two different points, preferably at different intersection points of the grid.

- If a borehole casing is located within the substation, it should be bonded to the substation.

- Buried conductors such as water and gas pipes within the substation should be bonded to the grid. (If possible, the substation site should be selected to avoid water and gas pipes.)

- If the soil has a very high resistivity, or if the area is prone to conditions such as severe freezing or drying that can cause large increases in resistivity, ground rods should be driven at the intersection points of the grid and connected to the grid.

- All buried conductors must be corrosion resistant. Copper must never be mixed with steel or aluminum. Conductors should be at least 2/0, but 4/0 conductors are preferred.

The entire ground mat should be buried about 45 cm to 60 cm below grade. The perimeter cable that extends about 1 m beyond the fence should be buried deeper, to prevent hazardous step potentials close to the perimeter wire. A denser grid pattern should be used near any operating handles to provide additional protection against touch potentials. A gravel surface, approximately 10 to 15 cm thick, should be used in the substation and outside the substation for at least 1.5 m beyond the fence to increase the contact resistance between a person and the earth. The entire substation area should be well drained to avoid any accumulation of water. Figure 27.11 shows a plan view of a typical ground mat for a mine substation.

Substation Surge Arresters   Surge arresters are very important components of a mine substation, serving to automatically divert any abnormal transient overvoltages to ground. The source of these transients generally includes lightning strokes and switching surges.

Although many configurations for surge arrester design are possible, common construction consists of a spark gap in series with a nonlinear resistance. This construction gives the surge arrester the desired characteristics for diverting surges: a high impedance to low voltages, and a low impedance to high voltages. The nonlinear resistor is typically composed of silicon carbide blended with a ceramic binder and fired in a kiln. The nonlinear resistor is typically called the valve block (Ohio Brass).

Surge arresters are connected between line and ground, and the arrester should be located as close as possible to the terminals of the equipment being protected. For example, surge arresters used to protect the main transformer in the substation may not protect the transformer if they are placed more than a meter away. If the transformer has primary fuses (which is most frequently done), the surge arresters can be placed on either side of the fuses; however, the most common practice is to place the surge arresters at the transformer terminals because this location provides the highest degree of protection for the transformer. Surge arrester leads should be as short and straight as possible. The leads must never be coiled or have any sharp bends.

Safety Ground Bed

As previously mentioned, the mining industry typically uses two separate ground beds. The second ground bed to be discussed, called the safety ground bed, is the one to which the frames of mining equipment are connected. Because of this connection, the potential at the frame of each piece of mining equipment is essentially equal to the potential of the safety ground bed (with respect to infinite earth). Consequently, the most important requirement for a safety ground bed is low resistance to earth, since the potential of the bed, and, more importantly, all connected equipment, will be elevated by fault current flow through the resistance of the ground bed.

Resistivity and Ground Rod Resistance   The resistance of the ground bed is primarily a function of the soil resistivity; however, soil is not a particularly good conductor compared with copper or aluminum. The earth becomes a good conductor by virtue of its immense size. To understand this mechanism better, consider the ground electrode shown in Figure 27.12. The total resistance of the soil is the sum of the resistances of a series of virtual shells progressing outward from the rod. The shells closest to the rod have the highest resistances because of their relatively small size, while the shells further from the rod have much lower resistance. At some distance from the rod, the resistance of the virtual shells effectively becomes zero (IEEE Std. 142 1991).

To illustrate the magnitude of this effect, consider a typical ground electrode 3 m long with a 15-mm diameter, in which a distance of 7.5 m represents 100% of the total electrode resistance. For this situation, 25% of the total resistance is accounted for within 30 mm of the rod, and 68% of the total resistance is accounted for within one-third of a meter! In other words, most of the total resistance of a ground rod occurs very close to the rod. Therefore, if any soil treatments are used to reduce resistance, they will be most effective close to the rod. It is important to recognize, however, that this relationship is valid only for a single rod, or for rods placed very far apart. Placing multiple rods close together reduces the effectiveness of the system because the current of each rod raises the potential of the others. Consequently, a ground bed composed of multiple rods close to one another is much less effective than one with rods spaced far apart.

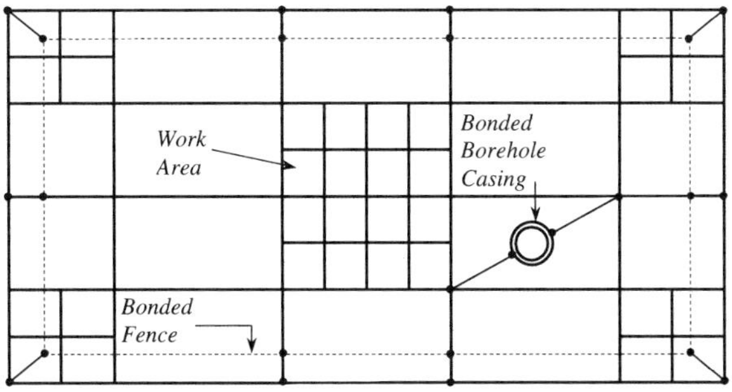

Figure 27.11 Plan view of a typical ground grid for a mine substation (after Cooley and King 1980)

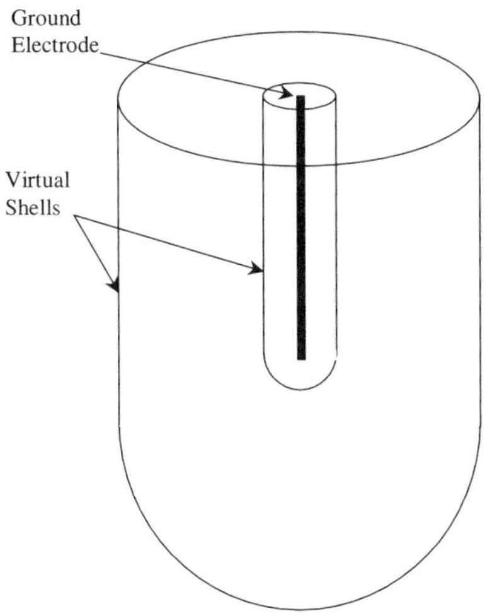

Figure 27.12 Ground electrode resistance concepts

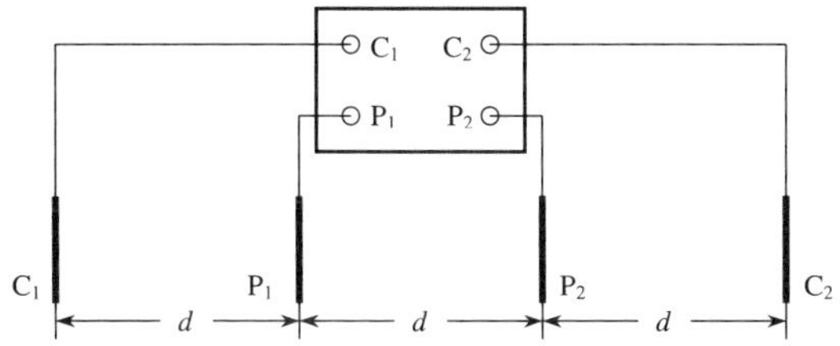

Figure 27.13 Wenner array used to measure soil resistivity

Safety Ground Bed Design Proper design and construction of a safety ground bed involves four distinct steps:

1. Measuring the soil resistivity
2. Choosing a bed design based on the soil resistivity
3. Constructing the ground bed
4. Measuring the bed resistance.

Soil resistivity measurements are frequently conducted with a resistivity meter connected in a Wenner array, as illustrated in Figure 27.13. Four electrodes are driven into the ground along a straight line, with an equal spacing, *d*, between each electrode. Current, *I*, is passed between the two outer electrodes (called current electrodes) C_1 and C_2, and the resulting voltage, *V*, is measured between the inner electrodes (called potential electrodes) P_1 and P_2. The soil resistivity, ρ, is computed as:

$$\rho = 2\pi d \frac{V}{I}$$ (EQ 27.9)

It should be noted that different devices may provide different formulas for computing resistivity, or they may display other values (e.g., resistance instead voltage and current). It is also imperative to use a resistivity meter designed for soil resistivity measurements and not simply a battery and voltmeter. Significant errors will be caused by polarization effects caused by an applied DC.

Four measurements are made in determining soil resistivity at a particular site.

1. Measurements with the electrodes at a 2-m spacing along a selected baseline. If possible, the baseline should be selected to follow any natural geologic features in the area, for example, if there is a stream nearby, the baseline should be oriented parallel to the stream

2. Measurements with the electrodes at a 6-m spacing along the baseline

3. Measurements with the electrodes at a 2-m spacing perpendicular to the baseline

4. Measurements with the electrodes at a 6-m spacing perpendicular to the baseline.

Using the results of the resistivity measurements, the resistance of a single rod can be estimated from the resistivity measurements and the rod dimensions:

$$R = \frac{\rho}{2\pi L} \ln\left[\frac{2L}{r}\right]$$ (EQ 27.10)

where
L = rod length
r = rod radius.

The grounding resistance of multiple-rod systems can be approximated by dividing the single-rod resistance by the total number of rods used, and multiplying this result by an appropriate multiplying factor. This factor is necessary because, as previously mentioned, placing rods close together increases the grounding resistance of the individual rods. Table 27.1 provides multiplying factors for the case in which 3-m long, 15-mm diameter rods are placed 3 m apart along a straight line, in the shape of a hollow triangle, hollow square, or hollow circle. Generally, a grounding resistance of 2–5 Ω is considered to be adequate. King et al. (1978) describes a more detailed method for determining specific rod configurations.

Caution must be exercised to be sure that consistent units are used in this formula. For example, if the soil resistivity is measured in Ohm-meters, the rod dimensions must be expressed in meters. It is important to note that this formula is valid for soil of homogeneous resistivity; in other words, the resistivity values along the baseline should be close to the values perpendicular to the baseline. Procedures for dealing with inhomogeneous soil are provided by King et al. (1978).

Once a particular rod configuration has been determined, the rods are driven into the ground and connected to one another by a connecting wire. Several types of rods are available, including iron, steel, copper, and copper-clad steel. Copper-clad steel provides high strength for driving the rod into the ground and permits copper-to-copper connections with the ground wire and connecting wire. Bare copper wire is typically used to connect the ground rods. The connecting wire should be kept slack to allow for thermal expansion and settling, and the entire system should be below the surface. Several methods for connecting the rods are used, including mechanical fittings, welding, and compression fittings.

Once the bed is constructed, the grounding resistance must be checked for acceptance—a resistance of 2–5 Ω. Existing beds should also be checked periodically to detect any changes in the resistance, especially when the soil is dry or the weather is cold. Several methods exist for measuring ground bed resistance, including the three-point method, the fall-of-potential method, and the ratio method. Of these three methods, the fall-of-potential is probably the most widely accepted. For this reason, we will describe only the fall-of-potential method here.

TABLE 27.1   Multiplying factors for multiple rod systems (after IEEE Std. 142 1991)

Number of Rods	Multiplying Factor
2	1.16
3	1.29
4	1.36
8	1.68
12	1.80
16	1.92
20	2.00
24	2.16

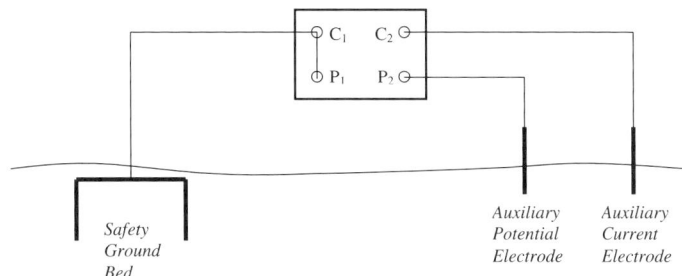

(a) Electrode configuration.

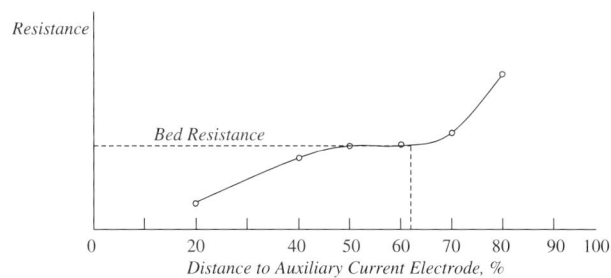

(b) Characteristic shape of resistance values.

Figure 27.14   Electrode configuration for fall-of-potential measurement

Figure 27.14 illustrates the electrode placement for the fall-of-potential measurement. Current is passed between the bed and the auxiliary current electrode and the potential difference between the ground bed and auxiliary potential electrode is measured as shown in Figure 27.14(a). The current electrode is driven into the ground a distance, D, from the center of the ground bed, where D is five times the longest straight-line dimension of the ground bed. If the longest straight-line dimension is less than 3 m, D should be 15 m. At least six measurements are made with the auxiliary potential electrode driven into the ground at the following distances from the center of the ground bed: $0.2D$, $0.4D$, $0.5D$, $0.6D$, $0.7D$, and $0.8D$. The measured resistance values should have the general shape shown in Figure 27.14(b). If so, the bed resistance is the value at $0.618D$. (Note that in certain situations, the resistance versus distance shape shown in Figure 27.14(b) will not be obtained. There are many reasons for this to occur, with the most common ones being that the soil is inhomogeneous or the auxiliary current electrode is located too close to the bed. Solutions for these types of situations are beyond the scope of this book.)

If a low-resistance ground bed cannot be obtained by normal means, soil treatment can be used to reduce soil resistivity. In fact, soil resistivity may be reduced by 15% to 90%, depending on the soil type and texture (Jones 1980). Chemicals are generally applied in a circular trench around an electrode to prevent direct contact with the electrode. Saturating the ground with water accelerates the effectiveness of the treatment. It is important to remember that chemical treatment is not permanent;

therefore, treatment must be renewed periodically, depending on the nature of the chemical and the soil. Common salt and magnesium sulfate are the most commonly used chemicals. As a result, corrosion protection of the grounding electrodes must be considered.

Ground Bed Separation

As previously described, the purpose of the station ground bed is to protect personnel in and around the substation and to protect substation equipment from severe electrical stress during faults, lightning strokes, or switching transients. The safety ground system (i.e., ground bed, grounding conductors, grounding resistor, and so forth) is designed primarily to control equipment frame potentials and provide a low-resistance path for ground current during a ground fault.

As shown in Figure 27.15, the station ground bed is separated from the safety ground bed. The purpose for this electrical isolation is to prevent hazardous potentials that result from faults or lightning strokes at the substation from being impressed onto the frames of the mining equipment. Probably the best way of clarifying the need for ground bed separation is to consider the situation illustrated in Figure 27.15. In this figure, a lightning stroke at the substation is used to illustrate the need for bed separation. (Faults can create similar types of hazards.) As the lightning stroke is diverted to ground by means of surge arresters, the current flow through the resistance of the earth elevates the potential of the station bed. If the safety bed is connected to the station bed, as shown in this figure, the frames of the mining equipment will be elevated as well. Because this equipment is normally located far from the substation, the potential of the earth at the equipment location would not be elevated; therefore, anyone coming in contact with the equipment could be exposed to lethal voltages.

Separating the station ground bed from the safety ground bed, at least in theory, prevents the frames of mining equipment from being elevated as a result of faults at the substation. However, in practice, simply isolating the two beds is often not sufficient. Consider Figure 27.16, in which the two beds are separated by a short distance. In this case, the current flow through the earth elevates the potential of the safety bed because the two beds are separated by an insufficient distance. Even though they appear to be electrically isolated, the two beds are coupled by the earth. Note, however, that the substation bed is still performing its primary and secondary functions because the potential of the entire bed is elevated while the potential *gradient* throughout the substation is maintained at a low value.

Because of the hazards associated with bed coupling, federal regulations require a bed separation of at least 25 ft for coal mines. However, strong evidence suggests that this distance is often insufficient, depending on soil resistivity and the size and shape of the two ground beds. For example, Cooley and Hill (1984) show practical situations in which the coupling between beds can exceed 30%, and in extreme situations, more than 90%. In addition to coupling by insufficient separation, beds can also be inadvertently coupled by conducting intermediaries such as water lines or faulty wiring.

Additional problems and remedies associated with ground bed coupling are difficult to detect and analyze, and are beyond the scope of this chapter. Cooley (1977) and Cooley and Hill (1984) are very good sources for additional information.

ELECTRICAL SAFETY PROGRAMS

This section summarizes several MSHA-recommended safe job procedures as they relate to electrical safety. Note that these descriptions are not intended to provide detailed instruction, rather, they are intended to serve as representative examples and to familiarize the reader with the most common electrical hazards and basic recommended safe job procedures for several common job functions. The first section describes basic procedures that apply to most pieces of electric equipment. The second section summarizes procedures for a coal mine shuttle car operator. Finally, equipment lockout procedures are summarized. See MSHA's "On-The-Job Training Modules" for additional details (MSHA 1985a; MSHA 1985b; MSHA 1986a; MSHA 1988a; MSHA 1988b).

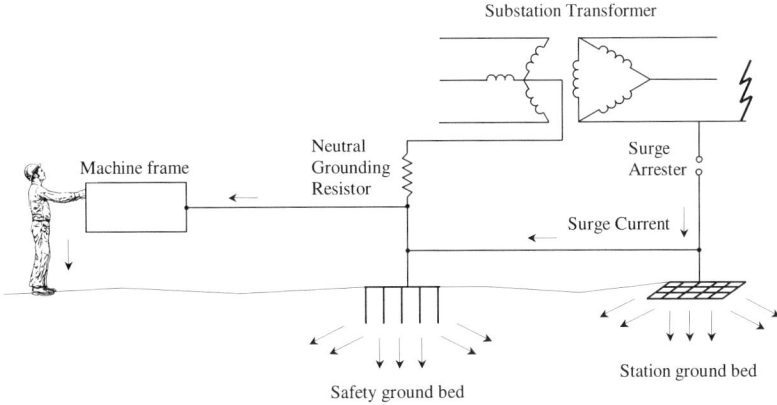

Figure 27.15   Shock hazard produced by lightning stroke and ground bed connection

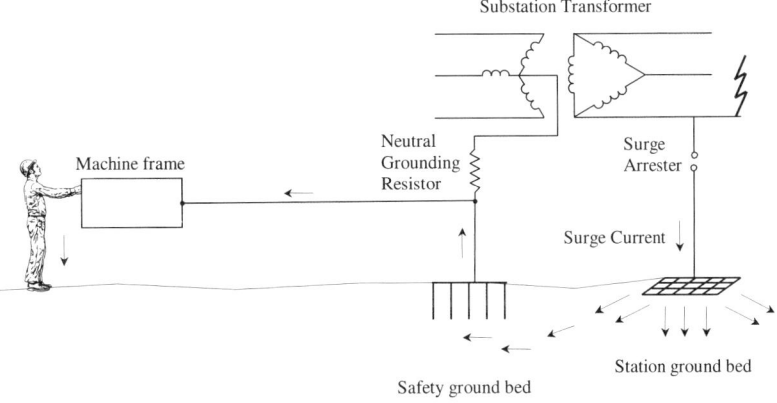

Figure 27.16   Shock hazard produced by lightning stroke and insufficient ground bed separation

Electrical Procedures for Nonelectricians Operating Electric Equipment

The general procedures for safe operation of equipment are divided into three basic steps: (1) remove power from the cable and equipment, (2) conduct a preoperational check of the equipment, and (3) operate the equipment safely.

Removing power from the cable and equipment first requires that the operator identify the correct cable coupler and circuit breaker (or other appropriate disconnecting device) at the power distribution center for the particular piece of equipment. This important step should not be overlooked. If an operator is careless, or if the equipment is not clearly marked, he or she could easily energize (or deenergize) the wrong piece of equipment. Once the proper circuit breaker has been identified, the operator should inspect it for cracks or other signs of damage. While standing on an insulated mat, the operator should set the switch to the OFF or ON position, as appropriate.

The preoperational equipment check should be performed by the operator with the power removed from the cable and piece of equipment. After removing power, the operator should check the cable, especially splices, for signs of damage. At the machine, the company permissibility checklist should be used to check enclosure and other permissibility requirements. Switches, lights, motors, guards, and so forth should also be checked to ensure that they are properly mounted on the machine. Grease, oil, and other combustible materials should be removed from the machine.

While running a piece of equipment, the operator should be aware of and avoid situations where electrical components can be damaged by ribs or pieces of equipment. If damage to electrical components or the power cable is suspected, the operator should check the component. Equipment operators must be careful not to run over or pinch cables with mining equipment. When possible, cables should be deenergized before shoveling or other activities are performed near them. Energized high-voltage cables must not be handled except under special provisions listed in Title 30 CFR (MSHA 1986b).

Cable-Reel Shuttle Car Haulage

When the operator first arrives at the section, he or she should proceed to the shuttle car power source and make sure that the power to the shuttle car is OFF. (Because there are typically multiple shuttle cars at a section, the operator must be careful to ensure that the proper cable coupler and circuit breaker have been identified.) The operator should next proceed to the shuttle car, following the trailing cable and inspecting it for physical damage. Splices should be checked for mechanical strength and flexibility and insulation integrity. The trailing cable anchor (or snub) should be examined to make sure that it is fastened securely. Upon reaching the shuttle car, the operator should check that the motor control switch is in the OFF position; the brakes should be set and the wheels blocked. The operator should check all electrical contactor cases and motor housings to make certain that the covers are properly fastened. Electrical conduits and cable guards should be checked for damage and loose or missing clamps. Headlights should be checked for cracked or broken lenses, lens tightness, and installation of seals. All packing glands should be checked to be sure that they are tight and properly packed. The cable reel assembly should be inspected to ensure that the sheave wheel turns freely and will not damage the cable when the cable is spooled out or reeled in.

The operator should check the haul road, making sure that cables are properly suspended across roadways and placed as close to ribs as possible. After the operator returns to the power distribution center, he or she should check the coupler to ensure that it is securely plugged into the receptacle. After identifying the proper circuit breaker, and examining it for signs of damage, the switch can be set to the ON position. If the power does not remain on, a danger sign should be attached and the condition should be reported to the foreman (MSHA 1986c).

Equipment Lockout Procedures

Serious injuries and deaths have occurred when an individual energizes a piece of equipment while another individual is performing maintenance on that piece of equipment. As a result of these injuries and fatalities, and the hazards associated with working on equipment that can become energized unexpectedly, various federal mining regulations require that lockout procedures be followed before any work is performed on electrical components. Lockout procedures are also recommended when work is performed on mechanical components so that employees can be protected against injuries sustained from exposure to moving parts caused by the unexpected startup of equipment.

Lockout procedures consist of disconnecting the power supply from the piece of equipment and "locking out" the disconnecting device so that the equipment cannot be inadvertently energized. An identification tag must also be attached to the disconnecting device that identifies the individual who has locked out the disconnecting device. The individual who is working on the equipment must carry out this procedure; if more than one person is working on the piece of equipment, each one should apply his or her own lock and tag.

Although the equipment lockout procedure is fairly straightforward to follow, several circumstances do require additional consideration. First, locking out only the control circuit on a piece of equipment is not sufficient. Although this practice may seem to prevent the equipment from being energized, it is an unreliable procedure. For example, a fault in the control circuit may energize the equipment.

Another situation where caution must be exercised is when equipment is energized from more than one point. (A good example is a DC trolley line in which rectifiers supply the trolley wire at various points along the trolley.) In these types of situations, all possible sources of electricity must be recognized and all disconnecting devices must be locked and tagged.

When a lockout must proceed from one shift to a later shift, transfer procedures must be conducted. The incoming employees must lock and tag the appropriate disconnecting device, and the departing employees must remove their locks and tags (MSHA 1986d).

SUMMARY

Electric-powered equipment continues to play a key role in the mining industry. Compared to 10 or 20 years ago, equipment is more powerful, efficient, and reliable and these improvements have helped to increase mineral production and productivity. In addition, improvements in safety features, such as sensitive ground fault protection for high-voltage coal mine longwall faces, have helped to reduce hazards associated with electricity use. Improved hazard awareness and safety training programs have undoubtedly helped to reduce the incidence of injuries and fatalities. With continued advances in equipment and training, electric-powered machinery will continue to provide safe and economic mineral production.

REFERENCES

Bridges, J.E. 1981. An investigation of low impedance, low voltage shocks. *IEEE PAS Transactions* 100(4): April.

——. 1986. *Cable-Reel Shuttle Car Haulage*. Publication IG 47, No. 4. MSHA National Mine Health and Safety Academy.

Cooley, W.L. 1977. Design considerations regarding separation of mine safety ground and substation ground systems. *Conference Record of the 1977 IEEE/IAS Annual Meeting*. Chicago, IL.

Cooley, W.L., and H.W. Hill. 1984. Coupling of mine grounds to surface grounds. *Conference Record of the 1984 IEEE/IAS Annual Meeting*. Chicago, IL.

Cooley, W.L., and R.L. King. 1980. *Guide to Substation Grounding and Bonding for Mine Power Systems*. USBM Information Circular 8835. USBM.

Dalziel, C.F. 1954. Threshold of perception currents. *Electrical Engineering* 73.

——. 1956. Effects of electric shock on man. *Institute of Radio Engineers Transactions on Medical Electronics*. May.

Dalziel, C.F., and J.B. Lagen. 1941. Effects of electric current on man. *Electrical Engineering* 60.

Dalziel, C.F., and W.R. Lee. 1969. Lethal electric currents. *IEEE Spectrum*. February.

——. 1986b. *Electrical Procedures for Non-Electricians*. Publication IG 47, No. 11. MSHA National Mine Health and Safety Academy.

——. 1986d. *Equipment Lockout Procedures*. Publication IG 47, No. 10. MSHA National Mine Health and Safety Academy.

Dalziel, C.F., and T.H. Mansfield. 1950. Effect of frequency on perception currents. *Electrical Engineering* 69.

Ferris, L.P., B.G. King, P.W. Spence, and H.B. Williams. 1936. Effect of electric shock on the heart. *Electrical Engineer*. May.

Gross, T.A. 1979. People-protecting three-phase ground fault current interrupters. *Plant Electrical Systems*. October/November.

——. *How Does a Distribution Class Surge Arrester Work?* Mansfield, OH: The Ohio Brass Company.

——. 1986. *IEEE Guide for Safety in AC Substation Grounding*. ANSI/IEEE Std 80-1986. New York: IEEE.

——. 1991. *IEEE Recommended Practice for Grounding of Industrial and Commercial Power Systems*. IEEE Std. 142-1991. New York: IEEE.

Jacimovic, S.D. 1982. *Allowable Values of Step and Touch Voltages*. IEEE Preprint CH1740-0/82/0000-0095. New York: IEEE.

Jones, W.R. 1980. Bentonite rods assure ground rod installation in problem soils. *IEEE PAS Transactions* Vol. PAS-99, No. 4. July/August.

Keesey, J.C., and F.S. Letcher. 1970. Human threshold of electric shock at power frequencies. *Archives of Environmental Health* 21.

King, R.L., H.W. Hill, Jr., R.R. Bafana, and W.L. Cooley. 1978. *Guide for the Construction of Driven-Rod Ground Beds*. USBM Information Circular 8767. USBM.

Kouwenhoven, W.B., R.W. Chesnut, G.G. Knickerbocker, W.R. Milnor, and D.J. Sass. 1959. AC shocks of varying parameters affecting the heart. *Transactions of the AIEE*.

Langworthy, O.R., and W.B. Kouwenhoven. 1931. The importance of point contact in electric injuries. *Journal of Industrial Hygiene* 13(5).

Lee, W.R., and S. Zoledziowski. 1964. Effects of electric shock in respiration in the rabbit. *British Journal of Industrial Medicine* 21.

Lee, W.R. 1966. Death from electric shock. *Proceedings IEEE* 113.

Maclachlan, W. 1930. Electric shock: interpretation of field notes. *Journal of Industrial Hygiene* 12(8).

———. 1992. *Mine Electricity–Coal Surface and Underground Entry Level Training*. Publication CI 7. MSHA National Mine Health and Safety Academy.

———. 1999. *Mine Electricity–Metal and Nonmetal Entry Level Training*. Publication CI 8. MSHA National Mine Health and Safety Academy.

MSHA. 1985(a). *On-the-Job Training Modules–Cement*. Publication IG 42, Nos. 1–15. MSHA National Mine Health and Safety Academy.

———. 1985(b). *On-the-Job Training Module–Sand, Gravel, and Crushed Stone*. Publication IG 40, Nos.1–19. MSHA National Mine Health and Safety Academy.

———. 1986(a). *On-the-Job Training Module–Underground Coal*. Publication IG 47, Nos. 1–13. MSHA National Mine Health and Safety Academy.

———. 1988(a). *On-the-Job Training Module–Anthracite and Bituminous Coal Preparation Plants and Shops*. Publication IG 49, Nos. 1–16. MSHA National Mine Health and Safety Academy.

———. 1988(b). *On-the-Job Training Module–Underground Anthracite*. Publication IG 50, Nos. 1–7. MSHA National Mine Health and Safety Academy.

Novak, T. 1998. Analysis of very-high resistance grounding in high-voltage longwall power systems. St Louis, MO: *Conference Record of the 1998 IEEE/IAS Annual Meeting*.

———. 1999. The effects of very-high resistance grounding on the selectivity of ground-fault relaying in high voltage longwall power systems. Phoenix, AZ: *Conference Record of the 1999 IEEE/IAS Annual Meeting*.

. . . .
Acronyms

ABIH	American Board of Industrial Hygiene
AC	alternating current
ACGIH	American Conference of Governmental Industrial Hygienists
AIHA	American Industrial Hygiene Association
ALJ	Administrative Law Judge
AMS	acute mountain sickness
AMSP	Associate Mine Safety Professional
AN	ammonium nitrate
ANFO	ammonium nitrate/fuel oil
ANSI	American National Standards Institute
ASP	Associate Safety Professional
ASSE	American Society of Safety Engineers
ATF	Bureau of Alcohol, Tobacco, and Firearms
ATRS	automated temporary roof support
ATS	American Thoracic Society
AWS	American Welding Society
BCOA	Bituminous Coal Operators' Association
BCSP	Board of Certified Safety Professionals
BEI	Biological Exposure Indices
BHP	Broken Hill Properties Limited
CAD	computer-aided design
CAOHC	Council for Accreditation of Occupational Hearing Conservation
CFR	*Code of Federal Regulations*
CG	computer graphics
CIH	Certified Industrial Hygienist
CM	coupling multiplier
CMSP	Certified Mine Safety Professional
CO	carbon monoxide
CO_2	carbon dioxide
COHST	Certified Occupational Health and Safety Technologies
CSB	Chemical Safety and Hazard Investigation Board
CSIR	Council for Scientific and Industrial Research

437

CSIRO	Commonwealth Scientific and Industrial Research Organization
CSP	Certified Safety Professional
CWP	coal workers' pneumoconiosis
CYA	cover your anatomy
dB	decibels
DC	direct current
DO	designated occupations
DOI	Department of the Interior
DOT	Department of Transportation
DPM	diesel particulate matter
DST	dry systems technology
EPA	Environmental Protection Agency
ESP	efficiency, safety, and productivity
FCAW	flux core arc welding
FM	frequency multiplier
FMSHRC	Federal Mine Safety and Health Review Commission
FRA	Federal Railroad Administration
FSV	free-steered vehicle
GC	gas chromatograph
GFCI	ground-fault current interrupter
GMAC	gas metal arc welding
GTAW	gas tungsten arc welding
HAZWOPER	hazardous waste operations
HCN	hydrogen cyanide
HCP	hearing conservation program
HEPA	high efficiency particulate air
HIV	human immunodeficiency virus
HMD	head-mounted display
HPS	Hantavirus Pulmonary Syndrome
HSE	Health and Safety Executive
IA	Interagency Agreement
IARC	International Agency for Research on Cancer
IEEE	Institute of Electric and Electronics Engineers
IHIT	Industrial Hygienist in Training
ILO	International Labor Office
IME	Institute of Makers of Explosives
IR	incident rate
IR	infrared
ISEE	International Society of Explosives Engineers

ISMSP	International Society of Mine Safety Professionals
ISO	International Standards Organization
JSA	job safety analysis
LCL	lower control limit
LD	Legionnaires' disease
LHD	load-haul-dump (units)
MAG	metal active gas
MESA	Mine Enforcement and Safety Administration
MIG	metal inert gas
MMA	manual metal arc
MOU	memorandum of understanding
MRS	mobile roof support
MS	mass spectrophotometer
MSDS	Material Safety Data Sheet
MSHA	Mine safety and Health Administration
NAS	National Academy of Science
NEC	National Electric Code
NFDL	nonfatal days lost
NFPA	National Fire Protection Agency
NG	nitroglycerin
NIHL	noise-induced hearing loss
NIOSH	National Institute for Occupational Safety and Health
NMA	National Mining Association
NO	nitrogen oxide
NO_2	nitrogen dioxide
NOSA	(South Africa's) National Occupational Safety Association
NSC	National Safety Council
NSW	New South Wales
NTSB	National Transportation Safety Board
OSHA	Occupation Safety and Health Administration
OSM	Office of Surface Mining Reclamation and Enforcement
PAH	polycyclic aromatic hydrocarbon
PAW	plasma arc welding
PEL	permissible exposure limit
PLUS	positive leadership upgrades safety
PMF	progressive massive fibrosis
PPE	personal protective equipment
PTS	permanent threshold shift

RCRA	Resource Conservation and Recovery Act
RFID	radio-frequency identification
RFP	request for proposal
ROI	return on investment
RWL	recommended weight limit

SAW	submerged arc welding
SHARE	Safety Helps And Recognizes Everyone
S&S	significant and substantial
SHE	Safety, Health, and Environment
SIMRAC	Safety in Mines Research Advisory Council
SM	severity measure
SMAC	shielded metal arc welding
SMCRA	Surface Mining Control and Reclamation Act
SME	Society for Mining, Metallurgy, and Exploration, Inc.
SME	subject matter expert
SOP	standard operating procedure
STEL	short-term exposure limit

TAC	total accident control
TACT	Total Accident Control Training
TB	tuberculosis
TIG	tungsten inert gas
TLV	threshold limit value
TTS	temporary threshold shift
TWA	time-weighted average

UCL	upper control limit
UL	Underwriters' Laboratory
USBM	U.S. Bureau of Mines
USC	*U.S. Code*
U.S. EPA	U.S. Environmental Protection Agency

| VPP | Voluntary Protection Program |
| VR | virtual reality |

| WBGT | wet bulb globe temperature |

Index

. . . .

Note: f. indicates figure; t. indicates table.